AF709998

FAST FACTS for Critical Care®

The Chapters

1 CV
2 Hemodynamics
3 ACLS
4 Stat Meds
5 Med Facts
6 Drip Tables
7 ECG
8 Pacing
9 Respiratory
10 Neuro
11 Renal/Endo
12 Lab/IV's/Blood

The Specialty Chapters (Optional)

13 Trauma
14 IABP
15 Pedi Acute Care
16 Cardiac Surgery

Fast Facts for Critical Care®

Produced in the United States of America by
Kathy White Learning Systems
PO Box 41113
Mobile, Alabama 36640

The Author
Kathleen M. White, RN, MSN
Critical Care Nurse, Educator, Consultant, Author, Publisher

Printing and Order Fulfillment
Gwin's Printing
957 Springhill Ave
Mobile Alabama 36604
800-940-0895 or 251-438-2175

To order the printed version
Toll free: 1-800-940-0895
Local phone: 251-438-2175
Fax number: 251-438-1959
Internet address: http://www.kathywhite.com

To purchase the iBook version for the Apple® iPad:
go to Apple, Inc. App Store and search "Kathy White"
Apple iBook version will be available in mid-2016

Disclaimer
The author, reviewers, and publisher have made a conscientious effort to ensure that the information, medications, and treatment schedules in this book are correct and accurate, and compatible with standards generally accepted at the time of publication. Nevertheless, many medications, treatment protocols, and diagnostic regimens are the subject of ongoing research, may be controversial, and are subject to frequent change. As new information becomes available, changes in diagnostic and treatment protocols and in the use of drug therapy become necessary. In view of the possibility of human error or changes in the medical sciences, neither the authors nor the publisher nor any other party who has been involved in the preparation of the publication of this work warrants that the information contained herein is in every respect accurate or complete and they disclaim all responsibility to any errors or omissions or for the results obtained from the use of the information contained in the work. The reader is strongly advised to consult the instructions, information, and warnings included in the package insert (prescribing information) of each medication or therapeutic agent before administration, and to consult accepted and published textbooks, journals, and standards of clinical practice for more detailed explanations, recommendations, and instructions on diagnostic and treatment regimens. The author, reviewers, and publisher disclaim all responsibility for any liability, loss, injury, or damage incurred as a consequence, directly or indirectly, of the use and application of any of the contents of this volume.

The list of references for *Fast Facts for Critical Care* is available on line at www.kathywhite.com.

ISBN International Standard Book Number
2016 edition: **978-1-889125-00-8**

Table of Contents

Section	Topic		Page
Cardiovascular	Head to toe/Systems assessment	CV	1
	CV assessment/Heart sounds		3
	Lipid profile & Cardiac biomarkers		5
	Acute Coronary Syndrome (ACS)		6
	UA/NSTEMI Assessment & Treatment		8
	STEMI Assessment & Treatment		9
	RV Infarction		15
	PCI (PTCA, Stents, Atherectomy, Vascular Access)		16
	Acute Heart failure		20
	Implanted Cardioverter/Defibrillator		23
	Pericarditis/Effusion/Tamponade		25
	Pericardiocentesis/Pericardial Catheter		27
	Deep Vein Thrombosis		29
	Arterial Thrombosis		32
	Acute Aortic Dissection		33
Hemodynamics	Pressure Monitoring Line Set-up	Hemo	1
	Arterial Pressure Monitoring		2
	Central Venous Pressure Monitoring		3
	Noninvasive Cardiac Output (NiCOM)		4
	PA Catheter Insertion		5
	PA Pressures, Waveforms, and Accuracy		6
	Cardiac Output Measurement		8
	The Determinants of Cardiac Output (CO)		10
	Shock and the Sympathetic-Adrenal Response		11
	Cardiogenic Shock		12
	Hemorrhagic Shock		14
	Sepsis and Septic Shock		16
	Hemodynamic and Pulmonary Parameters		21
ACLS	BLS by Healthcare Providers	ACLS	1
	Algorithm: VFib or Pulseless VT		2
	Defibrillation		3
	Asystole, PEA, Bradycardia Algorithms		4
	Transcutaneous Pacing		5
	Endotracheal Intubation		7
	Emergency Cricothyrotomy		8
	Post Cardiac Arrest -Therapeutic Hypothermia		9
	Tachycardia, Atrial Fibrillation		12
	Acute Ischemic Stroke		15
	Activase (r-tPA) for Acute Ischemic Stroke		16
	Summary of BLS given by Healthcare Providers		19
Stat Meds	Quick Drips	Stat Meds	1-2
	Emergency IV Meds Guide (A - Z)		3
	α & β Receptors, Agonists, and Antagonists		26
Med Facts	ACE inhibitors and ARB's	Med Facts	1
	Analgesia (Intravenous)		2
	Beta Blockers		3
	Calcium Channel Blockers		4
	Clotting/Lysing Cascades		5
	Clot Inhibitor: Heparin (LMWH and UFH) and		6
	Heparin Induced Thrombocytopenia (HIT)		8
	Clot Inhibitor: GP IIb/IIIa Receptor Antagonists		9
	Clot Inhibitor: Warfarin		11
	ClotBusters: Alteplase, Reteplase, Streptase		12
	Delirium		15
	Epidural Analgesia		16
	Insulin and Glycemic Control		18
	Neuromuscula Blockade		19
	Peripheral Nerve Stimulator, Train-of-four Testing		22
	Sedation		24
	Seizure Meds		26
Drip Tables	Infusion Tables A-Z		1-24

Table of Contents

Section	Topic	Tab	Page
ECG	The Normal ECG	ECG	1
	Basic ECG Analysis		2
	Lead Placement - 3 Leads, 5 Leads		3,4
	Dysrhythmias		5-14
	12 - Lead ECG to Localize Infarction		15
	Axis and Axis Deviation		16
			17
	ST-Segment Monitoring		19
Pacing	Pacing Classifications	Pacing	1
	Ventricular Pacer Controls		2
	Transvenous Pacing Indications and Insertion		3
	Ventricular Pacing: Connections		4
	Emergency Pacing		5
	Setting a Pacer for Demand Pacing		6
	Ventricular Pacing		7
	Troubleshooting		8
	AV Sequential Pacemaker		9
	AV Sequential Pacing: Connections		10
	AV Sequential Pacing: Start-up and Thresholds		12
	Complications of Pacing		11
Respiratory	Respiratory Assessment/Breath Sounds	Resp	1,2
	Oxygenation, Causes of Hypoxemia		3,4
	O2 Delivery Devices		5
	Oxygen Delivery, Supply/Demand Balance, SvO2		6-8
	Acid-Base Imbalance		9,10
	The Endotracheal Tube		11
	Modes of Ventilation		12-16
	Acute Respiratory Distress Syndrome (ARDS)		17
	Preventing Ventilator Associated Events		19
	Weaning from Mechanical Ventilation		21
	Pulmonary Embolism		23
	Pleural Effusion		25
	Pneumothorax and Chest Tubes		26-29
Neuro	CNS Structure and Function	Neuro	1
	Cerebral Circulation		2
	Cranial Nerve Assessment		3
	Neuro Assessment		4
	Neuro Map of Increased ICP		7
	Treatment of Increased ICP		8
	ICP Monitoring - Bolt and fluid filled column		9
	ICP Monitoring - IVC and fluid filled column		10
	ICP Monitoring - Fiberoptic catheters		11
	Interpreting ICP Waveforms		12
	PbtO2 (Brain Tissue Oxygen) Monitoring		13
	Subarachnoid Hemorrhage		15
	Spontaneous Intracerebral Hemorrhage		17
	Status Epilepticus		19
	Delirium Tremens		21
	Criteria for Brain Death		22
	Care of the Organ Donor after Brain Death		23
Renal/Endo	Acute Kidney Injury and Treatment	Renal/Endo	1-5
	Continuous Renal Replacement Therapy		6-10
	Potassium and Magnesium		11
	Potassium Administration		12
	Sodium and Chloride		14
	Calcium and Phosphorus		15
	Adrenal Insufficiency and Crisis		16
	Diabetic Ketoacidosis		17
	Hyperthyroid and Thyrotoxicosis		19
	Hypothyroid and Myxedema Coma		20
Lab, Fluids, Blood, and Charts	Lab Values	Lab	1-3
	Crystalloids/Colloids		4-5
	Blood Products/Massive Transfusion		6-7
	Fahrenheit/Celsius and Inches/Centimeters		8
	Lbs - Kgs, and BSA		9-10

α	alpha
AAL	Anterior axillary line
abd	Abdominal
AbdCS	Abd compartment syndrome
ABC	Airway, Breathing, Circulation
ACA	Anterior cerebral artery
ACC	American College of Cardiology
ACCP	American College of Chest Physicians
ACE	Angiotensin converting enzyme
ACEI	ACE Inhibitor
ACLS	Advanced cardiac life support
ACS	Acute coronary syndrome
ACT	Activated clotting time
ACTH	Adrenocorticotrophic hormone
ACV	Assist control ventilation
AD	Aortic dissection
ADH	Antidiuretic hormone
AID	Automatic internal defibrillator
AFib	Atrial fibrillation
AFlut	Atrial flutter
Alb	Albumin
AHA	American Heart Association
AHF	Acute Heart Failure
ALI	Acute Lung Injury
AMI	Acute myocardial infarction
APACHE	Acute physiologic and chronic health evaluation
AP	Arterial pressure
APC	Activated protein C
APRV	Airway pressure release ventilation
aPTT	Activated partial thromboplastin time
ARB	Angiotensin Receptor Blocker
ARDS	Acute Resp. Distress Syndrome
ARF	Acute Renal Failure
AS	Aortic stenosis
ASAP	As soon as possible
ASHP	American Society of Hospital Pharmacists
ASVD	Arteriosclerotic vessel disease
ATLS	Advanced trauma life support
ATN	Acute tubular necrosis
AV	Atrio-ventricular
AVB	Atrio-ventricular block
AVF	Augmented voltage of the feet
AVL	Augmented voltage of the left
AVR	Augmented voltage of the right
AVSP	Atrial-ventricular sequential pacing
β	beta
BB	Beta blocker
BBB	Bundle branch block
BD	Base deficit
BG	Blood glucose
BiPAP	Bi-level positive airway pressure
BNP	Brain natriuretic peptide
BP	Blood pressure
bpm	Beats per minute
brady	Bradycardia
BUN	Blood urea nitrogen
C	Centigrade
Ca	Calcium
CA	Coronary artery
CABG	Coronary artery bypass graft
CAD	Coronary artery disease
CAM	Confusion assessment method
CaO2	Oxygen content of arterial blood
CCB	Calcium channel blocker
CCL	Cardiac Catheterization Lab
CHF	Congestive heart failure
CHO	Carbohydrate
CI	Cardiac index (also Continuous Infusion)
Cl	Chloride
CK	Creatine phosphokinase
CMV	Control mode ventilation
CN	Cranial nerve
CNS	Central nervous system
CO	Cardiac output
Conc	Concentration
COP	Colloid osmotic pressure
COPD	Chronic obstructive pulmonary disease
Cor PP	Coronary perfusion pressure
CPAP	Continuous positive airway pressure
CPB	Cardiopulmonary bypass
CPK	Creatine phosphokinase
CPK-MB	CPK myocardial biomarker
CPP	Cerebral perfusion pressure
Cr	Creatinine
Cr Cl	Creatinine clearance
CRRT	Continuous renal replacement therapy
Cryo	Cryoprecipitate
CS	Cardiogenic shock
CSF	Cerebrospinal Fluid
CT	Computed tomography
CV	Cardiovascular
CVAH	Continuous arterial to venous hemofiltration
CvO2	Oxygen content of venous blood
CVP	Central venous pressure
CVVH	Continuous venous to venous hemofiltration
CVVHD	CVVH with dialysate
CVVHDF	CVVD with filtration
d	day
DBP	Diastolic blood pressure
DC	Discontinue
DCC	Direct current cardioversion
DDAVP	Desmopressin acetate
Defib	Defibrillator
DI	Diabetes insipidus
Dias	Diastolic

Abbreviations

DKA	Diabetic ketoacidosis
dL	deciliter
DOO	Dual chamber fixed rate pacing
DO_2	Oxygen Delivery
DP	Dorsalis pedis
2,3 DPG	2,3 Diphosphoglycerate
DTI	Direct thrombin inhibitor
DVI	Dual chamber pacing with ventricular inhibition
DVT	Deep vein thrombosis
EBL	Estimated blood loss
ECG	Electrocardiogram
Echo	Echocardiogram
ECMO	Extracorporeal membrane oxygenation
EF	Ejection fraction
EMG	Electromyelogram
EPS	Electrophysiology study
ET	Endotracheal
ETOH	Ethanol
F	Fahrenheit
FDA	Food & DrugAdministration
FeNa	Fractional excretion of sodium
FF	Filtration fraction
FFP	Fresh frozen plasma
FiO_2	Fraction (%) of inspired O_2
FM	Face mask
Fr.	French
FRC	Functional residual capacity
FUN	Filtrate urea nitrogen
fx	Fracture
g	gram
G	Ground
GCS	Glasgow coma scale
GCSE	Generalized convulsive status epilepticus
GFR	Glomerular filtration rate
GI	Gastrointestinal
GP	Glycoprotein
GPRA	Glycoprotein receptor antagonist
GSW	Gunshot wound
h	hour
hr	hour
HA	Headache
Hct	Hematocrit
HF	Heart failure
HFJV	High frequency jet ventilation
Hg	Mercury
Hg	Hemoglobin
H/H	Hemoglobin/Hematocrit
HIT	Heparin-induced thrombocytopenia
HITT	HIT with thrombosis
HNAD	Hyperosmolar Nonacidic Diabetes
HR	Heart rate
HOB	Head of bed
HS	Hypertonic saline
Hx	History
IABP	Intra-aortic balloon pumping
ICD	Implanted Cardio-defibrillator
ICH	Intracerebral hemorrhage
ICP	Intracranial pressure
ICS	Intercostal space
I:E	Inspiration:Expiration
IJ	Internal jugular
IL-1	Interleuken 1
IMA	Internal mammary artery
IMV	Intermittent mandatory ventilation
INR	International normalization ratio
IO	Intraosseous
IRV	Inverse ratio ventilation
ITA	Internal thoracic artery
IV	Intravenous
IVC	Inferior vena cava
IVP	Intravenous push
j	Joule
JCAHO	Joint Commission on the Accreditation of Health Organizations
JVD	Jugular venous distention
K	Potassium
kg	kilogram
lb	pound
L	Liter
LA	Left arm
LAP	Left atrial pressure
LAD	Left anterior descending
LBBB	Left bundle branch block
LDH	Lactate dehydrogenase
LDUH	Low dose unfractionated heparin
Lido	Lidocaine
LL	Left leg
LLL	Left lower lobe
LMWH	Low molecular weight heparin
LOC	Level of consciousness
LOS	Length of stay
LPM	Liters per minute
LR	Lactated Ringers
Lt	Left
LUQ	Left upper quadrant
LUL	Left upper lobe
LV	Left ventricle
LVEDP	Left ventricular end-diastolic pressure
LVEF	Left ventricular ejection fraction
LVHF	Left ventricular heart failure
LVSWI	Left ventricular stroke work index
mA	Milliamp
MAOI	Monoamine oxidase inhibitor
MAP	Mean arterial pressure
MAT	Multifocal atrial tachycardia
max	maximum
MCA	Middle cerebral artery

mcg	microgram
MCL	Midclavicular line
MCL1	Modified chest lead I
MDO_2	Myocardial oxygen delivery
m^2	square meter
mEq	milliequivalents
mg	milligrams
Mg	Magnesium
MIDCAB	Minimally Invasive Direct Coronary Artery Bypass
min	minute
mL	milliliter
mm	millimeter
mm^2	cubic millimeter
MODS	Multiple organ dysfunction syndrome
MOF	Multiple organ failure
mOsm	milliosmoles
MPT	Minimum pacing threshold
MR	Mitral regurgitation
MS	Morphine sulfate
mV	millivolt
MV	Minute ventilation
MVO_2	Myocardial oxygen demand
Na	Sodium
NA	Not applicable
NC	Nasal cannula
NCR	Nasal cannula reservoir
NCSE	Nonconvulsive status epilepticus
ng	nanogram
NG	Nasogastric
NIBP	Noninvasive blood pressure
NIH	National Institutes of Health
NMB	Neuromuscular blockade
NMBA	Neuromuscular blocking agent
NS	Normal Saline
NSAID	Nonsteroidal antiinflammant
NSR	Normal sinus rhythm
NSTEMI	Non ST-elevation myocardial infarction
NTG	Nitroglycerin
N/V	Nausea/Vomiting
NYHA	New York Heart Association
OD	Overdose
OER	Oxygen extraction ratio
OPCAB	Off-Pump coronary artery bypass
OPC	Organ procurement coordinator
OPO	Organ procurement organization
PA	Pulmonary artery
PAC	Premature atrial contraction
PAD	Pulmonary artery diastolic
PAI	Plasminogen activator inhibitor
PAM	Pulmonary artery mean
PAO_2	Partial pressure O_2 alveolar air
PaO_2	Partial pressure of O_2 in arterial blood
PAP	Pulmonary artery pressure
PAS	Pulmonary artery systolic pressure
PAT	Paroxysmal atrial tachycardia
Pb	Barometric pressure
$PbtO_2$	Oxygen dissolved in brain tissue
PCI	Percutaneous coronary intervention
PCT	Pleural chest tube
PCWP	Pulmonary capillary wedge pressure
PDEI	Phosphodiesterase inhibitor
PE	Pulmonary embolism
PEA	Pulseless electrical activity
Peep	Positive end-expiratory pressure
$PetCO_2$	Partial pressure of end-tidal carbon dioxide
P/F	ratio of PaO_2 to FiO_2
Phos	Phosphorus
PMI	Point of maximal impulse
PRBC's	Packed red blood cells
PSA	Phlebostatic axis
PSV	Pressure support ventilation
PSVT	Paroxysmal Supraventricular Tachycardia
PT	Prothrombin time
PTCA	Percutaneous transluminal coronary angioplasty
PTT	Posterior tibial
PVC	Premature ventricular contraction
PVD	Peripheral vascular disease
PvO_2	Partial pressure of O_2 in venous blood
PVR	Pulmonary vascular resistance
Q	Blood flow, perfusion, or cardiac output
QS/QT	Shunted flow/total flow
RA	Right arm
RAP	Rapid atrial pacing
RBC	Red blood cell
RL	Ringer's Lactate
RLL	Right lower lobe
RML	Right middle lobe
RSBI	Rapid shallow breathing index
RSI	Rapid Sequence Intubation
Rt	Right
r-tPA	recombinant tissue plasminogen activator
RUL	Right upper lobe
RUQ	Right upper quadrant
RV	Right ventricle
RVEDF	RV end-diastolic volume
RVEF	RV ejection fraction
RVHF	Right ventricular heart failure
RVMI	RV myocardial infarction
Rx	Treatment
SA	Sino-atrial
SAH	Subarachnoid hemorrhage
SaO_2	Arterial oxygen saturation

SBP	Systolic blood pressure
SBT	Spontaneous breathing trial
SC	Subcutaneously
SCCM	Society Critical Care Medicine
SCD	Sequential compression device
SCI	Spinal cord injury
SCIWORA	SCI without radiologic abnormality
SCUF	Slow continuous ultrafiltration
$ScvO_2$	Central venous O_2 saturation
SE	Status epilepticus
sec	Second
SGOT	Serum glutamic-oxaloacetic transaminase
SHI	Severe head injury
SIMV	Synchronized intermittent mandatory ventilation
SIRS	Systemic inflammatory response syndrome
$SjvO_2$	Oxygen saturation of jugular venous blood
SK	Streptokinase
SL	Sublingual
SpO_2	Pulse oximetry of arterial oxygen saturation
S & S	Signs and symptoms
SSS	Sick sinus syndrome
STBI	Severe traumatic brain injury
STEMI	ST-elevation myocardial infarction
SV	Stroke volume
SVG	Saphenous vein graft
SvO_2	Mixed venous O_2 saturation
SVR	Systemic vascular resistance
SVT	Supraventricular tachycardia
Sx	Suction
Sys	Systolic
TAFI	Thrombin activatable fibrinolysis inhibitor
TAT	Thrombin-Antithrombin
TBI	Traumatic brain injury
TBV	Total blood volume
TCP	Transcutaneous pacing
TdeP	Torsades de pointes
TEE	Transesophageal echocardiogram
TIMI	Thrombolysis in Myocardial Infarction
TNF	Tumor necrosis factor
TnI	Troponin I
TnT	Troponin T
t-PA	Tissue Plasminogen Activator
TRH	Thyrotropin releasing hormone
TSH	Thyroid stimulating hormone
TV	Tidal volume
TVP	Temporary ventricular pacing
UA	Unstable Angina
U	Unit
UF	Ultrafiltrate
UFH	Unfractionated Heparin
UK	Urokinase
UO	Urinary output
UrCl	Urea clearance
VAP	Ventilator associated pneumonia
VC	Vital capacity
Vent	Ventricular
VF	Ventricular fibrillation
VFib	Ventricular fibrillation
VKA	Vitamin K Antagonist
V/Q	Ventilation/perfusion
VSD	Ventricular septal defect
VT	Ventricular tachycardia
VTach	Ventricular tachycardia
VTE	Venous Thromboembolism
VOO	Ventricular fixed rate pacing
VO_2	Oxygen consumption
VP	Ventriculo-peritoneal
VVI	Ventricular demand pacing
WBC	White blood cell
WPW	Wolf-Parkinson-White
Xa	Activated clotting factor X
yo	Years old

Trauma

Trauma

Trauma Assessment

The Primary Survey:

- Among all individuals involved in an MVA, 75% will be injured.
- 50% of deaths occur at the scene or within the first hour.
- 70% of MVA deaths occur in rural areas.
- Injury and death rates have improved with better auto safety, but have been made worse by distracted and/or under the influence driving.

<u>% of pts who will have these injuries</u>

Head	70 - 80 %
Neck/spine	5 - 10 %
Chest	35 %
Upper extremities	29 %
Abdomen, pelvis	15 %
Lower extremities	40 %

<u>There are 3 Mortality Peaks</u>

1. Immediately, due to apnea or massive hemorrhage.
2. Minutes to several hours later, due to major hemorrhage or head injury.
3. Days to weeks later, due to severe head injury, sepsis, or organ failure.

Assume C-spine injury (especially if decreased LOC, injury above the clavicle, multisystem injury) until otherwise disproven.

ABCDE	Assessment	Action
Airway	Look, listen, feel for air movement, look for chest wall movement. Look for facial, mandibular, tracheal, laryngeal fractures, presence of edema, foreign bodies, secretions, blood. Listen for stridor. Determine if the patient can protect his airway.	Immobilize the C-spine (which requires head and torso restraint). Chin lift, jaw thrust, suction if needed Intubate if: apnea, unconscious, GCS ≤ 8, respiratory distress, or threat of upper airway obstruction. Emergency cricothyrotomy if: • Oral/nasal attempts fail • Penetrating neck not amenable to oral/nasal approach • Significant maxillofacial trauma
Breathing	Look for chest defects, palpate for crepitus and pain. Assess respiratory rate/depth and character of respirations. Listen for breath sounds. SpO_2 to assess oxygenation. $PaCO_2$ and/or $EtCO_2$ to assess ventilation. Reassess frequently.	Oxygen at high flow rate. May use ventilation with bag-valve-mask, but can cause rapid deterioration in presence of pneumothorax. Emergency chest tube for tension pneumo or large hemothorax. Gastric tube with suction to prevent vomiting (place tube orally if there is possible fracture of cribriform plate)
Circulation	Assess pulses, HR, rhythm, blood pressure, heart sounds, neck veins, skin color/temp. Sources of bleeding: chest, abdomen, extremities, back. Beware the absence of ↑ HR in aged pts on rate-limiting med.	Direct pressure to external bleed. Insert two large bore upper extremity IV catheters. Give crystalloid rapidly. Start blood if hypotension is unresponsive to crystalloid. Urethral cath unless contraindicated. Keep urinary output > 0.5 mL/kg/hr.
Disability (Neuro)	Assess LOC, Determine GCS. Assess pupils size, equality, reaction to light. Check motor ability/strength. Assess sensory status.	Protect from secondary injury: prevent hypothermia, hypoxemia, hypercapnea, hypotension, hypoglycemia, volume excess. Neuro consult if signs of ↑ ICP or SCI.
Exposure	Remove all of pt's clothing. Check front, back, all orifices, haired areas.	Inspect for any missed injuries. Apply warming blankets, prewarm the IV fluids (39°), ↑ room temp. It is critical to prevent hypothermia.

"AMPLE" Quick History	Adjuncts
A Allergies **M** Meds (Beta-blocker, steroid, NSAID, warfarin) **P** Past history, Pregnancies **L** Last Meal, Last menstrual period **E** Environment and Events related to injury	• ABGs, pulse oximeter • Exhaled CO_2 monitor • Chest and C-spine X-ray • Consider Abd X-ray, DPL, FAST, ECG, CT scan

The Secondary Survey

Structure	Assessments	Considerations
Head	Inspect and palpate skull for lacerations, bruises, fractures. Assess level of consciousness (GCS), abnormal breathing pattern, posture. Check for absence of sensation, or level of pain. Score the level of pain if possible (pain scale 1 - 10).	Scalp lacerations Focal vs diffuse brain injury Expanding intracranial mass Severity of brain injury: GCS ≤ 8 Severe = 9 - 12 Moderate = 13 - 15 Minor
Eyes	Check pupil size & reaction to light, presence of contact lenses, raccoon sign, abnormal eye movement.	Eye injury, injury to cranial nerves II - VI, orbit fracture, basilar skull fracture
Ears	Look for Battle's sign, CSF leak, hemotympanum.	External/internal ear injury Basilar skull fracture
Nose	Check for defects, pain, CSF leak, bleeding, presence of soot.	Caution: no nasal tubes if CSF rhinorrhea or Nosebleed
Mouth	Risk of aspiration, integrity of tongue, teeth, palate, presence of dentures or foreign objects.	Injury to tongue, teeth, gums, palate, surfaces of oral cavity Airway injury or threat
Maxillo-Facial	For defects, deformity, pain, jaw malocclusion, asymmetry, bleeding, inability to protect airway.	Facial fracture, Airway threat, Cranial nerve injury Uncontrolled bleeding
Neck	Palpate for pain, tenderness, hematoma in area of C-spine. Inspect for hematoma, jugular vein (flat vs full), penetrating injury. Palpate for swelling, mass, thrills, crepitus, position of trachea.	C-spine vertebral fracture, dislocation, ligament tear, Cervical nerve root injury, Laryngeal injury, Vascular injury, Hematoma or edema may threaten the airway.
Chest	Check for dyspnea, hypoxia. Assess chest wall expansion, pain, wounds, deformity, asymmetry, hematomas, sternal retraction. Palpate ribs, sternum, clavicle. Locate PMI. Note pulse deficits. Listen to heart and breath sounds.	Rib fractures, flail chest Spinal cord injury Bronchial or esophageal injury Hemo/pneumothorax Pulmonary contusion Aorta or cardiac injury Pericardial tamponade
Abdomen	Look for distention, asymmetry, mass, penetrating wound, hematoma, flank bruise, periumbilical bruise. Listen for bowel sounds. Palpate for pain, crepitus, pelvic instability. √ external rotation of limb.	Abdominal wall injury Abdominal organ injury Vascular injury Retroperitoneal bleeding Pelvic fracture Compartment syndrome
Perineum	Inspect for blood at the meatus, scrotal or perineal hematoma. Rectal exam for anal sphincter tone, blood, prostate position. Vaginal exam for wall integrity. Check urine for blood.	Renal, ureteral, bladder, or urethral injury Spinal cord injury Gynecologic injury Prostate/genital injury
Extremities	Look for bruises, abrasions, lacerations, hematomas, asymmetry, abnormal posture, lateralizing signs, motor/sensory deficits. Palpate for tenderness, pain, crepitus, deformity, bruit, pulse strength, capillary refill, joint range of motion.	Cranial or spinal cord injury Fracture vs dislocation Soft tissue injury and edema Peripheral nerve injury Vascular injury, ischemic threat (irreversible in 3 - 4 hr) Joint dislocation
Lab	T&C, ABG, CBC, H/H, Electrolytes, BG, PT/PTT, Blood alcohol, urine for blood, pregnancy test.	The "triad of death": Acidosis, Hypothermia, Coagulopathy.
Diagnostic Tests	FAST (Focus Assessment with Sonography in Trauma), DPL (Diagnostic Peritoneal Lavage), CT (Computerized Tomography), MRI (Magnetic Resonance Imaging), Arteriogram.	

Hemorrhagic Shock

Please refer to "Hemorrhagic Shock" in the Hemo chapter to review the hemodynamic effects of hemorrhage on blood pressure and oxygen delivery, and to estimate the amount of blood loss using the 4 levels of shock described by the American College of Surgeons ATLS (Advanced Trauma Life Support, 2012).

The MultiSystem Response to Hemorrhagic Shock:

Sympathetic/Adrenal response:

- Tachycardia may temporarily compensate for falling SV, to maintain CO. This compensatory mechanism, however, is absent in patients who have a pacemaker or those who take rate-limiting medications
- The adrenal glands release norepinephrine and epinephrine (to produce vasoconstriction and tachycardia), stimulate glycogenolysis (raising the blood sugar), and release aldosterone (to promote renal conservations of Na).
- Circulating epinephrine inhibits insulin release, to promote increased BG.
- Glucagon prompts the liver to convert stored glycogen into glucose.
- Vasoconstriction temporarily sustains MAP, but it also diverts blood away from nonvital organ systems (e.g., the skin, muscle, kidneys, intestines) and toward vital organs (brain, heart, lungs).
- The SA response can sustain BP until up to 30% of blood volume is lost.

Metabolic response:

The SA response, tachycardia, increased respiratory rate, vasoconstriction, and pain, all increase metabolic rate and the demand for O_2 and substrate.

The Inflammatory response:

- Inadequate blood pressure, decreased blood volume, and hampered oxygen delivery stimulate an inflammatory response that releases Histamine,
- Cytokines, Prostanoids and other chemicals that significantly increase vascular permeability. Capillary leaking is a second source of volume loss.

Coagulation:

Resuscitation with room temperature crystalloid can cause hypothermia, which hampers clotting mechanisms, while also diluting all clotting factors.

Prolonged shock:

Prolonged hemorrhage culminates in anaerobic metabolism, causing base deficits, coagulation failure, and failure to maintain compensatory tachycardia and vasoconstriction.

This is "a rude unhinging of the machinery of life" Samuel Gross 1862

Multi-System Assessment of Hemorrhagic Shock:

Neuro:	The early stages of shock may be expressed as thirst, anxiety, abusive language, or combative behavior. Level of consciousness slowly ↓ as severity of shock increases. Loud/repeated verbal stimuli may be required to arouse patient. The sympathetic response causes pupil dilation. Class IV shock produces unconsciousness. Head injury confounds all of the above indicators of shock.
Cardio-vascular:	HR > 130, SBP < 90, CVP < 3 mm Hg represents severe shock. Signs of sympathetic-adrenal response to significant blood loss: cold, clammy skin, tachycardia, tachypnea, slow capillary refill. CVP increase of > 3 - 5 mm Hg in response to 100 mL fluid bolus suggests limited cardiac reserve. Distended neck veins and/or CVP > 12 mm Hg suggests impaired cardiac filling due to pericardial tamponade or tension pneumo.
Respiratory:	Tachypnea is an early response to sympathetic discharge. Later in shock, tachypnea works to compensate for metabolic acidosis. Dyspnea accompanies rib fracture, flail, hemo or pneumothorax.
Abdomen:	Abdominal distention is an indicator of intraabdominal bleeding. Retroperitoneal bleeding produces few physical signs.
Renal:	↓ urinary output and ↓ urinary Na are early responses to ADH and Aldosterone, as compensatory efforts to conserve volume. Rust colored urine may represent myoglobin from muscle injury or hemoglobin from transfusion reaction.
Hematology	Consumption of coagulation factors is present in up to 30% of severely injured pts on admit. PT, PTT, platelet count are valuable.

Hemorrhagic Shock

Patient History Relevant to Hemorrhage:

- B-blocker or Calcium Channel blocker
- Anticoagulants, or taking NSAIS
- Implanted pacemaker or Cardiodefibrillator
- Diabetic patient, with insulin deficit or excess
- History of cardiac insufficiency
- Patient is an athlete, who may be able to effectively increase cardiac output, maintaining MAP longer than most.

Estimate Fracture-Related Blood Loss:	
Humerus:	250 mL
Tibia:	500 mL
Femur:	1000 mL
Pelvic:	2000 mL

Initial Management of Hemorrhage:

1 Volume Replace with Isotonic Crystalloid:

Warm (37°- 39° C) Ringer's Lactate (RL) is the preferred isotonic crystalloid. Give 1 - 2 L (20 mL/kg for pedi pts) as rapidly as possible, using a pump. The goal is to improve cardiac output, blood pressure, urinary output.

2 After 2 L of resuscitation fluids, hemorrhage is serious if:

- BP improves only briefly or not at all
- Base deficit remains ≥ 6 mEq/L
- CVP remains < 3 mm Hg
- Hgb falls more than 2 g/dL

3 Time to Transfuse:

- If the patient's MAP is stabilized, but Hgb declines to < 7 g/dL, oxygen carrying capacity should be restored by infusion of blood.
  In pts without cardiac or cerebral vascular disease, target Hgb > 7 g/dL.
  Pts with active coronary or cerebral vascular disease, target Hgb = 10 g/dL.
- If MAP remains < 65 mm Hg and the amount of administered RL is > 30 mL/kg, start blood. Optimal ratio of RL to blood is 3:1.

4 Scrutinize fluid resuscitation techniques:

- Aggressive fluid administration can lead to tissue swelling with ↑ pressure in the head, chest, abdomen, extremities (multi-compartment syndrome).
- Large volume fluid resuscitation dilutes the patient's clotting factors and reduces the oncotic force needed to sustain blood volume.
- Crystalline and colloid solutions do not carry oxygen.
- Ringer's Lactate provokes the inflammatory response, ↑ chance of ARDS.
- Cold fluids contribute to hypothermia induced coagulopathy.
- Esophageal or bladder temp offer accurate clinical measure of core temp.
- Aggressive fluid resuscitation can promote bleeding. Hypotensive resuscitation (MAP maintained at 65 mm Hg) is recommended prior to emergency surgical repair, EXCEPT for patients with severe head injury.
- MAST suit does not ↑ venous return, it ↑ SVR, restricts respiration, and causes compartment syndrome. MAST suit is not recommended.

5 Prevent the Triad of Death: Acidosis + Coagulopathy + Hypothermia

- Apply warming blankets. Warm all fluids and blood. Warm the room.
- Minimize acidosis by supporting the 3 components of oxygen delivery: Cardiac output, Hemoglobin, and Arterial oxygen saturation.
- Deficit of 2,3 DPG in old blood increases the affinity of hemoglobin for oxygen, thus impairing the unloading of oxygen at the tissue level.
- Activate **Massive Transfusion Protocol** if needed (**see next page**) ---->

6 Continued Hemorrhage in the ICU:

PA catheter is recommended. Continue fluids to ↑ PCWP to 15 mm Hg.
Goals: CI ≥ 3.8 L/min/m2, DO_2I > 400 - 500 mL/min/m2, SvO_2 > 60%.
If total fluid volume exceeds 10 L or PRBC's exceed 10 units, monitor for abdominal compartment syndrome (bladder pressure ≥ 25 mm Hg).
If Low CI + adequate PCWP + High SVR: Dobutamine is recommended, starting at 5 μg/kg/min, increased in increments of 2.5 μg/kg/min to a maximum of 20 μg/kg/min. Dopamine may also be used.
An inotropic agent with vasoconstrictive effects may be needed to keep MAP ≥ 60 mm Hg and improve myocardial contractility. Consider Norepinephrine starting at 0.05 μg/kg/min, increased in increments of 0.05 μg/kg/min. Maximum Norepinephrine dose is 0.2 μg/kg/min.

Massive Transfusion (MT)

Facts:

- MT is the replacement of a patient's total blood volume in less than 24 hrs, or the administration of > 50% of the patient's estimated blood volume per hour.
- Coagulopathy of trauma is non-surgical bleeding of wounds, mucosal lesions, and vascular access sites. Coagulopathy is present in 25% of trauma patients on admission to the ED, affects 35% of all patients with severe head injury, and is associated with a 5-fold increase in mortality.
- FFP and platelets are critical to prevention/management of coagulopathy.
- Massive Transfusion Protocol (MTP) has been shown in multiple studies to improve patient outcome and reduce the cost of massive transfusion.
- Coagulopathy may complicate severe brain injury; increases death risk 10-fold
- Presume coagulopathy if Base Deficit > 6 + hemorrhage + significant injury.

Causes of Coagulopathy:

1	**Acidosis** When pH $\leq$ 7, most clotting factor activity is reduced such that clot formation time is increased by more than 150%. At its 6-week expiration date, the pH of stored blood is < 7. Even without hypothermia, acidosis in combination with injury severity score (ISS) is linked to coagulopathy.
2	**Hypothermia** Caused by cold blood, cold fluids, environment, and open body cavities. Hypothermia 32° C results in same effect as pH = 7 (clotting time ↑ > 150%). Each 1° C decrease in body temp reduces clotting factor activity by 10%.
3	**Fewer clotting factors** Crystalloids have no clotting factors and dilute those that remain. Blood older then 24 hours is deficient in functional platelets. Stored blood is absent clotting factors V and VIII.
4	**Hyperfibrinolysis** Surgery and some resuscitation fluids trigger the inflammatory response, which initiates fibrinolysis (the breakdown of clot).

Trauma that may need MT	Proceed with MT
Penetrating torso trauma Severe blunt torso trauma Severe pelvic fracture Major vascular injury	As determined by the surgeon, or SBP $\leq$ 90, HR $\geq$ 120, positive FAST, pH $\leq$ 7.24, or if pt given $\geq$ 4 units PRBC over 1 hour, or if pt given $\geq$ 10 units in 24 hr

Example Massive Transfusion Protocol (MTP)

1. Physician activates MTP.
2. Blood Bank is notified. Stat blood sample is sent for type and crossmatch.
3. A "Blood Box" is prepared (if at all possible, type specific) containing 1:1:1 ratio of components (some recommend higher ratios).

PRBC	5 units
FFP	5 units
Platelets	5 units

   If hemorrhage is immediately life-threatening, the first Box will contain untyped O negative blood. Subsequent Boxes should be crossmatched.
4. Some protocols require a Box every 20 minutes until the MTP is cancelled by the physician. Others deliver additional Boxes as ordered.
5. Lab is notified. Stat blood samples are sent.
   PT, PTT, fibrinogen, thrombin time, d-dimer, CBC, H/H, chemistry, ABG.
6. Employ heat lamps, thermal caps, heated respiratory gases, prewarmed fluids
7. All blood components and fluids must be warmed.
8. Every 30 minutes, assess Hgb, INR, Plt count, PT, PTT, and fibrinogen levels.

If Hemoglobin is < 7g/dL:	PRBC's are given.
If INR > 1.5:	4 units FFP. Repeat until INR controlled.
If Plt count < 100,000/dL:	Platelet concentrate (1 pack/10 kg). 1 platelet pack should ↑ plt count by 25 - 50 k
If Fibrinogen < 100 mg/dL:	Cryoprecipitate (10 units)
If ongoing bleeding:	Tranexamic acid is considered (see next page)

   In the OR, abdominal or thoracic cavities may we irrigated with warm fluids.

Antifibrinolytics for Hemorrhage?

No to Novoseven:

- Blood loss not only produces hypovolemia, it also wastes clotting factors.
- In addition, hemorrhage activates the inflammatory response, which increases clot lysis (see "Med Facts" chapter, topic "Clotting and Lysing").
- In critical trauma patients, surgical repair alone may not stop the bleeding.
- Hopes once hinged on the use of Factor VIIa (Novoseven RT), a plasminogen inhibitor used to control bleeding in patients with hemophilia.
- Studies found that Factor VIIa, when used to stem bleeding in critical trauma patients, did not reduce the death rate, and carried the real risk of causing thromboembolism.
- Recommendations for the use of Factor VIIa in the treatment of coagulopathy of Trauma have been withdrawn.

Tranexamic acid (Cyklokapron)

Warning: Tranexamic acid is Not FDA approved for Hemorrhagic Shock.

Tranexamic acid is FDA approved for "patients with hemophilia for short-term use (2-8 days), to reduce or prevent hemorrhage and reduce need for replacement therapy following tooth extraction."

Description

- Tranexamic acid inhibits the activation of plasminogen and plasmin, to slow fibrinolysis (the lysis of clots).
- Has been used in liver transplantation and cardiac surgery to reduce blood loss and transfusion requirement.
- A randomized, controlled trial that included over 20,000 trauma patients with hemorrhagic shock showed that "Tranexamic acid given to patients with traumatic bleeding within three hours of injury significantly reduced mortality with no apparent increase in adverse thrombotic events."
- Tranexamic acid reduced the odds of death from bleeding by about 30% and reduced the odds of thrombotic events by about 30%. (see reference 1)
- Tranexamic acid binds more strongly than aminocaproic acid (Amicar).
- In bleeding trauma patients, Tranexamic acid is given as early as possible. The optimal effect occurs when given within the first 3 hrs of bleeding.
- For trauma patient admitted late after injury (> 3 hours), tranexamic acid may increase bleeding and should not be given.
- The benefits of tranexamic acid may be greatest in older trauma patients, who have a higher baseline risk of death from hemorrhage and from thrombotic events due to cardiovascular disease.
- Trials of tranexamic acid in patients undergoing cardiac surgery have found no evidence of increased risk.
- The World Health Organization (WHO) added Tranexamic acid to the "List of Essential Medicines."

Preparation: 100 mg/ml in 5 mL and 10 mL ampule

Dose for Adult Hemorrhage: 1 g over 10 min, then infusion of 1 g over 8 hr

Actions:

- Inhibits plasminogen.
- Actions are similar to aminocaproic acid (Amicar)
- No influence on platelet count, coagulation time, or various coagulation factors in blood.
- Does not bind to serum albumin.

1. The CRASH-2 collaborators. The importance of early treatment with tranexamic acid in bleeding trauma patients. The Lancet. Published online March 24, 2011.

2. Roberts I, Perel P, Prieto-Merino D, et al. Effect of Tranexamic acid on mortality in patients with traumatic bleeding: prespecified analysis of data from randomised controlled trial. BMJ 2012;345 Sept 2012.

Severe Traumatic Brain Injury

Facts:

- Severe Traumatic Brain Injury (STBI) is head injury with GCS ≤ 8.
- The implementation of evidence-based protocols (on treatment of intracranial hypertension and prevention of secondary neurologic injury) has reduced mortality due to STBI from 50% to 25%.
- 4 - 8% of patients with head injury also have spinal cord injury.

Risk Factors for Poor Outcome:

- Age > 40 years
- Patient takes warfarin
- Development of coagulopathy
- Intraventricular hemorrhage
- Obesity
- Episode of ↓ BP or ↓ PO_2
- Pupils remain unreactive
- Lower GCS score
- ↑ ICP or CT evidence of ↑ ICP (cerebral edema, compressed or absent basal cisterns, midline shift, major intracranial hemorrhage).
- Delay from neurologic deterioration to neurosurgical treatment.

Patho-physiology:

Mechanisms of traumatic injury:
1. Acceleration/deceleration of the brain inside the skull may: Produce shearing forces that disrupt axons and capillaries. Tear bridging veins between the brain surface and dura. Contuse the frontal lobes as they slide over the orbital plate. Cause the temporal lobe to impact the sphenoid ridge. Avulse the olfactory tracts from the cribriform plate. Close the spinal fluid pathways and venous drainage systems. 2. Skull fracture may lacerate underlying blood vessels, causing hematoma and/or direct injury to dura and brain parenchyma. 3. Penetrating trauma introduces infection and risk for seizures.
Response of the brain to injury:
1. Stage of **ischemia**: Immediately post injury, cerebral vasoconstriction reduces cerebral blood flow (CBF) as much as 50 - 60%. At its lowest 4 - 6 hours post injury, CBF may approach ischemic threshold (< 20 mL/100g brain tissue/min) (normal = 50 - 55 mL) 2. Stage of **hyperemia**: The inflammatory response to injury results in the release of chemicals which vasodilate and increase capillary permeability, causing cerebral edema. 3. Stage of **acute ischemia**: Release of chemical mediators from the CNS and vasoactive metabolites from lysed clots cause vasoconstriction, reducing oxygen delivery to the brain.
At the cellular level:
1. Ischemia and hypoxia allow progressive influx of calcium into the cells, culminating in disintegration of neurons. 2. The increased intracellular calcium is due to: release of excitatory amino acids (glutamate and aspartate) and release of intracellular stores of calcium.
Mechanisms of secondary brain injury ("the 2nd hit"):
1. Systemic causes: Hypotension, Anemia, Hypoxemia, ↑↓ BG, ↑↓ $PaCO_2$, Hyperthermia, Inflammatory response syndrome. 2. Intracranial causes: Hematoma, Infection, Cerebral edema, Seizures, Cerebral vasospasm, CSF outflow obstruction.

↑ ICP: (Increased Intracranial Pressure)

Increased ICP occurs in 25 - 45% of patients with severe head injury. The size of the 3 intracranial components must be reduced:

1. Cerebral blood volume: Spontaneous hyperventilation reduces CO_2 to effect vasoconstriction. Unfortunately, vasoconstriction reduces cerebral blood flow (CBF).
2. CSF volume: Therapeutically, an intraventricular catheter (IVC) may be used to remove CSF. See Neuro chapter for details.
3. Brain volume: Can be reduced with osmotherapy and with surgical removal of clot or contusion.
   When these fail, sustained intracranial hypertension causes cerebral ischemia, injury, herniation syndromes, death.

Types & Mechanisms of Head Injury

Contusion:	A bruise to the parenchyma, usually to the temporal or frontal lobes. Present in 20 - 30% of STBI. Often there is early progression (the first 24 hours post injury) due to edema or bleeding (intracerebral bleeding occurs in almost all pts with abnormal PTT or high INR). Refractory ↑ in ICP may require surgical decompression or removal. Coup/Contrecoup mechanism of injury: Accelerative/decelerative energy can cause contusions on opposite sides of the brain.
Concussion and DAI:	Transmission of energy to the brain results in diffuse axonal disruption (DAI). Examples include shaken baby syndrome, violent head rotation, or deceleration/whiplash in MVA. Also known as "shearing" injury. Usually presents in coma with no CT evidence of structural injury, then biochemical cascade results in cerebral edema. 90% who present in coma never regain consciousness.
Epidural hematoma:	Occurs in 1% of all head trauma. Hematoma forms between the dura and the skull, most commonly in the temporal/parietal area. Caused by laceration of the middle meningeal artery (but in 10% of cases, bleeding is venous). Intracerebral contusion is common. In 9%, the hematoma progresses in size over the first 24 hours. A classic presentation occurs in 1/3 of pts: loss of consciousness, followed by lucid interval, then neurologic decline. Mortality rate increases with the delay to surgery. Posterior fossa epidural is very rare, with few warning signs, presenting as "Talk, then Die" patients

Fig. 13.1 Fig. 13.2

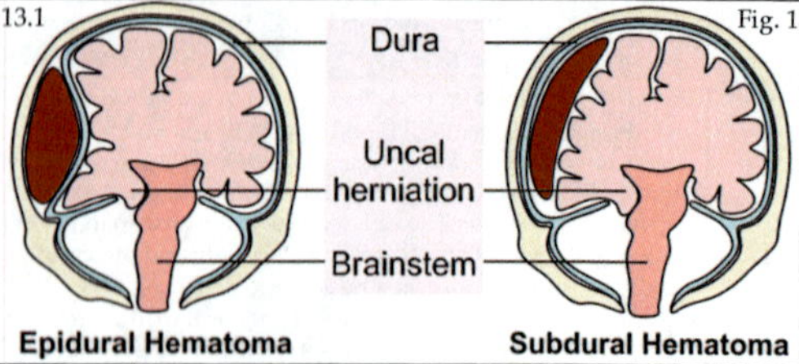

Subdural hematoma:	Occurs in about 1/3 of pts with severe head injury. Caused by disruption of bridging veins between brain surface & dura sinus 50% are simple (no underlying brain injury), with low mortality. 50% are complicated (there is contusion or laceration of brain).
Supratentorial hematoma:	Any hematoma located above the tentorium*; within or around the cerebrum. Expansion can lead to herniation syndrome.
Intraventricular hemorrhage:	Blood in the ventricles. STBI is very severe, prognosis is poor. Obstructed CSF outflow or impaired CSF reabsorption requires intraventricular catheter drainage.
Intracerebral hemorrhage	Hemorrhage into the parenchyma. Hemorrhage progression occurs in 32%. Permanent neurologic injury is common.
Basilar skull fracture:	Associated with brain and/or cranial nerve trauma, and sometimes CSF leak (which carries a 25% risk of meningitis as well as risk of tension pneumocephalus).

Fossa	Houses the	Evidence of Basilar Skull Fracture
Anterior	Frontal lobes	Altered eye movement, CSF rhinorrhea, epistaxis, periorbital ecchymoses ("Raccoon Eyes")
Middle	Temporal lobes	Hemotympanum, tinnitus, CSF otorrhea, hearing loss (8th CN), facial nerve paralysis (7th CN)
Posterior	Cerebellum, Brainstem	Bruise behind the ear ("Battle sign"), impaired gag, inability to rotate head.

* Tentorium separates the cerebrum from the cerebellum.

Brain Herniation Syndromes

Brain Herniation Syndromes:

- In patients with severe head injury, intracranial pressure is increased by intracranial bleeding, brain swelling, and/or hydrocephalus.
- If ICP increases enough, regions of the brain may herniate into adjacent compartments, resulting in compression, distortion, shifting, hemorrhage, obstructed blood supply, obstructed CSF circulation.
- In some patients, the herniation may be reversed by prompt reduction of cerebral edema or by removal of intracranial clot (craniotomy).
- Emergency Burr Holes seldom allow sufficient drainage.
- The ACS Committee on Trauma strongly recommends that emergency craniotomy be done only by neurosurgeon or neurosurgeon-trainee.

Transtentorial Herniation:

A. Central Herniation

Tentorium is the dura between cerebrum and cerebellum, supporting the occipital lobes. The diencephalon and parts of both temporal lobes of the cerebral hemispheres are squeezed downward through the tentorial notch (the opening in the tentorium through which the brainstem passes).
The compression progressively descends upon the diencephalon and then brainstem (midbrain, pons, medulla), producing progressive deterioration in neurologic signs:

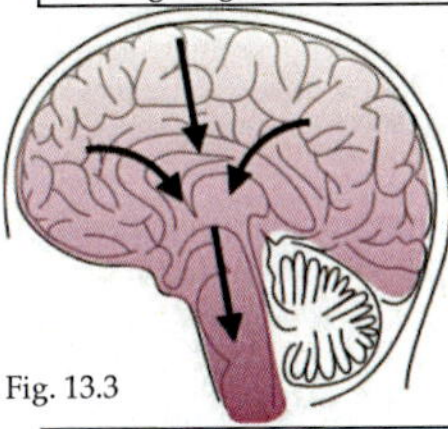

Fig. 13.3

Diencephalon: ↓	↓ LOC, decorticate posture, ↑ breathing rate, hemiparesis.
Midbrain: ↓	Pupils unreactive to light, size midposition or dilated, decerebrate posture, coma, spontaneous hyperventilation.
Pons: ↓	Flaccid posture, pinpoint pupils, apneustic breathing, coma.
Medulla: ↓ Death	Flaccid posture, dilated pupils, hemodynamic instability, cardiac and respiratory arrest.

B. Uncal Herniation

A lateral mass displaces the brain on one side and pushes the uncus of the temporal lobe medially over the tentorial edge (compressing the brainstem) and into the posterior fossa (compressing the cerebral artery, which may cause occipital lobe infarction). May advance to central herniation.

- Ipsilateral pupil is midposition or dilated, unreactive to light
- Contralateral posturing or paralysis
- Rarely, hemiparesis and unreactive pupil occur on the same side as the mass (Kernohan's notch syndrome)
- Spontaneous hyperventilation
- Eventually, signs of central herniation

Tonsillar Herniation:

Cerebellar mass causes downward displacement of the cerebellar tonsils through the foramen magnum, compressing the lower brainstem and upper spinal cord. The herniation can be precipitated by lumbar puncture. Few warning signs precede the rapid neurologic deterioration.

CT Classification	Description of Severity of Injury
Diffuse Injury I	No visible pathology seen on CT
Diffuse Injury II	Cisterns are present with 0 - 5 mm shift No high- or mixed-density lesion > 25 mL May have bone fragments or foreign bodies
Diffuse Injury III	Cisterns compressed or absent Shift 0 - 5 mm, no high- or mixed density > 25 mL
Diffuse Injury IV	Shift > 5 mm, no high- or mixed density lesion > 25 mL
Mass Lesion	High- or mixed density lesion > 25 mL
Evacuated Mass	A lesion has been surgically evacuated

Treatment of Severe Head Injury (GCS 3 - 8)

Treatment Plan:
Stabilize BP, maintain normal MAP
Prevent/Treat intracranial hypertension
Maintain adequate and stable CPP
Prevent secondary brain insults
Optimize cerebral hemodynamics
Optimize oxygenation
Prevent complications

Beware Obscured Neuro Signs:
Conditions that may conceal the presence of head injury: drugs, hypotension, other injuries.
Seizure: patient responsiveness will be worse for minutes to hours after.
Sedation: Avoid unless there is risk of injury. Short acting agents only.

1. **Oxygenate & Ventilate**
   - Monitor oxygenation, avoid hypoxia ($PaO_2 < 60$ or $SaO_2 < 90$).
   - An episode of hypoxia can increase mortality rate by as much as 50%, and worsen the outcome of those who do survive. Intubate if GCS ≤ 8.
   - Critical to maintain $PaCO_2$ 30 - 35 mm Hg.
   - In patients who have no signs of increased ICP, using hyperventilation to prevent increased ICP is not recommended.
   - During the first 24 hours, cerebral blood flow is often critically low (50% of normal). $PaCO_2 < 30$ mm Hg is therefore especially dangerous.

2. **Support Cerebral Perfusion by supporting MAP**
   - Prevent/quickly treat a SBP < 90 mm Hg.
   - Low GCS may improve with improvement in blood pressure.
   - A single episode of hypotension increases morbidity and can double mortality. Hypoxia + Hypotension = mortality of 75%.
   - Hypotension in patients with STBI is usually due to extracranial causes. It is critical to the neuro outcome to find and control the source of bleeding
   - Unless contraindicated by hypotension, elevate HOB 30°.
   - Maintain neutral neck position. Avoid compression of the jugular vein.

3. **Attend to Neuro Deterioration/Increased ICP**
   - Neither mannitol nor hypertonic saline will lower ICP in hypovolemic pts.
   - Temporary (15 - 30 minutes) hyperventilation to PCO_2 = 28 - 30 mmHg
     $PCO_2 < 30$ -> causes cerebral vasoconstriction
     $PCO_2 > 45$ -> causes cerebral vasodilation and increased ICP
   - Mannitol:
     For rising ICP: Mannitol 0.25 - 1 g/kg over 15 - 20 minutes.
     For acute neurologic deterioration: Mannitol 1 g/kg over 5 minutes.
   - If unresponsive to Mannitol, Hypertonic saline 2 mL/kg may be used, but there is risk of rapid shift in Na, causing pontine demyelination, or pulmonary edema in cardiac patients.

4. **Stat Surgery if CT Reveals Midline Shift ≥ 5 mm**

5. **Temperature**
   - Aggressively treat Temp > 38° C.
   - Maintaining temp (usually at 37° C) for > 48 hrs may decrease mortality.
   - Prophylactic hypothermia (35°) may offer marginal benefit.

6. **Blood Glucose**
   - Hypo and hyperglycemia can cause secondary insult.
   - Resuscitation fluids <u>must</u> be void of glucose.
   - Insulin may be needed to keep BG < 150 mg/dL.

7. **Stop Seizures**
   - Risk Factors for Seizures:
     GCS < 10, cortical contusion, depressed skull fracture, cerebral hematoma, penetrating head injury, seizures within 24 hrs of injury.
   - Phenytoin 15 - 20 mg/kg IV over 30 minutes, followed by 100 mg q 8 hrs, titrated to plasma level, for 7 days.
   - Barbiturate coma: do not use in presence of hypotension or hypovolemia, Barbiturates are not used in the acute resuscitation phase.
   - 3 factors are linked to development of late epilepsy: seizures during the first week, intracranial hematoma, depressed skull fracture.

8. Coagulopathy

- Occurs in > 35% of all STBI patients. Those at highest risk: GCS ≤ 8, ISS ≥ 16, presence of cerebral edema, subarachnoid hemorrhage, midline shift. Increases ICU length of stay, and death risk 10-fold.
- Look for Platelet count < 100,000 mm^3, elevated INR.
- Patients > 6 years old and on low dose aspirin therapy have higher risk for intracranial hemorrhage. Even those with mild head injury require repeat CT in 12 - 24 hr and observation x 48 hr.

9. ICP Monitor

- Brain swelling and ↑ ICP develop in 25 - 45% of STBI patients.
- ICP monitoring is instituted in all salvageable patients with STBI if:
  1. CT is abnormal and GCS is 3 - 8 after resuscitation, or
  2. GCS 3 - 8 and presence of any 2: age > 40, SBP < 90 mm Hg, unilateral or bilateral motor posturing.
- ICP monitor can be used to detect worsening intracranial pathology, calculate and manage cerebral perfusion pressure (CPP), allow therapeutic CSF drainage, permit continuous monitoring of ICP, and detect and restrict ICP reduction therapies that are ineffective.
- Ventricular catheter to external transducer is the simplest, most accurate, lowest cost, and most reliable method and permits therapeutic drainage of CSF.
- Complications of ICP monitoring include infection, hemorrhage, obstruction, malfunction, malposition, inaccurate values.

Normal ICP:	< 10 mm Hg
Upper limit:	= 15 mm Hg
Start treatment when:	> 20 mm Hg, or
based on clinical signs + ICP + CT results	

ICP, mm Hg	Mortality
< 20	18%
20 - 39	45%
40 - 59	74%
> 60	100%

10. Cerebral Perfusion Pressure

- Target a CPP of 50 - 70 mm Hg (CPP = MAP - ICP)
- Avoid CPP < 50 mm Hg (some say < 60 mm Hg).
  Low CPP is associated with cerebral ischemia, ↑ ICP, worsened outcome.
- Avoid aggressive attempts to maintain CPP > 70 mm Hg using fluids and pressors, because of the risk of fluid excess, increased cerebral edema, and pulmonary edema.

	Management of Refractory Intracranial Hypertension (develops in 10 - 15% of pts with STBI; mortality rate is 85 - 100%)
Barbiturate:	When all other medical and surgical treatments fail, high dose barbiturate can control ICP, but should not be used if the patient is hypotensive or hypovolemic. Pentobarbital: load with 10 mg/kg over 30 minutes, then 5 mg/kg every hour x 3 doses, then maintain at 1 mg/kg/hr, to achieve serum Pentobarbital level of 3-4 mg/dL or EEG pattern of burst suppression. Inducing "Burst suppression EEG" with barbiturate as a means of ***preventing*** intracranial hypertension is not recommended.
Propofol:	Propofol is recommended for control of ICP, but high dose (> 5 mg/kg/hr or any dose for > 48 hr) can cause significant morbidity (hyperkalemia, acidosis, myocardial or renal failure).
Hyperventilation:	$PaCO_2$ 28 - 30 mm Hg is discouraged during the first 24 hours. If used, should be guided by $SjvO_2$ or $PbtO_2$ monitoring. $PaCO_2$ < 28 mm Hg is not recommended.
Therapeutic Hypothermia:	Studies suggest that targeting a lower temp (32° - 35° C) for more than 48 hours may improve GCS and decrease mortality rate.
Extreme Measures:	Decompressive craniotomy has been used in Level I Trauma centers, with favorable outcome in 30% of patients. Laparotomy for abdominal compartment syndrome may be needed in pts with combined severe head and abdominal trauma.

Severe Traumatic Brain Injury (STBI)

Treatment Guidelines (cont'd)

Sympathetic Storm:	• Incidence is 15 - 30% of patients with STBI. • Characterized by agitation, diaphoresis, increased posturing, ↓ in LOC, ↑ BP, ↑ HR, ↑ RR, ↑ Temp, arrhythmias (AFib, Bradycardia, SVT), pupil dilation (due to sympathetic stimuli) • Places patient at risk for secondary brain injury. • Can occur within first 24 hrs and up to weeks later. • The syndrome duration averages 74 d. Mechanism is unknown. • Appears unprovoked (but may be triggered by suctioning, turning, alarms, fever), can last hours, ends abruptly. • Try Morphine, Fentanyl, Midazolam. Doses may be extreme. • Beta-blocker is given if MAP > 120, unless contraindicated. • Nipride poses risk of vasodilation and hypotension.
Nutrition:	• Attain full caloric replacement by day 7 (25 kcal/kg/day). • In pts with severe head injury, metabolic rate may ↑ 120 - 250%. • Even with paralysis, energy expenditure remains ↑ by 20 - 30%. • Starved TBI patients lose 15% of weight per week. • Two weeks of undernutrition -> significant ↑ in mortality rate. • Enteral feeding is the most common and desired route.
Steroids:	• Have not been shown to improve outcome or reduce intracranial pressure in STBI. • Some studies have shown that steroids ↑ mortality rate and are therefore contraindicated. However, surveys indicate that many physicians still routinely prescribe steroids for head injury.
Seizure treatment and prevention:	• Seizures occur in 15% of STBI patients. • Early seizure of brief duration is not linked to worse outcome. But subsequent seizure/s are likely. • Seizures lasting > 30-60 mins can cause secondary brain injury. • Anticonvulsant may be given, but is generally contraindicated during acute phase, due to hypotensive effects. • Phenytoin 1 g IV no faster than 50 mg/min loading dose, then maintenance dose of 100 mg/8 hours, titrated to serum levels. • Add Diazepam or Lorazepam for prolonged seizures. • NMBA is given <u>after</u> anti-seizure therapy is initiated. • Anticonvulsants may also be given to prevent early seizure. It is not recommended to use anticonvulsants beyond week 1. • Risk factors for post traumatic seizures: GCS < 10 — Any type of intracranial hematoma Cortical contusion — Depressed skull fracture Penetrating head wound — Seizure within 24 hr of injury
DVT prevention:	• Without prevention, risk of developing DVT is about 20%. • Graduated compression stockings or intermittent pneumatic compression are recommended (unless contraindicated by lower extremity injury) and continued until pt is ambulatory. • LMWH or low dose UFH should also be used, although risk for intracranial hemorrhage is increased.
Infection prevention:	• Antibiotics before or after intubation, and early tracheostomy help to reduce days of mechanical ventilation. However, length of stay, nosocomial pneumonia rate, and mortality rate will not be affected. • Early extubation is encouraged (to ↓ the risk of pneumonia). • Infection rate due to ICP monitoring can be as high as 27%. • Routine ventricular catheter exchange or prophylactic antibiotic use for IVC placement is not recommended. • Risk of external ventricular drainage infection is increased by: duration of use, prophylactic antibiotics, presence of subarachnoid or intraventricular hemorrhage, presence of other infection, open skull fracture, CSF leak, ICP catheter leak.

Spinal Cord Injury

Facts:

- Complete spinal cord injury (CSCI) is defined as the absence of sensory and motor function below a certain segment of the cord.
- Spinal shock ("stunned cord") presents as CSCI plus absence of reflexes, and can interfere with nerve transmission for 1 - 2 weeks, delaying the diagnosis of CSCI until reflexes return.
- Neurogenic shock: In patients with SCI above T6, impairment of the descending sympathetic pathways results in bradycardia, hypothermia, and peripheral vasodilation with hypotension.
- CT has replaced plain x-ray as the primary imaging technique.

Patho-physiology:

- There is a 6-fold increase in glutamate and aspartate (enough to destroy neurons) for 1 hour after injury.
- Inflammatory response releases leukotriene and thromboxane, which reduce cord perfusion 40 - 55% for up to 18 hrs.
- ↑ capillary permeability and vasodilation cause cord edema.
- ↑ Intracellular Na & Ca produce cell swelling and disintegration.
- Cysts or scars form at the site of blocked signal transmission

Neurologic level: The most caudal level that has normal motor/sensory function. Example: A patient has absent motor and sensory function from C6 down. "He's at C5" means that C5 is intact and functioning.

It's all about Location:

- All nerves emerge ABOVE their corresponding vertebra, except nerve C8, which emerges between vertebrae C7 and T1.
- SCI above C6 can cause partial or total loss of respiratory function
- Injury to C1-C8 segments of the cord result in quadriplegia.
- Injury to cord segments below T1 is paraplegia.
- Fracture/dislocation of thoracic spine almost always causes CSCI.

Motor Score: American Spinal Injury Association (ASIA) — Score 0-5, Rt & Lt

	Motor neuron	Motor response	Pt's Rt	Pt's Lt
C5	Biceps	flex elbow	0 - 5	0 - 5
C6	Wrist Extensors	dorsiflex hand	0 - 5	0 - 5
C7	Triceps	extend elbow	0 - 5	0 - 5
C8	Flexor Digitroum Profundus	flex middle distal phalanx	0 - 5	0 - 5
T1	Hand Intrinsics	abduct little finger	0 - 5	0 - 5
L2	Iliopsoas	flex hip	0 - 5	0 - 5
L3	Quadriceps	extend knee	0 - 5	0 - 5
L4	Tibialis Anterior	dorsiflex foot	0 - 5	0 - 5
L5	Extensor Hallucia Longus	dorsiflex big toe	0 - 5	0 - 5
S1	Gastrocnemius	plantarflex foot (point toes)	0 - 5	0 - 5

5 Normal contraction, full ROM against gravity and full resistance
4 Active movement, full ROM agains gravity and moderate resistance
3 Active movement, full ROM against gravity
2 Active movement, full range of motion (ROM) with gravity eliminated
1 Palpable or visible contraction
0 Absent muscle contraction
The maximum total score is 100

Sensory Assessment on next page ->

Partial Spinal Cord Injury (PSCI):

Fig. 13.4

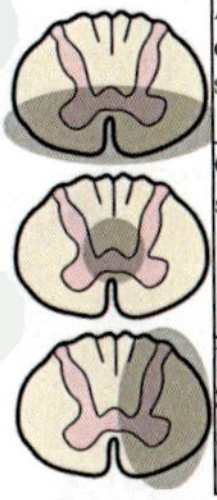

Type of SCI	Location of Injury	Physical Findings
Anterior cord syndrome	Loss of corticospinal + spinothalamic paths, with preservation of posterior column function	Loss of motor, pain, and temp sense. Position sense is preserved. Has the worst prognosis of the 3 PSCI's.
Central cord syndrome	Injury to centrally located fibers serving upper limb motor and spinothalamic function.	Upper extremities are weaker (at least 10 points on ASIA Motor Score) than lower extremities. Variable effect on sensory function.
Brown-Sequard syndrome	Injury to one side of the cord, due to penetrating trauma. Some recovery is usually seen.	Ipsilateral loss of motor and position sense + Contralateral loss of pain and temp sensation

Sensory Levels (Dermatomes)

American Spinal Injury Association (ASIA) Dermatome Assessment: Sensitivity to Rt/Lt touch and prick on a key point in each of 28 dermatomes.

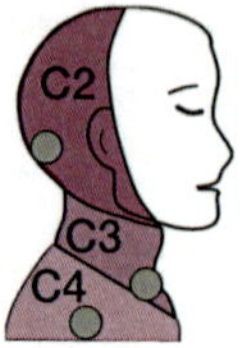

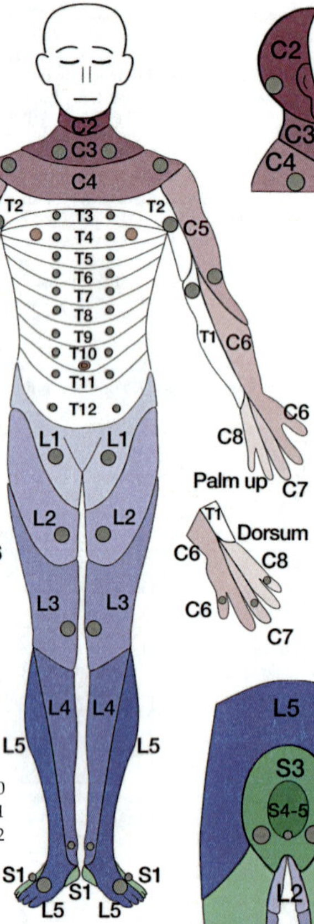

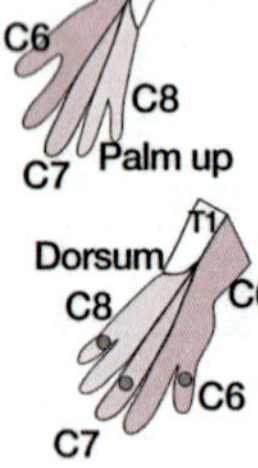

Sites for testing dull vs sharp sensation

Absent sensitivity:	0
Hypo or Hypersensitivity:	1
Normal sensitivity:	2

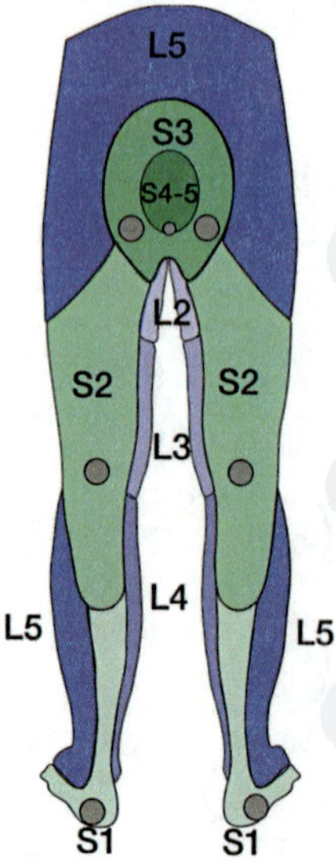

Begin by testing light touch of the feet, then move up the body.

adapted from: The American Spinal Injury Association. International Standards for Neurological Classification of Spinal Cord Injury. Chicago IL: 2011
http://www.asia-spinalinjury.org/elearning/ISNCSCI_Exam_Sheet_r4.pdf

Spinal Cord Injury

Some claim (but some question) "the C-spine is clear and x-rays are NOT required" if *all* of the following are present:

- Fully alert and oriented
- No drugs or alcohol on board
- No abnormal neurologic signs
- No fracture or significant other injury
- No head injury
- No neck pain

Presume SCI and unstable spine in all trauma patients with:

- Altered LOC, or
- Shock, or
- Pain in the spine or neck, or
- Any degree of paralysis, or
- Any degree of sensory loss

> Beware that transected spinal ligament/s produce spinal instability without fracture.

Assessment:

- History of any type of blunt, penetrating, or deceleration trauma.
- Subjective numbness, paresthesia, weakness.
- Pain/tenderness at site of injury. Paraspinous muscle spasm.
- Cervical or high thoracic SCI adversely affects vital capacity:
  C1, C2: vital capacity is 5 - 10% of normal, cough is absent.
  C3-C6: vital capacity is 20% of normal, cough weak, ineffective.
  T2-T4: vital capacity is 30 - 50% of normal, cough is weak.
  T-11: vital capacity is normal, cough is strong.
- Anal sphincter: decreased/absent tone. No voluntary contraction
- Motor and sensory loss as described on previous 2 pages.
- Loss of sensation may mask potentially serious injury elsewhere.
- In pts with SCI above T6, bradycardia combined with hypotension that fails to respond to fluids suggests neurogenic shock.

Treatment of Acute Spinal Cord Injury:

1	Spine immobilize	Rigid cervical collar; spine board is removed as soon as possible, then cervical traction, emergency MRI to detect cord compression Stat decompression and stabilization surgery (within first 24 hrs instead of usual 48 hr - 2 weeks) may improve outcome.
2	Airway:	Naso- or orotracheal intubation with head/neck traction. Fiberoptic guided orotracheal intubation has been used. Cricothyrotomy or Tracheostomy are emergency options.
3	Breathing:	Prevent acid-base imbalance and hypoxemia, which are causes of "second hit" injury to the spinal cord. Mechanical ventilation, treatment of chest injuries. Mobilize ASAP to prevent atelectasis. Gastric tube to reduce aspiration risk. Prevent DVT/PE with anticoagulants, SCD's, rotating bed.
4	Circulation:	ICU monitoring allows early detection of cardiac disturbance, hemodynamic instability, pulmonary dysfunction, hypoxemia. Beware that loss of pain perception may mask other injuries. Prevent secondary insults that cause spinal ischemia: ↓ MAP, ↓ HR (use Atropine), ↓ CO, arrhythmias, thrombosis. Maintain MAP 85 - 90 mm Hg for 7 days after acute SCI, and CVP 4 - 8 mm Hg. Blood is given to keep Hgb at least 10 g/dL. Neurogenic shock is managed with phenylephrine, dopamine, or norepinephrine.
5	Steroid:	No longer recommended. Offers not benefit and can cause harm (infection, respiratory compromise, GI hemorrhage, death).
6	Temp:	Early in the patient's course, prevent hypothermia and poikilothermia (patient assumes the temperature of the room). Use warming blankets. Later, *Aggressive* control of fever.
7	Surgery for:	Persistent spinal compression, unstable/deformed spine, ligament injury, or unreducible dislocation.
8	Nutrition:	Must be started early, due to acceleration of metabolic rate.
9	Skin:	Aggressive skin care, growth factor, anabolic steroid

Ongoing Problems:

Deep vein thrombosis	Constipation	Urinary infection
Pulmonary embolism	Hyperreflexia	Urinary calculi
Aspiration/pneumonia	Skin breakdown	Pain

Chest Trauma

Facts:

- Blunt thoracic injuries are directly responsible for 20 - 25% of all trauma deaths. Chest trauma contributes to death in 50% of trauma deaths.
- 85% will require a chest tube; but < 15% will need thoracic surgery.
- Many types of chest trauma are lethal, while the chest wall conceals the extent of injury. Signs may be subtle, may progress slowly, or may be delayed. Index of suspicion must remain high.

Chest Trauma Alters The Mechanics of Breathing:

1. Loss of negative intrathoracic pressure impairs the "thoracic pump" that facilitates venous return to the chest, especially during inspiration. Less cardiac filling results in ↓ CO, ↑ SVR, and eventual hypotension.
2. Loss of negative intrathoracic pressure defeats the patient's effort to establish the pressure gradients needed for inhalation and exhalation. Hypoxemia, hypercapnea, acidosis, and increased work of breathing result.
3. Blood in the chest interferes with lung expansion.
4. Diaphragm and/or phrenic nerve injury lessens the degree of diaphragm contraction during inhalation.
5. Splinting of chest muscle due to fracture pain causes hypoventilation.
6. SCI at or above the thoracic spine causes respiratory muscle paralysis.

Emergency ED Thoracotomy to:	**Operating Room Thoracotomy if:**
Relieve tamponade	Massive hemothorax
Directly control bleeding	Widened mediastinum on x-ray
Perform cardiac massage	Major injury to diaphragm
Cross-clamp the descending aorta to increase perfusion above the clamp	Major air leak
	Major anterolateral flail

Video-guided Repair: Thoracotomy incurs anesthesia risks, pulmonary and surgical wound complications, greater immobility, longer LOS. In the following patients, surgery may be avoided with use of video guided thoracoscopic repair.

1. Prolonged chest tube bleeding in hemodynamically stable pt. (intercostal vessel injury is likely)	3. Minor diaphragm injury 4. Pleural effusion 5. Delayed empyema
2. Prolonged air leak	6. Clotted hemothorax

Rib Fractures

1. 10% of trauma patients have rib fracture (ribs 4 - 10 the most common sites).
2. Rib fractures are often accompanied by some degree of pulmonary contusion, can produce hemothorax by lacerating intercostal or intrathoracic vessels, or cause pneumothorax or tension pneumo by lacerating pleural membranes.
3. In patients with rib fracture, 20% will have hemothorax, 25% will have pneumothorax, 30% will have both.
4. Fractures of ribs 8-12 raises the risk of injury to the diaphragm, spleen, liver.
5. First rib fracture suggests the patient received severe blow/force. 15% of these patients will have aortic injury. Sometimes there is bronchial injury.
6. Although rare, coronary artery laceration can be caused by a fractured rib.
7. Pain may induce the patient to splint and hypoventilate, resulting in progressive atelectasis, pneumonia, impaired gas exchange, especially if the patient has preexisting pulmonary disease or is elderly.
8. In patients older than 80 years, mortality rate is 20% due to pneumonia.

Assessment	Management
• Chest wall bruises, abrasions, wounds • Crepitus over the site • Local tenderness • Pain with breathing • Labored yet restricted respirations • Signs and symptoms of hemo/pneumothorax or pulmonary contusion	• Aggressive pain control, without causing respiratory depression: 1. Thoracic epidural analgesia, or 2. Continuous bupivacaine infusion through thoracic paravertebral block, or 3. Intercostal nerve block q d x 3 d, with 0.5% Bupivacaine 3 - 4 mL (effects last 24 hrs), or 4. Intrapleural Bupivacaine 5. Patient controlled IV analgesics • Aggressive pulmonary care. • Surgical fixation.

Flail Chest

Description:
1. Two or more adjacent rib fractures, producing a segment of ribs that moves paradoxically (opposite) to the rest of the rib cage. Separation of the ribs from their attachments to cartilage (costochondral separation) can also cause flail chest. Flail represents the loss of stability of the thoracic cage. 2. The force necessary to produce a flail usually causes other severe injuries. 3. If the patient splints respirations to reduce pain, or if the patient is intubated and mechanically ventilated, paradoxic motion may not be visible. 4. Often associated with hemopneumothorax and sometimes tension pneumothorax, requiring emergency chest tube insertion. 5. The severity of underlying injury directs the critical care. Some patients have minimal disruption in pulmonary function, others have incapacitating respiratory insufficiency due to progression of pulmonary contusion. 6. The goal of treatment is to avoid intubation and mechanical ventilation but in some, aggressive analgesia and mechanical ventilation may be needed. 7. Compression of the chest (e.g., steering wheel injury) increases intrathoracic pressure to such an extent that venous outflow from the head may be obstructed, causing congestion of the veins of the head, face, and neck (known as traumatic asphyxia or vena cava syndrome). These patients present with facial petecchiae and edema. Sternal flail may be present. 8. Heart injury may accompany sternal flail. 9. Mortality rate for large flail requiring mechanical ventilation may exceed 50%.

Fig. 13.5

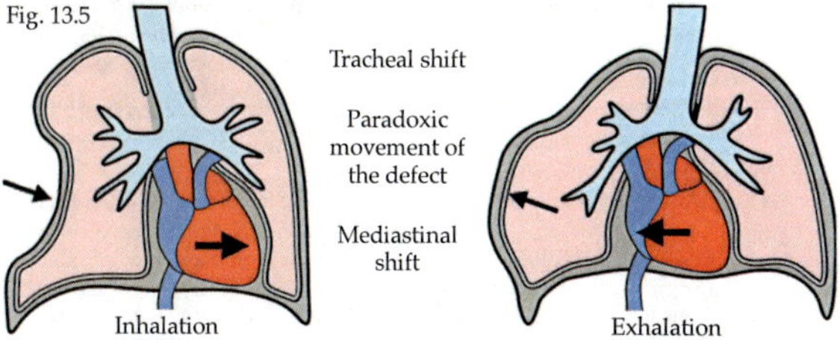

Assessment	Management
• Tachypnea, notable ↓ in resting TV. • Chest contour may be asymmetrical. Breathing appears restricted. • Chest pain, dyspnea, splinting, labored breathing, ↓ breath sounds • Hypoxemia and respiratory failure may develop, either immediately or over 24 hrs • Agitation, anxiety due to ↓ PO_2. • Tachycardia, ↓ BP if cardiac output is affected by hemothorax or by ↓ venous return. • Crepitation may be present. • Deformity and/or paradoxic motion of the chest wall. • If the patient is mechanically ventilated, overinflation raises the risk of producing pneumothorax in the other lung. • Monitor breath sounds and SaO_2 as measure of effectiveness of aggressive pulmonary care.	• Supply 100% O_2. • Assess for possible hemo/pneumo and prepare for chest tube insertion. • Judicious use of fluids, to avoid worsening pulmonary edema. • Aggressively manage pulmonary contusion (see next page). Avoid intubation and mechanical ventilation if at all possible. • If respiratory insufficiency occurs ($PaO_2 < 60$, $PaCO_2 > 60$, dyspnea, PaO_2/FiO_2 ratio < 300) or severe chest wall deformity is present, mechanical ventilation is required. • Surgical fixation may shorten the duration of intubation and length of stay, and reduce the incidence of post injury disability. • To protect injured lung from over-inflation, or if there is bronchial injury, double-lumen ET tube with a ventilator for each lung may be necessary.

Simple Pneumothorax

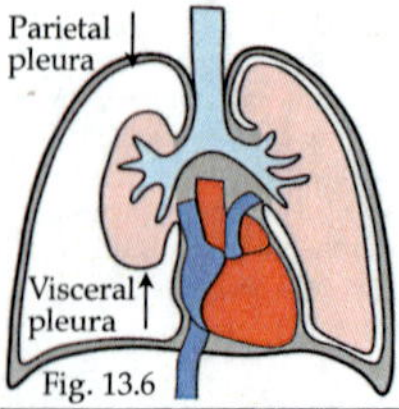

Fig. 13.6

Description:

1. A tear in the visceral pleural membrane that allows air to leak into the pleural space. The defect is caused by rib fracture, or by a blunt force that causes sudden ↑ in intrapulmonary pressure.
2. Loss of negative intrapleural pressure allows the lung to recoil.
3. The air leak occurs at the time of insult, and usually does not continue to leak.

Assessment	Management
• 80% have Dyspnea • 90% have chest pain • ↓ breath sounds on affected side Hyperresonant percussion note, unless there is also a hemothorax. • ↓ SpO_2 and cyanosis if the pneumothorax is large. • Ultrasound can speed diagnosis. • Air that leaks from the pt's lung injury can be detected using the air leak indicator of some chest drainage units.	• No anesthesia, no positive pressure breathing, no air transport until chest tube is inserted. • If pneumo > 20%, pleural chest tube will be inserted at 4th or 5th ICS, just anterior to the midaxillary line. • Post insertion chest x-ray is used to check tube placement, resolution of the pneumo, presence of iatrogenic injury. • Many require -20 cm H_2O added suction. • Persistent pneumothorax can be resolved with stapling or application of gel sealant under guidance of video-assisted thoracostomy.

Open Pneumothorax

Description:

1. A chest wall injury and tear in the parietal pleura that allows air from the atmosphere to enter the pleural space, causing total pneumothorax.
2. If wound size exceeds airway diameter, preferential movement of air into the wound rather than into the airway -> severe alveolar hypoventilation.
3. A large defect may result in shifting of the mediastinum and its contents. This shift and the loss of negative pleural pressure cause ↓ venous return.
4. Tension pneumothorax can result if clothing or an occlusive dressing obstruct the chest wound while the visceral pleura continues to leak.

Fig. 13.7

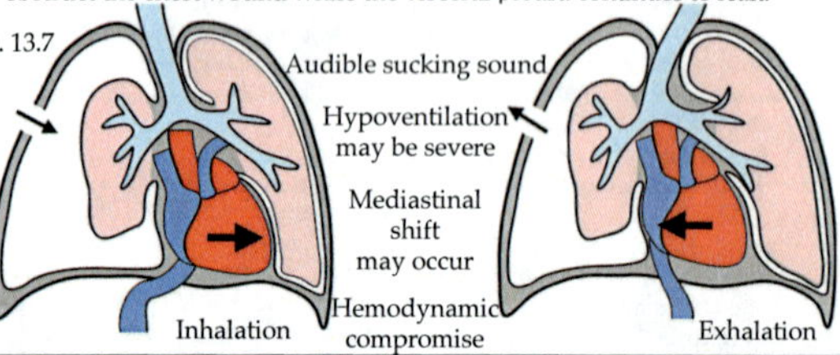

Assessment	Management
• Obvious chest wall wound with audible sucking sound. • Dyspnea, ↑ resp rate, hypoxemia, respiratory distress. • Anxiety, agitation driven by the feeling of suffocation. • ↓↓ or absent breath sounds. • ↓ BP, tachycardia, ↓ SaO_2. • Associated hemothorax is likely, assess the degree of blood loss.	• At end-expiration, sterile semi-occlusive "flutter valve" dressing is applied: Vaseline gauze over the wound, then gauze, securely tape three (3) sides, leaving untaped the 4th side, which serves as a vent for trapped air. • Prepare for chest tube insertion, possible added suction. • Surgery may be necessary to close the chest wall defect.

Tension Pneumothorax

Description:

1. A defect in the trachea, bronchus, visceral pleura or chest wall which acts as a one-way valve that allows air to enter the pleural space during inspiration, but prevents its escape during expiration. With each breath, both intrathoracic pressure and the size of the pneumothorax increase.
2. Increased intrathoracic pressure causes ↓ venous return and ↓ CO, shifts the mediastinum away from the affected lung, thus compressing the unaffected lung. Progressive hypotension and hypoxemia may lead to cardiac arrest.
3. Tension pneumo can develop slowly, can occur spontaneously, or expand rapidly, especially if the patient is receiving positive pressure breathing.

Fig. 13.8

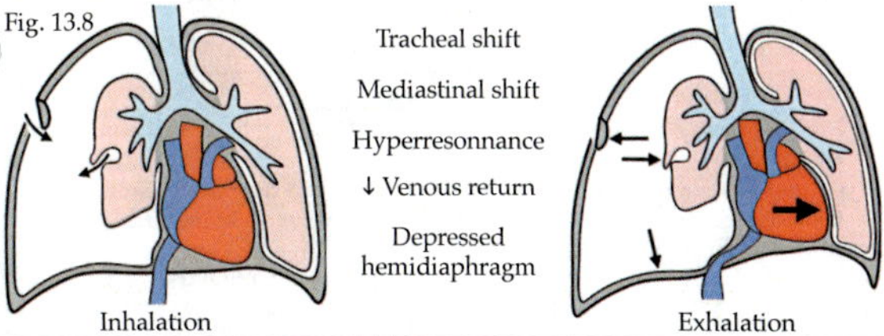

Assessment	Management
• Tachycardia, tachypnea, air hunger. • Chest pain, progressive dyspnea, agitation, respiratory distress. • Severely diminished to absent breath sounds on one side. • Hyperresonant to percussion. • ↑ pressure required to ventilate, high pressure alarm on ventilator. • Abdominal distention due to downward, displaced hemidiaphragm. • Signs of central venous obstruction (distended neck veins, ↑ CVP). • Shift of trachea or PMI (occurs late) • CXR - collapsed lung, displaced hemidiaphragm, mediastinal shift • Distinguished from pericardial tamponade by the absence of breath sounds and presence of hyperresonance on the affected side. • ↓ SaO_2, ↓ BP, shock, ↓ LOC. Pulseless Electrical Activity (PEA) precedes death.	• 100% Oxygen, elevate head of bed • Ultrasound for rapid diagnosis • Needle thoracostomy with 14 - 16 g IV catheter inserted at 5th ICS just anterior to the midaxillary line. • Beware: needle thoracostomy can be life-saving, but also can cause unintended injury. Also, a needle-catheter length of 2" (4.5 cm) may not penetrate the chest wall in 10 - 35% of patients.). A needle 8 cm in length is recommended. Pleural chest tube insertion follows. • Added suction, manually or with equipment set at 20 - 30 cm suction. • If defect is large, continued air leak may require surgical repair. • Some stop the leak by applying PEEP to the chest tube. • Jet ventilation sometimes used for persistent leak. • 15% will redevelop pneumothorax after chest tube removal, and 3 - 4% of these pts require repeat chest tube.

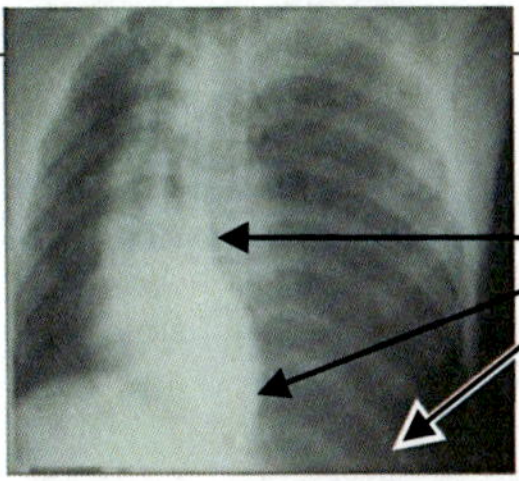

"The most common cause of tension pneumothorax is mechanical ventilation with positive-pressure ventilation in patients with injury to the visceral pleura." American College of Surgeons. ATLS 2012, Chicago IL

Pulmonary Contusion

Description:

1. The most common and potentially lethal chest injury.
2. Injury to the lung parenchyma, leading to edema, bleeding into alveolar spaces, loss of normal structure and function. At 24 hrs, there is massive accumulation of inflammatory cells. At 48 hrs, fibrin, cell debris, and granules of type II alveolar cells are present. The lymphatics are dilated and filled with protein. 50% of patients develop ARDS, which may affect only one lung.
3. Near-side lateral impact greatly increases the risk for pulmonary contusion.
4. A major contributor to ↑ morbidity/mortality in patients with chest trauma.
5. Aggressive pulmonary care can reduce need for intubation/ventilation from 100% to 23% and can reduce mortality rate from 40% to 7%.
6. Fluids must be carefully controlled so that the edema is not made worse.

Assessment	Management
• Gradual onset of dyspnea, ↑ PCO_2, ↑ work of breathing, decreased pulmonary compliance. • ↑ airway resistance; bloody sputum • 20 - 30% have increase in heart rate. • ↓ breath sound in affected areas • If PaO_2 < 65 mm Hg or SaO_2 < 90% on room air, intubation and mechanical ventilation are needed. • Fall in PaO_2/FiO_2 (P/F ratio) to < 300 correlates with severity. • ↑ pulmonary vascular resistance doubles the RV afterload. • Chest x-ray initially underestimates the extent of injury, often lagging behind the clinical picture by 12 - 48 hr.	• Intensive pulmonary care: 1. Judicious use of fluids, guided by CVP monitoring 2. Albumin to mobilize edema 3. Diuretics 4. Bronchodilators 5. Secretion removal 6. Mobilize patient ASAP 7. Deep breathing/coughing • CPAP or BiPAP to avoid intubation • Mechanical ventilation with PEEP • Double-lumen endotracheal tube if unilateral injury causes over-ventilation of the uninjured lung. • Management of RV dysfunction

Fig. 13.9

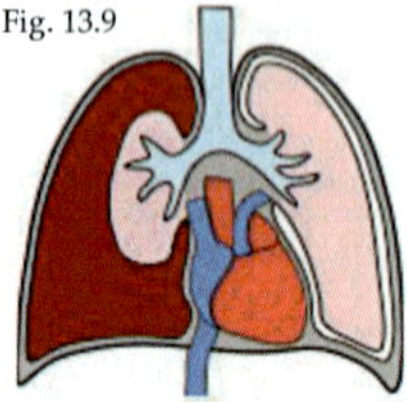

Hemothorax

Description:

1. Injury to pulmonary parenchyma, intercostal vessels, internal mammary, or heart and great vessels, with bleeding into the pleural space.
2. Pulmonary compression impairs oxygenation and ventilation. Blood loss can be severe.
3. In high risk complex patients, angiographic embolization is preferred over surgery.

Assessment	Management
• History of blunt or penetrating trauma • Rib fractures may be present. • If < 300 mL, there will be little or no evidence of hemothorax on exam or on CXR. • If > 350 mL, expect varying degrees of ↓ or absent breath sounds, shortness of breath, dull percussion note, ↓ PaO_2, flat neck veins, pain on affected side. • Upright CXR shows air/fluid interface. • If > 1500 mL, hemothorax is massive. Hemorrhagic shock can be profound. Patient may require massive transfusion and surgery.	• RL/albumin/PRBC's; auto-transfusion may be employed. • 36 - 38 Fr. chest tube, 5th ICS, just anterior to the midaxillary line. Multiple chest tubes may be required. • Surgery required if: > 1500 mL immediate blood loss > 200 mL/hr for 2 - 4 hours Blood transfusions required. • Despite chest tubes, hemothorax may fail to drain in 3 - 8% of pts. • Intensive respiratory care is crucial to restoring pulmonary function.

Blunt Cardiac Injury

Description:

1. Cardiac injury occurs in 10 - 15% of patients with blunt chest trauma.
2. Acute compression of the heart can increase intracardiac pressure, tearing the valves (often the tricuspid), the septum, papillary muscle, right atrium, or right ventricle.
3. Right ventricular contusion can cause RV dysfunction and dysrhythmias.
4. Contractility and conduction are impaired in 20% of patients. Dysrhythmias most often occur within 24 hrs and are the most common cause of death.
5. Pericarditis, pericardial effusion, conduction disturbance may develop later.

Assessment	Management
• Possible precordial bruise/abrasion. • Sternal fracture implies serious injury. • RBBB, SVT, dysrhythmias (AFib, SVT, VT, VF), or Right axis deviation. • Possible ST segment elevation. • If there is friction rub, gallop, or murmur, suspicion should be raised for valve injury, septum injury, or pericardial tamponade. • If severe, there may be chest pain, ↑ HR, SOB, MI, AV dissociation, heart failure. • Troponin I poorly predicts complications. • Ultrasound is useful in detecting effusion or tamponade. • Echocardiogram is best diagnostic test. • If the patient has no tachycardia, no dysrhythmia, and is normotensive, myocardial contusion is unlikely.	• 100% Oxygen. • Dysrhythmia management. • Unless contraindicated by other injuries, anticoagulation to prevent mural thrombus. • Fluids to maximize cardiac performance (maintain PCWP = 15 - 17 mm Hg). • Pericardiocentesis if there is tamponade (see CV chapter for procedure) • Inotropic agents if cardiac output is inadequate to sustain blood pressure. • Emergency surgery for valve tear or dysfunction and for septal rupture.

Penetrating Cardiac Injury

Description:

1. Most are fatal, found dead at the scene. 6% reach the hospital alive.
2. If the patient arrives without a pulse, mortality rate is 100% despite treatment. Resuscitation and open thoracotomy should not be performed.
3. If the path of penetrating injury traverses the mediastinum, injury to major structures is probable.
4. Some have pericardial tamponade (which likely "saved" the patient from exsanguination), or hemorrhagic shock, or both. If signs of tamponade are present on arrival to ED, survival rate is 50%.
5. Up to 90% of SWs, but few GSWs, develop tamponade.
6. If the mediastinum is traversed, major structures may be injured: great vessels, tracheobronchial tree, esophagus, heart. Thoracotomy is likely.

Location of Injury:

40% have right ventricle injury — 30% have left ventricle injury
24% have right atrial injury — 3% have left atrial injury
5% have injury to valve, papillary muscle, coronary artery, or septum.

Emergency considerations:

1. "Scoop and run" is an absolute prehospital principle.
2. ED Thoracotomy is done to:
   relieve tamponade
   control exsanguination
   perform cardiac massage
   cross-clamp the descending aorta to reduce distal bleeding and to increase perfusion of the brain and heart
3. Open thoracotomy requires abduction of the left arm, to allow the surgeon access to the 5th ICS. Once the chest is open and retractor applied, aortic cross clamping is done. A search for cardiac and great vessel wounds is made and digital control of hemorrhage is maintained to the OR.
4. Suspect air embolism if precipitous onset of arrhythmias or cardiac arrest, especially if penetrating injury is to low-pressure chambers.

Fig. 13.10

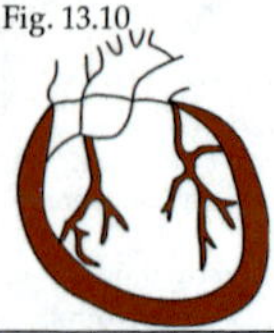

Pericardial Tamponade

Description:
Bleeding from the heart, great vessels, or pericardial vessels into the pericardial space. The collection of 50 - 200 mL of blood impedes cardiac filling, causing inadequate cardiac output and hemodynamic crisis.

Assessment	Management
• Beck's Triad: 1. Dilated, engorged neck veins, ↑ CVP. 2. Muffled heart sounds. 3. Hypotension resistant to fluids. • Breath sounds and percussion note are unaffected (not so in tension pneumo). • P & QRS alternans is specific to tamponade. • CXR may not be helpful, it takes 250 mL tamponade to enlarge the heart on xray. • FAST (Focused Assessment with Sonography in Trauma) can be 90% accurate in detecting pericardial fluid. • See CV chapter for pericardiocentesis.	• Pericardiocentesis is urgently needed. But the effort may fail if pericardial blood has clotted. • Stretching of the pericardium may incite vagally mediated bradycardia. Atropine is used. • Withhold positive pressure breathing, especially PEEP, which can acutely ↓ cardiac output. General anesthesia also increases intrathoracic pressure and can cause catastrophe if tamponade isn't relieved first.

Aortic Injury

Description:

Fig. 13.11

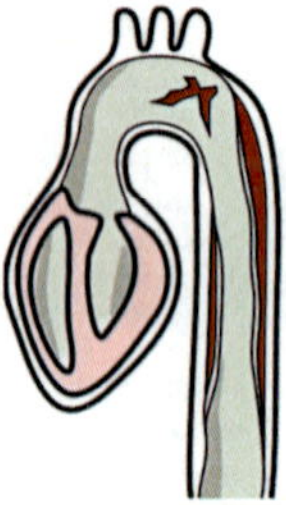

1. Aortic tears most often result from deceleration trauma, due to auto collision or a fall from a significant height.
2. Severe impact can increase intra-aortic pressure from 100 mm Hg to as much as 350 - 600 mm Hg.
3. 15% survive to hospital because of incomplete tear or bleeding contained by adventitia or by hematoma.
4. Risk is high for delayed rupture, exsanguination, death.
5. 50% have little or no evidence of injury on exam. 25% have normal CXR. But the mechanism of injury will determine if other significant deceleration/impact trauma exists, such as head injury, spine fracture, rib or scapula fracture, sternal fracture.
6. In some patients, surgery can be delayed while other life-threatening injuries are managed.
7. Tears of the ascending aorta are often accompanied by lethal cardiac injury.

Assessment	Management
• History of deceleration, blunt trauma, lateral near-side impact in MVA. • May have a first rib fracture. • Weak/absent pulses in any extremity. • BP difference between right & left arm • Back or shoulder pain, angina-like. • Patient may express impending doom. • If aneurysm compresses the laryngeal or pharyngeal nerve, hoarseness and/or dysphagia may be present. • Many show signs of significant hemothorax and hemorrhagic shock. • 3 findings on CXR have a sensitivity of 86%: Widened mediastinum Obscured aortic knob Displaced left paraspinous line	• To prevent dissection/rupture it is critical to control BP. Beta blocker Labetalol is preferred: Maintain: SBP = 100 - 120, MAP = 60 - 70, HR = 60 - 80. • Aortogram, Transesophageal echocardiogram (TEE), or CT are used in diagnosis. Future choice will be Helical CT. • Following surgery, a dreaded complication is paraplegia (the result of shock + aortic clamping). • Endovascular stent repair has been used for nonemergency cases. Compared to conventional surgery, mortality rate and the incidence of paraplegia are less.

Abdominal Trauma

Facts:

- Abdominal (abd) trauma is present in 7-10% of trauma patients
- 70% of pts with blunt abdominal trauma have other injuries.
- Mortality rate for blunt trauma = 10-30%; for penetrating = 5%.
- Two major autopsy studies showed that 20 - 36% of trauma deaths that were not related to CNS injury were preventable and were due to delay in diagnosing intraabdominal bleeding.
- Retroperitoneal injuries are easy to miss. Mortality rate is 20-40% and half of those who survive will have major complications.

Frequency of Organs Injured due to Blunt vs Penetrating Trauma:

	Liver	Spleen	SB	Diaphr	Colon	Abd vessel	Retro hem
Blunt	35 - 45%	40 - 55%	5 - 10%	rare			15%
SW	40%		30%	20%	15%		
GSW	30%		50%		40%	25%	

Mechanism of Injury:

- Organ injury associated with these fractures:
  - left lower ribs -> 25% have spleen injury
  - right lower ribs -> 55% have liver injury
  - pelvis -> 10% have bladder injury
  - L1 -> kidney injury
- Blunt force can shear/compress organs which lay over the vertebral column (liver, pancreas, bowel, mesentery).
- Blunt force may compress/rupture hollow organs (e.g., bowel).
- Cavitation by gunshot wound causes stretching/tearing of blood vessels and solid organs (liver, spleen).
- Shearing force can tear organs from their blood supply (kidney from the renal pedicle) or from points of fixation (bladder from the urethra).

Assessment:

- Obtain history to identify possible wounding mechanisms.
- Note presence of fractures that ↑ risk for abd organ injury.
- Assess degree of shock. Patient may require damage control.
- Look for bruise, abrasion, signs of intraabdominal bleeding: distention, pain on palpation, dullness to percussion.
- Conditions that complicate abdominal assessment:
  1. Significant blood loss into the abdominal cavity may not change its appearance or cause peritoneal irritation.
  2. Abdominal signs may develop insidiously or late.
  3. Shock, ETOH, head injury, drugs can obscure the pain.
  4. Pain of associated injuries may overcome the patient's recognition of abdominal pain.
  5. Expanding solid organ hematoma may rupture later.
  6. Spinal cord injury may render the abdomen anesthetic.
  7. Retroperitoneal injury (duodenum, pancreas, kidney, major vessels) may not be detectable on physical exam.
- The peritoneal membrane, which lines the abdominal wall and encapsulates most of the abdominal organs, will develop capillary leak, cell swelling, third spacing, and pain if shock or leaked organ enzymes produce injury.
- Look for peritoneal signs:
  1. Pain and tenderness on palpation or percussion
  2. Decreased or absent bowel sounds
  3. Involuntary guarding (a reliable sign of peritoneal irritation).
  4. Rebound tenderness (release of deep palpation causes pain)
  5. Splinting of respirations
  6. Abdominal distention, rigidity
  7. Pain on coughing or on moving legs
  8. Pt avoids abdominal breathing (it requires contraction of the diaphragm, causing movement of abdominal organs)
  9. Intrascapular pain suggests peritoneal or diaphragmatic irritation.
- Absence of dull percussion note over solid organs may indicate presence of free air.
- Rectum is checked for blood, rectal tone, prostate position.

Abdominal Trauma

Other Clues:

- Grey-Turner's Sign: flank ecchymosis, along with loss of psoas shadow on x-ray, are signs of retroperitoneal injury.
- Cullen's sign: bluish umbilicus suggests hemoperitoneum.
- Blood at the meatus or perineal or scrotal hematoma are associated with urethral injury. Do not insert urinary catheter.
- Lap belt mark is sign of deceleration/compression force. 20 - 30% of these patients have mesenteric or intestinal injury.
- Fracture of lower thoracic ribs: possible liver or spleen injury.

Diagnostic Tools:

- FAST - **F**ocused **A**ssessment **S**onography for **T**rauma is fast, accurate, portable, noninvasive way to detect free fluid.
  1. Offers rapid identification of the abdomen as the probable source of bleeding in patients too unstable for CT scan.
  2. A quick screening tool in stable patients with suspected abd trauma. Has almost replaced Diagnostic Peritoneal Lavage.
  3. Not helpful in patients with major pelvic fracture.
- Abdominal **CT**
  1. Only for ***stable*** pts. Time requirement and restricted patient access make this study too risky for unstable patients.
  2. CT may miss injury to hollow organs or to the mesentery.
  3. Is the only method for detecting retroperitoneal injury.
- Diagnostic Peritoneal Lavage (**DPL**) for unstable patients, or those with multisystem injuries and confounding findings.
  1. Unless contraindicated, gastric tube to suction and urinary catheter to drainage are required before DPL to prevent accidental puncture of bladder or bowel.
  2. Warm NS or RL infused per intraabdominal catheter into the abdominal cavity, then drained and analyzed. Adults: Instill 20 mL/kg warm NS or RL, up to 1 liter. Children: Instill 10 - 15 mL/kg
  3. Must return at least 200 mL for testing to be accurate.
  4. To reduce the chance of bowel or hematoma perforation in patients with obesity, pregnancy, pelvic fracture, past abd surgery, "open" technique for catheter insertion is used.
  5. DPL is positive if: > 100,000 RBC/mm^3, > 500 WBC's/mm^3, presence of amylase, bacteria, or bile.
  6. DPL is highly accurate in detecting intraabdominal bleeding.
  7. However, it is itself a form of penetrating trauma, not only affecting all subsequent assessments of abdominal pain, but also risking accidental intra-abdominal injury (perforation of bowel, bladder, intraabdominal vessel). Except for the detection of hollow viscus injury, FAST is preferred.
  8. Both FAST and DPL fail to evaluate retroperitoneal and diaphragmatic injuries.

Lab:

WBC > 15,000/mm^3	Elevated serum amylase
Hematuria	Blood in stool or NG aspirate
Falling Hgb/Hct	Elevated liver enzymes

X-ray: Free intraperitoneal air

Diagnostic Strategy:

If patient in severe shock, abdomen distended, go to OR
If remains in shock despite fluids, maybe FAST, then go to OR
If stabilizes with fluids -> FAST, then CT
If stable -> FAST, DPL, then CT

Retroperitoneal organs:

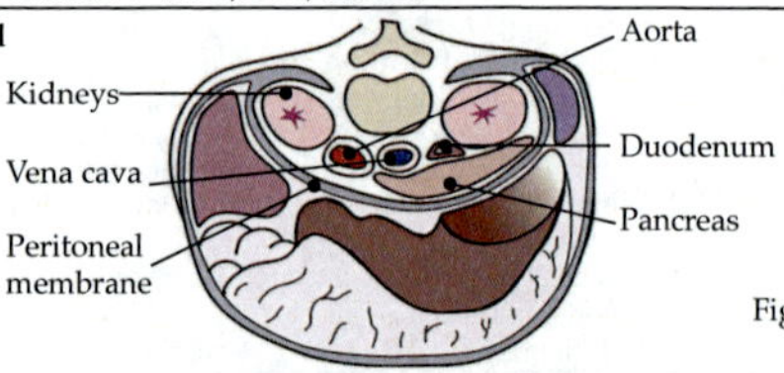

Fig. 13.12

Damage Control

Description:	• Damage control attempts to salvage patients who have suffered physiologic insult from hemorrhage, resuscitation, and surgery and who spiral toward the "Triad of Death:" Hypothermia, Acidosis, Coagulopathy (see page 7). • Bleeding and contamination control, physiologic stabilization, and patient salvage become the only surgical priorities. • Repair of individual injuries is postponed. • In 23% of abd. trauma pts who undergo damage control, the abdomen is left open to prevent abd. compartment syndrome. • After an abbreviated surgery, the patient is taken to ICU where metabolic derangements are corrected and the pt. is stabilized. • Repeat laparotomy is performed in 24-48 hrs to remove packing and devitalized tissue and to perform definitive repairs.
Who Needs Damage Control:	• Exsanguinating patients (> 10 units RBC's in the first 24 hrs). • Post resuscitation pH < 7.3, Temp < 35° C, Platelets < 95,000. • Massive intraabdominal hemorrhage or retroperitoneal bleed.
Limit the Time in Shock:	1. In patients bleeding from penetrating trauma, prehospital response time is limited to 10 minutes to "scoop and run." 2. Some say prehospital fluids should not be given; others say fluids should be limited to 250 mL hypertonic saline. 3. Resuscitation time in ED is resricted to < 20 minutes. The probability of death increases 1% for each 3 minutes in the ED. 4. OR time is restricted. Bleeding is controlled with simple ligation, abdominal packing, angiographic embolization. 5. The patient is transferred ASAP to ICU for stabilization.
ICU Stabilize:	• Warm the environment and all IV fluids. • FFP and platelets are essential to correcting the coagulopathy. • Pulmonary artery catheter is suggested. • Mechanical ventilation and hemodynamic support to achieve adequate O_2 delivery ($DO_2I > 500$ mL/min/m^2) as well as acid-base balance. • Electrolyte imbalances must be promptly corrected. • Monitoring of intraabdominal pressure is recommended. • Goals: Hgb > 7 g/dL, Fibrinogen > 100 mg/dL, Platelets > 95,000, PT < 16 seconds
Repeat laparotomy:	• For definitive delayed repair of intraabdominal organ injuries. • If the fascia cannot be closed, a vacuum assisted abdominal wound management system may be used: 1. A foam dressing is placed in the wound. 2. A biologic drape is placed over the foam and also over a 3 - 5 cm border of intact tissue around the wound. 3. Tubing placed through the drape is attached to continuous suction at 75 - 175 mm Hg. 4. The abdominal dressing is changed q 48 hrs in the OR, where gradual closure of the fascia is performed each time. 5. Complete closure is accomplished in about 10 days.
Complications:	1. Delayed organ repair increases infection risk. 2. Open abdomen is source of heat loss and increases infection risk 3. 8% develop enterocutaneous fistula, of which 60% fail to close spontaneously. Surgical closure will be required.
From the Military:	• Better outcome has been achieved with: Limiting fluids in the field to only sustain SBP at 90 mm Hg. In the OR, limiting crystalloid to "keep lines open" and giving RBC's:Plasma ratio of 1:1 or 2:1. Giving fresh warm whole blood to the most severely wounded. • Most patients arrive in ICU warm, euvolemic, with normal pH, and minimal edema. Patients are more easily ventilated and more quickly extubated. Further study is needed.

Abdominal Compartment Syndrome (ACS)

Definition:	• Normal IAP = 5 - 7 mm Hg (9 - 14 mm Hg in the morbidly obese) • Intra-abdominal hypertension (IAH) is defined as sustained increase in intra-abdominal pressure (IAP) ≥ 12 mm Hg. • ACS is defined as sustained or repeated increase in IAP that is > 20 mm Hg that is associated with new organ dysfunction. • ACS adversely affects hemodynamic function, mesenteric and renal perfusion, respiratory mechanics, and cerebral blood flow.
Facts:	• 35% of pts who require damage control surgery develop ACS. • Early abdominal decompression can ↓ the incidence MOF. • Negative pressure wound therapy decreases the incidence of ACS, ARDS, fistula, and sepsis and speeds wound closure. • ACS can recur in pts treated with expanded abdomen techniques
Patho-physiology:	1. **CV & Hemodynamics:** IAH interferes with venous return, undermines preload and CO (SVR may be very high), reduces perfusion of all organs, perpetuates hypotension, and increases risk for DVT. If IAH impedes diaphragmatic excursions, intrathoracic pressure may increase, requiring higher peak ventilatory pressures, and falsely elevating pulmonary artery pressures & CVP, producing a confusing hemodynamic picture. To use CVP as a guide to volume status, it must be corrected: Corrected CVP = (measured CVP - 0.5) x IAP. 2. **Renal:** reduced perfusion affects the kidneys more than other organs. IAH is an independent risk factor for renal failure. 3. **Pulmonary function:** IAH impedes diaphragmatic excursions, causing decreased functional residual capacity, pulmonary shunting and hypoxemia. In the early stage, this mimics ARDS, but can be reversed with abdominal decompression. 4. **Neuro:** elevation in CVP impedes cerebral venous return, which increases the ICP. Decreased CO threatens cerebral blood flow. 5. **GI:** poor perfusion may cause intestinal ischemia, interfering with nutrient absorption and increasing the risk for bacterial translocation and sepsis. 6. **Abdominal wounds:** poor perfusion threatens wound healing, abdominal wall tension may cause wound dehiscence.
Patients at Risk for ACS:	• Reduced abdominal wall compliance (e.g., burn eschar) • Increased peritoneal cavity contents (e.g., hematoma, seroma, ascites, interstitial edema, abdominal packing) • Increased intestinal contents • Excess fluid resuscitation in the presence of capillary leak. a. Injury, shock, fluids, burns, physiologic stress, infection all incite the inflammatory response, causing capillary leaking and interstitial edema. Rising IAP perpetuates the process. b. In the presence of capillary leak, the administration of > 5 L fluid in 24 hours is likely to cause increased IAP.

Abdominal Perfusion Pressure (APP):	Grades of IAH:
APP = MAP - IAP > 60 mm Hg, survival is improved < 50 mm Hg, mortality is increased (MAP is lower in children, therefore normal APP for pedi patients is lower)	Grade I: 12 - 15 mm Hg Grade II: 16 - 20 mm Hg Grade III: 21 - 25 mm Hg Grade IV: > 25 mm Hg

Other Factors that Increase IAP:

- Positive pressure ventilation
- Coughing
- PEEP > 15 mm Hg, particularly when baseline IAP is > 12 mm Hg
- 30° HOB elevation may ↑ IAP by 4 mm Hg
- 45° HOB elevation may ↑ by 9 mm Hg
- Prone position

Intraabdominal Pressure

Intra-abdominal Hypertension (IAH) Assessment Findings:

- Tense and/or distended abdominal wall.
- Hypoxemia, Elevated peak airway pressure (> 45 cm H_2O).
- ↑ CVP, jugular vein distention, ↓ CO, ↑ SVR, ↓ BP.
- Elevation of the diaphragm on x-ray.
- Oliguria (< 0.5 mL/kg/hr), progressing to renal failure.
- Physical assessment usually fails to detect IAH early.

Fig. 13.13

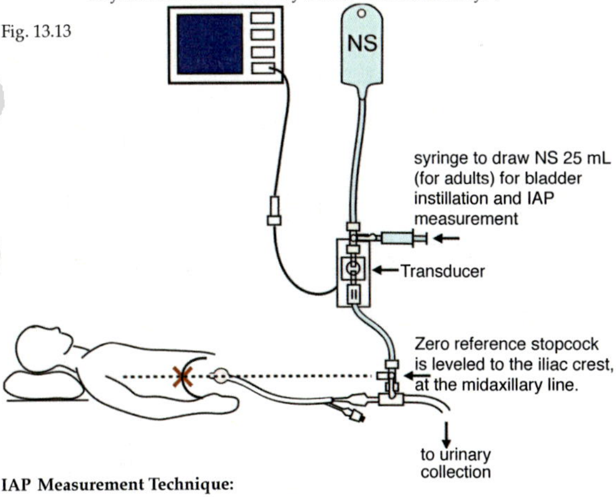

IAP Measurement Technique:

1. Place patient supine for measurement.
2. Zero transducer to the iliac crest at the level of the mid-axillary line.
3. Clamp off the drainage of urine to the urinary drainage bag.
4. Fill bladder with no more than 25 mL sterile normal saline (in Pediatric patients, instill 3 mL total).
5. Wait 30 - 60 seconds to allow bladder detrusor muscle to relax.
6. With lumens open from the foley to the transducer, and at end-expiration, and in the absence of abdominal wall contraction, record IAP in mm Hg.
7. Reestablish urine flow from foley to urinary drainage bag.
8. Repeat measurement every 1 - 2 hours.
9. The goal is Abdominal Perfusion Pressure > 60 mm Hg (APP = MAP - IAP).
10. IAP can also be measured with an indwelling abdominal cavity catheter.

Methods of Reducing IAP:

1. Reverse Trendelenberg is better than head of bed elevation.
2. Remove intestinal contents with cathartics, enemas, rectal tubes.
3. Promote GI motility by correcting ↓ K, ↓ Mg, ↓ Phos, ↑ Ca.
4. Provide sedation and pain control in patients with pain or agitation.
5. Neuromuscular blockade may further relax the abdominal wall.
6. CRRT to continuously remove fluid excess, particularly in the presence of capillary leak syndrome.
7. Drainage of ascites or large retroperitoneal fluid collection.
8. Reduce edema with colloid infusion and continuous hemofiltration.
9. Surgical decompression is the last resort, but is needed when ACS occurs.

Beware: sudden decompression of ACS can release the products of ischemia into the circulation, causing acidosis, vasodilation, cardiac dysfunction, cardiac arrest. Treatment includes crystalloid, mannitol, dopamine or milrinone.

Liver Injury

Facts:
- The most often injured abdominal organ.
- Most are managed without surgery, but the risk for delayed bleeding, missed injuries, and complications remains.
- Up to 14% of hepatic hematomas rupture and bleed later. Time delay to rupture ranges from 8 hours - 6 weeks.
- Patients with grade IV and grade V liver injuries face 85% mortality rate, due mainly to hemorrhage, but also infection, sepsis, biliary leak, hepatic necrosis.

Assessment:
- History of injury to right upper quadrant, fracture right ribs 7-9
- Abdominal distention, RUQ pain, guarding, abdominal rigidity
- Varying degrees of hemorrhagic shock
- X-rays shows elevated right hemidiaphragm

General Approach:
- If the patient is unstable, then diagnostic peritoneal lavage.
- If > 2000 mL needed to maintain BP, then direct transport to OR.
- If pt is stable, CT is usually followed by nonoperative treatment.
- If nonoperative patient bleeds, then surgery is mandatory.

Hepatic Injury Scale:

Grade	Description	Size	Depth/Length
I	Subcapsular hematoma	< 10% surface area	< 1 cm deep
II	Subcapsular hematoma	10 - 50% surface area	1 - 3 cm deep
	Intraparenchymal hematoma	< 10 cm diameter	< 30 cm long
III	Subcapsular hematoma	> 50% surface area	> 3 cm deep
	Intraparenchymal hematoma	> 10 cm or expanding	> 30 cm long
IV	Parenchyma disruption involving 25 - 75% hepatic lobe		
V	Parenchyma disruption involving > 75% hepatic lobe; major venous injury		
VI	Hepatic avulsion (the liver has been torn away from its attachments)		

Treatment:

1. Nonoperative treatment includes observation, laparoscopy, or angiographic embolization (AE).
   Careful ongoing hemodynamic and abdominal assessment, and monitoring of Hgb/Hct are critical to detecting delayed bleeding.
   Coagulation defects are aggressively corrected.
   25% of those managed nonoperatively will require treatment for complications:

Delayed bleeding	Hemobilia
Other abd organ injuries are missed	Bile Leak
Abscess/Sepsis	Biliary duct stenosis

2. Angiography followed by embolization (AE): Gelfoam particles or stainless steel coils are deployed to embolize and thrombose the identified bleeding artery. Very effective in controlling bleeding. Has dramatically decreased the number of immediate surgeries. But complications rate is high (Grade III: 19%; IV: 66%; V: 100%) due to liver or gallbladder necrosis, abscess, sepsis, bile leak.
3. Diaphragm rupture is rare and is easy to miss. Raise suspicion if there is history of deceleration, or if splenic or pelvic fracture exist. 70% are left hemidiaphragm tears, 30% occur on the right. Rarely, the liver herniates into the chest.
4. Hemobilia (blood in the gallbladder) results from a connection between an intrahepatic blood vessel and the biliary tract. Classic symptoms include abdominal pain, jaundice, GI bleeding. Treatment options include angiographic embolization, fibrinolytic therapy, endoscopic stenting or surgical exploration of the common bile duct, or cholecystectomy.
5. Other strategies include endobiliary stenting, CT guided drainage of bilomas and abscesses, laparoscopic intra-abdominal washout, Argon laser and "tissue welding."
6. Liver fracture with severe hemorrhagic shock is managed with Damage Control, and return to OR in 24 - 48 hrs.

Spleen Injury

Facts:
- Very vascular organ, in the LUQ, near the tail of the pancreas.
- Blunt forces cause hematoma, laceration, or fracture.
- Deceleration may tear the organ from its point of fixation, (i.e., avulsion from the splenic nerves and vasculature).
- Delayed rupture (usually within 2 weeks) can result from expanding subcapsular hematoma or from pseudoaneurysm. Nonoperative management is now attempted in 80% of patients, but failure rate is 10 - 20%. There is concern regarding its use in higher grade injuries, where failure rate is 50 - 100%.

Functions of the Spleen:
- Immunologic: makes antibodies, houses macrophages.
- Filter: of old RBCs (erythrocytes) and platelets.
- Blood reservoir: contraction of the spleen during shock contributes 150 mL blood to the central circulation.

Assessment:
- History of deceleration, or blunt injury to the LUQ.
- LUQ or diffuse abdominal pain and rebound pain are likely.
- 25% of pts with spleen injury have fracture of left lower ribs.
- Kehr's sign (left shoulder tip pain) in 50% of cases, caused by referred pain from subdiaphragmatic nerve irritation.
- Abdominal distention, guarding of the left upper quadrant.
- X-ray: left hemidiaphragm elevation, gastric displacement.
- Leukocytosis of 15,000 - 25,000 and falling serial Hgb/Hct.

G	Characteristics	Laceration	NOF
I	Subcapsular < 10% surface area	< 1 cm parenchymal depth	0%
II	Subcapsular 10% - 50% surface area Intraparenchymal < 5 cm in diameter	1 - 3 cm parenchymal depth does not involve trabecular vessel	0%
III	Subcapsular > 50% surface area or expanding; Parenchymal hematoma ≥ 5 cm or expanding	> 3 cm parenchymal depth or involves trabecular vessels	24%
IV	Major devascularization (> 25% of the spleen)	Laceration involving segmental or hilar vessels, causing major bleed	53%
V	Completely shattered spleen	Completely shattered spleen	100%

G: Grade of Injury **NOF**: Non-operative failure rate

Treatment:
- Hemorrhage and shock require emergency surgery. Patients who do not improve with 2 L fluid are also managed surgically. If hemorrhage is protracted or there are other serious injuries, threshold for splenectomy is low.
- In high grade injuries, damage control may be needed.
- Splenic lacerations can be repaired with argon gas, fibrin "glue," or High Intensity Ultrasound.
- Due to the immunologic functions of the spleen, the goal in stable patients is splenic preservation using less invasive means. But the risk of occult or delayed hemorrhage remains, whether treatment is observational, surgical, or post angioembolization.
- Of those who fail nonoperative treatment, 95% fail during the first 72 hours. Careful monitoring is critical.
- Risk factors for failure: age > 55, hypotensive on admission, large hemoperitoneum, higher grade injury, higher injury score.
- Repeat CT in 24 - 48 hrs may offer early detection of pseudoaneurysm (believed to be the cause of "delayed rupture"), arteriovenous fistula, and occult vascular injury.
- Complications of splenic angioembolization include delayed hemorrhage, abscess, splenic infarct. Up to 8% of embolized patients have delayed bleeding and require laparotomy.
- Lab test for the absence of Howell-Jolly bodies in blood indicates the repaired spleen is able to clear old RBC's.
- If splenectomy is necessary, beware:
  1. Subphrenic abscess rate is 1 - 13%.
  2. Post op thrombocytosis places patient at risk for DVT. 1/3 of pts in one study had platelet count > 370,000). Lifetime anticoagulation may be required.
  3. Splenectomy confers lifetime risk for OPSI (see next topic). Immunologic advantage of spleen salvage is being questioned

Spleen Injury (cont'd)

Overwhelming Post Splenectomy Infection (OPSI)

1. Asplenic patients have a 5% lifetime risk for rapid onset, fulminant infection.
2. Starts as a flu-like syndrome with fever and muscle aching, progresses to septic shock, respiratory failure, anuria, DIC, death.
3. Incidence is < 1% in adults, < 5% in children, but mortality is 50 - 70%. 70% of incidents occur in the first 7 years following splenectomy. More than 50% die within 48 hours of hospitalization.
4. Lab test: presence of Howell-Jolly bodies suggests the patient is asplenic.
5. After splenectomy, patients can be 70% protected by combo vaccine:
   Streptococcus pneumoniae vaccine (Pneumovax) 0.5 mL IM, and
   Meningococcus vaccine 0.5 mL IM, and
   Hemophilus influenza B vaccine 0.5 mL IM.

   Given immediately after emergency splenectomy or given 2 weeks before elective splenectomy. Revaccination should occur every 5 years.
6. **Patient education is critical**. 10 - 50% of asplenic patients are unaware they have no spleen. These patients should have antibiotics on standby at all times.

Kidney Injury

Facts:
- Usually due to significant blunt trauma, and often accompanied by serious associated injuries that may mask its presence.
- Renal fracture or disrupted blood supply can cause significant hemorrhage, sometimes hidden in the retroperitoneal space.

Assessment:
- In blunt trauma, CVA (costovertebral angle) tenderness, flank mass, Grey-Turners sign (flank ecchymosis) may be present.
- Fracture of lumbar vertebrae or posterior lower rib is common.
- Hematuria is present in 95% of patients.
- CT reveals extravasation of contrast. Serial CT's are important.
- The mechanism of injury, need for transfusion, and increased BUN and Cr are indications for surgery.

Renal Injury Scale:

Grade 1: Contusion or subcapsular hematoma, no laceration
Grade 2: < 1 cm laceration, no hematoma or urinary extravasation
Grade 3: > 1 cm laceration, no violation of the collecting system
Grade 4: Parenchymal laceration involving collecting system, expanding hematoma, injury to renal artery or vein
Grade 5: Shattered kidney, avulsed renal artery, no blood supply

Treatment:
- Injury Grades 1 - 3 are usually treated conservatively. Risks include delayed bleeding, missed injury, infection.
- Leaking or thrombosed renal artery can be repaired angiographically. Renal vein injury requires emergency surgery.
- Grade 5 injury may require damage control strategy, including nephrectomy, renal packing, hemostatic gelatin.
- Critical to maintain patency of collecting system drainage tubes.

Pancreatic Trauma

Facts:
- Penetrating injury or severe blunt force may cause contusion, hematoma, transection, pancreatic duct disruption, or injury to nearby structures (aorta, vena cava, spleen, duodenum).
- Detection is difficult due to retroperitoneal location & presence of other injuries. Delay in diagnosis results in high morbidity.

Assessment:
- With isolated pancreas injury: pain, tenderness, guarding.
- Look for lap belt mark, flank ecchymoses, multiple organ injury.
- Serum amylase is a poor indicator, may even be normal. Increased amylase in DPL fluid is a fairly sensitive indicator.
- CT (only for stable pts) may reveal retroperitoneal air or fluid.
- Pancreas injury in exsanguinating pt is diagnosed at surgery.

Treatment:
- Patients with minor injuries may be observed for 72 hours.
- Hemorrhaging, multi-organ injury may require damage control.
- Severe trauma requires pancreatic resection, pancreatic duct repair, or wound suction to remove pancreatic enzymes.
- 20 - 40% have complications, which include formation of fistula, abscess, or pseudocyst, acute or chronic pancreatitis, ARDS.

Small Bowel Injury (SBI)

Facts:	• Most often injured abdominal organ in penetrating trauma. • High energy blunt trauma is required to injure the small bowel. Compression against the vertebral column with abrupt increase in intraluminal pressure can cause rupture. Deceleration forces can cause stretching/tearing of bowel loops at points of fixation. • Diagnosis is difficult. Initial CT, FAST, and lab may be normal, while associated injuries obscure the assessment. • In the past, SB perforation was typically an incidental finding during laparotomy for solid organ injuries. Now that most pts with solid organ injury are managed nonoperatively, the rate of missed SBI's is expected to increase. Mortality rate is 4% if repaired in < 24 hr, and is 18% if repaired at 48 hrs.
Assessment:	• Abdominal seat belt mark is highly suggestive of blunt SBI. • Pain, tenderness, evolving peritoneal signs, abdominal distention. Absent bowel sounds in most, but not all patients. • Frequent assessment and repeat CT is critical detection. • Free fluid, free air, and bowel wall thickening on CT, however CT is not helpful in localizing the exact location of SBI. • As a retroperitoneal organ, duodenum may produce few early signs of injury. 30 - 50% develop hypotension, 6 - 18% have upper GI bleeding. Reconstructive repair can be complex.
Treatment:	• Laparoscopic repair, instead of laparotomy, is done if free air and abdominal pain are localized. • Laparotomy is needed in patients with diffuse free air, increasing pain, or have signs of peritonitis. • Since blood supply to the small bowel is good, resection and suture reanastomosis is usually done. • Complications include bleeding, failed anastomosis with leaking of bowel contents, intra-abdominal abscess, acute renal failure, ARDS, sepsis, pneumonia, DVT, wound dehiscence.

Colon Injury

Facts:	• Frequently caused by penetrating trauma, rarely by blunt trauma • Blunt colon injury requires significant force. Other serious injuries are likely and complicate the management. • Compression against the vertebral column may cause rupture. • If the patient requires damage control, colon and small bowel repair is delayed, which significantly increases infection risk. • Diaphragmatic tear allows herniation of colon into the chest. Following repair, morbidity is 35%, mortality rate is 3 - 15%
Assessment:	• Development of peritoneal signs • Blood on rectal exam is sensitive indicator • X-ray shows free intraperitoneal air • Grade I: Isolated colon injury, no shock, minimal contamination Grade II: Perforation, laceration, moderate contamination Grade III: Tissue loss, devascularized, heavy contamination
Treatment:	• Current trend is toward primary repair, no diverting colostomy. Anastomosis failure and leak are the major postop concerns. Risk factors for postop leak: shock prior to surgery, received 4 - 6 units PRBC's, fecal contamination, > 12 hr delay to surgery. • Leak rate after primary repair is 5 - 10%. • Diverting colostomy is performed in Grade III injury. Diverting colostomy may be closed in < 6 weeks in less severe injuries, if contrast enema shows healing, no leaking. Late closure (> 3 months after injury) is done for more serious, heavily contaminated trauma.

Late increase in WBC, fever, abdominal pain, tachycardia, need for fluids to support BP and UO suggest missed small or large bowel injury.

Complex Pelvic Fracture

Facts:
- Hemorrhaging pelvic fracture carries a mortality rate > 40%.
- Sources of pelvic hemorrhage include the vasculature (venous plexus, internal iliac artery), sacroiliac (SI) joint, fractured bone surface, liver, spleen. Average transfusion requirement: 20 units PRBC, 20 units FFP, 20 units platelets.
- Since deceleration forces are often the cause of "Open Book" injury, the presence of aortic dissection should be questioned.
- Isolated iliac wing fracture seems minor, but serious associated injuries (organs, vasculature, neurologic) may threaten life.
- Genitourinary injury should raise suspicion for other injuries.

Assessment:
- External rotation of lower extremity or unequal limb length.
- Presence of pelvic asymmetry. X-ray presence of separated SI joint or symphysis pubis, or iliac crest fracture (a cadaver study showed that only a portion of the maximal displacement that occurs at the time of injury is seen on initial x-ray).
- Manual compression of the iliac crests or posterior compression of pubic symphysis elicits tenderness, pain, crepitus. Because this test aggravates bleeding, it is performed only once.
- Lower extremities should be tested for sensory/motor function.
- Associated GU injury (bladder or urethral tear) is manifested by hematuria, blood at the meatus, scrotal or perineal ecchymoses.
- Look for presence of hemorrhagic shock, positive FAST or DPL. CT is sensitive and specific, but shock state limits its use.

Young-Burges Classification for Pelvic Trauma (OTA Classification):

LC 60 - 70% of pelvic fx pts	Lateral compression	I Sacral compression on side of impact II Iliac wing fracture on side of impact III LCI or LCII injury on side of impact and contralateral open-book injury
APC 15 - 20% of pelvic fx pts	Anterior-posterior compression ("Open Book")	I Slight widening of pubic symphysis or anterior part of SI joint, with intact SI ligaments II Widened SI joint with disrupted anterior and intact posterior SI ligaments III Complete disruption of SI joint
VS 5 - 15%	Vertical shear	Vertical displacement, disrupted SI joint, separated symphysis pubis.

Treatment: In stable pts and those with Mild (Class I) blood loss, options are:
- To OR for abdominal organ injury repair and pelvic fixation.
- Angiographic embolization of arterial bleeding (the cause of bleeding in 10 - 15% of patients).
- If transport is necessary, the unstable pelvis must be stabilized externally with a pelvic binder.

In multi-trauma patients with exsanguinating pelvic fracture:
- Angiographic embolization of arterial bleeding can be effective, but must follow surgery for abd. organ or thoracic bleeding, and sometimes must be repeated. Complications include necrosis of the gluteal muscle, bladder wall, femoral head.
- Some perform "crash lap," using pelvic packing and external stabilization for immediate control of hemorrhage, then 1-2 days of ICU resuscitation, followed by definitive surgical repair. Infection rate is 30%, DVT risk is high.
- Infrarenal intra-aortic balloon inflation has been used as a life-saving method to temporarily stem the bleeding until embolization procedure or surgery can be performed. Complications include lower extremity ischemia, compartment syndrome, amputation.

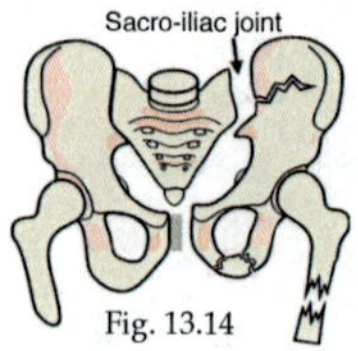

Fig. 13.14

Gunshot Wounds

Facts:
- GSW's are the second leading cause of trauma-related death.
- Gunshot wounds account for 31,000 deaths/year in the US and 25% of all deaths between the ages 15 - 24, 55% of which are suicide, 41% are homicide, 2% are accidental.
- The #1 cause of death for black males age 10 - 34.
- Cost of GSW's: $21,700/GSW fatality in the ED, $28,000 per hospitalized GSW, $6,500/treated and released GSW (1994 data)
- More teens die from GSW than from all other causes.
- Firearms in the home increase the chance of homicide three-fold and suicide five-fold.

Wounding Mechanism:
1. Direct tissue laceration/destruction by the bullet.
2. Vessel penetration and embolization of the bullet.
3. Temporary cavity formation due to high energy bullets.

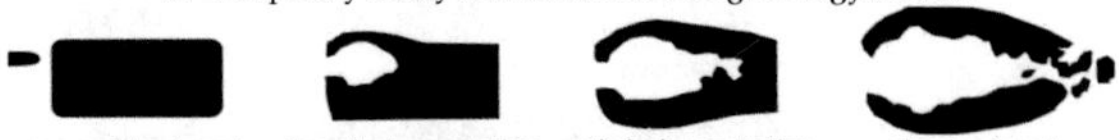

Fig. 13.15

- As the bullet penetrates tissue, energy transmitted from bullet to tissue propels tissue away from the bullet track.
- The temporary cavity lasts 5 - 10 milliseconds, its size can exceed bullet diameter by 10 - 15 times, and it can have an intracavity pressure as high as 1000 lb per square inch.
- High energy bullets have more mass or higher speed (rifle bullets, or magnum handgun bullets).
- The actual transmission of the kinetic energy to the tissue and thus increased severity of injury depends on: whether the ammunition deforms, the yaw of the bullet at the time of impact, and density/elasticity of the tissue.
- Dense and inelastic tissue, such as bone, spleen, liver suffer greater injury than do elastic tissues such as skin or bowel.
- Tissue, vessels, and bone not in the direct path of the bullet may be destroyed, lacerated, or fractured.

High energy bullets are those with mass and speed:

$$\text{Kinetic energy} = \frac{\text{mass x velocity}^2}{2}$$

4. Combustion of gunpowder (discharged at the end of the gun barrel) in the tissue or body cavity.
   - A factor in wounding when the gun is held in contact with the victim. Shotgun contact wound is devastating.
   - Effects on the skin (powder soot, powder burns) are important to the Medical Examiner in estimating distance from weapon to victim at time of wounding.
   - Soot on the hands of the victim may indicate the wounds were self-inflicted.

The ME:
1. The medical examiner or coroner needs accurate description of the wound/s at the time of admission, and description of wounds inflicted by the surgeon in the course of treatment.
2. Retrieved bullets, the patient's clothing, soot on the hands, need to be preserved as evidence. Photographs should be taken before soot is removed during treatment.

Shotguns Wounds:
- Pellet diameter ranges from 0.08 - 0.33 inches.
- The number of pellets in a shotgun shell varies from 9 to 450.
- Pellets produce a crushing, macerating injury.
- All contact wounds are severe (and often fatal), since the pellets enter as one mass, along with a cloud of combusting gunpowder.
- If < 3 yards from victim to weapon, wound will be severe.
- Since the pellets are not aerodynamic, they do not tend to penetrate deeply enough to exit.
- Pellets that penetrate vessels can embolize.

Severe Burns

Pathophysiology:

- Burns > 15% TBSA incite the systemic inflammatory response, which infuses the circulation with chemical mediators that increase capillary permeability. There is widespread intravascular loss of water, sodium, albumin, and RBC's
- Evaporative water loss from the burns contributes to the hypovolemia and is also a cause of hypothermia.
- Fluid resuscitation is critical and must be aggressive, despite mounting edema, which may increase the tissue pressure enough to:
  - threaten blood flow to affected extremities
  - threaten the airway in patients with face or neck burns
  - restrict ventilation in patients with burns of the chest wall
  - cause abdominal compartment syndrome.
- Burn injury to vasculature interrupts blood flow, consumes clotting factors.
- Microvascular reactions in the surrounding dermis may extend the injury.
- Nephrons obstruct with myoblobulin and hemoglobin
- Sympathetic-adrenal response results in:
  - Tachycardia, intense vasoconstriction
  - Accelerated gluconeogensis, insulin resistance, hyperglycemia.
  - Hypermetabolism, with 50 - 100% increase in resting energy expenditure.
- The risk of infection, sepsis, and septic shock increases with the % TBSA burn
- Multi-system organ failure is a common final pathway to late burn mortality.

FIRST PRIORITY is **STAT Intubation for:**	• Apnea • Presence of stridor • Circumferential burns of the neck

Quick Assessment of % TBSA Burn:

The Adult "Rule of 9's"

Body part	% of TBSA
Head & Neck	9%
1 entire Arm	9%
Posterior trunk	18%
Anterior trunk	18%
1 entire Leg	18%
Perineum	1%

1. Do not include 1° burns in the assessment of % TBSA burn.
2. Estimate how much of each area is burned.
   Example of adult patient, with burns on:
   1/3 of the arm = 3 %
   2/3 of the leg = 12 %
   1/2 of anterior chest = 9 %
   24 %TBSA burns
3. Reassess later with the more accurate Lund/Browder chart.

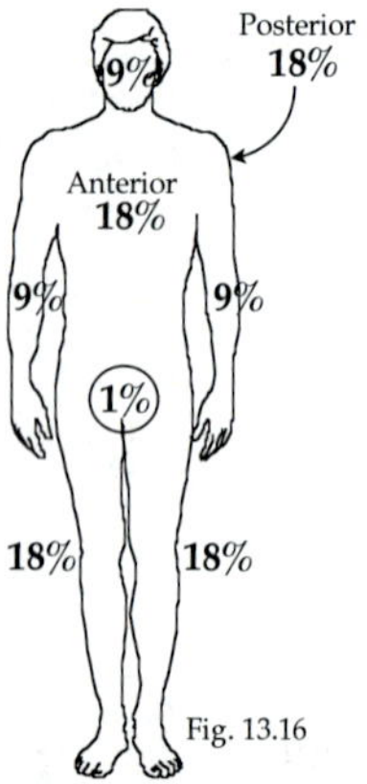

Fig. 13.16

Depth of Burn Injury:

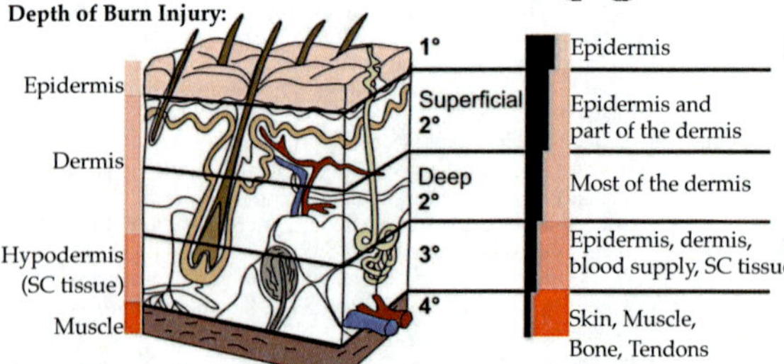

Fig. 13.17

Severe Burns

Depth	Affected Structures	Description of the Burn Wound	Initial Wound Care and What to Expect
1°	Epidermis (Do not include 1° burns in your estimate of % TBSA burn)	Pink or red, "sunburn." Blanches with pressure. Painful, no blisters. If blisters develop later, reclassify as 2° burn.	Moisturize, keep clean. Pain resolves in 3 - 5 days, epidermis sloughs in 1 - 2 weeks.
Superficial Dermal 2°	Epidermis and part of dermis. "Scald" injury	Blisters present, painful. Wet, pink, very weepy, capillary refill and sensation intact.	Cleanse, apply petroleum gauze or synthetic skin substitute (seals the wound, decreases pain). To face or perineum burn apply bacitracin or neomycin ointment, bid. Heals in 10 - 14 days.
Deep Dermal 2°	Only the skin appendages in the hair follicles remain.	Blisters present. Exposed dermis is pale, white, or yellow. Capillary refill is absent. Pain sensation is diminished.	Gentle washing with antibacterial soap. Silver sulfadiazine with a closed dressing, or Silver impregnated dressing. Usually requires excision and grafting.
Full thickness 3°	Epidermis, dermis, and subcutaneous tissue. No skin appendages remain (hair follicles, sweat glands, sebaceous gland)	Dry, leathery, may be red, pearly white, or black, may have thrombosed veins, marked edema, reduced distal circulation. Painless due to destruction of nerves. Hair falls out. Skin is dead.	Gentle washing with antibacterial soap. Cover with Silver sulfadiazine and a closed dressing, or Silver impregnated dressing. Requires excision and grafting or skin substitute.
4°	Skin, muscle, tendon, bone	Black, dry, charred, bone may be visible, no pain, becomes gangrenous.	Requires excision, graft, or skin substitute, and sometimes amputation.

Circulation:
- Priority is very high to establish large-bore IV access and start fluid resuscitation (3 - 4 mL/kg/% TBSA per hour).
- Those with inhalation injury sometimes require 30 - 40% more fluids (close to 5.7 mL/kg/% TBSA).
- Central line placement should be accomplished early, before edema obscures landmarks.
- When burn size approaches 15 - 20% TBSA, shock will occur if hypovolemia is inadequately treated.
- Hypovolemia will continue to incite the inflammatory response.
- Underresuscitation can convert a 2° superficial dermal burn into deep dermal or full-thickness burns.

	Parkland Formula:	Modified Brooke Army Formula:
First 24 hr:	Lactated Ringer's 4 mL/kg/% burn Half is given within the first 8 hours after the burn, and the other 1/2 over the next 16 hours.	Lactated Ringer's 2 mL/kg/% burn + Plasma 0.5 mL/kg/% burn + D5W 2000 mL Half is given within the first 8 hours after the burn, and the other 1/2 over the next 16 hours.
Second 24 hr:	Colloid: 0.3 - 0.5 mL/kg/% burn + D5W to maintain UO, and serum Na at 140 mEq. (about 2,000 mL D5W per 24 hrs)	Lactated Ringer's 0.75 mL/kg/% burn + Plasma 0.25 mL/kg/% burn + D5W 2000 mL

Severe Burns: Treatment

Beware that the calculated fluid requirement may not be enough in some patients (causing the consequences of hypovolemia), and will be too much in others (causing excessive tissue edema, compartment syndromes, pulmonary edema).

1. Remember the first 24 hours starts **AT THE TIME OF BURN**.
2. Colloid may be avoided in the first 24 hrs, due to capillary leak.
3. Catecholamines can support BP, even while hypovolemia exists.
4. PA cath is suggested if hemodynamic stability can't be achieved.
5. Base deficit > 5 mEq/L reflects inadequate oxygen delivery.
6. Third-spacing peaks at some point 6 - 12 hours postburn as the capillary barrier begins to regain integrity.
7. Capillary leak continues for 24 hrs and beyond in patients with large injury, inhalation injury, or delay in resuscitation.
8. Often within 48 hours, fluid replacement can be given enterally.
9. Myocardial depression may require inotropic support.

The Goals of Fluid Resuscitation
Patient is arousable, UO is 0.5 - 1 mL/kg/hr Warm extremities, full peripheral pulses Base deficit < 2, SBP > 100 mm Hg, HR < 120 Serum albumin > 2.5 gm/dL, Hgb ≥10 g/dL

Planned Intubation:	• History of being confined in a burning environment • Explosion with burns to head and torso • Singed eyebrows, eyelashes, nasal hairs • Carbon deposits in the mouth, nose, or sputum • Burns or inflammation inside the mouth • Hoarseness, wheezing • > 20% TBSA burn, and plan to transport patient to a burn center
Pulmonary:	• Oxygen to maintain SpO_2 > 90%. • Pt is carbon monoxide toxic if carboxyhemoglobin level is > 10%. • To prevent vomiting/aspiration, gastric tube if: TBSA > 20%, or nausea/vomiting, or pt is intubated, or plan to air transport. • Anticipate need for chest escharotomy if circumferential burns of the chest wall inhibit adequate ventilation.
Disability:	• Compare current neuro status to that reported at the scene. • Exclude head injury and SCI; maintain low threshold for CT scan • Check for peripheral nerve dysfunction as edema progresses. • Neck burns may need escharotomy to aid cerebral venous outflow.
Exposure:	• Evaporative water loss can be significant: on average, 1.5 - 3.5 mL/kg/% TBSA burn. • Cover burns to protect from contamination, to decrease pain caused by airflow, and to reduce evaporative water loss. • Prevent hypothermia: Set room temp 28-33°C — Use heat shield — No ice Warm IV fluids — Eliminate drafts — No wet dressings Use warm blankets — Wrap pt's head — No cold wash • Larger burns cause greater heat loss. • Maintain patient temp at 37° - 38°.
Eyes:	• Check for corneal burn before eyelid swelling compromises the ability to examine. • Eyelid edema may retract eyelids. Protect with lubricating drops.

Severe Burns: Treatment

Extremities:	Elevate HOB (if patient is stable) and affected extremities ASAP. Edema fluid consists of water, electrolytes, protein, fibrinogen, making a gel-like substance, poorly drained by lymphatics. Increasing tissue pressure may threaten blood flow to burned extremities, increasing the depth of tissue injury. An early sign of compromised blood flow is "painful passive extension" - assess for pain upon extending digits and toes. Monitor for distal pain, pallor, paresthesia, weakness/paralysis, weak or absent pulse (use doppler), polar (cold). Escharotomy is needed if tissue pressure exceeds 25 mm Hg. Burned + fractured limbs are immobilized with external fixation. Physical Therapy is critical to preventing contractures.
GI:	Expect ileus to develop in patients with large burn (> 20%); gastric tube and gastric suction should be Other GI developments include GI ulceration and hemorrhage, cholecystitis, pancreatitis, bowel ischemia.
Hematologic:	Hemoconcentration may cause initial elevation in Hct. Burn injury/destruction of RBCs often causes anemia. Maintain Hgb > 10 g/dL to support oxygen delivery to tissue. In some patients with TBSA > 50%, consumptive coagulopathy causes ↑ PT/PTT and ↓ platelets.
Immunologic:	Risk for infection is increased by lymphocyte dysfunction. Burn patients who receive transfusions are also at higher risk. Monitor for signs of sepsis, report temp elevation ASAP. Prophylactic antibiotics are not beneficial and are not given. Best prevention for wound sepsis is early excision of deep burns and biologic closure of the wounds. Assess need for tetanus prophylaxis.
Metabolism:	After resuscitation, there is marked increase in metabolic rate, by 50% in a 25% TBSA burn and 100% in burns greater than 40%. Catabolism causes severe fat and muscle wasting, anemia, poor wound healing, immune deficiency, and prolonged recovery. Some use beta-blockers to reduce the catabolic response. In most patients, enteral feeding can begin in 6-8 hours, given as 25 kcal/kg/day + 40 kcal/% TBSA burn/day, with 1-2 g/kg/day of the calories as protein. Early excision of the burn with immediate biologic closure will shorten the hypermetabolic phase and dramatically reduce pain.
Pain:	Use opioids liberally (within limits of patient safety) until burn excision and wound closure can be achieved (usually in 4-14 days)
Renal:	In electrical or deep thermal burns, pigmented urine is due to myoglobin and/or hemoglobin. Large volume crystalloid is used to aid renal elimination and reduce the threat of tubular necrosis.

Initiate Plan to Transfer to a Burn Center if:

- Partial thickness burns > 10% of TBSA in patients < 10 yrs or > 50 yrs.
- Partial thickness burns > 20% of TBSA in other age groups.
- 3° Burns in any age group.
- Burns involving the face, hands, feet, genitalia, perineum, or major joints.
- Electrical burns, Chemical burns, Lightning injury.
- Burns in patients with preexisting medical disorders that could complicate management, prolong recovery, or affect mortality rate.
- Burn patients with trauma (such as fractures) in which the burn injury poses the greatest risk of morbidity or death.
- Burn injury in children in hospitals without qualified personnel or equipment.
- Burn injury in patients who will required special social, emotional, or long-term rehabilitative intervention.

Some Important References

Used to update the 2011 edition of Trauma to 2014

American College of Surgeons. **Advanced Trauma Life Support (ATLS).** Chicago IL: 2012.

ANS/CNS Joint Guidelines Committee. Guidelines for the Management of Acute Cervical Spine and Spinal Cord Injuries. **Neurosurgery,** March 2013;72 (2): 1-259

ASA Committee on Blood Management. Smith CE, Bauer AM, MD, Pivalizza EG, et al., Massive Transfusion Protocol (MTP) for Hemorrhagic Shock. Amer Soc Anesthesiology.

Bougle A, Harrois A, Duranteau J. Resuscitative strategies in traumatic hemorrhagic shock. **Ann of Inten Care,** 2013;3(1):1-8.

Brown LM, Call MS, Margaret KM, et al. A normal platelet count may not be enough: the impact of admission platelet count on mortality and transfusion in severely injured trauma patients. **J Trauma 2011, 71:**S337-S342.

Crash-2 Collaborators. The importance of early treatment with transexamic acid in bleeding trauma patients. Lancet 377(9771):1096-1101

DuBose JJ, Scalea TM, Holcomb JB, et al. Open abdominal management after damage-control laparotomy for trauma. **J of Trauma and Acute Care Surgery:** January 2013;74(1):113-122.

Dutton RP: Resuscitative strategies to maintain homeostasis during damage control surgery. **Br J Surg,** 2012;99(Suppl 1):21-8

Dutton RP. Current Concepts in Hemorrhagic Shock. **Anesthesiology Clinics.** 2007;25:23-34.

Guang J, deMoya MA., Duggan M., et al Traumatic Brain Injury and Hemorrhagic Shock: **Shock,** July 2012; 38(1):49–56.

Haddad SH, Arabi YM. Critical care management of severe traumatic brain injury in adults. **Scan. J of Trauma, Resus and Emerge Med** 2012,20:12.

Hadley MN, Walters BC, Aarabi B, et al. Clinical Assessment Following Acute Cervical Spinal Cord Injury. **Neurosurgery**. March 2013(72):40-53.

Hoyt DB. How much fluid is enough? **J of Trauma and Acute Care Surg,** May 2013;74(5):1206.

Jin G, Duggan M, Imam A, et al. Pharmacologic resuscitation for hemorrhagic shock combined with traumatic brain injury. J Trauma Acute Care Surg, Dec 2012;73(6):1461-70.

Johansson PI, Stensballe J, Ostrowski SR, Current management of massive hemorrhage in trauma. **Scan J of Trauma, Resus and Emerg Med**. 2012; 20:47.

Mancini MC, Geibel J. Chest Trauma, Aug 2012, **emedicine.medscape.com**

Morrison CA, Carrick MM, Norman MA, et al. Hypotensive Resuscitation Strategy Reduces Transfusion Requirements and Severe Postoperative Coagulopathy in Trauma Patients. **J of Trauma,** March 2011;70(3):652-663.

Olthof DC, Joosse P, van der Vlies C, et al. **J of Trauma and Acute Care Surgery,** February 2013; 74(2):546-557.

Ryken TC, Hurlbert RJ, Hadley MN, et al. The Acute Cardiopulmonary Management of Patients With Cervical Spinal Cord Injuries. **Neurosurgery,** March 2013;72:p 84–92.

Savage, SA, Zarzaur BL, Croce MA, Fabian TC. Redefining massive transfusion when every second counts. **J of Trauma and Acute Care Surgery**. February 2013;74(2):396-402.

Oliver RI, Jde la Torre JI, Burn Resuscitation and Early Management. emedicine.medscape.com Feb 1, 2012.

Olthof DC, Peiter J, van der Vlies CH, et al. Prognostic factors for failure of nonoperative management in adults with blunt splenic injury. **J of Trauma and Acute Care Surgery,** Feb 2013;74(2): 546-557.

Neuro

Neuro

Central Nervous System

Structure & Function

Fig. 10.1

Cerebral Cortex:
Memory of:
- Sound and smell - the temporal lobe
- Sight - the occipital lobe
- Emotion and sensation - the parietal lobe

Frontal Lobe:
Willed movement (motor cortex)
Initiative, spontaneity
Personality
Mentation
Hand skills
Contralateral eye movements
Word formation (Broca's area)

The left hemisphere is the language center for all right-handed people and 85% of left-handed people.

Parietal Lobe:
Tactile sensations: touch, pressure, vibration
(Somatic sensory cortex)
Position sense
Pain sense
Heat vs cold
Taste
Emotion

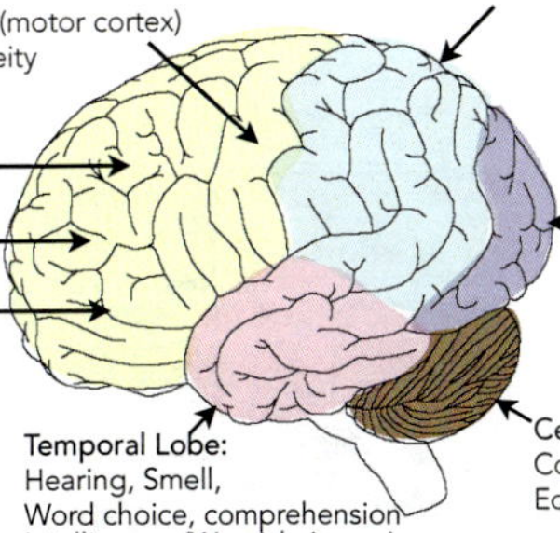

Occipital Lobe:
Vision

Temporal Lobe:
Hearing, Smell,
Word choice, comprehension
Intelligence (Wernicke's area)
Understanding language

Cerebellum:
Coordination
Equilibrium

Diencephalon (located between the cerebral cortex and brainstem):

Hypothalamus:
- Link to sympathetic and parasympathetic activity
- Link between psyche & soma
- Thermoregulation
- Control of wakefulness
- Control of appetite
- Control of the pituitary:
  - Anterior pituitary (Growth hormone, Thyroid stimulating hormone ACTH, Follicle stimulating and luteinizing hormones, Melanocyte stimulating hormone)
  - Posterior pituitary (Antidiuretic hormone, Oxytocin)

Thalamus:
- Links sensory impulses to cerebrum
- Part of arousal/alerting mechanism
- Part of reflex movements

Epithalamus

Subthalamus

Fig. 10.2

CSF Circulation:

From the choroid plexus, CSF enters the lateral and 3rd ventricles at a rate of about 20 mL/hr

CSF is reabsorbed by arachnoid villi.

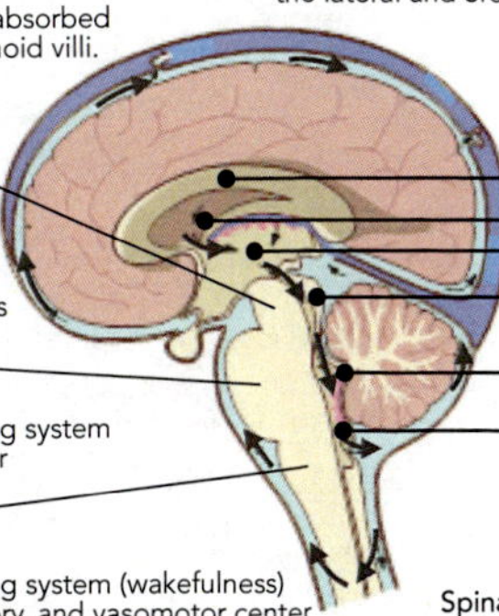

The Brainstem:

Midbrain:
CN 3 - 5
Reticular activating system (RAS)
Certain auditory and visual reflexes

Pons:
CN 5 - 8
Reticular activating system
Respiratory center

Medulla:
CN 9 - 12
Reticular activating system (wakefulness)
Cardiac, respiratory, and vasomotor center
Nonvital reflexes - sneezing, coughing, swallowing, hiccoughing, vomiting
Sensory/motor tracts connecting brain to spinal cord

CSF circulates:
Lateral ventricle
Foramen of Munro
Third ventricle
↓
Aqueduct of Sylvius
↓
Fourth ventricle
↓
Foramen of Luschka and Magendie
↓
Spinal cord and meninges

Cerebral Arteries

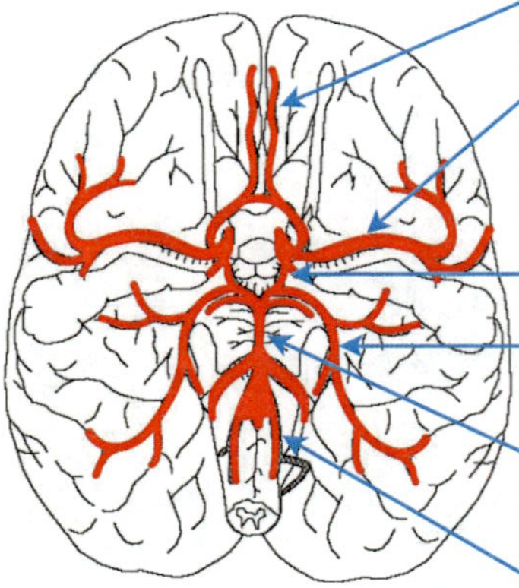

Fig. 10.3

Artery	Supplies
Anterior cerebral (ACA)	Surface of frontal & parietal lobes, anterior 4/5 of corpus callosum, parts of anterior basal ganglia, internal capsule.
Middle cerebral (MCA)	Most of the cerebral hemisphere (not the occipital lobe), internal capsule & basal ganglia, anterior temporal lobe.
Posterior commun-icating	Connects anterior and posterior cerebral arteries to form the circle of Willis. Also supplies the midbrain.
Posterior cerebral (PCA)	Inferior temporal lobe, occipital lobe, posterior circle of Willis, thalamus, hypothalamus, hippocampus.
Basilar	Main blood supply to the brainstem, branches to the cerebellum, connects to the circle of Willis.
Vertebral	Spinal cord, part of the cerebellum, posterior 2/5 of the cerebrum, brainstem.

Cranial Nerves

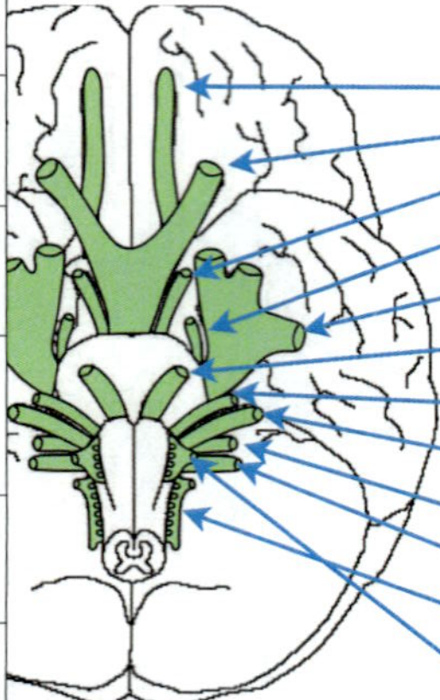

Fig. 10.4

	Cranial Nerve	Origin
1	Olfactory	Olfactory Lobe
2	Optic	Thalamus
3	Oculomotor	Midbrain
4	Trochlear	Midbrain
5	Trigeminal	Midbrain, Pons
6	Abducens	Pons
7	Facial	Pons
8	Acoustic	Pons
9	Glosso-pharyngeal	Medulla
10	Vagus	Medulla
11	Spinal accessory	Cervical cord
12	Hypoglossal	Medulla

Cranial Nerves

# Cranial Nerve	Origin	Function	How to Test	Abnormal Findings
1 Olfactory	Upper 1/3 of nasal septum	Sensory: Smell	Present odors for patient to identify. Test each nostril separately.	Decreased or absent smell Incorrect identification of a smell
2 Optic	Lateral geniculate body	Sensory: Vision	Bring hand quickly to eye. Have patient identify and count objects.	No response to visual threat Can't identify or number the object/s
3 Oculomotor	Midbrain	Sensory: Pupil constriction to light Motor: Elevation of upper eyelid, With CN 3, 4, 6 controls eye movements	Direct light into pupil of each eye. Note position of upper eyelid and eye. Note pupil size. Test for consensual reaction to light.	Pupil constriction is slow or absent Ptosis (eye turns down and out) Abnormal pupil size (< 2 or > 3 mm) Consensual reaction is absent
4 Trochlear	Midbrain	Motor: Moves the eyes down	Ask patient to look down and out.	Cannot move eyes down and out
5 Trigeminal	Pons	Sensory: Corneal reflex Sensation of cheeks, lips, chin Motor: Masseter and oral muscles	Touch cornea with cotton. Test sensory for cheeks, chin, lips. Ask patient to "bite down and chew."	No blink when cornea touched. Reduced or absent sensation of cheeks, lips, chin. Can't approximate or clench teeth
6 Abducens	Pons	Motor: Abducts the eye	"Look to the right, look to the left."	Can't move Lt eye to left, or Rt to right
7 Facial	Pons	Motor: Muscles around the eyes, forehead, mouth Sensory: Taste of anterior 2/3 of tongue	"Wrinkle your forehead, squint, purse your lips, frown, show your teeth, whistle, puff your cheeks, smile."	Weakness, asymmetry, paralysis of face Eyes stay open Weak of absent sensation of taste
8 Acoustic	Acoustic	Sensory: Hearing and equilibrium	Clap hands near ear. Place tuning fork to forehead.	Decreased or absent hearing
9 Glossopharyngeal	Medulla	Motor: control of swallowing Sensory: Taste of posterior 1/3 of tongue	Test with Vagus nerve.	See Vagus
10 Vagus	Medulla	Sensory: Pharynx and larynx Motor: Pharynx and larynx Movement of soft palate and uvula With CN 9, 10, 11 speak clearly	Inspect soft palate. "Say ah" Touch back of tongue; swallow water. Note articulation of words.	Sagging of soft palate. Uvula fails to elevate, or deviates to one side Absence of gag reflex Poor articulation of words
11 Spinal Accessory	Medulla	Motor: Trapezius and Sternocleidomastoid	Raise shoulders against resistance. Turn head against resistance.	Weakness or paralysis of neck and shoulder muscles
12 Hypoglossal	Medulla	Motor: Tongue "Stick out your tongue"	"Push your tongue into your cheek," against the resistance of your hand.	Tongue deviates toward the weak side Muscle atrophy of the tongue

Neuro Assessment

Overview: You must know the structures and functions of the central nervous system (see page 1) in order to understand the origin and significance of abnormal neurologic signs.

Assessment must be systematic and objective.

Establish a baseline, against which neuro change can be compared.

Abnormal neurologic signs are generally classified as: indicative of injury to a particular structure (localizing signs), or indicative of diffuse injury.

Abnormal neurologic signs are produced by any or all of these:

- ischemia due to clot, plaque, leak, high pressure, ↓ BP, trauma
- hypoxemia
- electrolyte imbalance
- hypoglycemia
- hyperthermia, hypothermia
- chemical toxicity
- infection

When abnormal neuro signs are present, often it isn't known if those signs represent reversible or irreversible insult. Only over time, and with the patient's improvement (or lack thereof), can the extent of permanent insult begin to be known.

History:

Headache:	Character, location, time of onset, intensity, duration, frequency, aggravating factors, associated symptoms (e.g., nausea, vomiting, vision changes, vertigo).
Vertigo:	A feeling of moving or the room moving, association with nausea, vomiting, change in hearing, vision, gait.
Vision:	Right versus left acuity, blind spots, field of vision, abnormal objects or flashes of light, photosensitivity.
Hearing:	Right versus left acuity, ringing, deafness.
Motor:	Paralysis, atrophy, involuntary movements, gait, ability to chew and swallow.
Sensory:	Paresthesias, pain, hyperesthesia, numbness.
Autonomic:	Control of urination and bowel function, sweating, heat/cold intolerance.
Seizures:	Character, precipitating factors, aura, duration, distinguishing features, frequency.
Meds:	Currently taken for headaches, vertigo, seizures, blood pressure, pain, diabetes.

The Components of Neuro Physical Assessment

1. Level of Consciousness
   - Considered the most sensitive indicator of neurologic change.
   - Controlled primarily by reticular activating system.
   - The key to accurate assessment is to use progressively stronger stimuli, in the hopes of eliciting a purposeful response.
   - Coma is defined as ***"no purposeful response to any type of stimuli."***
   - Assess LOC with the Glasgow Coma Scale or with these classic definitions:

Level	Stimulus	Response
Awake & alert	Verbal	Prompt response, aware, cognizant.
Lethargic	Verbal	Sleepy, but verbal stimulus does elicit an appropriate response. Some spontaneous movement.
Obtunded	Physical (but not painful)	Responds inconsistently to voice. Physical stimulus (e.g., gently shaking the patient) is required to elicit a sluggish but purposeful response. Less spontaneous motor activity.
Stuporous	Painful	Painful stimulus is required to elicit a purposeful response, which tends to be simplified and repeated each time. No spontaneous purposeful activity.
Semi-coma	Painful	Painful stimulus sometimes elicits purposeful response, sometimes it doesn't.
Coma	Painful	Pain consistently fails to elicit a purposeful response. Patient either postures or is flaccid.

Neuro Assessment

Glasgow Coma Score:

Parameter	Stimulus	Response	Score
Eye Opening	Spontaneous: To speech: To pain: To pain:	Opens eyes on own Opens eyes when asked to Opens eyes to pain Does not open eyes	4 3 2 1
Best Motor Response	To command: To pain: To pain: To pain: To pain: To pain:	Follows simple commands Pulls away from pain Withdraws to pain Flexes (decorticates) to pain Extends (decerebrates) to pain No response to pain	6 5 4 3 2 1
Best Verbal Response	Can carry on a conversation, is oriented to time, place, and person Converses, but pt may be confused/disoriented Replies with inappropriate words Makes only incomprehensible sounds Makes no verbal response		5 4 3 2 1

2. Pupillary light reflex:
   - Tests Cranial Nerve III (the Oculomotor Nerve) and its site or origin (the midbrain), which is the highest structure in the brainstem.
   - Normal pupil size, 2 mm, and reactive to light imply intact brainstem.
   - Pupil size is affected by medications and by sympathetic response.

     Mydriasis (pupillary dilation) is caused by catecholamine, atropine.
     Miosis (pupillary constriction) is caused by opioids, benzodiazepine.
   - Pupil size and unreactivity may reveal location of brainstem dysfunction:
     3 mm (Midposition) + unreactive = CN III (Midbrain) compromise.
     1 mm (Pin-point) + unreactive = Pontine compromise.
     5 mm (Dilated) + unreactive = Medullary compromise

3. Motor Function/Posture:
   - Test the Motor strip (located in the frontal lobe), the motor pathways through the spinal cord, and ending with peripheral motor neurons.
   - A typical scale for quantifying motor strength:
     5 Complete motion against gravity and full resistance, normal strength.
     4 Complete motion against gravity and some resistance
     3 Barely complete motion against gravity
     2 Complete motion with gravity eliminated (limb lays on bed)
     1 Slight contractility (palpable or visible), but no joint motion
     0 No evidence of contractility/paralysis
   - Abnormal posture may reflect the location of insult:

Posture	Description	Dysfunction of
Gegenhalten	Resists movement	Diencephalon
Decorticate	Arms flexed, legs and feet extended	Diencephalon
Decerebrate	Arms extended, internally rotated. Legs and feet extended.	Midbrain
Opisthotonus	Arms and legs are extended, back is arched. A severe form of decerebrate posturing.	Midbrain
Flaccid	Limp, no movement	Pons, Medulla, or Spinal Cord

4. Abnormal Breathing Patterns:

Pattern	Description	Dysfunction of
Cheyne Stokes	Crescendo-Decrescendo-Apnea	Diencephalon
Central Neurogenic Hyperventilation	Hyperventilation, both in depth and in respiratory rate	Midbrain
Apneustic	Inspiration is prolonged	Pons
Cluster	Periods of apnea	Lower Pons
Ataxic	Patternless, long periods of apnea	Medulla

Neuro Assessment

5. Sensory Function

Function	How to Test	Responses
Pain	Have pt close eyes. Use dull and sharp ends of an opened paperclip to elicit sensation. Ask pt to describe	Increased (hyperalgesia) Reduced (hypoalgesia) Absent (analgesia)
Tactile sense	With patient's eyes closed, use gauze to lightly stroke symmetric points	Increased (hyperesthesia) Reduced (hypoesthesia) Absent (anesthesia) Tingling (paresthesia)
Temperature	Distinguish between hot/cold	Present or absent
Position	Flex patient's finger or toe and ask patient to state new position	Correct or incorrect response
Vibration	Ability to sense vibration of tuning fork set on a boney prominence	Present or absent

Sensory Dermatomes

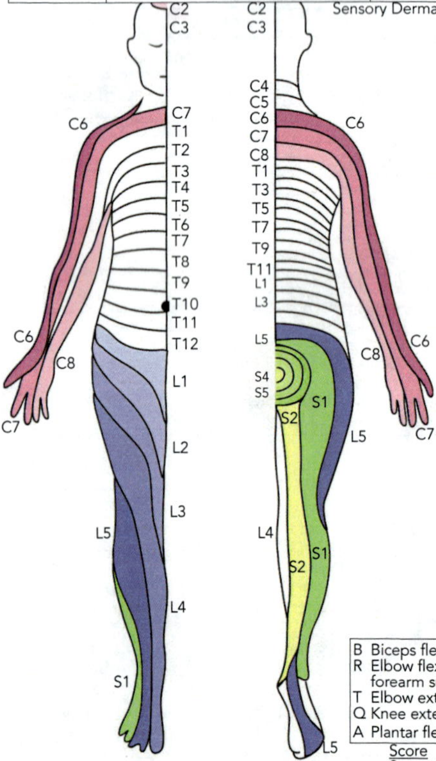

Fig 6. Deep Tendon Reflexes

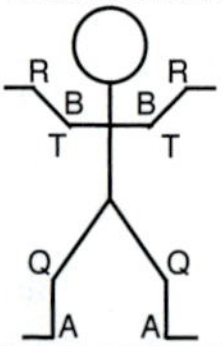

B	Biceps flexion	C5 - C6
R	Elbow flexion and forearm supination	C6
T	Elbow extension	C7 - C8
Q	Knee extension	L2 - L4
A	Plantar flexion	L5 - S2

Score	Response
0	Absent
+	Diminshed
++	Normal
+++	Hyperactive
++++	Clonus

Neuro Map to Assess Rising ICP

Fig. 10.6

If ↑ ICP progresses to downward herniation of the brain, compression and ischemia of the following structures will produce characteristic signs:

Structure	Level of Consciousness (LOC)	Breathing Pattern	Motor Movement/Posture (may be unilateral or bilateral or opposite the side of an injury)	Pupils	Other
Cerebral Cortex Motor Strip	Awake Lethargic Obtunded Stuporous	Normal	Weakness/paralysis	Normal size React to light	Specific dysfunction according to affected structure
Diencephalon	Semi-coma Coma	Cheyne-Stokes (Crescendo-descresendo-apnea)	Gegenhalten (resists movement) Decorticate (arms flexed, legs extended)	Normal size React to light	Diabetes insipidus Fever
Midbrain	Coma	Central Neurogenic Hyperventilation (Deep, rapid, can't be controlled unless neuromuscular blocking agent used)	Decerebrate (arms and legs are extended, arms are internally rotated) Opisthotonus is the extreme form of decerebration	Midposition Unreactive to light (CN III originates in the midbrain)	Ptosis (one or both eyes is down and out)
Pons	Coma	Apneustic (prolonged inspiration) Cluster (various patterns with periods of apnea)	Flaccid	Pinpoint Unreactive to light	
Medulla	Coma	Agonal, Ataxic (patternless, long periods of apnea)	Flaccid	Dilated Unreactive to light	Absent Doll's eyes, No response to caloric stimulation, Cushing Reflex

As ICP rises, the pressure descends → Trans Tentorial Herniation → Herniation at the Foramen Magnum

Increased Intracranial Pressure

Definition: Intracranial hypertension is an ICP ≥ 20 mm Hg for ≥ 5 minutes.

Normal ICP	=	5 - 15 mm Hg
If ICP	>	20 mm Hg, time to treat
If sustained ICP	>	40 mm Hg, prognosis is poor
If sustained ICP	>	60 mm Hg, almost always fatal

Causes of ↑ ICP: Inadequate oxygen delivery to the brain due to O_2 deprivation, reduced cerebral blood flow, or direct injury.
Interstitial edema due to increased capillary permeability.
Mass effect, due to intracranial hematoma or hydrocephalus.

Pathophysiology: When ICP ↑, compensatory responses include (in this order):

1. Reduction of CSF volume by contraction of the ventricles.
2. Reduction of blood volume in the cranium by means of:
   a. hyperventilation to ↓ $PaCO_2$ → cerebral vasoconstriction
   b. Cushing's reflex (a late development) → ↑ BP and ↓ HR
3. Displacement of brain matter (herniation).

Treatment of Increased ICP	
No "2nd Hit"	• Hypotension, hypoxemia, and i cerebral perfusion pressure are important causes of additional (secondary) brain injury.
O_2 and CO_2	• Endotracheal intubation and mechanical ventilation. • If possible, avoid PEEP. Target $DO_2 \geq 600$ mL/min/m^2 • Maintain $PaCO_2$ = 35 - 40 mm Hg. Since sustained $PaCO_2$ = 30 causes cerebral ischemia, reserve aggressive hyperventilation for treatment-resistant episodes of ↑ ICP,
Maintain CCP	• Think CPP = MAP - ICP at all times. Keep CPP > 60 - 70 mm Hg by keeping SBP > 90 mm Hg, supporting with inotrope if needed, and minimizing increases in ICP. • Maintain SBP > 90 mm Hg. Do not use D_5W. Fluid type is controversial: NS (0.89 %), Hypertonic Saline (3.5% or 7%), Albumin, Hespan, FFP, or 7% Saline in 6% Dextran 70. • Carefully monitor Intake & Output for fluid excess or deficit
Decrease O_2 demand	• Aggressively treat fever. Do not allow shivering. May use controlled hypothermia to reduce core temp of 92° F. • Sedation with Propofol is recommended, to lessen the ↑ in ICP caused by agitation, suctioning, coughing, fighting ventilator. • Sedation also reduces cerebral metabolic rate and O_2 demand • Propofol has short half-life, allows frequent neuro assessment. • Avoid opioids due to their hypotensive effect.
Control ICP	• Promote venous outflow by elevating head of bed 30 - 45° (but beware of BP) hypotension), prevent neck or hip flexion, beware tight cervical collar or tight tracheostomy ties. • Minimize noxious stimuli. Prevent ↑ intra-abdominal pressure. • Allow ICP to recover from positioning and procedures. • Careful suctioning technique. Some give Lidocaine to prevent further ↑ in ICP. Preoxygenate with 4 breaths of 100% O_2, limit suction to ≤ 10 seconds, make only 1 or 2 suction passes. • Mannitol 0.25 - 1 g/kg IV. Monitor serum osmolality, maintaining at 305 - 320 mOsm/L (normal = 270 - 290). • Lasix 0.5 - 1 mg/kg is sometimes given to i CSF production. • Maintain colloid osmotic pressure by maintaining serum albumin = 4 g/dL (low albumin is a cause of cellular edema). • Aggressive hyperventilation should be guided by jugular vein O_2 saturation ($SjvO_2$) monitoring. • If there are signs of herniation, begin hyperventilation to reduce $PaCO_2$ to 30 - 35 mm Hg. Then hyperventilate to achieve a reduction in ICP. Use ventilator, avoid using ambu bag, which may inadvertently apply PEEP • Barbiturates are considered if ↑ ICP is refractory to treatment; • Monitor EEG, cardiac output (may need inotropes) and $SjvO_2$.

ICP Monitoring

ICP monitoring is indicated if:

- Traumatic head injury with GCS 3 - 8 and with abnormal CT, or with GCS 3 - 8 and with normal CT, but with 2 or more of the following: age > 40, SBP < 90, unilateral or bilateral posturing.
- Subarachnoid hemorrhage, hydrocephalus, tumor, stroke, encephalitis

Benefits of ICP monitoring:

Facilitate the detection of expanding mass
Help limit the use of unnecessary interventions
Allow prompt treatment, to improve outcome
Drain and sample CSF
Estimate prognosis
Analyze ICP waveforms

Subarachnoid Bolt, Fluid Filled Column, Transducer

This method has the easiest set-up and the lowest infection rate, but the bolt sometimes obstructs with debris, blood, or brain tissue, and does not allow removal of intraventricular CSF. This method is used when the ventricles are collapsed and cannot be cannulated.

Set-up: Head of bed should be elevated 30°.
Use ICP monitoring kit, that includes transducer, pressure tubing, stopcocks, but **no** flush device and **no** administration set.
Flush the system with *preservative-free* sterile Normal Saline.
Use bubble-free technique to connect monitoring tubing to ICP bolt.
Dry, occlusive dressing (no antibiotic ointment) should be applied.
Level the end of the bolt to the stopcock near the transducer.

Fig. 10.7 Zero the system

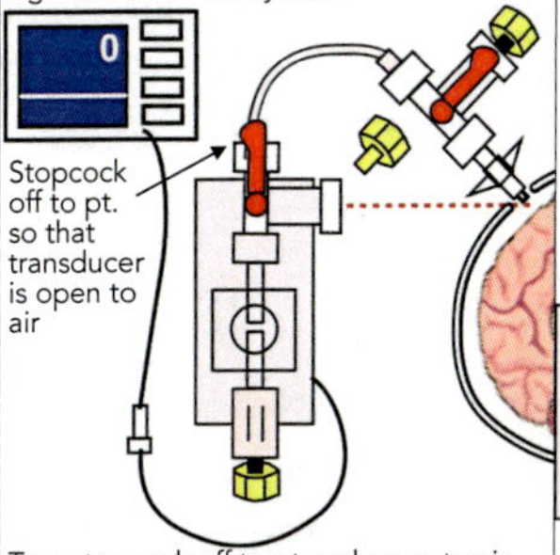

Turn stopcock off to pt and open to air.
Press "zero" on the pressure monitor.
Return stopcock to monitoring position.

Fig. 10.8 Remove bubble in monitoring line

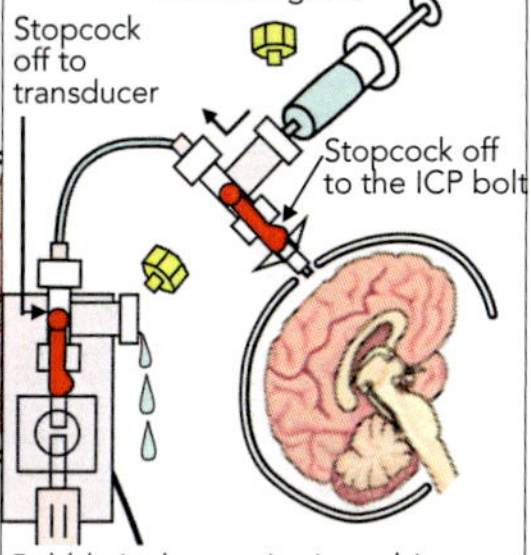

Bubble in the monitoring tubing: Using sterile technique, flush tubing with preservative-free sterile NS

Obstruction in the ICP bolt: (In some institutions, only physicians may perform this procedure): Using sterile technique, **flush with < 1 mL of preservative-free, sterile normal saline.**

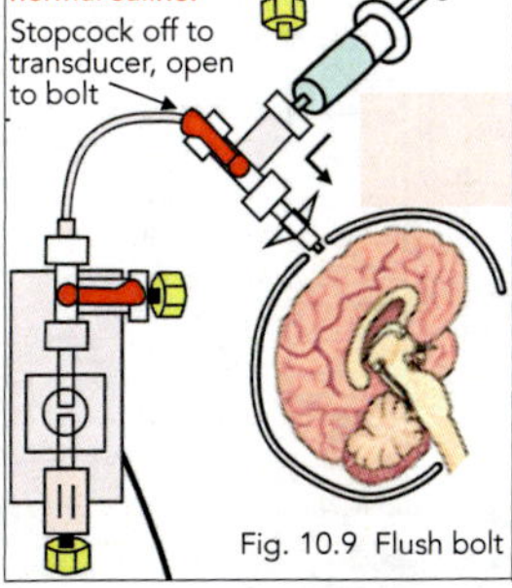

Fig. 10.9 Flush bolt

Fig. 10.10 Stopcocks in the monitoring position

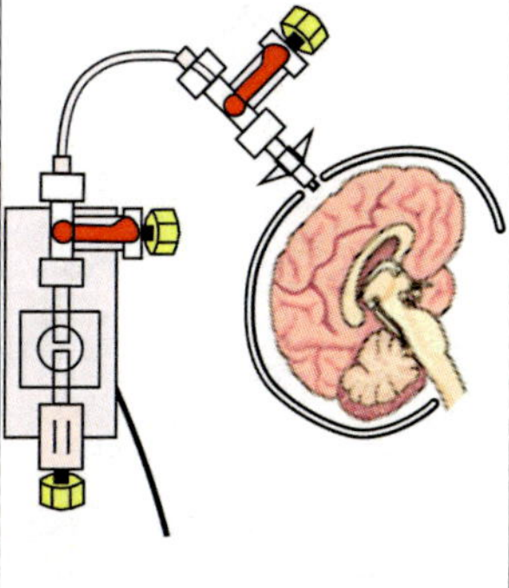

ICP Monitoring: Intraventricular Catheter (IVC)

Description:.

- An IVC allows drainage of CSF as a means of controlling intracranial pressure.
- The catheter is inserted anterior to the coronal sutures, 3 - 4 cm off the midline, and positioned in the anterior horn of the lateral ventricle.
- The catheter is connected to a closed, sterile drainage system, which is usually positioned 15 cm above the ventricle.
- If ICP increases to > 15 cm, CSF drains into the system, preventing any further increase in intracranial pressure.
- This level **must** be carefully maintained as long as the system is open to CSF drainage. If **for any reason** the patient's position must be changed, halt CSF drainage by turning stopcock nearest the IVC to the "off" position. When pt positioning complete, reopen the IVC stopcock to restore CSF drainage.

Set-up:

1. Using preservative-free sterile saline, prime the pressure tubing, the transducer, and tubing to the collection system. Secure connections
2. Head of bed elevation should be secured at 30° - 45°.
3. Connect IVC to the pressure tubing.
4. Physician will order the "pressure level," the distance the collection chamber is to be positioned above the patient (usually 15 cm).
5. Measure from the pt's zero reference point (see below)) up to the point where the drainage tubing enters the collection chamber.
6. If the patient's ICP increases to 15 cm H_2O, CSF will overflow into the chamber, preventing further increase in ICP.
7. If the patient's ICP remains < 15 cm H_2O, no CSF will drain.
8. Secure the position of the drainage system.
9. If the drainage system is placed too low, excess CSF may drain. (rapid CSF removal can result in tearing of bridging veins)
10. If the drainage system is placed too high, CSF decompression will not occur until a higher ICP is reached.
11. Filtered air vent must be kept dry. Wet filter prevents CSF drainage.

Measure ICP:

1. Check that the transducer is properly leveled and zeroed.
2. Turn stopcock to open IVC to the transducer. Record pressure.
3. Return stopcock to the position that permits CSF drainage.

The "pressure level" is the distance (cm) above the tip of the catheter (the zero reference point) to which the intracranial pressure must climb before CSF drains into the collection system.

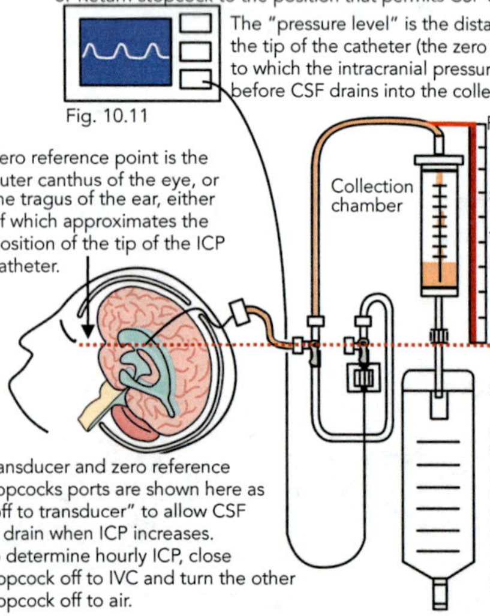

Fig. 10.11

Zero reference point is the outer canthus of the eye, or the tragus of the ear, either of which approximates the position of the tip of the ICP catheter.

Usually, drainage system is raised 15 cm H_2O above the zero reference point.

CSF collection bag

Bright red CSF drainage suggests new bleed and may obstruct the IVC with clot. Report immediately to physician.

Transducer and zero reference stopcocks ports are shown here as "off to transducer" to allow CSF to drain when ICP increases. To determine hourly ICP, close stopcock off to IVC and turn the other stopcock off to air.

Complications: Infection, Bleeding, Excessive or inadequate drainage of CSF, ICP elevation due to poor positioning of the drainage system.

ICP Monitoring: Fiberoptic Catheter

A miniature fiberoptic pressure transducer is on the tip of an intracranial catheter, which can be placed through a bolt or tunneled under the scalp, through the skull, and positioned under the dura, in the brain parenchyma, or in the ventricle.

1. The problems of a fluid-filled system (e.g., clotting, air bubbles, catheter occlusion) are eliminated.
2. With fewer manipulations, contamination risk may be lower.
3. There tends to be less artifact in the pressure waveform.
4. The catheter is zeroed once, at the time of insertion. Cannot be rezeroed thereafter. Zero drift of the transducer is about 1 - 2 mm Hg per day, considered by some to introduce significant error after 3 - 5 days.
5. Ventricular drainage and ICP monitoring may be done simultaneously.
6. Extreme catheter bending or kinking can damage the fiberoptics.
7. Technically easier, but more costly than a fluid filled system.

Fiberoptic Catheter, subdural and intraparenchymal (CSF drainage not possible)

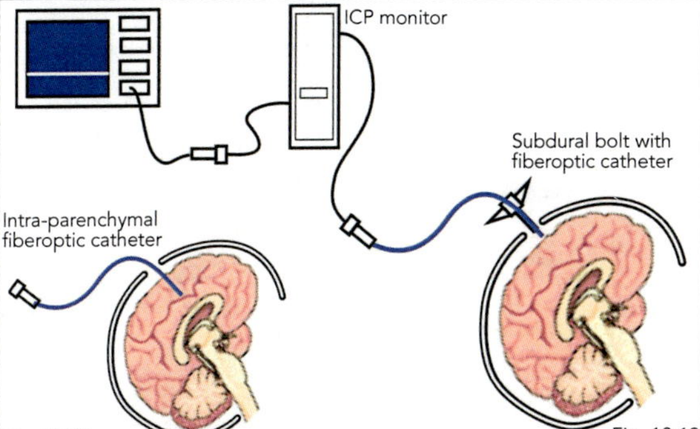

Fig. 10.12 Fig. 10.13

Intraventricular Fiberoptic Catheter

Fig. 10.14

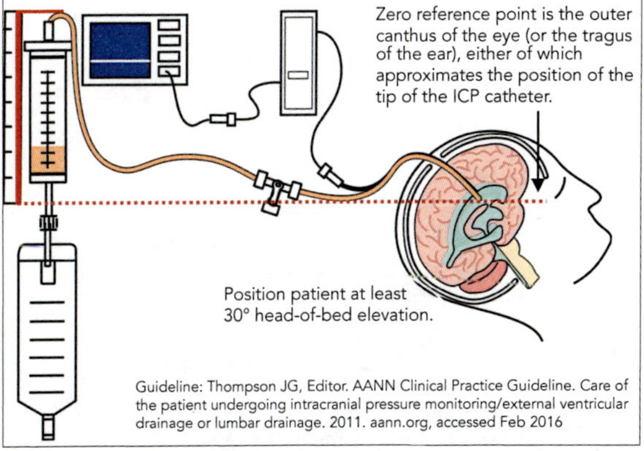

Guideline: Thompson JG, Editor. AANN Clinical Practice Guideline. Care of the patient undergoing intracranial pressure monitoring/external ventricular drainage or lumbar drainage. 2011. aann.org, accessed Feb 2016

Interpreting ICP Waveforms

Real time waves:

- P1 Percussion wave: A reflection of the systolic impulse.
- P2 Tidal wave: Occurs in systole, before closure of the aortic valve (the dicrotic notch on the ECG). As ICP rises, the amplitude of P2 exceeds P1, indicating reduced cerebral compliance and possibly a rapidly expanding mass.
- P3 Dicrotic wave: Occurs after aortic valve closure (after the dicrotic notch appears on the ECG).

Normal ICP waveform

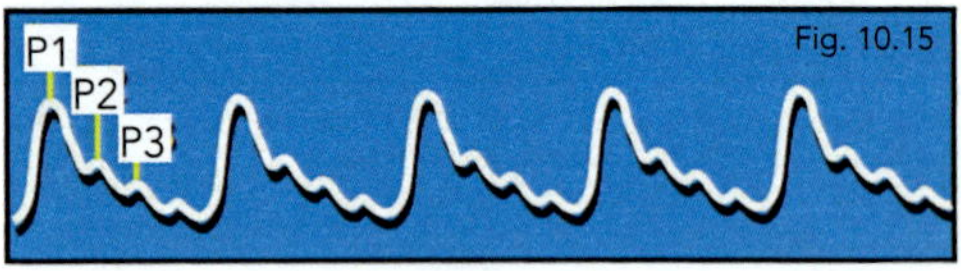

Fig. 10.15

The ICP waveform is influenced by cerebral blood volume, arterial blood pulse inflow, venous outflow, intracranial volume, and cerebrovascular resistance.

Trended waves: Can be seen only on a monitor with slow trend capability.

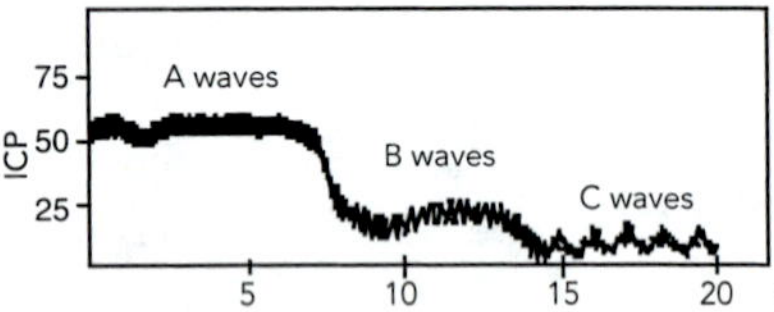

Fig. 10.16

A waves

- Also called plateau waves.
- Characterized by rapid onset, rapid resolution.
- A sharp rise in ICP, as high as 30 - 70 mm Hg (or > 50 mm Hg over baseline) lasting 5 - 20 minutes.
- Implies marked decrease in intracranial compliance and low cerebral perfusion pressure.
- Requires immediate and aggressive intervention.
- Causes include any condition that increases cerebral blood volume, CSF volume, or tissue mass or any condition that reduces venous outflow (such as increased intrathoracic or intra-abdominal pressure).

B waves:

- Repeated episodes of increased ICP up to 50 mm Hg (or 10 - 20 mm Hg above baseline) lasting 30 seconds to 2 minutes, followed by normal ICP.
  Creates saw-toothed spikes on trend recording.
- B waves have a high amplitude (increased difference between peak and trough pressure), reflecting compensatory action by the brain to decrease ICP.
- Because they frequently precede A waves, may be early indication of intracranial decompensation.
- Patient's treatment should be evaluated.

C waves

- Small waves, with pressure up to 20 mm Hg, that correspond to normal changes in systemic blood pressure and to changes in intrathoracic pressure during breathing.
- Occur 4 - 8 times/minute. Are clinically insignificant.

Report to physician:

1. ICP > 20 mm Hg.
2. CPP < 60 mm Hg (CPP = MAP - ICP).
3. Appearance of new blood in CSF drainage.
4. CSF leak around the insertion site.
5. CSF drainage > 500 mL/24 hr.
6. Signs of infection at the insertion site.

$PbtO_2$ (Brain Tissue Oxygen) Monitoring

Description:
- An intraparenchymal PO_2 probe, placed through an introducer and subdural bolt, is used to continuously monitor brain tissue oxygenation ($PbtO_2$).
- The probe is inserted approximately 35 mm below the dura, into the white matter of the brain, on the injured or uninjured side, but not directly into a lesion.
- Multi-lumen introducer allows additional monitoring probes for:
- Brain temperature (normally 0.5 - 1 C° higher than core temp)
- Intracranial pressure (ICP) (treated if > 20 mm Hg)

Indications: Patients at risk for developing cerebral hypoxia or ischemia due to head trauma, cerebral aneurysm, subarachnoid hemorrhage, stroke

Fig. 10.17

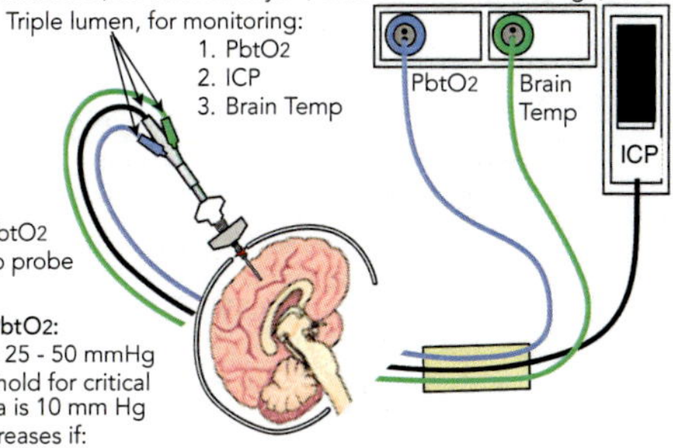

Double lumen introducer is available for:
1. Combined $PbtO_2$ + Brain Temp probe
2. ICP

Assessment of $PbtO_2$:
Normal $PbtO_2$ = 25 - 50 mmHg
The $PbtO_2$ threshold for critical cerebral ischemia is 10 mm Hg
Risk of death increases if:
- $PbtO_2$ < 15 mm Hg for 30 minutes
- $PbtO_2$ < 10 mmHg for 10 minutes
- $PbtO_2$ < 5 mmHg very high mortality
- $PbtO_2$ < 2 mmHg neuronal death

Prevent injury or displacement.
Secure the lines/cables.
Protect the bolt.

Studies have shown:
- Despite aggressive therapy to maintain ICP/CPP at normal levels, some patients still experience brain hypoxia.
- Some interventions once thought to improve tissue oxygenation may improve ICP and CPP, but actually decrease $PbtO_2$.
- In patients with traumatic brain injury who are adequately resuscitated (i.e., ICP < 20 mm Hg and CPP > 60 mm Hg), severe brain hypoxia (defined as $PbtO_2$ < 10 mm Hg) may still be present in nearly one third of patients.
- 1° Celsius change in brain temperature can alter cerebral metabolism by 5% - 13%, causing altered cerebral blood flow and abnormal ICP.
- Some warn that even a good $PbtO_2$ must be scrutinized. If neurons fail to uptake O_2 (due to cytotoxic edema, or mitochondria dysfunction), "an acceptable looking" $PbtO_2$ may be the result.

Contraindications: acute or chronic infection, infection at the site of insertion, coagulopathy (e.g., due to hypothermia, thrombocytopenia, liver disease).

Complications:
Intraparenchymal monitoring: infection, hematoma.
intraventricular monitoring: complication rate is 5 - 10%.

Low $PbtO_2$ is caused by:
- Decreased oxygen delivery, due to:
  1. Decreased cerebral blood flow due to vasoconstriction or decreased cardiac output.
  2. Decreased oxygen content due to hypoxemia or decreased hemoglobin.
- Increased cerebral oxygen demand, due to many causes:
  1. Pain, shivering, agitation, seizures, fever, injury.
  2. Following severe head injury, cerebral metabolic rate can be increased as much as 40 - 100%.

Pascual JL, Georgoff P, Maloney-Wilensky E, et al. Reduced brain tissue oxygenation in traumatic brain injury. J of Trauma, 2011;70:535-546.

Protocol for $PbtO_2$ Monitoring

Insertion Site should be:

- At least 14 mm away from an intraventricular drain.
- Near a lesion, when the goal is to monitor O_2 availability to damaged tissue.
- Away from a lesion, when the goal is to monitor good tissue at risk for injury.
- Away from areas of infarct or hematoma.
- For safety reasons, placed in the right frontal region rather than the left because speech function is located in the left hemisphere.
- Should not be placed through a craniotomy bone flap.
- Special Considerations:
  1. Subarachnoid Hemorrhage (SAH): the probe is placed in the brain near area of suspected vasospasm (determined by the distribution of subarachnoid blood on CT scan and by aneurysm location).
  2. Anterior communicating artery aneurysm: placement is on the right
  3. Right posterior communicating artery, internal carotid artery or middle cerebral artery aneurysm: placement is on the right.
  4. Left posterior communicating artery, internal carotid artery or middle cerebral artery aneurysm: placement is on the left.
  5. Basilar aneurysm: placed on the right
  6. Traumatic Brain Injury (TBI)
     a. Placement should tend toward the area of greatest injury seen on head CT scan.
     b. Diffuse axonal injury (DAI): If no asymmetry seen on head CT, placement is on the right.
     c. Asymmetry observed on head CT: Probe is placed on same side of maximum pathology (e.g. edema, contusion, subdural hematoma)
     d. Subdural, extradural or intracerebral hematoma: Probe placed on the same side as pathology.
     e. If the patient has undergone a craniotomy: Probe is placed on same side as the injury if the craniotomy flap permits.

(adapted from the Hospitals of the University of Pennsylvania)

Careful with the Equipment:

The probes are sophisticated physiologic monitoring devices.
They must not be kinked, pulled, clamped, cut, or twisted.
The cables are also critical to accurate monitoring. Protect them from damage.
Prior to insertion, make any cable connections and perform calibrations required by the manufacturer. Also, computer warm-up time may be significant (up to 3 h)

Insertion Procedure:

- Head of bed up 45° and bed at a level comfortable to the surgeon.
- Shave head to a diameter of about 2 - 4 cm off midline, just anterior to the coronal suture. Prep with Iodine.
- Using strict sterile procedure, deliver sterile supplies to the field.
- The physician will anesthetize the area and incise the skin with a scalpel, drill through the skull, and using a #11 blade make an opening in the dura.
- The bolt is threaded into the opening. The skin is sutured around the bolt.
- The triple lumen introducer is inserted into the bolt as far as possible.
- The compression cap is turned to secure the introducer loosely to the bolt.
- Guide wires are removed from the introducer, any unused ports are capped.
- The compression cap is tightened to firmly secure the introducer to the bolt.
- ICP catheter, $PbtO_2$, and Temp probes are inserted and calibrated if necessary.
- Secure sterile dressing is placed around the bolt. Secure the cables. Allow no tension on the probes. Protect probe/cables during care, treatments, patient positioning, patient transport, and diagnostic studies.
- Initial $PbtO_2$ readings are affected by the tissue trauma incurred by probe insertion. For the first 30 to 120 minutes after insertion, the $PbtO_2$ values will not be stable and will not reflect the patient's cerebral oxygenation.
- Responsiveness of the O_2 probe may be tested by administering 100% O_2 for several minutes and noting an increase in the displayed value for $PbtO_2$.
- $PbtO_2$ values usually remain accurate for up to 5 days.

Subarachnoid Hemorrhage

Description: Bleeding into the subarachnoid space (which ruptured cerebral aneurysm, or leaking AV malformation.
Risk factors: hypertension, smoking, heavy alcohol consumption, history of SAH in first-degree relatives, atherosclerosis.
10 - 15% die before reaching hospital; > 50% die within 6 months.

Neurologic complications:

- 50 - 70% of patients who rebleed, die. Aggressive control of blood pressure and urgent surgical or endovascular obliteration are mainstays of prevention.
- Hydrocephalus occurs in 20 - 30% of pts and causes increased ICP in > 50%. Can be treated with CSF drainage by intraventricular catheter (which itself may cause bleeding), so is reserved for those with deteriorating neuro signs.
- Vasospasm occurs in 2/3 of pts, and may cause cerebral ischemia/infarction.

Sentinel pain or leak:	At the time of or after aneurysm rupture:
40% of pts have unusual HA, sometimes with nausea, vomiting, photophobia, nuchal rigidity, 10-20 days prior to aneurysm rupture.	Violent "explosive," "cataclysmic" headache. 50% have decreased level of consciousness, Cranial nerve deficit, N/V, Hyperventilation Hemiplegia, Hemiparesis.
If aneurysm is expanding: HA, Visual-field defects, Extraocular muscle palsy, Eye pain, Face pain.	Meningeal irritation: Stiff neck, neck pain, positive Kernig's and Brudzinski's signs, photophobia, blurred vision, irritability, restlessness May occur during exertion or valsalva
If vasospasm or embolism: Motor or sensory deficits.	25% have a seizure at onset 50% have ↑ BP, or labile BP if ICP ↑

Severity of SAH: the Hunt-Hess Grade	Mortality Rate
I Asymptomatic, minimal HA, slight nuchal rigidity	30 %
II Moderate to severe HA, nuchal rigidity, cranial nerve palsy	40 %
III Lethargic, confused, mild focal neurologic deficit	50 %
IV Stupor, hemiparesis, possibly decorticate posturing	60 %
V Coma, decerebrate posturing, moribund	90 %

Diagnostic Tests: Urgent CT/MRI (but results will be negative in 10 - 15%).
Cerebral angiography (will be negative in 10 - 20%).
Transcranial doppler daily in ICU, to detect vasospasm.
CSF analysis (spinal tap is contraindicated if ICP is increased).

During Treatment It is imperative to avoid insults such as hyperglycemia, acidosis, electrolyte fluctuations, hypoxia, and hyperthermia

O_2 and $PaCO_2$: If Grade > III or GCS ≤ 8, intubate to protect the airway.
Maintain PaO_2/SaO_2 to minimize cerebral ischemia.
Keep $PaCO_2$ 35 - 40 mm Hg. If ↑ ICP and signs of deterioration, may increase ventilator rate/volume to achieve $PaCO_2$ = 30 - 35.
Anemia is linked to poor outcome, transfusion may offer benefit.
Keep Hgb at least 8 g/dL, unless there is ongoing cerebral or cardiac ischemia, then keep Hgb ≥ 10 g/dL.

Control Blood Pressure: NS to maintain normovolemia (keep CVP = 6 - 12 mm Hg).
Critical to control hypertension, the primary cause of rebleeding.
Labetalol 10 - 40 mg IV q 15 - 30 mins to keep SBP < 150 mm Hg, DBP < 80, MAP < 110. Esmolol or Nicardipine are also used.
Avoid Nitroprusside, which tends to ↑ ICP; toxicity is also a threat.
In hypotensive patients, Dobutamine to keep SBP > 120 mm Hg and maintain CPP > 60 - 70 mm Hg.

Anti-Fibrinolytic: Recent studies showed tranexamic acid (see "Stat Meds" chptr) when combined with prevention of cerebral vasospasm and given immediately after diagnosis of SAH, reduced rebleeding rates.

Reduce Stimuli: Morphine 1 - 4 mg IV q 1 h for headache, pain, or stress.
Sedate with Propofol 5 mcg/kg/hr.
Quiet/dim room, visitor restriction, minimal physical activity.
HOB elevated 30°. No valsalva. Provide stool softeners.
Minimize coughing, avoid sneezing if possible.

Connolly ES, Rabinstein AA, Carhuapoma JR, et al. Guidelines for the management of aneurysmal subarachnoid hemorrhage. AHA, Stroke.ahajournals.org; June 2012;43: (accessed 2/22/16)

Seizure Prophylaxis:
- Seizures occur in 10 - 25%, usually in the first 24 hours.
- Seizure risk is increased by: rebleeding, intraoperative retraction of temporal lobe, vasospasm, middle cerebral artery aneurysm.
- Seizures can cause rebleeding, hypertension, hypoxia.
- Although seizure prophylaxis is common, it is now called into question because of side effects and questionable benefit.

Cerebral Vasospasm:
- Cerebral infarction due to vasospasm is cause of early mortality.
- Unless BP is < 120 mm Hg, cerebrovasodilator Nimodipine is given as 60 mg enterally q 4 h x 21 days.
- Focal constriction of cerebral arteries adjacent to the site, possibly due to chemical mediators (serotonin, prostaglandin, catecholamines) or due to vasoactive metabolites released as the clot lyses. Causes cerebral ischemia or infarction
- Symptoms occur in 20 - 40% of patients. Incidence and extent correlate with the amount of blood in the subarachnoid space.
- Vasospasm occurs in almost all patients with clot size ≥ 5 x 3 mm Threat begins in 3-4 days, peaks in 7-14 days, resolves in 28 d.
- Lethargy with or without focal neurologic deficit is considered vasospasm until proven otherwise -> Stat transcranial doppler.
- Progressive deterioration (confusion, ↓ LOC, motor weakness, sensory deficit, visual/speech deficits) requires STAT angiogram

Manage Cerebral Vasospasm:
- Triple H Therapy (Hypervolemia, Hemodilution, Hypertension) is an option, although a supporting evidence is scant.
- Hemodilution (to a Hgb < 10 g/dL) may well increase cerebral blood flow, but at the expense of oxygen delivery.
- NS 1 mL/kg/hr, and albumin q 2 hrs if needed is given to maintain CVP ≥ 5 mm Hg.
- After obliteration of the aneurysm, vasopressors are given to maintain SBP > 100 mm Hg if needed. But if signs of cerebral ischemia develop, systolic blood pressure target is 180 - 220 (hypertensive therapy is delayed in pts with hydrocephalus).
- If technically feasible, balloon angioplasty of spastic vessels.
- Intraarterial Nicardipine, Verapamil, Nimodipine, or Milrinone, given for vasodilatory effects.
- Magnesium continuous infusion x 14 days may reduce cerebral ischemia due to vasospasm by as much as 34%.
- Large volume hypotonic fluids are avoided.

Location of Vasospasm:
If legs are weak - suspect anterior cerebral artery
If speech disturbance - suspect middle cerebral artery
If facial weakness, cranial nerve deficit - posterior cerebral artery

Definitive Treatment:
Best outcome is achieved when complete obliteration of the aneurysm is achieved as early as possible:
Clipping usually done early (within 24 hrs) on Grades I - III.
Aneurysms located in the Circle of Willis are inoperable.

GDC:
Guglielmi **D**etachable **C**oil embolization - transarterial placement of microcoils into the aneurysm to prevent bleeding.
GDC is able to completely occlude only half of aneurysms treated.
Ischemia and aneurysm perforation complicate 2 - 8% of GDC pts.

Non-neurologic complications:
50 - 80% develop one or more major medical complications which are as likely to cause death as either rebleeding or vasospasm. Listed in order of frequency:
1. Acute hypertension; Acute left ventricular dysfunction.
2. Pulmonary insufficiency (accounts for up to 50% of medical mortality)
3. Hyponatremia (can cause seizures; too rapid correction -> demyelination)
4. Hyperglycemia (BG > 180 mg/dL is associated with ↑ risk of vasospasm)
5. Arrhythmias (occur in 90% of patients, but life threatening in < 5%)

Diringer MN, Bleck TP, Hemphill JC, et al. Critical care management of patients following aneurysmal subarachnoid hemorrhage. NeuroCritCare, 2011;15:211-240.
Bederson JB, Connolly ES, Batjer HH, et al. Guidelines for the management of aneurysmal subarachnoid hemorrhage, Stroke,2009;40:994-1025.

Spontaneous Intracerebral Hemorrhage

"Hemorrhagic Stroke"

Description:

- Bleeding into the brain usually due to ruptured intracranial vessel. Can lead to brain disruption, compression, displacement, ischemia, cerebral edema.
- Accounts for 15% of all strokes and is more likely to cause disability/death.
- In 30%, the hematoma continues to expand during the initial 6 hours. (more likely to occur in patients who are hypertensive or anticoagulated).
- Intraventricular hemorrhage (IVH) occurs in 30 - 50%, carries high mortality. In addition to obstructive hydrocephalus and intracranial hypertension, the release of hematoma-associated factors cause thrombin generation, inflammation, oxidative stress, excitotoxicty, and global brain dysfunction, compared to the more focal process that occurs in ICH without IVH.
- Only 50% survive the first year. Most survivors are functionally dependent.

Classic Presentation:	• Many (40%) have headache, nausea, decreased LOC (which is • uncommon in ischemic stroke), 50% have vomiting. • 90% have ↑ BP. There may also be fever, cardiac arrhythmias, nuchal rigidity, retinal hemorrhages. Seizures occur in 6 - 7%. • 55% have slow progression of focal neurologic deficit. • 35% have sudden maximal (sometime clinically devastating) symptoms at onset.

Deficits: Incidence of hematoma location and the focal neurologic signs:

40 - 50%	Basal ganglia - Contralateral hemiparesis, contralateral conjugate gaze paresis, or confusion
20 - 50%	Lobar - Contralateral hemiparesis or sensory loss, contralateral conjugate gaze paresis, homonymous hemianopia, apathy, aphasia, neglect, or apraxia
10 - 15%	Thalamus - Contralateral hemiparesis, sensory loss, and conjugate gaze paresis. Also homonymous hemianopia, myosis, aphasia, or confusion
5 - 10%	Cerebellum - Ataxia, usually beginning in the trunk, ipsilateral facial weakness, ipsilateral sensory loss, gaze paresis, miosis, or ↓ LOC. Vomiting is common.
1 - 5%	Brain stem - Quadriparesis, facial weakness, ↓ LOC, gaze paresis, ocular bobbing, myosis, or autonomic instability. Pontine or other brainstem hemorrhage carries a mortality rate of 75% at 24 hours.
	Putamen - Contralateral hemiparesis, sensory loss, and conjugate gaze paresis. Also homonymous hemianopia, aphasia, neglect, or apraxia.

Diagnostic Studies: CT clearly differentiates hemorrhagic from ischemic stroke. Cerebral angiography should be done if CT suggests AVM. MRI and/or MRA are sometimes superior to CT.

Treatment of ICH:	
Airway	• ET intubation if $PaO_2 < 60$, $PaCO_2 > 50$, GCS ≤ 8. • Delay in intubating can cause secondary brain injury due to hypoxemia, aspiration, hypercapnea. • Elective tracheostomy is recommended if the patient remains intubated for than 2 weeks.
Control BP:	• To minimize ongoing bleed, hypertension must be controlled. • But there is concern that excessive BP reduction could cause cerebral ischemia (remember CPP = MAP - ICP). • Goal is to cautiously lower BP to MAP < 130 mm Hg. • If SBP > 230 or DBP > 140, use Nitroprusside (has rapid onset, but may cause excessive fall in BP). • If SBP 180 - 230 or DBP 105 - 140, Labetalol or Esmolol is given. (Nicardipine is a cerebro-selective vasodilator, but can cause hypotension). • If SBP < 180 and DBP < 105, defer antihypertensive therapy. • If ICP monitor available, keep CPP > 70 mm Hg.

cont'd on next page ➡

Spontaneous Intracerebral Hemorrhage (cont'd)

Prevent ↓ BP:
Fluids (isotonic saline or colloid) to maintain euvolemia:
- Target a CVP = 5 - 12 mm Hg, PCWP = 10 - 14 mm Hg.
- Fluid-in should = Fluid-out (daily urinary output + 500 mL insensible loss + 300 mL/each 1° fever)

If SBP remains < 90 or MAP remains < 80, consider:
- Phenylephrine 2 - 10 mcg/kg/min, or
- Dopamine 2 - 20 mcg/kg/min, or
- Norepinephrine titrated from 0.05 - 0.2 mcg/kg/min.

Sedate, ↓ cerebral O2 demand:
- Propofol, benzodiazepine, or morphine may prevent excessive elevation in BP, reducing the risk of hematoma expansion.
- Do not allow ET suctioning to cause ↓ PaO_2/SaO_2, ↑ ICP, ↓↑ BP, or arrhythmias. May need neuromuscular blockade.
- If temp > 38.5° C acetaminophen 650 mg or surface cooling.

Correct clotting:
Correct any identifiable coagulopathy with fresh frozen plasma, Vitamin K, Protamine, or Platelet transfusion.

Seizure prophylaxis:
Most seizures occur in the first 24 hours.
Phenytoin is recommended to prevent or treat seizure activity.

Intra-ventricular Catheter:
- Intraventricular catheter (IVC) may be used to monitor ICP and to drain CSF.
- Studies indicate that instilling low dose tPa (Alteplase 2 - 4 mg) into the ventricles for 1 hour may speed the restoration of CSF circulation and can significantly reduce ICP.

Prevent DVT/PE:
The ACCP recommends use of IPC (Intermittent Pneumatic Counterpulsation) device early in the course of care.
In stable patients, ACCP recommends low-dose SC heparin as soon as the second day after onset of the hemorrhage.

Manage ↑ ICP:
If ↑ ICP or clinical deterioration occurs, due to mass effect:
- 20% Mannitol 0.25 - 1 g/kg q 4 - 6 hr for ≤ 5 days, and measure serum osmolality bid, maintaining 310 - 320 mOsm/L. Furosemide 10 mg q 2 - 8 h may be given simultaneously.
- Corticosteroid is controversial. Used if there is evidence of large amounts of vasogenic edema and mass effect.
- Hyperventilation (TV = 12 - 14 mL/kg; $PaCO_2$ = 30 - 35 mm Hg) lowers ICP 25 - 30% in most patients.
- Reducing the ICP to target may take up to 30 minutes.
- If hyperventilation fails to ↓ ICP, prognosis is grave.
- Neuromuscular blockade with sedation may ↓ elevated ICP by preventing coughing, straining, fighting the ventilator.
- If ICP remains refractory, barbiturate coma (with pentobarbital or thiopental) may be used to impose EEG silence.

Surgery:
- Surgical reduction of the hematoma may decrease the mass effect, lessen ICP, and limit the potential for edema/cell death.
- Surgery, however, subjects the patient to surgical risks, brain manipulation, and anesthesia.
- Surgery is reserved for those with:
  - Moderate GCS
  - Moderate hematoma volume
  - No intraventricular hemorrhage
- Patients presenting in a coma, with a large hematoma volume and IVH or hydrocephalus usually die, regardless of therapy.

No to factor VIIa
NovoSeven "reduced growth of intracerebral hematoma, but did not improve survival or functional outcome"

Mayer SA, Brun NC, Begtrup K, et al. Efficacy and safety of Recombinant Factor VII for acute intracerebral hemorrhage. MEJM, May 2008;358:20.

Status Epilepticus

Description of a Grand Mal Seizure:

- A typical generalized convulsive seizure lasts about 1 - 2 minutes. It begins with a **Tonic Phase:** continuous muscle contraction with extension of the back and neck, followed by extension of arms and legs, loss of consciousness, abnormal deviation of the eyes. Laryngeal spasm causes apnea. HR and blood pressure increase, and there is profuse sweating and tracheobronchial hypersecretion. The tonic phase is usually brief, lasting 10 - 20 seconds.
- The **Clonic phase** follows: the muscle spasms relax intermittently, producing phases of atonia, followed by repeated violent flexor spasms. Each spasm is accompanied by pupillary contraction and dilation.
- Finally there is an atonic periods lasting about 30 seconds., during which apnea and motionless continue, and after which breathing resumes.

What is Status Epilepticus (SE)?

- Status epilepticus is a Grand Mal Seizure lasting longer than 10 minutes.
- Brain ischemia develops after 10 minutes of convulsive activity.
- If the seizure lasts longer than 60 minutes, in-hospital mortality is 32%.

Non-convulsive SE (NCSE):

NCSE is a rare cause of unconsciousness. Like visible seizures, NCSE dramatically increases cerebral metabolic rate. EEG should be considered if:

- A patient with convulsive history presents in an unresponsive state.
- Treatment ends convulsions, but the patient fails to regain consciousness

One study found that 8% of ICU patients in coma were in NCSE.

Causes of SE:

- CNS trauma, neoplasm, hemorrhage, ischemic stroke, infection.
- CNS drug toxicity (ETOH, Theophylline, Lidocaine, Cocaine)
- CNS drug withdrawal (ETOH, benzodiazepines, barbiturates).
- Metabolic disorder, such as
  ↓ or ↑ blood glucose, Acid-base imbalance, End stage liver disease
  Electrolyte Imbalance (↓ or ↑ Na, ↓ Phos., rarely ↓ Ca, ↓ Mg)
  Post liver transplantation (seizures are the most common postoperative neurologic complication in these patients)
- CNS hypoxic injury (severe hypoxemia, prolonged cardiac arrest)

Pathophysiology:

- Excessive neuronal activity results in:
  1. increase in intracellular Ca level to toxic levels
  2. activation of cell autolytic enzyme systems
  3. production of toxic O_2 radicals
  4. generation of nitric oxide, which enhances excitation
  5. increase in extracellular K, which propagates more seizures
- Diaphragmatic and chest muscle spasm results in ineffective respirations, hypoxemia, cyanosis, and lactic acidosis cause further brain injury and ↓ the patient's responsiveness to anticonvulsants.
- ↑ Cerebral and total body demand for oxygen results in:
  1. increased CO_2 production → respiratory acidosis
  2. anaerobic metabolism → metabolic acidosis
  3. ↓ skin blood flow + heat production → hyperthermia
     (a 2° F increase in half the pts; as high as 107° in a few patients)
- Catecholamine surge results in ↑ BP, ↑ HR, arrhythmias (in more than half of patients), pupillary dilation, ↑ PAP (some develop pulmonary edema), ↑ SVR, hyperglycemia. With prolonged SE, blood pressure will eventually fall.

CT Scan:

62% of ICU patients have a vascular, infectious, or neoplastic reason for the seizure. CT Scan, followed by CSF analysis, are usually considered.

Lab:

- Blood glucose, urea, electrolytes, arterial blood gases,
- Serum creatine kinase to exclude rhabdomyolysis.
- Epileptic drug levels, Toxicology.

cont'd on next page →

Status Epilepticus: Treatment

Protect the airway:	Padded tongue blades are not recommended. If needed, suction to clear airway of saliva/blood/vomitus. Turn patient onto side until suction is available.
Oxygenate, Ventilate:	O_2 by nasal cannula, 4 LPM if possible. Given the risk for aspiration and for respiratory depression due to anticonvulsants, plan for intubation and ventilation.
Maintain BP:	Establish 2 IV's, for anticonvulsants and for inotropic agents. If ↓ BP, start with volume replacement. About 1/3 of patients will require vasopressor. If ↑ BP, delay antihypertensives until SE is controlled.
Test BG:	Perform rapid blood glucose determination. If BG < 80, give Dextrose 1 mg/kg (may also give Thiamine 100 mg because glucose ↑ risk of Wernicke's encephalopathy in some patients).
Medicate:	See "Seizure Meds" in Med Facts chapter for dosing details: • Lorazepam is preferred as the first line agent. • Fosphenytoin is given when a second drug is needed. • If intravenous access cannot be established, loading dose of Fosphenytoin IM or rectal diazepam 0.5 mg/kg may be given. • Midazolam (Line 2 med) may resolve refractory SE. • Phenobarbital, Pentobarbital, Propofol are 3rd line agents. • Valproate acid is also a 3rd line agent. It is associated with hepatic and pancreatic toxicity. • All seizure medications cause respiratory depression and may mandate mechanical ventilation. • If meds fail, there is probably extensive underlying brain injury. Anesthesia (Isoflurane) may be considered.
Check ABG:	If the pH is < 7 (metabolic + respiratory acidosis), may give sodium bicarbonate 100 mEq in 1 liter of 0.25 NS. If $PaCO_2$ > 60 mm Hg, increase ventilatory rate.
Check Lab:	If serum Na < 125 mmol/L, 3% NaCl may be given. If creatinine elevated, rehydrate with 0.9% NaCl. If history of ETOH abuse, Thiamine 100 mg IV may be given
Control ↑ Temp:	Tylenol suppositories. Hypothermia unit may be necessary. Cooling peritoneal lavage has also been done.
Reassess:	If SE resolves spontaneously (no anticonvulsants were given) expect patient to awaken in 15 - 20 minutes. But continued unresponsiveness may represent nonconvulsive (subclinical) SE. Patient needs emergency EEG. Those patients treated with anticonvulsants and NMBA require EEG to rule out subclinical SE.
EEG:	Invaluable in identifying the location and the type of seizure. Used to test for subclinical status epilepticus or SE in patients under the influence of both neuromuscular blocking agents and sedatives.
Problems:	Rhabdomyolysis is common, may lead to renal failure; treatment involves vigorous saline diuresis. Other complications include compression fractures, joint dislocations, tendon avulsions. Memory and behavioral problems are common. Cerebral edema and ↑ ICP may occur. Having had SE lowers the threshold for subsequent seizures.

For EMS: (see http://www.midazolam.net/midazolam-nasal-spray)
Midazolam nasal atomizer: Easy to give, no IV required, pt response is rapid. The median time from medication administration to seizure cessation was 1.3 minutes less for inhaled midazolam compared with rectal diazepam.

Delirium Tremens

Facts:

- 5% of those who withdraw from alcohol progress to DT's, a state of mental delirium, intense sympathetic activity, fluid and electrolyte imbalance, fever, and seizures.
- Mortality is as high as 35% if untreated, < 5% if recognized and treated early. DT's are considered a medical emergency.
- Death is usually due to hyperadrenergic state (arrhythmia) or due to respiratory failure.

Pathophysiology: Persistent ethanol intake leads to down-regulation of the benzodiazepine-GABAa-chloride complex. Ethanol withdrawal results in a decrease in the inhibitory neurotransmitter GABA. This results in an unopposed increase in sympathetic activity.

Clinical Presentation: Alcohol withdrawal symptoms may start several hours after decreased or halted ethanol intake. Alcohol withdrawal symptoms include tremors, irritability, insomnia, anorexia. DT's usually begin 2 - 10 days after the last drink, persist 2 - 3 days, are characterized by confusion, hallucinations, delusions, seizures, and sympathetic hyperactivity (↑ HR, ↑ RR, ↑ BP, ↑ temp, diaphoresis, hyperreflexia, mydriasis, incontinence).

Missed Diagnosis?

- The recognition of DT's may be missed if the signs of autonomic activity are attributed to injury, hemorrhage, or anxiety and if the index of suspicion is low. Perform risk assessment using CIWA scale (go to www.agingincanada.ca/CIWA.HTM).
- On the other hand, pts who are known to abuse alcohol may be subject to a premature diagnosis of "DT's," before other causes of delirium and hyperadrenergic state are considered (such as PE, CVA, hypo or hyperglycemia, hypoxemia).
- DT's should be a diagnosis of exclusion.

ECG: AFib is most common. Also AFlutter, PAC's, SVT, PVC's.

Lab Findings:
Blood glucose: Often low due to chronic glycogen depletion
CBC reveals: Leukocytosis, anemia, thrombocytopenia
Liver enzymes: ↑ AST, ↑ ALT, ↑ GGT, ↑ bilirubin
PT, PTT: ↑ due to Vitamin K deficiency
ABG & lactic acid: Metabolic acidosis may be present

Treatment:

- O_2 per nasal cannula at 2 - 4 LPM
- Glucose 1 ampule of 50 mL $D_{50}W$ IV
- D_5NS to rehydrate (may need 4 - 10 L in 24 h) and to prevent hypoglycemia.
- Thiamine 100 mg IV q d x 3 days
- Folic acid 1 mg IV
- $MgSO_4$ 2 g in 50 mL D_5W over 20 mins IV
- Electrolytes (DT patients often have ↓ Ca, ↓ Mg, ↓ Phos, ↓ K)
- Benzodiazepine is the medication of choice for the delirium. Onset is rapid, duration of effect is long. Dose needed will vary tremendously among individuals. If 10 mg Diazepam fails to control agitation for at least an hour, hourly doses may be escalated up to 100 - 200 mg of a diazepam equivalent. If agitation is not controlled for at least an hour, then barbiturate is preferred.
- Barbiturates may be required for patients with benzodiazepine-resistant agitation. Beware ↓ BP and respiratory depression. Phenobarbital in hourly escalating doses of 65, 130, 260 mg have been used.
- There are reports that the need for mechanical ventilation can be reduced if agitation is treated with a protocol of escalating doses of diazepam and phenobarbital.
- If Diazepam and Phenobarbital fail to control severe agitation, then Propofol 20 mg bolus + infusion + mechanical ventilation are required.
- Haldol has also been used.
- Beta-blockers may be used to treat the hyperadrenergic, hypertensive state.

Brain Death Criteria

Prerequisites (all must be checked)
- Coma, irreversible and cause known
- Neuroimaging explains coma
- CNS depressant drug effect absent (if indicated toxicology screen; if barbiturates given, serum level <10 mcg/mL)
- No evidence of residual paralytics (electrical stimulation if paralytics used).
- Absence of severe acid-base, electrolyte, endocrine abnormality
- Normothermia or mild hypothermia (core temperature > 36° C)
- Systolic blood pressure $\geq$ 100 mm Hg
- No spontaneous respirations

Examination (all must be checked)
- Pupils nonreactive to bright light
- Corneal reflex absent
- Oculocephalic reflex absent (tested only if C-spine integrity ensured)
- Oculovestibular reflex absent
- No facial movement to noxious stimuli at supraorbital nerve, temporomandibular joint
- Gag reflex absent
- Cough reflex absent to tracheal suctioning
- Absence of motor response to noxious stimuli in all 4 limbs (spinally mediated reflexes are permissible)

Apnea testing (all must be checked)
- Patient is hemodynamically stable
- Ventilator adjusted to provide normocarbia ($PaCO_2$ 34 – 45 mm Hg) Patient preoxygenated with 100% FiO_2 for > 10 minutes to PaO_2 > 200 mm Hg
- Patient well-oxygenated with a PEEP of 5 cm of water
- Provide oxygen via a suction catheter to the level of the carina at 6 L/min or attach T-piece with CPAP at 10 cm H_2O
- Disconnect ventilator
- Spontaneous respirations absent
- Arterial blood gas drawn at 8 –10 minutes, patient reconnected to ventilator
- $PCO_2 \geq$ 60 mm Hg, or 20 mm Hg rise from normal baseline value OR:
- Apnea test aborted

Ancillary testing (only 1 needs to be performed; to be ordered only if clinical examination cannot be fully performed due to patient factors, or if apnea testing inconclusive or aborted)
- Cerebral angiogram
- HMPAO SPECT (Cerebral scintigraphy)
- EEG Electroencephalogram
- TCD Transcranial Doppler

Wijdicks, EFM, Varelas PN, Gronseth GS, Greer DM. Evidence-based guideline update: Determining brain death in adults. Neurology June 8, 2010 vol. 74 no. 23 1911-1918, Current guideline (June 2010) Reaffirmed on April 30, 2014 and endorsed by the American College of Radiology, the Association of Organ Procurement Organizations, the Child Neurology Society, the Neurocritical Care Society, the Radiological Society of North America, and the Society of Critical Care Medicine.

Care of the Organ Donor after Brain Death

Facts:
91,000 Americans are awaiting organ transplantation.
Only 40% of those waiting will ever receive a transplant.
Organs can be donated by individuals aged newborn to 75.
Contraindications: HIV, Hepatitis B & C, Malignancy.

Transplantable Organs/Tissues: Heart, Lungs, Skin, Ligaments, Fascia, Kidney, Pancreas, Bone, Heart valves, Cartilage, Liver, Dura, Veins, Eyes/Corneas

Referral and Consent:
1. Notify OPO (organ procurement organization) of potential donor before brain death has occurred.
2. The OPO will assess patient for suitability.
3. Family is more likely to consent to donation if approached by OP coordinator in collaboration with hospital staff.
4. If consent obtained, notify ME/coroner for approval.

Routine Care:
1. Q 1 hr monitor Vital Signs, SaO_2, CVP, PAP, Intake/Output.
2. Insert 2 large bore IV catheters and an arterial line.
3. Suction q 2 hr, reposition patient q 2 hr.
4. Gastric decompression with NG tube to low suction (80 - 120 mm Hg). Check placement and output q 2 hrs.
5. Discontinue meds except pressors and antibiotics.

Goals	History needed by the transplant team	Notify OPC if:
SBP > 90 mm Hg	Heart disease, chest pain	SBP < 90
CVP = 6 - 8 mm Hg	Hypertension	CVP < 4 or > 11
PCWP = 8 - 12 mm Hg	Diabetes	HR < 70 or > 120
CI > 2.4 L/min/m^2	Smoking	UO < 1 mL/kg/hr
SVR = 800-1200	Alcohol	UO > 3 mL/kg/hr
UO > 1 mL/kg/hr	Drug Abuse	Na > 150 mEq/L
PaO_2 > 100 mm Hg	High risk behaviors	PaO_2 < 90
SpO_2 > 97%	Episodes of hypoxemia	SpO_2 < 95%
Hgb > 10 gm /dL	Episodes of hypotension	Hgb/Hct < 10/30
pH = 7.35 - 7.45	Episodes of arrhythmia	PT > 14 seconds
temperature > 34°C	Cardiac arrest and duration	PTT > 28 seconds

Problems of Donor Maintenance

Hemodynamic Instability:
- Brain death produces a catecholamine surge in > 60 % of pts, precipitating vasoconstriction (SBP as high as 200 mm Hg), HR > 140 bpm, myocardial ischemia, tachyarrhthmias. Duration is 30 minutes to 6 hours (avg 1.2 hrs). and may threaten heart procurement. Esmolol or Nicardipine may be used.
- Hypotension follows, due to hypovolemia, cardiac dysfunction, vasodilation.
- Hypovolemia is related to prior fluid restrictions, diuretics, mannitol for increased ICP. Posterior pituitary dysfunction with diabetes insipidus, and hyperglycemic-induced osmotic diuresis also contribute to volume deficit.
- Loss of vasomotor tone precipitates pooling of blood volume.
- A Central Venous Catheter should be placed; all fluids should be warmed.
- Volume status must be supported with RL to a CVP 6 - 8 mm Hg.
- Concern must also be directed toward protecting the lungs from excess fluid administration, one of the greatest reasons for lung unsuitability.
- Dopamine at ≤ 10 mcg/kg/min. is the inotrope of choice. Dobutamine causes unwanted tachycardia and increased myocardial oxygen demand.
- The use of high-dose Dopamine (> 10 mcg/kg/min), Dobutamine (> 10 mcg/kg/min), Epinephrine (> 0.05 mcg/kg/min), and Norepinephrine (> 0.05 mcg/kg/min) are linked to poor function of the transplanted organs.
- Some have used Glucose-insulin-potassium infusion to improve ventricular function, without incurring the tachycardia seen with Dobutamine.
- Hormone replacement (thyroxine, steroid, vasopressin, insulin) can decrease the catecholamine requirement.
- PRBC's should be used to maintain Hct 30%.

cont'd on next page ➞

Problems of Donor Management (cont'd)

Bradycardia, Cardiac Arrest

- Brain death causes cardiac unresponsiveness to atropine. Use Epinephrine 0.05 - 0.1 mg IV for hemodynamically significant bradycardia.
- Cardiac arrest occurs in 25% of all donors during the maintenance phase and should be treated according to ACLS protocols.

↓ Temperature

Ischemic damage to the hypothalamus and pituitary → loss of thermoregulation. Hypothermia can lead to cardiac irritability and depression, coagulopathy, and reduced oxygen delivery to tissues. Hypothermia also precludes the certification of brain death. Donor core temperature must be maintained at > 34° C.

- humidified, heated ventilator gases
- warmed IV fluids
- warming blankets
- heat lamps

Pulmonary injury

- Minimize atelectasis/infection risk with aggressive tracheobronchial care.
- Maintain PaO_2 between 70 - 100 mm Hg, use TV of 6 - 8 ml/kg, $FiO_2 < 60\%$, PEEP < 7.5 cm H_2O, keeping $PaCO_2$ within normal range.
- If PaO_2 is < 70 mm Hg, increase FiO_2 and Peep to maintain $SaO_2 > 95\%$.
- Minimize barotrauma risk by monitoring Peep effect on cardiac output. Keep peak inspiratory pressure < 30 cm H_2O.

Oliguria

- If UO < 1 ml/kg/hr after adequate volume loading, use loop diuretics (furosemide), or osmotic diuretics (mannitol).
- Avoid nephrotoxic drugs (aminoglycosides) and agents that adversely affect renal perfusion (e.g., NSAIDs).

Diabetes Insipidus (DI)

Occurs in > 70% of brain-dead donors, results from insufficient blood levels of ADH from posterior pituitary. Look for polyuria along with hypernatremia, hyperosmolality, and diluted urine (urine osmolality < 300 mOsm/L).

- Once U/O exceeds 300 ml/hr or 4 ml/kg/hr, may give desmopressin, or give vasopressin 0.01 - 0.04 units/min.
- Common practice is to replace the previous hour's UO with a hypotonic fluid (5% Dextrose in 0.45% NaCl), and closely monitor electrolytes. Elevated serum Na is linked to poor function of grafted organs.

Electrolyte Imbalance

- If Na < 140, Switch to $D_5 1/2$NS , $D_5 1/4$NS or 0.45 NS
  If Na > 170, switch to D_5W.
- 90% of patients develop hypokalemia, due to diuretics, polyuria, alkalosis. If K < 3.2 mEq/L, KCl 20 mEq in 100 mL D_5W over 1 hr x 3 doses. May add KCl 20 - 40 mEq to 1 L of IV solution.
- Mg, Ca, and Phos are replaced as needed.

Hyperglycemia

Following brain-death, ↑ BG may be due to stress, catecholamine-induced insulin resistance, steroid administration for treatment of cerebral edema, or infusion of large amounts of dextrose-containing IV fluids. Hyperglycemia leads to osmotic diuresis and electrolyte imbalances.

- Insulin infusion to achieve normoglycemia
- Beware that lowering BG may result in ↓ K and ↑ Na.

Coagulopathy

Ischemic brain tissue releases thromboplastin, fibrinogen, tissue plasminogen, resulting in consumptive coagulopathy. Clotting factors and platelets are diluted by fluid administration. Hypothermia also prolongs clotting times. Cryoprecipitate, FFP, and or platelets may be given.

Ischemia-Reperfusion Injury: High dose steroid may protect the organs.

Transport to OR: With ambu bag and 100% O_2, PEEP valve, infusions, transfusions, cardiac and hemodynamic monitoring.

These efforts may result in life for a transplant patient.

CV

CV

Quick Head to Toe Assessment

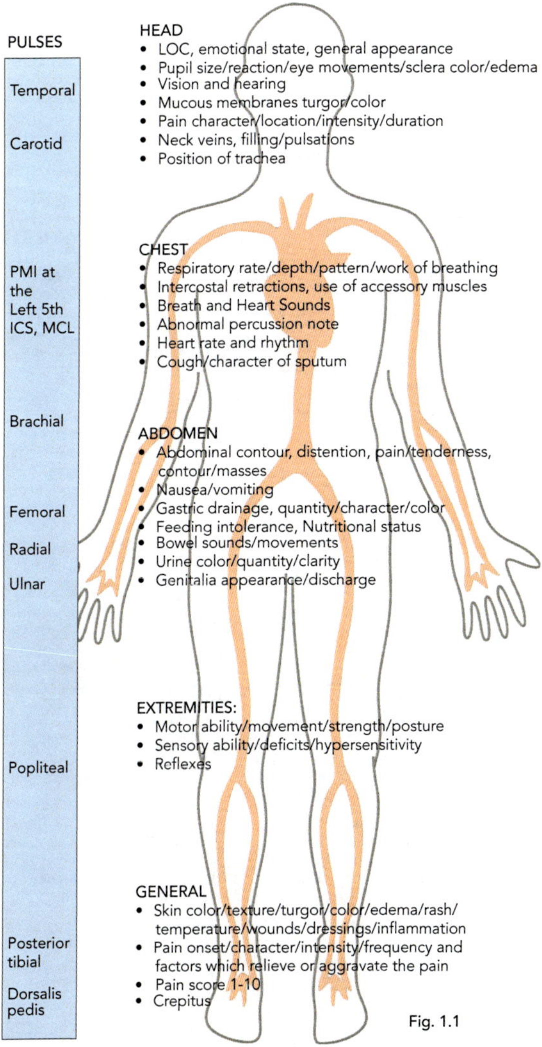

Fig. 1.1

Systems Assessment

	Usual Assessments	Additional Assessments
NEURO	Level of consciousness, orientation Motor ability, strength, ROM Speech, clarity, appropriateness Pupillary light reflex, eye movement Presence of confusion or delirium Breathing pattern, work, depth Temporal pulses, quality Headache, vision/hearing deficits Paresthesias, Reflexes (grade 0-4+) Pain, intensity and perception of	Restraints, immobility, devices Use of hypothermia Monitoring device Abnormal eye movements Peripheral nerve stimulator Sedative use/level of sedation Use of paralyzing agents Foot support/boots Epidural catheter PCA device, BIS monitor
CARDIO-VASCULR	Pulses: (grade 0 - 3+) Radial Femoral Dorsalis pedis Ulnar Popliteal Posterior tibial Brachial Cardiac thrill Capillary refill time: < or > 2 sec. Edema (grade 0 - 3+) Heart sounds, murmurs, thrills Neck veins, Location of PMI ECG, Dysrhythmias, ST Segment Presence/description of chest pain Activity tolerance	Patient's position Vascular access, Cardiac output, $ScvO_2$ Pressure monitoring Pacemakers settings & function Mediastinal tubes, dressings Intra-aortic balloon catheter Transcutaneous pacemaker Implanted Cardiodefibrillator Lower extremity compression stockings or device
RESP	Depth, rate, rhythm of breathing Use of accessory muscles Cyanosis, central/peripheral Sputum, character and amount Effectiveness of cough Audible wheeze, stridor Breath sounds, Lt and Rt Percussion note, Lt and Rt Position of trachea Suctioning frequency and tolerance	FiO_2, patient's SpO_2 Artificial airway, size, position Mechanical ventilator, settings Thoracotomy dressings Pleural chest tube/s and suction Transtracheal catheter Pulse oximeter End-tidal CO_2 monitor Apnea monitor/alarm In-line suction catheter
GI/GU and RENAL	Abd. pain, tenderness, guarding Abd. distention, wall contour Tolerance to eating, feeding Nutritional status Character of vomitus and stool Status of mucous membranes Presence of nausea/vomiting Bowel sounds in the 4 quadrants Urine amount/quality Status of urinary catheter Status of/problems with genitalia	Feeding tube type, size, site Feeding formula, rate, residuals GI tubes - patency/drainage Hyperalimentation line/site Abdominal sumps/drains Surgical dressings Ostomies Dialysis shunt or catheter Peritoneal dialysis Continuous renal replacement.
SKIN	Color, texture, turgor, temp Rashes, abrasions, wounds, burns, bruises, inflammations Status of boney prominences Discomfort (itching, burning)	Patient's position Type bed/mattress/pt tolerance Dressings, wounds, ulcers Protective aids Hypo/hyperthermia unit
EXTREM	Limitation in movement Deformities, Contractures Evidence of ischemia: Pain, pallor, paresthesia, paralysis, pulseless, polar (cold)	Arterial and venous catheters Anti-embolism stockings Casts, splints, restraints Sequential compression device
PSYCH	Emotional state, Coping ability Available support systems Communication ability Sleep/rest deficits	Emotional support Patient/family teaching needs Social service needs Transfer/Discharge planning

CV Assessment

History:	Palpitations	Character, frequency, precipitating factors, associated symptoms
	Dyspnea	Exertional, at rest, nocturnal, positional, or associated with cough
	Chest pain	Character, location, onset, duration, intensity, what aggravates/relieves it, relation to breathing
	Extremities	Muscle aching, pain while walking, ankle swelling, cramps, weight gain
	Other	Nausea, vomiting, dizziness, fainting, sweating, fever, weakness, fatigue
	Hx of illness	Rheumatic fever, diabetes, hypertension, angina, heart failure, valve disease, CAD, medications
	Psycho/Social	Personality type, occupation, physical activity, smoking, diet, current stress level
Inspect:	Skin	Color, mottling, pallor, petechiae, bruises
	Neck veins	• At 45° HOB elevation, venous pulse should be < 3 cm above the sternal notch. • Venous pressure should not rise when abdomen is compressed (+ Hepatojugular reflux is due to liver congestion associated with heart failure and with tricuspid regurgitation). • Lying flat, neck veins should be full.
	Apex	Apical impulse (normally at 5th ICS, MCL)
	Lt Sternal border	Visible lift implies right ventricular strain.
	Extremities	Capillary refill (should be prompt, < 2 seconds). Ulcers/lesions, hair loss, varicosities
	Pitting edema	0 - 1/4" = 1+ 1/4 - 1/2" = 2+ 1/2 - 1" = 3+
Palpate:	Apex	Point of Maximal Impulse (PMI) at the 5th ICS, MCL. Chest wall thrill (vibration due to valve dysfunction or ventricular septal defect)
	Lt sternal border	Lifting pulse associated with RV hypertrophy
	Precordium	Vibrations caused by aortic insufficiency or stenosis, pulmonary stenosis, ventricular septal defect.
	Trachea	Normal midline position vs. shift to one side
	Epigastric area	Aortic pulsations
	Skin	Temperature, sweating vs dry, turgor, color
	Peripheral pulses	0 absent 1+ weak, thready, decreased 2+ normal 3+ bounding, increased

Palpation of Right Posterior Tibial pulse

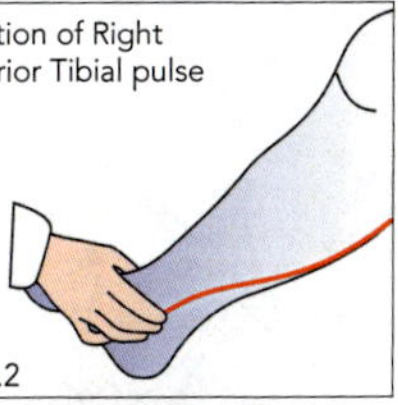

Fig. 1.2

Palpation of the Left Dorsalis Pedis pulse

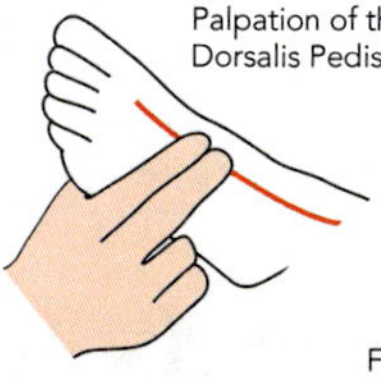

Fig. 1.3

Percuss: Distance of liver edge (cm) below right costal margin
Location of left and right borders of cardiac dullness.

Auscultate: The heart sounds, the carotid artery, subclavian artery, abdominal aorta, femoral artery, popliteal artery.

Heart Sounds

Stethoscope Placement:

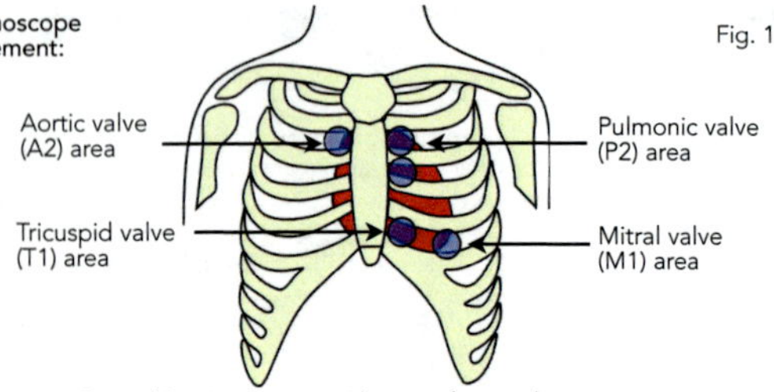

Fig. 1.4

S1: the Start of Systole	Caused by simultaneous closure of two valves: Mitral - whose sound is called M1, heard best at apex. Tricuspid - whose sound is called T1, heard best at the lower left sternal border (LLSB). Equated to "lub" of "lub-dub." The sound signals the beginning of systole. Heard best when using the diaphragm of the stethoscope. The S1 sound may "split" (because M1 & T1 do not always occur simultaneously) due to Right or Left Bundle Branch Block. Systolic Murmurs: Aortic Stenosis - high flow/intensity, blowing Mitral Regurgitation - low flow murmur
S2: the Start of Diastole	Caused by simultaneous closure of two valves: Aortic - whose sound is called A2 Pulmonic - whose sound is called P2 Equated with the "dub" of "lub-dub." The sound signals the beginning of diastole. Heard best on either side of the sternum, 2nd ICS. Normally split (A2 & P2) on inspiration. Abnormal splitting of S2 may be caused by: Right Bundle Branch Block (RBBB), pulmonic stenosis, atrial septal defect. Diastolic Murmurs: Mitral stenosis - High intensity, high flow Aortic Regurgitation - Blowing, low flow
S3: in early Diastole	Caused by decreased ventricular compliance. Heard best at apex, with patient recumbent or turned to left side. Use the bell of the stethoscope. The tempo sounds like "Kentucky." Generally implies ventricular failure or volume overload.
S4: in late Diastole	Caused by vibrations due to forceful atrial contraction. Heard best at apex, during inspiration, with patient recumbent. Use the bell of the stethoscope. Tempo sounds like "Tennessee." Possible causes: LV Hypertrophy Ventricles are stiffer than usual. May occur in the normal adult.

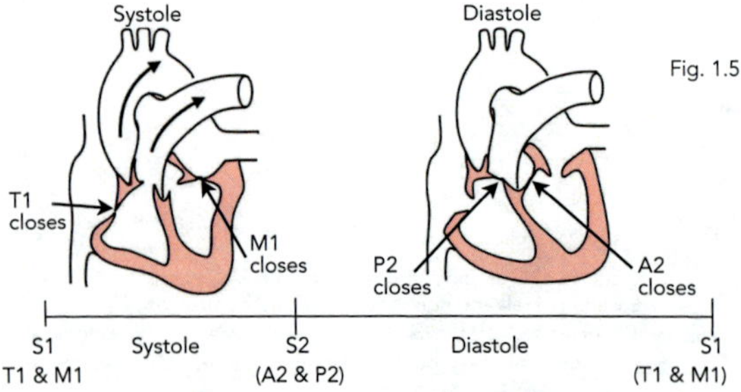

Fig. 1.5

Lipid Profiles and Cardiac Biomarkers

Cholesterol	ideal < 200 mg/dL borderline = 200 - 239 high > 240
Triglycerides	normal < 150 mg/dL borderline = 150 - 199 high = 200 - 499 very high > 500
Homocysteine	normal = 5 - 15 μmol/L moderately high = 16 - 30 intermediate = 31 - 100 severe > 100
High density lipoprotein (HDL)	normal (men) = 40 - 50 mg/dL normal (women) = 50 - 60 mg/dL desirable > 60 mg/dL
Low density lipoprotein (LDL)	optimal < 100 mg/dL near optimal = 100 - 129 borderline = 130 - 159 high = 160 - 189 very high ≥ 190
Cholesterol Ratio (Cholesterol:HDL)	keep below = 5:1 optimal = 3.5:1

See p. 9 "High sensitivity" cardiac biomarkers in the diagnosis of acute MI.

Cardiac Biomarkers:	Elevated cardiac biomarkers may indicate myocardial cell injury. Biomarkers that are slow to elevate may still be within normal range if lab work is drawn soon after symptom onset. Biomarkers that peak early may not be elevated if significant delay occurred from symptom onset to medical care.
Troponin hs-TnI	Found only in myocardial cells. Rises slowly after AMI, but the sensitivity is 100 % when tested 6 - 12 hrs after symptom onset. Elevated troponin is linked to increased risk for death. Slow return to normal makes it unusable for detection of reinfarction immediately after initial AMI.
Troponin T hs-TnT	Found in both skeletal and myocardial cells. Many conditions other than ACS may cause elevated troponin (e.g, myocarditis, heart failure, PE, renal failure, hypovolemia).
Myoglobin	Found in both skeletal and myocardial cells. Following AMI, the marker may be zero in patients who delay seeking medical care for more than a day. If the level does not rise within 24 hrs of symptom onset, AMI may be ruled out.
Creatine Kinase myocardium (CK-MB)	An early onset (3 - 6 hrs) marker. A value more than 2 times the upper limit of normal is specific for myocardial cell death. Rapid return to normal makes it insensitive 48 hours after AMI, but is superior in diagnosing reinfarct occurring < 48 hr after MI.
C-reactive protein, high sensitivity (hs-CRP)	A marker of inflammation, elevated C-reactive protein can be associated with coronary artery disease and risk for cardiac event. hs-CRP < 1 mg/L is low risk for CV disease, 1 - 3 is average risk, hs-CRP > 3 mg/L is high risk for CV disease.
BNP	Stretched myocardium releases Brain Natriuretic Peptide (BNP). Normal BNP is < 100 pg/mL. In patients with moderate heart failure, BNP is > 500 pg/mL. In patients with severe heart failure, BNP is > 900 pg/mL. BNP is predictive of 30-day survival in cardiogenic shock.

Jarolim P. High sensitivity cardiac troponin assays in the clinical laboratories. Clin Chem Lab Med, 2014;2-18. found @ www.quanterix.com.
Thygesen K, Giannitsis E, Mueller C, et al. How to use high-sensitivity Cardiac Troponins in acute cardiac care, Eur Heart J, 2012;33(18):2252-2257.

Acute Coronary Syndrome (ACS)

Acute Coronary Syndrome is the abrupt decrease in coronary artery blood flow.

The Chest Pain:
- Pressure type chest pain, usually starting in the retrosternal area, and lasting > 10 minutes.
- May radiate to one or both arms, shoulder, back, neck, jaw.
- Typically occurs at rest or with minimal exertion.

Other signs: May also experience diaphoresis, dyspnea, abdominal pain, nausea/vomiting, sweating, unexplained fatigue, syncope.

Risk is high if: Continuing chest pain, severe dyspnea, palpitations, syncope.

Pain that isn't myocardial ischemia:
- Pleuritic pain (occurs with respirations or cough)
- Primary location is in the middle or lower abdomen
- Localized by the tip of 1 finger, particularly at the LV apex
- Caused by movement or palpation of the chest wall or arms
- The episodes of pain are brief, lasting a few seconds or less
- The intensity of the pain was maximal at onset
- The pain radiates into the lower extremities.

If EMS is the first medical contact:
- Get a history for CAD or MI; particularly past and recent use of ASA or NTG.
- 12-lead ECG should be performed, assessed, reported to hospital. (Beware that normal ECG occurs in 1 - 6% of ACS patients)
- Determine if the patient has contraindications to fibrinolysis.
- If transport time is > 30 minutes, trained providers may give fibrinolytic. (Once fibrinolytic given, PCI must be delayed at least 3 hrs).
- Do not exceed 2 hours from first medical contact to reperfusion therapy (by either fibrinolysis or by PCI)

3 coronary syndromes:	UA Unstable Angina	NSTEMI Non ST-Elevation MI	STEMI ST Elevation MI
The ECG	Normal ST 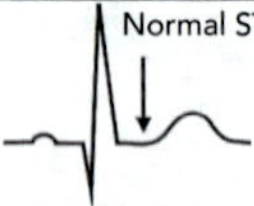 Partial thrombosis or vasospasm causes sudden unexpected chest pain due to reduced coronary blood flow (but no myocardial cell death). Comes as a surprise. May last longer than stable angina. Rest or medication usually do not help. Myocardial ischemia can worsen over time, and could progress to infarction.	Normal ST 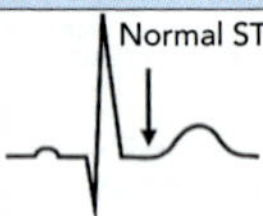 or the following may be present, but are not diagnostic: Inverted T 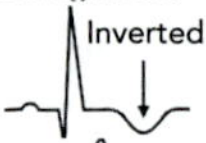 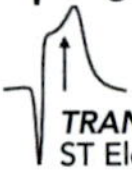 *TRANSIENT* ST Elevation or Depression 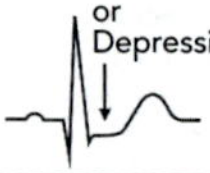	Persistent ST Elevation 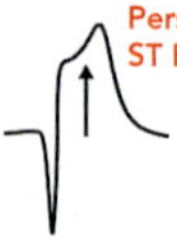 or evidence of posterior AMI, which includes New LBBB:→ 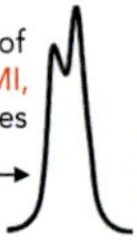 or ST Depression in anterior leads (V2, V3) 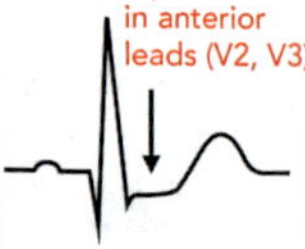
Cardiac Biomarkers Immediate and in 2 hours	Troponin **NEGATIVE** hs-cTNT and hs-cTNI is absent in ≥ 95% of patients who present with symptoms of ACS.	Troponin **POSITIVE** hs-cTNT and hs-cTNI rise within a few hrs of onset of symptoms and remain elevated a few days.	Troponin **POSITIVE** hs-cTNT and hs-cTNI rise within a few hrs of symptom onset and remain elevated a few days or up to 2 wks

Signs/symptoms of UA and NSTEMI are similar, but are more severe in NSTEMI.

O'Connor RE, Al Ali AS, Brady WJ, et al. Part 9: Acute Coronary Syndromes. 2015 AHA Guidelines for CPR and ECC, Circulation 2015;132(suppl 2):S483-S500.
Amsterdam EA et al. 2014 AHA/ACC Guideline for the Management of Patients With Non-ST-Elevation Acute Coronary Syndromes. J Am Coll Cardiol 2014;64:2645-2687.

Acute Coronary Syndrome (ACS)

- ACS occurs in > 780,000 individuals per year in the US.
- 70% of these will have Non-ST Elevation ACS (NSTE-ACS)
- NSTE-ACS typically have more comorbidities than patients with STEMI.

If Symptom onset **> 12 hrs**, but patient has:
- Hemodynamic instability
- Refractory pain
- ST elevation
- Heart Failure

Early PCI is recommended.

If Symptom onset ≤ 12 hr	TIMED GOALS (from time of admit)
Diagnosis/Immediate Rx	< 10 minutes
Fibrinolytic, if indicated	< 30 minutes
Chest X-Ray	< 60 minutes
PCI (Angioplasty)	< 90 minutes

Immediate Care by EMS or ED:

1. Vital signs, ECG monitor, SpO_2.
2. If breathless, signs of heart failure, or shock, start O_2 4 LPM to keep SpO_2 ≥ 94% (beware high-flow oxygen may cause harm).
3. 12-lead ECG, run continuously or repeat q 15-20 min. (AHA recommends against computer-assisted ECG interpretation due to "high false-negatives")
4. Quick, targeted medical history
   - Past history of angina, infarction or other cardiac diagnosis
   - Regular or recent use of ASA or NTG to relieve chest pain
   - Any contraindications to ASA
   - Any risk factors (see TIMI score below)
5. If no contraindications to aspirin (allergy, active peptic ulcer, active bleeding disorder, severe untreated hypertension, or severe hepatic disease): ASA 160 - 325 mg is given to chew (or 300 mg suppository for patients with nausea, vomiting, or GI intolerance to ASA).
6. Do not give any other NSAIDS (may cause harm).
7. One dose NTG, repeat q 3 - 5 min up to total of 3 doses, unless SBP < 90 mm Hg or ≥ 30 mm Hg below the patient's normal baseline. .Use extreme caution in patients with RV infarction - these patients need preload.

Additional Care by ED:

- Send blood for Troponin hs-cTnI STAT (repeated in 3 - 6 hrs), and as indicated by ECG changes. Send blood for electrolytes, renal function, coagulation.
- Identify contraindications to r-tPA. Brief physical exam is performed.
- Morphine if NTG does not resolve chest pain. Caution in pts with UA/NSTEMI
- The next step is fibrinolysis (if not already done by EMS) or PCI if indicated.

ED must accomplish all in < 10 mins

CXR within 30 mins of arrival, to identify other possible causes of chest pain.

TIMI Score: An Assessment of Patient Risk for Death, new or recurrent MI, or severe recurrent ischemia that reauires

	Score
Age ≥ 65	1
Patient has at least 3 of these risk factors: Family history of CAD Hypertension Diabetes mellitus Elevated cholesterol Current smoker Peripheral vascular disease Low LDL (< 40 mg/dL)	1
Aspirin use in last 7 days	1
≥ 2 anginal events in last 24 hrs	1
Elevated Troponin T or I	1
ST change ≥ 0.5 mm in contiguous leads	1
Known coronary artery stenosis ≥ 50%	1
Total the above for pt's TIMI Score:	

Timi	Score Total:
0 - 2	Low Risk
3 - 4	Moderate Risk
≥ 5	High Risk

TIMI Score	Percent risk that the pt will experience death, MI, or urgent revascularization for ischemia:
0 – 1	5 %
2	8 %
3	13 %
4	20 %
5	26 %
6 - 7	41 %

O'Connor RE, Al Ali AS, Brady WJ, et al. Part 9: Acute Coronary Syndromes. 2015 AHA Guidelines for CPR and ECC, Circulation 2015;132(suppl 2):S483-S500.
Amsterdam EA et al. 2014 AHA/ACC Guideline for the Management of Patients With Non-ST-Elevation Acute Coronary Syndromes. J Am Coll Cardiol 2014;64:2645-2687.

UA/NSTEMI Treatment

Early Hospital Care

Oxygen	Given only when $SaO_2 < 90\%$, respiratory distress, or other high-risk features of hypoxemia
Aspirin	162 - 325 mg is given as soon as possible after hospital arrival, followed by daily maintenance of 81 - 162 mg/day. NSAIDS should be discontinued.
Nitrates	Sublingual nitroglycerine q 5 mins x 3 for continuing ischemic pain. IV NTG for persistent ischemia, heart failure, or hypertension.
Morphine	Morphine may be given for pain. Morphine also venodilates, thus decreasing preload. Have fluids ready. If needed, the effects of morphine can be reversed with Naloxone.
Beta-blockers	• Should be started in the first 24 hrs UNLESS there is heart failure, low cardiac output, and AV block, asthma. • Sustained-release metoprolol, carvedilol, or bisoprolol is recommended for beta-blocker therapy with concomitant NSTE-ACS, stabilized HF, and reduced systolic function. • Those with initial contraindications to beta blockers should be reassessed periodically for resolution of those contraindications. • In patients with NSTE-ACS who have normal LV function, beta-blocker therapy can be continued.
IABP	• Intra-aortic Balloon Pumping is believed to improve coronary artery perfusion and reduce ventricular afterload and may be beneficial in bridging the patient to PCI. • When studied in rigorous RCTs, however, IABP failed to reduce MACE (Multiple Adverse Cardiac Events) in high-risk elective PCI, to decrease infarct size after primary PCI for acute STEMI, or to diminish early mortality in patients with cardiogenic shock complicating AMI.
Calcium Channel Blocker	• Verapamil or Diltiazem (dihydropyridine calcium channel blockers) should be given to patients who have contraindications to beta blockers. However, the patient must NOT have clinically significant LV dysfunction, increased risk for cardiogenic shock, PR interval greater than 0.24 second, or those with second- or third-degree AV block but do not have a cardiac pacemaker.
Anti-platelet	• Clopidogrel, when given in addition to ASA, reduces CV death, stroke, nonfatal MI. Loading dose is 300 - 600 mg, then 75 mg/day. Several hours are required for effect. Discontinue at least 5 days prior to surgery. • Ticagrelor 180 mg (2 tablets) loading dose, then 90 mg bid. A much faster-acting platelet inhibitor than Clopidogrel. When discontinued, effects diminish rapidly, which is an advantage if there are plans for surgery.
Anti-coagulant	• Enoxaparin, or • Bivalirudin, or • Fondaparinus, or • Unfractionated Heparin
ACE Inhibitor	Unless contraindicated, ACE inhibitor should be started and continued indefinitely in all patients with LVEF less than 40% and in those with hypertension, diabetes mellitus, or stable Chronic Kidney Disease (CKD). Those with contraindication to ACEI should be given Angiotensin Receptor Blocker (ARB).
Insulin	Insulin is recommended for treatment of hyperglycemia (BG > 180 mg/dL). As long as Insulin is given, monitor blood glucose to avoid accidental hypoglycemia

O'Connor RE, Al Ali AS, Brady WJ, et al. Part 9: Acute Coronary Syndromes. 2015 AHA Guidelines for CPR and ECC, Circulation 2015;132(suppl 2):S483-S500.
Amsterdam EA et al. 2014 AHA/ACC Guideline for the Management of Patients With Non-ST-Elevation Acute Coronary Syndromes. J Am Coll Cardiol 2014;64:2645-2687.

STEMI

STEMI (ST-Elevation Myocardial Infarction) is myocardial cell death (necrosis) due to coronary artery thrombosis. The extent of necrosis can be limited by prompt reperfusion therapy (Fibrinolysis, PCI, or CABG).

STEMI is diagnosed when all of the following are present:

1. The signs and symptoms of Acute Coronary Syndrome are present.
2. In at least 2 contiguous leads, there is new ST elevation at the J point:

	J-point elevation in Leads V2 and V3 is:	J-point elevation in other contiguous leads is:
men ≥ 40 years old:	≥ 0.2 mV (2 mm)	0.1 mV (1 mm)
men < 40 years old:	≥ 0.25 mV (2.5 mm)	0.1 mV (1 mm)
women:	≥ 0.15 mV (1.5 mm)	0.1 mV (1 mm)

   or, in either gender, Left Bundle Branch Block (LBBB) is present on ECG.
3. Giant hyperacute T Waves may precede the development of ST elevation.
4. Cardiac biomarkers (Troponin, and CK-MB) are elevated.
5. Usually Q-waves evolve (but 1- 20% are false and do not indicate infarction).

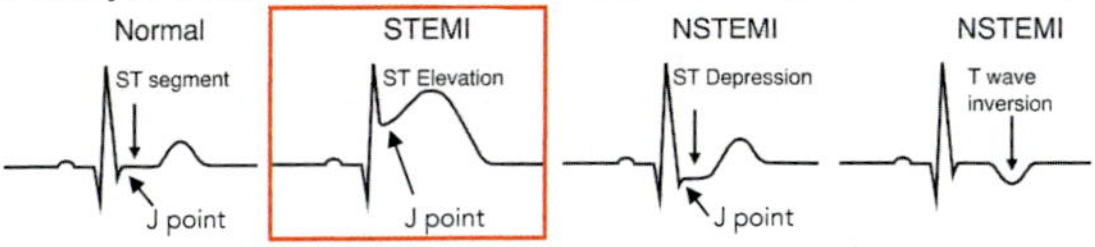

(J point is "the point where the QRS ends and the ST segment begins)

The presence of ST changes in specific leads reveals the location of AMI:

Area	Blood Supply	ST elevation	ST depression
Septum	Left Anterior Descending (LAD)	V1, V2	NA
Anterior wall	Left Anterior Descending (LAD)	V2 - V4	NA
Lateral wall	Circumflex	I, AVL, V5, V6	II, III, AVF
Posterior wall	Right CoronaryArtery (RCA) Posterior Descending Artery (PDA)	V7 - V9	V2 - V3
Inferior wall	Right Coronary Artery (RCA)	II, III, AVF	I, AVL
Right Ventricle	Right Coronary Artery (RCA)	V3R - V6R	AVL

Fig.1.6 The Coronary Arteries

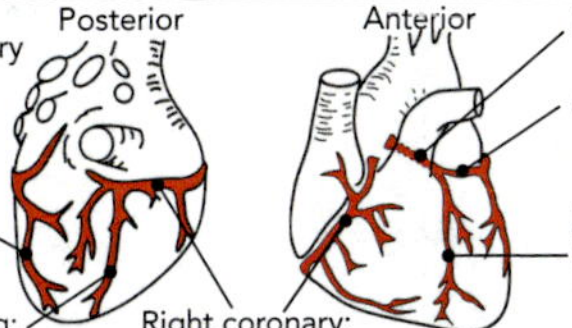

Left Main:
The entire LV

Circumflex:
Left atrium
Lateral wall

Left Posterolateral:
Lateral wall
Posterior wall

Left Anterior Descending (LAD):
Anterior wall
Anterior 2/3 of the septum
Anterior division of the Left Bundle Branch

Posterior descending:
Posterior and Inferior walls
Posterior 1/3 of the septum
Posterior division of the left bundle branch

Right coronary:
Right atrium
SA node (in 65 % of patients)
AV node (in 80 % of patients)
HIS bundle

Cardiac Biomarkers	Description	CP onset	Test result on admit is	Repeat test is	Implication
hs-cTnI	Better test for pts who present < 3 h from CP onset	< 3 h	< 5 ng/L	< 3 ng/L	May rule out AMI
			0.5-26 ng/L	elevated	Suspicious
			> 26 ng/L	elevated	Risk for MI/death
hs-cTnT	Better test for pts who present > 3 h	> 3 h	≤14 ng/L	< 3 ng/L	May rule out AMI
			≥ 52 ng/L	↑ ≥ 5 ng/L	Probable AMI
CK-MB	A marker of myocardial cell death.	>4 - 5 h	> 5 mcg/L	elevated	Peak: in 12 - 24 h Possible AMI
Myoglobin	Early onset. But may be zero if pt delays care > 1 d.	1 - 2 h	>100 mcg/L	NA	Peak: in 8 - 12 h Consider AMI Normal in: 24 h

Thygesen K, Alpert JS, Jaffee AS et, et al. ESC/ACCF/AHA/WHF Expert consensus document. Third Universal Definition of Myocardial Infarction. Circulation, 2013;126:2020-2035.

STEMI: ST-Elevation Myocardial Infarction

Facts:	• Frequency of thrombotic events is highest 6 am - 12 noon. • 20 - 30% have no chest pain. The average STEMI pt does not seek medical care for about 1.5 - 2 hrs after onset of pain. • 30% of STEMI patients are women. • About 5% of STEMI patients who survive to hospital will experience a cardiac arrest during hospitalization. • Mortality ↑ with the number of ECG leads with ST elevation. • Survival from VF is inversely related to the time interval between its onset and termination, with the odds of survival decreasing 7 - 10% for each minute of delay to successful defibrillation.
Patho-physiology:	• Injury to the coronary artery endothelium attracts platelets, white blood cells, fibrin, and lipids. • Macrophages infiltrate the damaged endothelium, become engorged, then die. A fibrous scar (or cap) forms, which narrows the lumen and secretes procoagulant factors. • When the fibrous cap ruptures (due to physical or hemodynamic stress), platelets are activated and secrete vasoconstrictive substances. The GP IIb/IIIa receptors on the platelet surface are activated and bind to fibrinogen, which forms a bridge between the platelets, collecting them in a growing mass. • 20 - 40 mins of occlusion → irreversible local myocardial damage. • 6 - 8 hrs of occlusion → death of most of the distal myocardium. • Catecholamines → ↑ HR, ↑ BP, ↑ SVR, ↑ volume → ↑ MVO_2. • Cell death → release of intracellular contents K, CK-MB, and lactate, which may stimulate ventricular arrhythmias. • SA & AV node Ischemia → conducting system arrhythmias. • Other causes of infarct: hypotension, hypoxemia, chemical toxin.
The Treatment Options:	• When emergency medical personnel attend to a patient who has signs/symptoms of STEMI, a 12-lead ECG should be done, followed by immediate transport to a PCI capable hospital. • Reperfusion, either by PCI or Fibrinolysis, must be performed within 12 hours of symptom onset. • The ideal time from "first medical contact" to PCI is ≤ 90 mins. • If PCI cannot be accomplished within the 12 hour timeframe, and the patient has no contraindications, fibrinolytic therapy should be given within 30 minutes of hospital arrival. • Urgent CABG is indicated in those with STEMI with coronary anatomy that is unsuitable for PCI, or produces ongoing or recurrent ischemia, cardiogenic shock, or severe heart failure. • In patients with STEMI and out-of-hospital cardiac arrest, neurologically intact survival rates have been improved with the use of therapeutic hypothermia.
The ECG of STEMI:	• ST-Elevation is greater than 1 mm, is present in two or more contiguous leads, or there is new LBBB. • In the very early phase of STEMI, giant hyperacute T waves may precede the development of ST elevation. • Subendocardial MI does not generate Q waves, but rather ST depression or inverted T waves, and is treated as NSTEMI. • Q waves indicate transmural infarction, but may take hours to develop (and 1-20% of Q waves are false and do not mean AMI). • If ECG is nondiagnostic, but suspicion for MI is high, ECG's at 5 - 10 minute intervals or continuous ST monitoring may be done. • Use Leads III and V_3 until 12-lead ECG reveals the location of the myocardial ischemia/injury.

O'Connor RE, Al Ali AS, Brady WJ, et al. Part 9: Acute Coronary Syndromes. 2015 AHA Guidelines for CPR and ECC, Circulation 2015;132(suppl 2):S483-S500.
Amsterdam EA et al. 2014 AHA/ACC Guideline for the Management of Patients With Non-ST-Elevation Acute Coronary Syndromes. J Am Coll Cardiol 2014;64:2645-2687. O'Gara PT, Kushner FG, Ascheim DD, et al. 2013 ACCF/AHA guideline for the management of ST-Elevation myocardial infarction: Executive Summary. Circulation, 2013;127:529-555.

STEMI: Treatment Plan

The best treatment outcome for STEMI is achieved with:

1. PCI (percutaneous coronary intervention), performed on
2. a STEMI patient that presents < 12 hrs from symptom onset, and
3. is completed within 90 minutes of hospital arrival, or within 120 minutes of first medical contact (i.e., EMS, or a non PCI hospital)

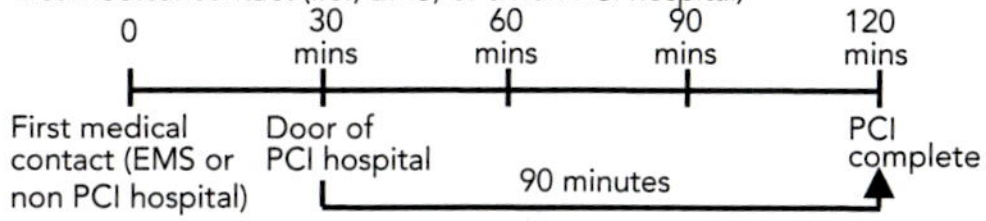

Only a minority of U.S. hospitals are capable of performing primary (urgent) PCI. When PCI is more than 30 minutes away, urgent fibrinolysis is the only option.

Symptom Onset — 12 h — 24 h

If < 12 hrs from symptom onset:	If > 12 hrs from symptom onset:
Fibrinolytic should be given within 30 minutes of arrival if: 1. PCI is unavailable, or 2. It is impossible to accomplish PCI within 2 hours (120 mins) of first medical contact (i.e., EMS or the emergency department), and 3. The pt has no contraindications to fibrinolysis (including shock or HF)	Fibrinolysis may be considered if: 1. PCI cannot be accomplished within 120 minutes (2 hours), and 2. The patient has a large area of myocardium at risk, and 3. The patient has no contraindications to fibrinolysis (especially shock or heart failure) If fibrinolysis is chosen, it should be given within 30 mins of arrival.

Anticoagulation prior to and during PCI
Aspirin 162 - 325 mg should be given before primary PCI, then Aspirin 81 - 325 mg/day should be continued indefinitely.
Platelet Inhibitor (ASAP, prior to PCI) A loading dose of a P2Y12 receptor inhibitor should be given ASAP or at the time of primary PCI. • Clopidogrel 600 mg, or • Ticagrelor 180 mg, or • Prasugrel 60 mg (but NOT if there is history of stroke/TIA) Platelet inhibitor may be continued for 1 year in STEMI patients who receive a stent (bare-metal or drug eluting). Doses are: • Clopidogrel 75 mg qd, or • Ticagrelor 90 mg bid, or • Prasugrel 10 mg qd (but NOT if there is history of stroke/TIA)
Heparin (Unfractionated), to achieve therapeutic ACT: If GP IIb/IIIa is planned: Heparin UFH 50 - 70 Units/kg bolus If GP IIb/IIIa is NOT planned: Heparin UFH 70 - 100 Units/kg bolus or Bivalirudin • In STEMI patients undergoing PCI who are at high risk of bleeding, bivalirudin anticoagulation may be given instead of the combination of UFH and a GP IIb/IIIa receptor antagonist. • 0.75 mg/kg IV bolus, then 1.75 mg/kg/hr infusion. • An additional bolus of 0.3 mg/kg may be given if needed. • If CrCl is < 30 mL/min, reduce infusion rate to 1 mg/kg/hr.
GP IIb/IIIa inhibitor is selected and given: • Abciximab: 0.25 mg/kg IV bolus, then 0.125 mcg/kg/min (max:10 mcg/min) • Tirofiban: (high-bolus dose): 25 mcg/kg IV bolus, then 0.15 mcg/kg/min. In patients with CrCl <30 mL/min, reduce infusion by 50% • Eptifibatide: (double bolus): 180-mcg/kg IV bolus, then 2 mcg/kg/min; a second 180-mcg/kg bolus is given 10 mins. after the first bolus. In patients with CrCl < 50 mL/min, reduce infusion by 50%. Avoid in patients on hemodialysis

Treatment of STEMI after PCI

Treatment Overview			
O_2	Heparin	Heparin	Pacing (maybe)
ASA	Clopidogrel (maybe)	ACEI or ARB	IABP (maybe)
No NSAIDS	GP IIb/IIIa inhibitor, maybe	Statin therapy	Morphine?
NTG?	Aldosterone antagonist?	Beta-Blocker	CCB (No)

Oxygen only if SaO_2 is < 90%

- Routine use is no longer recommended. O_2 can increase coronary vascular resistance. Compared to pts on room air, those given supplemental O_2 may have a higher risk of death.
- O_2 therapy is appropriate if the pt is hypoxemic (SaO_2 < 90%).
- Caution in those with COPD.

Aspirin

81 mg/day, continued indefinitely.
Should not be withheld before urgent CABG.

Say No to NSAIDS

- NSAIDS (e.g.,Ibuprofen) and COX-2 inhibitors (e.g., celebrex) increase the risk for reinfarction, hypertension, heart failure, renal insufficiency, hypertension, cardiac rupture, and death.
- Should not be given during the acute phase, and should not be taken by the patient thereafter.

Clopidogrel

75 mg daily after PCI. Should be discontinued at least 24 hrs before urgent on-pump CABG, if possible.

Beta-blocker

- Oral beta-blocker should be started in the first 24 hours and continued indefinitely unless contraindicated by:
  HR < 60 bpm, SBP < 100 mm Hg
  PR > 0.24 seconds, or 2° or 3° heart block
  Signs of heart failure
  Signs of peripheral hypoperfusion, or low cardiac output
  Asthma or reactive airway disease
- Beta-blockers reduce mortality in STEMI by opposing elevated catecholamines, thus decreasing the:
  1. size of the infarction
  2. frequency of life-threatening ventricular arrhythmias
  3. reinfarction rate in those who are given fibrinolytics
- Beta-blockers also prolong diastole, increasing the time for diastolic filling and coronary perfusion.
- STEMI patients who are hypertensive or have ongoing ischemia may be given intravenous beta-blocker Metoprolol 5 mg IV every 5 minutes as tolerated up to 3 doses.

ACEI

Unless contraindicated, an angiotensin-converting enzyme inhibitor should be given within the first 24 hrs to those with:

- Anterior STEMI
- Heart failure
- Post MI LV systolic dysfunction (Ejection fraction ≤ 40%)

ARB

If intolerant of ACEI's, then the patient should be given an angiotensin receptor blocker.

Aldosterone antagonist

Given to those with STEMI who are already receiving an angiotensin-converting enzyme inhibitor (ACEI) and beta blocker, but have an ejection fraction ≤ 40 %, as well as symptomatic heart failure or diabetes mellitus.

Pacing

Indicated for symptomatic bradycardia unresponsive to meds.

(cont'd on next page) →

O'Gara PT, Kushner FG, Ascheim DD, et al. 2013 ACCF/AHA guideline for the management of ST-Elevation myocardial infarction: Executive Summary. Circulation, 2013;127:529-555.
* O'Connor RE, Brady W, Brooks SC, et al. 2010 AHA Guidelines for CPR and Emergency Cardiovascular Care.Part 10: Acute Coronary Syndromes. Circulation 2010;122;S787-S817.
Kushner FG, Hand M, Smith SC, et al. ACC/AHA Guidelines for the manage-ment of patients with STEMI and guidelines on PCI. (Updates). Circulation,2009;120:2271-2306,

NTG

- Intravenous nitroglycerin is no longer routine, since it may limit the use of beta-blockers or ACEI's.
- NTG can cause profound hypotension. Do not give NTG if:
  1. BP < 90 or ≥ 30 mm Hg below baseline,
  2. tachycardia (> 100 bpm),
  3. possible RV infarction, or
  4. bradycardia (< 50 bpm).
- Do not give NTG if the patient took sildenafil within the last 24 hr or tadalafil in the last 48 hr. Doing so may cause ↓↓ BP.
- Intravenous nitroglycerin may be given for the first 48 hrs for persistent ischemia, pulmonary congestion, or hypertension.
- There is no reason for oral nitrates during convalescence.

Cardiac Surgery

- Emergency PCI is recommended in patients with cardiogenic shock due to pump failure after STEMI irrespective of the time delay from MI onset.
- Urgent CABG is indicated in STEMI patients when the coronary anatomy contraindicates PCI and the patient has ongoing or recurrent ischemia, cardiogenic shock, or severe heart failure.

Morphine

- The drug of choice for pain relief in patients with STEMI.
- Reduces work of breathing, reduces anxiety.
- The venodilatory effects can lessen ventricular preload, offering benefit to those with pulmonary edema. However, in patients with RV infarction, where higher filling pressure are required to maintain cardiac output, morphine must be withheld.
- Dose depends on patient age, body size, BP, and heart rate.
- Monitor closely, to avoid hypotensive episode.
- "Administration of morphine to ease STEMI pain appears to dampen the antiplatelet effects of newer P2Y12 platelet inhibitors in the hours after primary PCI," (Parodi G., et al) The effect was similar for both prasugrel and ticagrelor.

Calcium Channel Blocker?

- Does not minimize the size of an infarction.
- Does not reduce the incidence of reinfarction.
- "CCB may be useful to relieve ischemia, lower BP, or control ventricular rate in Atrial Fib in those intolerant of beta-blockers." (O'Gara)
- Caution is advised in patients with LV systolic dysfunction.
- Immediate-release Nifedipine is contraindicated in STEMI due to risk of hypotension and reflex tachycardia.

IABP

- Indicated in STEMI patients who have coronary anatomy that precludes PCI and who have ongoing ischemia, cardiogenic shock, severe heart failure, or serious mechanical defect.
- Mechanical circulatory support may be required for patients who remain hemodynamically unstable before, during, and after urgent cardiac surgery.

(go to the Hemo Chapter for the topic "Cardiogenic Shock")

Factors that Improve Outcome	Factors that Contribute to Poor outcome	
Early reperfusion is achieved.	Delay in reperfusion	Tachycardia
MI location is inferior wall.	Anterior infarction	Poor Renal function
ASA, β-blockers, ACEI given early.	Prior infarction	Diabetes mellitus
LV function is preserved.	History of smoking	↑ Biomarker level

Parodi G, et al. Myocardial Infarction. Circulation: Cardiovascular Interventions,2015;8.
O'Gara PT, Kushner FG, Ascheim DD, et al. 2013 ACCF/AHA guideline for the management of ST-Elevation myocardial infarction: Executive Summary. Circulation, 2013;127:529-555

Complications of STEMI

Cardiogenic Shock	• Patients with STEMI who develop cardiogenic shock should be managed with emergency PCI or CABG, Intra-aortic balloon counterpulsation (IABP) may offer immediate support if medication alone is insufficient to sustain the patient to PCI/CABG. • Patients who are unsuitable candidates for either PCI or CABG are assessed for Fibrinolytic therapy.
Marginal Cardiac Output	Serum potassium > 4 mEq/L supports myocardial contractility and reduces risk for arrhythmias.
Bradyarrhythmias	• Sinus bradycardia is common with inferior MI. • Atropine may be given. If the bradycardia persists and the patient is symptomatic, temporary pacing is indicated. 2° and 3° AV block and persistent bundle-branch block warn of worse short- and long-term prognosis, particularly in anterior/lateral MI because of the greater extent of myocardial injury.
Other Major Dysrhythmias	• Most episodes of VFib occur in the first 24 hours, with the highest incidence during the first 4 hrs. • AIVR is the most common reperfusion arrhythmia, is usually tolerated, often does not require treatment. • Bradycardia occurs frequently (represents 30 - 40% of AMI arrhythmias) and is often due to inferior MI or to reperfusion of the right coronary artery. • If magnesium level is < 1.5 mEq/L and ventricular arrhythmias occur, Magnesium should be given.
Pericarditis	• Aspirin is recommended for pericarditis after STEMI. • If aspirin, even in higher doses, proves to be ineffective, acetaminophen, colchicine, or narcotic analgesics are reasonable alternatives. • Nonsteroidal anti-inflammatory drugs and glucocorticoids are potentially harmful to patients with pericarditis after STEMI.
Pericardial effusion/ tamponade	Asymptomatic effusion is common, and usually ≤ 1 cm in width. If ≥ 1 cm or expanding, anticoagulation should be discontinued and the patient closely monitored for tamponade. If tamponade develops, presume free-wall rupture, or aortic dissection.
Mural Thrombus	For patients with STEMI and asymptomatic LV mural thrombi, anticoagulant therapy with a vitamin K antagonist may be given.
Formation of ventricular septal defect	Usually results in left-to-right intracardiac shunt, which can increase pulmonary blood flow as much as 4-fold, while significantly decreasing left ventricular cardiac output. Abrupt onset of acute heart failure and pulmonary edema may follow.
Papillary muscle dysfunction with mitral regurgitation	Sudden volume/pressure overload of the left atrium and pulmonary circulation cause pulmonary edema, while the fall in Left Ventricular output results in shock.
Recurrent ischemia and extension of the infarct	12-lead ECG reveals new ST-segment elevation, chest pain may recur, cardiogenic shock may follow.
Cardiac rupture	occurs in 1 - 4%, most often in transmural AMI.

* O'Connor RE, Brady W, Brooks SC, et al. 2010 AHA Guidelines for CPR and Emergency Cardiovascular Care.Part 10: Acute Coronary Syndromes. Circulation 2010;122;S787-S817
O'Gara PT, Kushner FG, Ascheim DD, et al. 2013 ACCF/AHA guideline for the management of ST-Elevation myocardial infarction: Executive Summary. Circulation, 2013;127:529-555.

Right Ventricular Infarction

Occlusion of the posterior descending right coronary artery interrupts blood flow to the inferior and posterior walls of the right ventricle, as well as to the posterior septum.

Consequences:

- Significant decrease in RV contractility results in impaired RV output.
- RV diastolic pressure increases significantly, while systolic function falters.
- Poor RV output leads to poor LV input, and thus poor cardiac output.
- Decreased blood flow to the AV node incites AV block, loss of AV synchrony.
- Elevation in Rt atrial pressure stimulates release of atrial natriuretic factor, which has potent vasodilating, diuretic, and aldosterone-inhibiting effects. Thus the patient becomes unusually sensitive to diminished preload.
- Ischemic injury of the chordae tendonae may cause tricuspid regurgitation.
- Ischemic injury to the septum may produce ventricular septal defect.

Assessment:

- Specific to RV dysfunction are hypotension, RAP > 10 mm Hg, Kussmaul's sign (↑ JVD during inspiration), and clear breath sounds.
- The hypotension responds to and depends on IV fluids.
- Hepatojugular reflux (CVP ↑ when firm pressure is applied to the RUQ of the abdomen) may be present.
- Paradoxic pulse occurs in 1/3 of patients with RV infarction.
- PCWP is often normal, PAP is often unchanged. But CVP is > 10.
- RV end-diastolic pressure is increased, RV systolic pressure often remains unchanged. Eventually peripheral edema develops.
- Tricuspid regurgitation produces holo-systolic murmur
- If RV failure is severe, expect ↓ CO, ↓ SV, ↑ SVR, ↓ LOC, ↓ urinary output.
- The higher the ST-segment, the more dysfunctional will be the right ventricle.

V4R is located: 5th ICS, MCL

Right vs Left ECG Chest Leads:

- ST segment elevated > 1 mm in V4R is 93% predictive of RV infarct with significant injury. ST segment elevation decreases in amplitude from V1-V5.
- In half of patients, ST segment elevation resolves within 10 hrs of symptom onset.
- AV block occurs in 50 % of patients.
- AV sequential pacing can significantly improve cardiac output.
- AFib occurs in 1/3 of patients.

Fig. 1.7

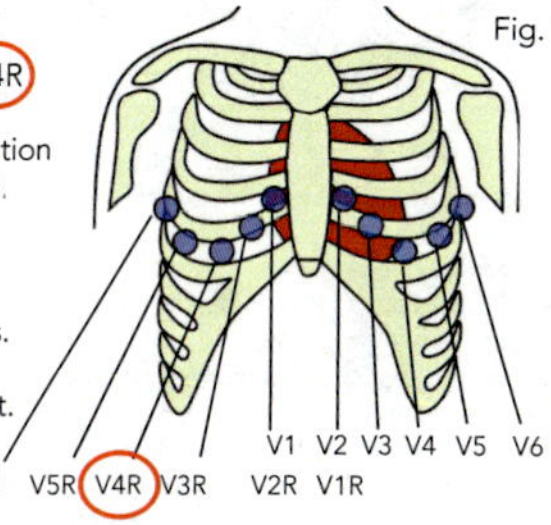

Treatment:

- If the jugular venous pressure is low or normal, 0.5 - 1 L NS over 8 hrs may be given to ↑ CVP to 10 - 15 mm Hg.
- Maintain AV synchrony. AFib, AFlutter, heart block can lead to ↓ RV preload, ↓ CO, and shock.
- Beware that positive pressure ventilation can also decrease preload.
- Avoid agents that ↓ preload, such as Lasix, Morphine, ACEI, NTG (one sublingual NTG can cause profound hypotension).
- Give standard treatment for STEMI.
- Early reperfusion with PTCA or, if indicated, fibrinolysis improves RV function and reduces incidence of heart block.
- Inotropic support (Dobutamine or Milrinone) is used for hemodynamic instability that is unresponsive to fluids.
- During AV block, AV Sequential pacing may be used to maintain RV preload.
- IABP reduces afterload, improves coronary artery perfusion.
- IABP of the pulmonary artery has been used to decrease RV afterload and support RV output.

Warning: Patients with extensive RV necrosis are at risk for RV perforation during insertion of pulmonary artery catheter or pacing wire.

Coronary Intervention

Description:

1. Coronary Intervention (PCI) refers to coronary reperfusion procedures performed in the Cardiac Cath Lab.
2. Percutaneous Coronary Angioplasty (PTCA) is temporary inflation of a small balloon inside a stenosed coronary artery, in order to restore blood flow.
3. Intra-coronary stent placement maintains patency of the affected artery.
4. Most stents are "drug-eluting," whereby anti-inflammatory and antiproliferative drugs are slowly released, to prevent redevelopment of plaque in the once stenosed artery.

Anatomy of a Stent:

- Most intracoronary stents are made of stainless steel, are either slotted or coiled in design, and are housed over an angioplasty balloon.
- Both the stent and the balloon are deflated, to allow smooth passage.
- Once directed into the vessel lumen, the balloon is inflated briefly to
  1. accomplish angioplasty
  2. deploy the stent
- As a foreign substance, metal can provoke inflammation, scarring, and thrombosis. Biodegradable or bioabsorbable stents are currently being studied.

Unfractionated Heparin During PCI:

- Without GP IIb/IIIa inhibitor: A weight-adjusted heparin bolus of 70 to 100 U/kg sufficient to produce an ACT of 250 - 350 seconds.
- With GP IIb/IIIa inhibitor: A weight-adjusted Heparin bolus of 50 - 70 U/kg to target ACT of 200 seconds is recommended.
- Heparin should be discontinued at the end of the procedure.

or Bivalirudin:

- Bivalirudin, a direct thrombin inhibitor, is used instead of heparin to anticoagulate patients with HIT (Heparin Induced Thrombocytopenia)
- Bivalirudin has a lower rate of bleeding complications and may be used in patients at high risk for bleeding.
- Bivalirudin is given as a 0.75 mg/kg bolus, then infusion of 1.75 mg/kg/hr during PCI. An additional bolus of 0.3 mg/kg may be given if needed.
- If estimated CrCl is < 30 mL/min, the dose is reduced to 1 mg/kg/hr.

Before PCI:

- Anticoagulants should be discontinued at least 3 days prior to an elective procedure.
- Aspirin 75 to 325 mg is administered within 24 hours prior to the PCI.
- Clopidogrel 300 mg po loading dose (best results if given 6 h prior to PCI), or Prasugrel loading dose of 60 mg. Because of bleeding risk, Prasugrel is contraindicated in elderly patients and those with history of stroke.

The PCI Procedure:

- The patient is heparinized and given vasodilators. Sedative is given.
- The femoral artery and vein are cannulated. A guide wire is advanced into the affected coronary artery. Angiogram is done to locate areas of stenosis.
- In STEMI patients, a guide wire is advanced beyond the stenotic lesion.
- A catheter may be inserted over this guide wire in order to aspirate any clot distal to the lesion.
- A catheter with a "stent-over-balloon" (in a deflated state) is inserted, and positioned within the stenotic area and inflated briefly, to stretch the wall of the artery, and partially disrupt and redistribute the intimal plaque.
- High-pressure (16 - 18 atm) dilations are often necessary to increase lumen diameter and to imbed the stent into the vessel wall.
- The stent "tacks up" intimal debris, seals off subintimal space, resists arterial elastic recoil, but may increase the risk for thrombosis.

Kushner FG, Hand M, Smith SC, et al. ACC/AHA Guidelines for the management of patients with ST-Elevation myocardial infarction and guidelines on percutaneous coronary intervention. 2009 Focused updates. Circulation,2009;120:2271-2306.

PCI-Related Care

The PCI Procedure (cont'd from previous page):

- The balloon is deflated, repeat angiogram performed, and the balloon angioplasty catheter and guidewire are removed.
- Intracoronary nitroglycerin may be given to control vasospasm of the affected coronary artery.
- The femoral introducer is secured and covered with a sterile dressing.
- Later, when the clotting studies are acceptable, the introducer is removed.

After Stent Insertion:

- A small degree of thrombosis between the struts of the stent provide an area for growth of endothelial cells. Up to 80% of the stent is covered with endothelium as soon as 72 hrs later.
- Intravenous heparin or synthetic heparin is given to inhibit clotting.
- Aspirin is given to prevent platelets from adhering to the artery wall.
- Nitrates and calcium channel blockers are used to minimize vessel spasm.
- 12 months of dual antiplatelet therapy required to prevent stent thrombosis.

Post PCI Complications:

Abrupt Closure is due to a combination of:	Individuals at increased risk:
1. Tearing of the inner lining of the artery	• Women
2. Thrombosis at the balloon site	• Those with unstable angina
3. Constriction or elastic recoil of the artery at the balloon site.	• Those with developing myocardial infarction

Abrupt coronary artery closure occurs in 5% of patients after simple balloon angioplasty, and accounts for most of the serious complications related to PCI.

At the end of PCI:

- Some institutions utilize vascular closure device at the end of PCI, to reduce time to ambulation.
- Heparin should be discontinued as soon as possible after the procedure, and may be restarted if needed 4 hrs after vascular catheters are removed.
- The use of a 12-hour continuous infusion of Nitroglycerin is common, but has been questioned.

Routine Post PCI Care:

- Bed rest, immobilize affected extremity (use restraint if necessary).
- Keep extremity straight, prevent hip flexion. HOB 10° max.
- Hourly Check:
  1. Vital signs, ECG
  2. Dressing over cath site
  3. Pedal pulses and foot color
  4. Motor/sensory of the feet
  5. Urinary output
  6. Development of chest pain or extremity pain.
- Reiterate the importance of leg immobility.
- Bed rest should be reduced from 6 hours to 3 hours.

> See 10-minute video: Martinelli M. St. Peter's Hospital. Albany, NY. Cardiac Cath with Angioplasty and Stenting. youtube.com

Risk Factors for PCI Complications:

Advanced age	Hypertension	Elevated C-reactive protein
Female gender	Hypotension/Shock	Left Main lesion
Diabetes	Intracoronary thrombus	LV dysfunction, ↓ EF, Heart failure
Renal disease	Multivessel disease	High risk UA/NSTEMI or STEMI

(see next page for complications) →

Ishikawa K, Aoyama Y, Hirayama H. Management of drug-eluting stent restenosis. J Invasive Cardiol,2012;24(4):178-182.

ACC/AHA/SCAI guidelines on percutaneous coronary intervention. 2009 Focused updates. Circulation,2009;120:2271-2306.

3D Medical Animation Library @Youtube.com. "Percutaneous Intervention Stenting." accessed 3/9/2016)

Complications of PCI

Complication	Considerations	Comments
Femoral access complications	Hematoma/Bleeding	Use of antiplatelet agents. Premature removal of femoral sheath.
	Pseudoaneurysm	Pulsatile mass over the puncture site with systolic bruit, normal distal arterial pulse. May require surgery.
	Thrombosis	Poor distal perfusion (↓ pedal pulses, ↓ motor/sensory).
	Infection	Contamination of access site. Use of vascular closure device.
Dysrhythmias	Are caused by myocardial ischemia, reperfusion, or vasovagal response	CA injury, thrombosis, vasospasm. Usually PVC's, short runs VT. Bradycardia when sheath removed
Chest Pain	Occurs in up to 50% of patients after PCI.	Monitor 12 - lead ECG for changes in the ST segment and the T wave.
Retroperitoneal Hemorrhage	Injury to the femoral artery above the inguinal ligament. and promoted by anticoagulant effect.	High vascular puncture site. Unexpected hypotension. bradycardia or tachycardia. Unexplained decrease in Hgb.
Nephropathy	Risk factors: preexisting renal disease, advanced age, diabetes,dehydration.	Preprocedure assessment of BUN/Cr and maintenance of hydration are critical.
Myocardial Infarction (occurs in 1% - 2%)	Abrupt occlusion, thrombosis, plaque embolization, vasospasm. Risk is higher in patients with LV dysfunction. Use of stents has reduced the incidence of PCI associated AMI.	Maintenance of antiplatelet therapy after PCI is critical. ECG is central to assessing post-PCI chest pain. Should check Troponin I or T (are always slightly elevated post PCI, but a 5-fold increase is significant for possible infarction).
CA perforation (occurs in < 1%)	Guidewire injury Atherectomy injury Risk is higher in females and the elderly.	Can result in pericardial tamponade, CV collapse, shock, death. Rescue CABG is required.
Thrombo-cytopenia	Use of heparin may cause HIT (Heparin induced thrombocytopenia)	Monitor platelet count post PCI. Bivalirudin will be used if the patient has history of HIT.
Hypotension	Consider causes: reaction to the contrast, excess nitroglycerin, opiate side effect, hypovolemia, coronary occlusion.	Assess ECG for ischemic pattern. Lower HOB, give IV fluids, stop nitroglycerin.
Stroke	Intracerebral bleeding	Careful neurologic monitoring.

Delayed Complications of the Access Site:	
Hematoma	Pain or burning at site, difficulty moving hip or leg, Red or purple discoloration of the skin.
Pseudoaneurysm	Groin pain or burning, back pain, swelling at site. Ecchymosis, pulsatile mass, bruit.
AV fistula	Swelling at groin site, development of leg pain. Possible tachycardia and decreased diastolic BP.
Retroperitoneal hematoma	Moderate to severe back pain, possibly pain in groin, flank, or lower-quadrant of the abdomen. Possible shock.
Arterial occlusion	Pain, pallor, paresthesia, paralysis, pulseless, polar (cold)
Neuropathy	Pain, tingling at groin site, numbness at site or distal leg. Motor dysfunction of the affected leg.

Removal of Vascular Access After PCI

Facts:

- Incidence of major complication following PCI is about 5%.
- Sandbags are ineffective in reducing the incidence of bleeding.
- 60% of patients suffer back pain, nausea, or vomiting after PCI (likely associated with conventional methods of sheath removal).
- After PCI, bed rest should be limited to 6 hrs; delayed removal of sheath increases risk of complications.
- Use of percutaneous closure device (insertion of a collagen plug directly over the artery, or percutaneous suture repair of the artery at the time of sheath removal) allows sheath removal at the end of PCI, eliminates need for 20 - 30 minutes of manual pressure at the insertion site, is better tolerated, allows earlier ambulation, but is not associated with lower bleeding rate.

ACT must be 150 - 180 seconds, before the femoral sheath may be removed.

Sheath Removal:

1. Some premedicate with analgesic or sedative. Some use subq lidocaine at the insertion site. Remove dressing and sutures.
2. Arterial sheath is removed first. Palpate arterial pulse about 1 inch proximal to (above) the skin insertion site.
3. Attach 10 cc syringe to arterial port and another to the venous port and aspirate 5 - 10 mL blood.
4. Using middle three fingers, apply firm pressure just above the sheath insertion site. Smoothly pull out sheath at the angle at which it was inserted. Apply firm pressure, but monitor the foot to insure you don't completely occlude blood flow. Use the free hand to reinforce the pressure on the insertion site.
5. Hold with strong pressure for 5 minutes, then gradually release pressure over next 15 minutes. If bleeding occurs, start over. Minimum hold time is 20 minutes.
6. Vasovagal response (diaphoresis, nausea, syncope, $\downarrow$ BP, $\downarrow$ HR) sometimes results from pain, fear, tissue injury. Usually treated with 20° leg elevation, fluids, Atropine.
7. Remove venous sheath using the same technique. Apply pressure x 5 minutes. Watch both sites for bleeding/hematoma.
8. Apply small sterile gauze pad. May elevate head of bed 15°.
9. Check site, motor/sensory, and distal pulses of extremity, ECG, HR, BP: q 15 mins x 4, q 30 mins x 2, q 60 mins x 1.
10. Instruct patient to: Remain on his back with leg straight x 1 hr.
    Avoid lifting head, coughing, sneezing, or valsalva.
    If any of these are unavoidable, support site with hand.
    Call for assistance for pain, or if the dressing becomes wet.
11. After 1 hour, may raise head of bed to 20°.
    Use reverse Trendelenburg for eating or voiding.
    Turn patient to side after 1 hour.
12. Wait 4 hours to ambulate.

Remodeling after PCI:

- All PCI's involve injury to the targeted vessel.
- Within minutes, platelets and fibrin adhere to the site.
- Within days, inflammatory cells infiltrate the site and vascular smooth muscle cells begin to hypertrophy.
- Over several months, remodeling of the vessel wall results in either negative remodeling (decrease in lumen diameter) or positive remodeling (increase in lumen diameter).
- After 6 months, the repair process stabilizes.

Delayed Restenosis:

- The use of stents has cut the rate of restenosis in half.
- Drug Eluting Stents have further reduced the restenosis rate.
- Recent studies indicate that the intima is slow to heal, requiring patients to continue clopidogrel indefinitely.
- Only 60% with restenosis will develop signs and symptoms.
- Patients who fail to comply with ongoing antiplatelet therapy are at high risk for coronary thrombosis.

The Future: Pharmacologic agents, radiation, and gene therapy are under investigation and may be beneficial in the treatment of restenosis.

Acute Heart Failure (AHF)

Description:

- Dysfunction of one or both ventricles impairs cardiac output.
- Failure of the heart to accommodate venous return may cause pulmonary, peripheral, and splanchnic edema.
- In patients with chronic heart failure, hypervolemia is usually the event that causes decompensation, manifested most often by pulmonary edema.
- About half of patients with AHF have LV Ejection Fraction > 40%.
- Less than 5% develop hypotension that requires an inotrope.

Causes of Heart Failure:

Patients may have Systolic HF or Diastolic HF; but most often they have both.

Systolic HF the heart is unable to provide sufficient blood flow	Diastolic HF the heart is unable to accommodate the return of venous blood flow
Reduced contractility caused by: • ischemic heart disease • chronic hypertension • idiopathic cardiomyopathy • valvular disease • toxin-induced cardiomyopathy	Impaired cardiac relaxation/filling due to: • left ventricular systolic dysfunction • right ventricular infarction • severe chronic tricuspid regurgitation • chronic hypertension • cardiomyopathy

Pathophysiology:

- Injury or stress on the myocardium leads to LV chamber dilation, myocyte cell proliferation (hypertropy), myocardial remodeling, and antinatriuresis (reduced urinary excretion of sodium), resulting in total body fluid excess.
- Activation of neuroendocrine system plays an important role in the severity of HF. Elevated levels of Epinephrine, Norepinephrine, Vasopressin, Angiotensin II, Aldosterone, and Endothelin cause ↑ HR, ↑ afterload, ↑ preload, ↑ heart work, as well as toxic injury to cardiac cells. Fibrosis ensues.
- Increased calcium entry into myocytes augments contractility and impairs myocardial relaxation, which increases myocardial energy expenditure and decreases cardiac output.
- The intracellular overload of calcium may also induce arrhythmias and can lead to Ventricular Tachycardia, Ventricular Fibrillation and sudden death.
- Decline in the effect of endogenous vasodilators (nitric oxide, prostaglandin, bradykinin, atrial and B-type natriuretic peptide), further stimulates vasoconstriction.
- Poor LV and RV emptying result in elevated pulmonary artery pressures and central venous pressures. Pulmonary edema may become severe.

ECG:

Must be scrutinized for myocardial ischemia, hypertrophy, dysrhythmia, prolonged QT, effect of abnormal electrolytes.

Echocardiogram:

2-D echo with Doppler flow studies are used to assess left ventricular size, Left ventricular ejection fraction (LVEF), wall thickness, and valve function.

NT-proBNP (N-terminal pro-brain natriuretic peptide):

- Secreted in response to changes in pressure that occur with heart failure.
- Levels rise when heart failure gets worse; levels fall when HF improves.

Age, years	NT-proBNP, pg/mL	Is HF likely?
Any age	< 300	No
< 50	> 450	Yes
50 - 75	> 900	Yes
> 75	> 1800	Yes

Yancy CW, Jessup ML, et al.. 2013 ACCF/AHA Guideline for the Management of Heart Failure. Circulation, 2013;128:e240-e327.

Kim Han-Na and Januzzi JL. Clinician Update Natriuretic Peptide Testing in Heart Failure. Circulation. 2011; 123(18): 2015-2019.

For the diagnosis of heart failure The Framingham criteria: includes the presence of either 2 major criteria, or 1 major and 2 minor criteria.

Major criteria:	Minor criteria include:
• Paroxysmal nocturnal dyspnea • Orthopnea • Neck vein distention • Rales, Acute pulmonary edema • Hepatojugular reflux • Cardiomegaly, S-3 gallop • CVP > 16 cm water • Circulation time of 25 seconds • Radiographic cardiomegaly • Pulmonary and visceral edema • Weight loss of 4.5 kg in 5 days in response to outpatient treatment	• Nocturnal cough • Dyspnea on ordinary exertion • A decrease in vital capacity by one third of the previously recorded maximal value • Pleural effusion • Tachycardia (rate of 120 bpm) • Hepatomegaly • Bilateral ankle edema

The Goals of Treatment:	The Pharmacotherapy
• Maintain oxygenation • Reduce volume excess • Reduce high afterload • Relieve pulmonary congestion • Control hypertension • Control symptomatic hypotension • Avoid adverse treatment effects	• Loop Diuretics • Vasodilators (Nitrates, ACEI or ARB) • Beta-blocker (unless hypotensive) • Aldosterone Receptor Antagonist • Hydralazine (Apresoline) • Aspirin as Anticoagulant • Inotropic agent

Treatment of Acute Heart Failure

Problem	Medical Rx	Need to know
Poor Oxygenation	O2 and NPPV	• If SaO2 is < 90%, oxygen therapy should be started. If more support is needed, Noninvasive Positive Pressure Ventilation (NIPPV) offers relief, while decreasing the rate of intubation, mechanical ventilation, and morbidity/mortality.
Excess Blood Volume	Nitroglycerin	• As a potent venodilator, NTG reduces venous return of blood flow to the heart, thus moderating LV preload, pulmonary vascular pressures, and peripheral edema.
	Loop Diuretics	• Loop diuretics (furosemide, bumetanide, torsemide) remain the cornerstone of treatment for acute heart failure. • In patients with hypertensive heart failure and mild fluid retention, thiazide diuretics are preferred because of their more persistent antihypertensive effects.
	Ultrafiltration	• If congestion is refractory to the above, renal ultrafiltration may be used.
Excessive Afterload	Nitroprusside	• As a potent arterial vasodilator, can cause severe hypotension. However, this agent is ideal for those with both severe pulmonary congestion and hypertension. • Caution. Nitroprusside can cause profound hypotension.
Coagulation, risk of VTE	ASA	To decrease the development of thromboembolism, due to these risk factors: immobility, atrial fibrillation, poor perfusion.
Hypertension and dyspnea	Clevidipine	This is the only CCB that may be given.

Yancy CW, Jessup ML, et al.. 2013 ACCF/AHA Guideline for the Management of Heart Failure. Circulation, 2013;128:e240-e327.

Acute Heart Failure Treatment

Problem	Treatment	
Excessive Neurohumoral response	ACEI or ARB	• Angiotensin Converting Enzyme Inhibitor (lisinopril, enalapril, or captopril), or • Angiotensin Receptor Blocker (valsartan or candesartan) if patient is intolerant of ACEI • Both reduce the neurohumoral response to low blood flow. • Both improve LVEF; Both improve survival.
	Hydralazine and Isosorbide dinitrate	• For those who cannot tolerate ACEI or ARB. • May also be to added to a ACEI or ARB. • Improves ventricular function, symptoms, and survival.
	Beta blocker	• Modifies the neurohumoral response to low blood flow, to improve cardiac function, ease pulmonary and peripheral edema, prevent arrhythmia, control ventricular rate. • Cannot be given, however, if the patient is hypotensive.
	Aldosterone Receptor Antagonist	• Spironolactone or eplerenone may be given, to those with moderate-to-severe symptoms, LV ejection fraction $\leq$ 35%. • Offers additional diuresis, symptom control, improved heart rate, decreased ventricular arrhythmias, reduced cardiac workload, improved LVEF, and improved survival. • However, if renal function is borderline (Cr > 2 mg/dL), risk for ↑ K^+ may outweigh benefit.
Hypo-perfusion	Dopamine or Dobutamine or Milrinone.	To restore perfusion and reduce congestion when unresolved by the above interventions. • Dopamine, Dobutamine, or Milrinone should be given to patients with hypoperfusion, ↓ BP, ↓ CO, or evidence of elevated cardiac filling pressure. • Use of these drugs warns of poor prognosis. • Milrinone is recommended in patients receiving a beta-blocker. Milrinone increases SV and CO more than Dobutamine, and is less likely to cause tachyarrhythmias. Milrinone is also the best choice for patients already maintained on beta-blocker.
Do Not Give:	CCB, except Clevidipine	• Calcium Channel Blockers, EXCEPT for Clevidipine, which is a vaso-selective calcium channel blocker that reduces blood pressure while improving dyspnea
	NSAIDS	• Anti-inflammatory drugs, NSAIDS (may make heart failure worse). • Most Antiarrhythmics have cardiodepressant effects and may promote arrhythmia; only amiodarone and dofetilide are safe for AHF. • Risks of digoxin outweigh its benefits.

Indications for Invasive Monitoring:

- Persistent symptomatic hypotension despite initial therapy
- Worsening renal function despite initial therapy or despite adjustment of recommended therapies
- Need for parenteral vasoactive agents after initial clinical improvement
- Cardiogenic shock requiring escalating inotrope and/or pressor therapy and mechanical support is being considered
- Advanced device therapy or transplantation is being considered.

Yancy CW, Jessup M, Bozkurt B. 2013 ACCF/AHA Guideline for the Management of Heart Failure. Circ, 2013;1228:1810-1852.

Implanted Cardioverter/Defibrillator (ICD)

Background:
- Each year in the US, 300,000 - 400,000 individuals experience sudden cardiac death. Only 5% survive to hospital.
- Mortality rate from sudden cardiac death can be decreased 30 - 55% with implantation of a cardioverter/defibrillator.
- The greatest benefit is realized in patients with LV dysfunction.
- Patients who receive multiple and frequent shocks often suffer psychological consequences (fear, stress, anxiety, depression).

AHA Class I Indications:
- Prior myocardial infarction with:
  LVEF ≤ 35% + NYHA class II or III + more than 40 d post MI
  LVEF ≤ 30% + NYHA class I + more than 40 d post MI
  LVEF ≤ 40% and inducible VT or VF
- Survivors of cardiac arrest due to VFib or hemodynamically significant VT that was due to an irreversible cause
- Structural heart disease, with spontaneous sustained VT
- Syncope with VT or VF, inducible by electrophysiology study.
- Nonischemic dilated cardiomyopathy, with LVEF ≤ 35% and NYHA Class II or III

ICD is Not Indicated if:
- Life expectancy, with acceptable function, is < 1 year.
- VT or ventricular fibrillation are incessant.
- Serious psychiatric illness that may be provoked by the device.
- NYHA Class IV patients with drug-refractory heart failure.
- Syncope of undetermined cause, with VT or VF that cannot be induced by EPS, and with no structural heart disease.

Description:
- The ICD pulse generator is placed in a pocket under the skin in the area below the clavicle. Inserted in the OR, CCL, or EPS lab, using local anesthesia and conscious sedation.
- Leads are inserted transvenously through the subclavian or cephalic vein (if defibrillation can't be achieved with the transvenous leads, a subcutaneous patch can be placed in the anterior chest wall to deliver energy more efficiently).
- These devices sense, pace, and cardiovert/defibrillate. Some also monitor atrial activity and store the ECG. Sophisticated algorithms minimize shocks for atrial fibrillation, sinus tachycardia, and other non–life-threatening SVT rhythms.
  1. If ventricular tachycardia is detected, "burst pacing" will pace the ventricle at a rate faster than the dysrhythmia.
  2. Minimum output of 0.1-0.2 joules allows painless cardioversion. Success rate for termination of VTach is > 90%.
  3. If anti-tachycardia pacing fails, low-energy (0.2-30 joules) synchronized (on the R wave) cardioversion is attempted. If that fails, high-energy (30-40 joules) defibrillation is used.
  4. Bradycardia prompts ventricular demand pacing.
  5. If VFib is detected, immediate defibrillation occurs.
  6. Battery life can be as much as 10 years.

Post Insertion Problems	
Related to the transvenous insertion:	Hemothorax, pneumothorax, hemoptysis, air embolism Subclavian artery injury, Brachial plexus injury RV perforation, pericardial tamponade
Related to the site:	Pocket hematoma, seroma, abscess
Related to the leads:	Lead fracture, dislocation, migration Diaphragmatic stimulation Venous thrombosis, pulmonary embolism
Related to generator malfunction:	Shocks on non-VTach Fails to deliver a shock or the shock is ineffective Battery failure
Post insertion care:	Immobilize arm in sling for 24 hours. Ambulate within 8 hours. Usually discharge in 24 hr. Minimal pain medication should be required. If inappropriate firing of ICD, assess rhythm, call Dr.

Implanted Cardioverter/Defibrillator (ICD) (cont'd)

To Deactivate:	• A magnet is placed over the pulse generator to suspend the detection of arrhythmias. The generator remains deactivated as long as the magnet is held in place. • Use of the magnet on most ICD's does not affect detection and pacing of bradycardia. • In some patients, magnet mode may be programmed "off."
Defibrillator Storm:	• Cluster of multiple shocks occurs in 10 - 20% of patients. • Inappropriate shocks may be delivered for atrial fibrillation, sinus tachycardia, and other types of SVT. • These patients describe a decline in quality of life due to stress, anxiety, fear, depression, anger. • ICD reprogramming/fine-tuning may eliminate the problem. • Amiodarone combined with a beta-blocker may reduce the incidence of ICD shocks and inappropriate shocks. • Patients benefit from psychological support and counseling.
Major ICD Malfunctions:	• Sensing and/or pacing failures, inappropriate cardioversion, ineffective cardioversion/defibrillation, device deactivation. • Operative failures are identical to those found in regular pacemakers.
If ICD patient arrests:	• Do CPR as usual. If you are touching the patient when the generator discharges, you may feel a slightly uncomfortable sensation. Rubber gloves can provide insulation. • If defibrillation necessary, place right defib pad as you would for implanted pacemaker (at least 1 inch from the device). • If defibrillation is unsuccessful, place defib pads in anterior-posterior position. • Do not try to time discharge to the firing of the ICD device.
Long Term:	• Many experience reduced psychological distress for 6 months after implantation, but perception of physical health declined during the 4 years after implantation. • Phantom shock (perception of a shock when none was delivered) has been reported in 7% of ICD patients.

Patient Teaching:

1. Arm movement may be restricted until wound heals.
2. Female patients may need to go without a bra until edema/soreness subsides. Clothes that fit tightly over the pulse generator should be avoided.
3. What the patient will feel when the device fires depends on the output of the generator. Low energy output may not be detectable. Progressively intense sensations may be felt. The lack of warning often generates anxiety. Dizziness, weakness, nausea, palpitation, chest soreness, and going limp and falling have also occurred.
4. Avoid:

Strong magnets	Large stereo speakers, CB or ham radio
MRI	TV or radio transmitting tower (stay 25 feet away)
Electrocautery	Cell phone held < 6 inches from generator
Security search wand	Arc and resistance welders
Security devices	Large motors, generators and power plants
Electrolysis	Industrial magnets (may be in amusement rides)
	Magnetic mattress or chair

5. Contact with microwaves, hair dryers, household appliances is OK.
6. Report to physician if signs and symptoms of infection, and if the device fires. Report what activities occurred before and after ICD fired.
7. Antiarrhythmia meds may still be needed.
8. No driving for 6 months after ICD insertion.
9. Wear a Medi-Alert bracelet or necklace. Family should attend CPR class.
10. Notify Dr. if travel out of town. Tell other Doctors/Dentist about ICD.

> If symptoms warn you of arrhythmia: Sit or lie down.
> If receive 1 shock and feel OK: Call Dr when able.
> If receive multiple shocks and feel awful: Call 911 or get to ER.

Pericarditis

Description: Pericardial inflammation, which may produce exudate, fibrosis, adhesions, pericardial effusion, tamponade, death.

Causes:	Noninfectious:	Trauma, cancer, irradiation, renal failure, post pericardiotomy, post STEMI, hypothyroidism,
	Infectious:	Viral (the most common cause), bacterial, fungal, tubercular, parasitic, rheumatic fever
	Drugs:	Anticoagulants, procainamide, hydralazine.
	Rheumatologic:	Lupus, scleroderma, rheumatoid arthritis,
	Medications:	Penicillin, isoniazid, phenytoin
	After STEMI:	Asymptomatic pericardial effusions are common.
Signs/ Symptoms:	Chest pain:	Varies in intensity from annoying to excruciating The pain is usually in the substernal area, may radiate to the neck, left shoulder, left arm, scapula, or trapezius. The pain may be aggravated by swallowing, coughing, inhaling, lying down, rotating chest left/ right, elevating arms. The pain must be distinguished from that of myocardial ischemia. Relieved by sitting up, leaning forward, with forearms rested on legs (Mohammed's sign).
	Pericardial friction rub:	Heard best at 4th or 5th ICS, with patient sitting and leaning forward, and breath-holding at end-expiration. The sound is high pitched, "squeaky like leather," and in synchrony with heart beat. If effusion develops, friction rub may disappear.
	Fever:	The course is severe when fever is > 38° C.
	Paradoxic Pulse:	During inspiration, systolic blood pressure falls more than 15 mm Hg.
	Heart sounds:	S2 may be louder than S1.

EKG: Usually sinus tachycardia, but sometimes AFib or AFlutter.
J-point elevation (↑ ST) in all leads except aVR and frequently V1.
J point elevation is greater in Lead II than in Lead III.

Stage	ECG Changes	Duration
Stage 1	ST ↑ in more than 1 region, concave ST, PR depression, no Q.	Lasts about 1 - 2 weeks
Stage 2	ST returns to baseline, T wave flattens in all leads except V6, aVL, aVR. PR is depressed.	Lasts about 2 weeks
Stage 3	T wave becomes inverted.	Lasts from a week to months
Stage 4	Return to normal	May take weeks to years

Diagnosis:
- Lab: Cardiac markers are usually normal, but may be slightly ↑. Also ↑ WBC, ↑ sedimentation rate, ↑ C reactive protein.
- CXR: Often normal.
- Echo: Can detect effusion as small as 15 mL, thickening of the pericardial sac, size of the cardiac chambers.

Treatment:
- ASA 650 mg q 4-6 hr for 2-5 d or Ibuprofen 400 - 800 mg q 4-8 h
- Indocin 75-200 mg po daily in 3 - 4 divided doses (avoided in the elderly due to its adverse effect on coronary blood flow).
- Colchicine 0.5 mg po bid (dose doubled for recurrent cases).
- Prednisone is reserved for patients intolerant or unresponsive to ASA, NSAID, and Colchicine. Steroid may ↑ risk for recurrence.
- If pericardial effusion develops or increases, anticoagulants must be discontinued immediately, to avoid pericardial hermorrhage.
- Pericardiectomy: only for refractory, highly symptomatic cases.

Pericardial Effusion/Tamponade

Description:
- Inflammatory exudate or blood in the pericardial space.
- The clinical effects depend on the rate of fluid accumulation.
- Rapid accumulation of as little as 80 mL can cause increased intrapericardial pressure with signs and symptoms, and a rapid collection of 200 mL can cause hemodynamic crisis and death.
- Slow accumulation of up to 2 L may produce no symptoms.

Causes:

Pericarditis	Uremia	Anticoagulation therapy
Trauma	Malignancy	Myocardial infarction
Myxedema	Aortic dissection	Injury during PCI

Transudate vs Exudate: Transudate results from increased hydrostatic pressure or decreased oncotic pressure.
Exudate results from increased capillary permeability or decreased lymphatic resorption due to inflammation, cancer, pancreatitis, or autoimmune processes.

Signs and Symptoms:
Esophageal compression with dysphagia
Laryngeal nerve compression with hoarseness
Tracheal-bronchial compression with cough
Phrenic nerve compression with hiccups
Chest pain, pressure, discomfort
Diminished or absent apical impulse
Muffled heart sounds
Previous pericardial friction rub disappears

ECG:
- ↓ QRS voltage (suggests large effusion)
- Electrical alternans (beat-to-beat variability in QRS height).

If there is Tamponade
- Neck veins distend on inspiration (Kussmaul's sign)
- Beck's Triad: ↓ BP, ↑ venous pressure, muffled heart sounds
- Pallor, diaphoresis, mottling, weakened peripheral pulses
- Narrowed pulse pressure (↓ SBP, ↑ DBP)
- Rule of 20's: CVP > 20 mm Hg, HR increased by 20 bpm
  Systolic BP ↓ 20 mm Hg, Paradoxic pulse > 20 mm Hg
- Slow forming tamponade may produce paradoxic pulse (pulse is weak/absent on inspiration), while Beck's triad may be absent.
- Tachypnea/dyspnea due to compression of lungs and airways, or to an increase in pulmonary artery pressures
- Breath sounds are clear (unlike CHF or Pneumothorax)
- Apprehension, lightheaded, syncope, deteriorating LOC.

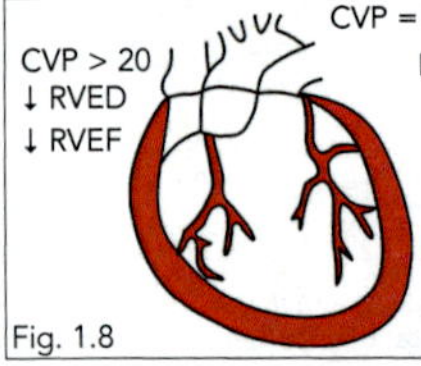

Fig. 1.8

CVP = PAD = PCWP = LAP

Beck's Triad:*
Hypotension
Rising jugular venous pressure
Muffled heart sounds

(Recent studies have shown that Beck's Triad is observed in a minority of those who have cardiac tamponade)

Diagnosis:

CXR:	Widened mediastinum if there is > 250 mL collection.
Ultrasound:	Is the most accurate method of diagnosis and to guide the advance and position of the needle.
Lab:	Lab values that suggest exudate, not transudate: Fluid specific gravity is > 1.015, LDH > 300 U/dL, and total protein > 3 mg/dL.

Treatment:
- ↑ HOB to 30° - 45 ° if vital signs allow.
- Discontinue anticoagulants immediately.
- IV Fluids to increase LV filling pressure may be helpful.
- PA catheter may be helpful in monitoring patients with mild tamponade in whom pericardiocentesis is deferred.
- Needle Pericardiocentesis (see next page), or Pericardial catheter (see page 28) to remove pericardial blood/fluid.

Pericardiocentesis

Description: Percutaneous subxiphoid aspiration of pericardial fluid to relieve the restriction on adequate cardiac filling.

Facts:

- Injury from a blind subxiphoid approach carries a morbidity rate of 50% and mortality rate of 6%.
- Ultrasound guided pericardiocentesis has decreased the complication rate to 5% and mortality rate to 0%.

Relative contra-indications:

Thrombocytopenia	Coagulopathy	Stable vital signs
Cardiac rupture	Aortic dissection	Tamponade d/t trauma

Prepare for the Procedure:

1. If vital signs allow, elevate HOB 30°- 45°.
2. Insert NG tube for gastric decompression.
3. Secure IV access, O_2, and resuscitation equipment.
4. Apply ECG limb leads, have V lead available.
5. Prep skin below the xiphoid.
6. Ultrasound monitor is placed in a subcostal position.
7. Provide anesthetic for skin, 22 g + Lidocaine 1%.
8. Provide sterile 50 mL syringe + 18 g cardiac needle + 3-way stopcock through which lidocaine or contrast is given.

Procedure:

1. If ultrasound is unavailable, ECG guidance is achieved by using a sterile alligator clip and wire connection from the needle to the V-lead of the EKG monitor.
2. The needle is inserted at a 45° angle, below the xiphoid, and directed toward the left shoulder. When the epicardium is encountered, ST elevation occurs. The needle is withdrawn slightly, until the ST segment returns to normal.
3. Contrast media can be injected into the pericardial space to confirm proper needle placement.
4. The depth of the needle is usually 2 - 8 cm.
5. Aspiration of pericardial fluid may result in ↑ ECG voltage.
6. With stopcock positioned between syringe and needle, drainage bag may be attached to the side port to allow aspirate to be drained, contained, and sent for analysis.
7. Large effusions should be drained slowly.
8. Operator may thread a catheter into the pericardial space and connect to a drainage system (see next page).

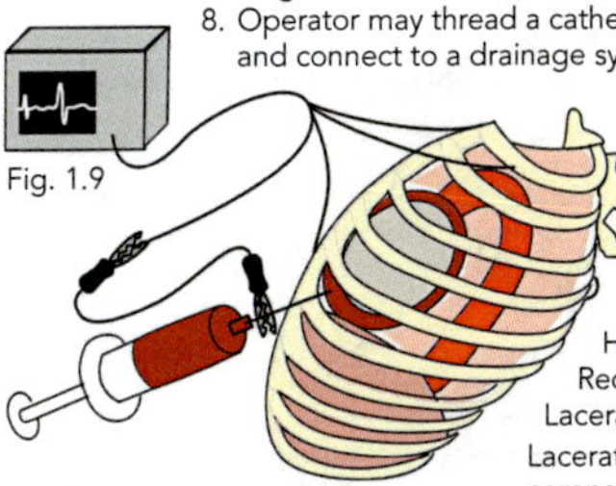

Fig. 1.9

Complications:
Vasovagal reaction
Pneumothorax
Pneumopericardium
Dysrhythmias
Infection
Hemothorax
Recurrence
Laceration of the diaphragm or liver
Laceration of the ventricle, septum, coronary artery or vein

Postprocedure Care:

- Assess for complications and recurrence
- Chest x-ray for pneumothorax, pleural effusion
- Observe for 24 hours in critical care unit

Other Approaches:

1. For recurrent malignant effusion, pericardial sclerosis may be safer and more effective than pericardiocentesis in reducing recurrence rates. Success rate is as high as 91%, but the procedure is painful and tends to generate dysrhythmias.
2. Subxiphoid pericardial window can be performed under local anesthesia and is associated with low morbidity, mortality, and recurrence rates. This procedure may replace pericardiocentesis as initial treatment for stable effusions.

Fitch MT, Nicks BA, Pariyadath M, et al. Emergency Pericardiocentesis. NEJM, 2013; 366:e17, March 22, 2012.

Pericardial Catheter

Description:

Placement of a catheter in the pericardial space in order to:
- evacuate recurrent pericardial effusions (50% of patients with pericardial effusion will experience recurrence).
- infuse heparin, antibiotics, or chemotherapeutic agents.

To avoid infection, catheter removal in 2-4 days is suggested.

Insertion:

Disposable trays are available.
1. The physician performs a pericardiocentesis.
2. The syringe is removed and a guidewire is inserted into the needle lumen. The needle is removed.
3. A dilator is advanced over the guidewire and removed.
4. The pericardial catheter is advanced and positioned in the pericardial space. The guidewire is removed.
5. A sterile 3-way stopcock is attached to the end of the catheter and to the drainage tubing and collection bag. Secure all connections; cover stopcock port with sterile cap.
6. Apply occlusive dressing of sterile gauze and tape.

Catheter Maintenance:

Maintain catheter drainage:
1. Position the drainage bag below the level of the patient.
2. Prevent kinks in the pericardial catheter.
3. Keep drainage tubing coiled on the bed and free of kinks, occlusion, and gravity loops.
4. Drainage is continued until volume falls to < 25 mL/day.
5. Do not apply suction in the effort to promote drainage.
6. Replace dressing if it becomes damp, loosened, or soiled:
   - Prep the site with antiseptic solution.
   - Apply sterile gauze and occlude dressing with tape.
7. When recording catheter output, subtract volume of medications and irrigants from the total volume of output.

Catheter obstruction:

Obstruction of drainage may lead to pericardial tamponade. If obstruction of pericardial drainage is suspected:
1. Check the entire system for catheter or tubing kink or occlusion, and for incorrect positioning of the stopcock.
2. Assess patient for signs of pericardial tamponade.
3. Notify physician. An echocardiogram may be ordered.

Upon physician order and according to hospital policy:
1. Attach syringe of 2.5 - 5 mL of heparinized or plain saline to the stopcock sideport. Turn off to the drainage bag.
2. Slowly inject the saline into the catheter. Turn stopcock off to the sideport to allow drainage into the bag.
3. If catheter still will not drain, replacement may be needed.

Infusion of Medications:

Upon physician order and according to hospital policy, medications may be instilled into the catheter.
1. Connect medication to the stopcock sideport.
2. Turn off to drainage bag, and slowly infuse medication.
3. If order is for medication to "dwell," follow the medication with 2.5 - 5 mL sterile saline, then turn stopcock off to the catheter for the prescribed dwell time.
4. Monitor patient for tamponade effect. If signs develop, immediately turn the stopcock to restore catheter drainage.
5. At the end of the prescribed dwell time, resume drainage by turning stopcock off to the medication port.
6. Record appearance of drainage and patient responses.

Complications		
Coronary artery laceration	Recurrent effusion/tamponade	Dysrhythmias
Pneumothorax	Abdominal organ injury	Infection
RV puncture	Catheter occlusion	Pain

Deep Vein Thrombosis/Venous Thromboembolism

Description:
- Death from DVT associated pulmonary embolism causes 300,000 deaths per year in the US, and represent more annual deaths than those from breast cancer, AIDS, and traffic accidents combined.
- Lower-extremity DVT is the source of 90% of acute PEs.
- Because critical illness often compromises cardiopulmonary reserve, VTE may pose a greater threat to ICU patients than to non ICU patients.
- The consequences DVT/VTE include prolonged mechanical ventilation, prolonged hospital and ICU stay, and death.

Causes: Virchow's triad describes 3 factors that result in DVT:
- Venostasis due to: vascular disease, pregnancy, crush injury, immobility, heart failure, obesity, pelvic tumor, shock.
- Hypercoagulability due to: decreased fibrinolytic activity (deficiency of antithrombin III, protein S or protein C) or high levels of plasminogen activator inhibitor 1.
- Injury/inflammation of vessel intima due to: surgery (especially orthopedic), trauma, burns, sepsis, IV catheters. 20% of clots propagate proximally.
  Until the thrombus organizes (organization starts in 5-10 days), the disorganized thrombus may propagate and/or embolize. Organized thrombus usually results in venous valve destruction.

Signs and Symptoms:
- Most non-ICU patients have extremity swelling, tenderness, pain. Some have venous distention, warmth, erythema, fever.
- Less than one third of patients will have positive Homan's sign (pain in the calf on forced dorsiflexion of the foot).
- In ICU patients, who are often mechanically ventilated, sedated, and unable to communicate, symptoms are rarely elicited.

Incidence of DVT if DVT prophylaxis is not provided:

Patient Diagnosis	DVT Incidence
Spinal cord injury:	60 - 80 %
Major Trauma:	40 - 80 %
Critical Care Patients:	15 - 80 %
Stroke:	11 - 75 %
Heart Failure:	20 - 40 %
Neurosurgery:	15 - 40 %
Major orthopedic surgery:	40 - 60 %
Major gynecologic surgery:	15 - 40 %

Chest 2008;133; pp. 381S-453S

ACCP Guidelines recommend that hospitals develop the following strategy:
- Perform DVT risk assessment on all patients.
- Develop a written DVT/VTE policy.
- Utilize computer decision systems, preprinted orders, and periodic audits.
- Provide ongoing staff education.

Risk Assessment:

Low risk for DVT	Moderate Risk	High Risk for DVT
Ambulatory, with no risk factors, & expected LOS is < 2 days	Patients who are not low or high risk, check for specific Risk Factors below:	Elective hip or knee surgery Acute spinal cord injury with paresis Multiple major trauma Surgery for Abd. or pelvic cancer.

Risk Factors for DVT

Age > 50 years	Sepsis	Prolonged (> 3 days) immobility
Stroke	Paralysis	Inflammatory bowel disease
Myocardial infarction	Previous VTE	Nephrotic syndrome
Heart Failure	Critical illness	Protein C or Protein S deficiency
Major Surgery	Obesity	Cancer or cancer therapy
Major Trauma	Pregnancy	Recent post-partum with immobility
Invasive Procedures	Estrogen therapy	Systemic inflammatory response
Central venous catheter	Varicose veins	Hypercoagulable state

Most patients have at least 1 risk factor. 40% have three or more.

DVT/VTE: Prevention and Treatment

Assess for contraindications to anticoagulants:

Absolute: Active bleeding of any type. In the previous 4 weeks, severe head or spinal cord trauma with hemorrhage.

Relative: Intracranial hemorrhage in the past year
Craniotomy within past 2 weeks
Active intracranial lesion/neoplasm
Hypertensive urgency/emergency.
Intraocular surgery in past 2 weeks.
Gastrointestinal or genitourinary hemorrhage within the last month.
Thrombocytopenia (< 50,000) or coagulopathy (PT > 18 seconds).
End stage liver disease.
Surgery that carries a high risk for postop bleeding is planned:

- Urologic surgery (prostate surgery, kidney biopsy, nephrectomy)
- Pacemaker/implantable cardioverter-defibrillator placement
- Surgery on blood-filled organs like the liver, kidney, and spleen
- Intracranial, cardiac, or spinal surgery

When the risk for DVT/VTE is high, the benefits of some anticoagulants may far outweigh their relative contraindications.

Debatable: Immune mediated heparin-induced thrombocytopenia (HIT)
Epidural analgesia with spinal catheter (present or planned).

When there are contraindications to anticoagulants, and the patient's risk for DVT is Moderate or Higher, use Compression:

- True gradient compression stockings (GCS)
  1. Provide a gradient of compression (30 - 40 mm Hg), which is highest at the toes, and gradually decreases to the thighs.
  2. Improperly fitted stockings can reverse the pressure gradient and are associated with higher incidence of DVT.
  3. Compression stockings may reduce the incidence of post-thrombotic syndrome (extremity pain, swelling, cramping, numbness, itching)
- Intermittent Pneumatic Compression Devices (IPC)
  1. Increase blood flow, reduce venous distention, enhance fibrinolysis.
  2. One study showed the risk of DVT decreased by 60%.
- Disadvantages of Compression Devices:
  1. No established standards for size, pressure, or physiologic features.
  2. Many mechanical devices have never been assessed in a clinical trial.
  3. There is greater effect in reducing calf DVT than proximal DVT.
  4. May reduce or delay the use of more effective anticoagulants..
  5. Proper use by patients and staff is often poor.
  6. There is cost associated with purchase, storage, dispensing, cleaning of the devices, as well as ensuring proper application and use.
- When the bleeding risk decreases and is believed to be low, the patient should be switched from mechanical to anticoagulant prophylaxis.

Patient's Risk for DVT	Prevention Strategy
Low Risk (< 10%)	• Early and aggressive ambulation (for mobile pts) • Aspirin is an option for patients with major orthopedic surgery. • Low risk patients should not receive pharmacologic or mechanical prophylaxis.
Moderate Risk (10 - 40%) and no contraindications:	Low Molecular Weight Heparin (LMWH), or Low Dose Unfractionated Heparin (LDUH)
High Risk (40 - 80%) and no contraindications:	• LMWH (preferred over LDUH) • Compression Device may be added.

Treatment Strategy
• If there are no contraindications, intravenous Heparin is given without delay. • Administration of thrombolytics is no longer recommended, due to bleeding complications, increased risk of death, and insignificant improvement in PTS (post thrombotic syndrome) • Percutaneous mechanical thrombectomy is faster and safer.

Bates SM et al. Diagnosis of DVT. Antithrombotic Therapy and Prevention of Thrombosis, 9th ed: ACCP Evidence-Based Clinical Practice Guidelines. Chest, 2012;141(2supp):351-418.

Acute Aortic Dissection

Description:

- Tearing of the intima (inner layer of the aorta) allows blood between the intima and the media (middle layer of the aorta), and ultimately to separation (or dissection) of the media from the adventitia (the outer most layer of the aorta).
- Aortic dissection produces a false lumen that parallels the true aortic lumen (few have associated aneurysm).
- Hypertension, which occurs in 45-80%, advances the dissection.
- Depending on the location of the aneurysm, affected organs may be threatened by poor perfusion and thrombosis.
- Astute assessment and prompt intervention is critical.
- If untreated, 50 - 70% of patients die in the first 48 hours.

> "The immediate mortality rate in aortic dissection is as high as 1% per hour over the first several hours. Early diagnosis and treatment is critical to survival." Braverman AC. Acute Aortic Dissection. Circulation, 2010;122:184-188.

Fig. 1.11

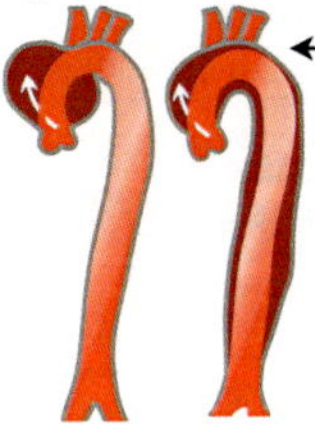

Stanford Type A (75% of cases)

Dissection starts in the ascending aorta. Associated with the most common fatal complications: tamponade, AMI, heart failure. Most require surgery.

Stanford Type B (20% of cases)

Dissection starts in the descending aorta, and propagates distally.
Unless there is hypotension or major complications, type B is treated medically

Fig. 1.12

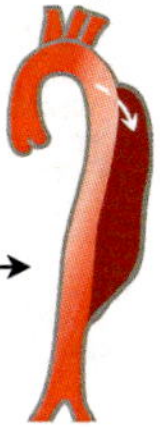

Risk Factors:			
	Hypertension	Family history	Pregnancy
	Aortic coarctation	Deceleration trauma	Cocaine use
	Age group 50 - 65	Connective tissue disease	Syphilis

Emergency Treatment of Hypertension:

- To reduce risk of aortic rupture, keep SBP = 100 - 120 mm Hg and HR < 70.
- In those with history of hypertension, reduce MAP to lowest tolerable level. Nitroprusside given with a beta-blocker (metoprolol, esmolol, or labetalol) is the most common first-line therapy.
- Refractory patients may require clonidine, or verapamil.
- Sedatives may help.

Diagnostics:

On CXR, mediastinum widened > 8 cm occurs in 25% of patients.

CXR may also reveal blunting of aortic knob, pleural effusion, hemothorax.

Angiography: highly accurate, but is associated with the risks of pt. transport, contrast media, and missed diagnosis if the false lumen is thrombosed.

CT and transesophageal echocardiography (TEE) are at least as accurate as aortic angiography and are more rapidly obtained.

Signs Produced by Either Type A or Type B Dissection:

- Sudden onset of precordial or interscapular pain, often described as tearing or ripping. Pain may radiate to the chest, neck, or jaw (may mimic ACS), lower back, abdomen, groin. May be accompanied by a cold sweat.
- Hypertension (more often in Type B than Type A Dissection) and ↑ HR
- Only about 20% of patients with aortic dissection have pulse deficits (defined as a difference between palpable pulse rate and audible apical rate)
- Peripheral nerve ischemia may cause numbness, tingling, pain, paralysis.
- Signs of hemorrhage may develop.
- Development of a vascular bruit (signifying turbulent blood flow).
- Anxiety, premonition of death.

Hallett JW. Aortic Dissection. Merck Manual Professional, Last full review/revision May 2014.
Braverman AC. Acute Aortic Dissection. Circulation, 2010;122:184-188.

Acute Aortic Dissection

Type A (Ascending aorta) vs Type B (Descending Aorta)

Type A (Dissection of the Ascending Aortic)

Signs/Symptoms (in addition to those previously described on previous page)

Chest pain: Anterior chest, neck, or jaw; may mimic ACS.

Murmur: Diastolic murmur of aortic insufficiency.

ECG: If dissection involves the coronary ostia, ischemic changes on ECG may occur (ST depression, T wave inversion) sometimes accompanied by elevated cardiac biomarkers.

Complications: Pericardial tamponade, Hemorrhage, Hemothorax, Myocardial infarction, Heart failure, Pleural effusion.

Description:

- Almost all patients with acute Type A dissection are treated surgically.
- The development of better grafts (woven Dacron, collagen-impregnated, gel-coated) has greatly enhanced the success rate.
- With profound hypothermic circulatory arrest (limited to < 45 minutes) and retrograde cerebral perfusion, mortality rate has been decreased to 10%.
- However, 10% of patients suffer significant neurologic complications.
- Aminocaproic acid (Amicar) or tranexamic acid (Cyklokapron) are sometimes used to reduce bleeding. (Aprotinin has been withdrawn from the market)
- If dissection extends into the aortic valve leaflets or into the coronary ostia, aortic valve replacement and/or coronary artery revascularization may also be needed.
- Up to 1/2 of Type A patients also have intimal tear located in the aortic arch or descending aorta, requiring repair of both (prognosis is much worse)
- With optimal medical and surgical methods, mortality is 5 - 30%.

Type B (Dissection of the Aortic Arch or Descending Aorta)

Signs/Symptoms (in addition to those previously described on previous page)

Pain: Anterior chest, neck, or jaw; may mimic ACS.
Diastolic murmur of aortic insufficiency.
If dissection involves the coronary ostia, ischemic changes on ECG may occur (ST depression, T wave inversion) sometimes accompanied by elevated cardiac biomarkers.

Ischemia: Mesenteric ischemia causes severe abdominal pain with minimal physical findings. But often there is bloody stool.
If the dissection involves the renal arteries, there may be hematuria, oliguria, elevation in BUN and creatinine.
Weak and/or unequal pulses. Recall the 6 P's of ischemia: pain, pallor, paresthesia, pulseless, paralysis, polar (cold).

Treatment:

- Uncomplicated descending dissections that are treated medically (by controlling BP) have the same or lower mortality rate as those treated surgically. Beta-blockade is started (Labetalol is preferred, for its alpha-blocking effect). If Beta-blocker is contraindicated, then verapamil or diltiazem are used.
- Nitroprusside is added for BP control. Rapid and significant reduction in BP and HR is the goal. Patients who remain stable and pain free may be moved from ICU in 24-48 hrs.
- Many malperfusion problems can be corrected with catheter-based stent.
- Surgical repair is associated with very high mortality and morbidity and thus reserved for complications related to poor perfusion and severe pain, which are indicative of aortic dilation, impending rupture, progressive dissection.
- Repair of the descending aorta is associated with a higher incidence of paraplegia than repair of other types of dissections because of interruption of blood supply to the spinal cord.
- With the use of profound hypothermic circulatory arrest and retrograde cerebral perfusion, the surgical morbidity/mortality rates have decreased.

Hemo

Hemo

Pressure Line Set-up

1 **Fill the Line:**
Insert administration set into outlet of the flush solution.
While holding the bag and drip chamber upside-down, squeeze the bag and squeeze the flush device in order to flush the line, stopcocks, and transducer free of air bubbles. Check for complete absence of air bubbles.

2 **Pressurize:**
Place bag in pressurization cuff.
Hang the bag on IV pole.
Pressurize bag to 300 mm Hg.

3 **Zero the transducer:**
Close the line "off to the patient" and "open" between the transducer and air.
Press "zero" on the monitor. (zeroing removes the effect of atmospheric pressure).
Return the stopcocks to "Off to Air, Open to patient."
The line is now ready to be checked for accuracy.

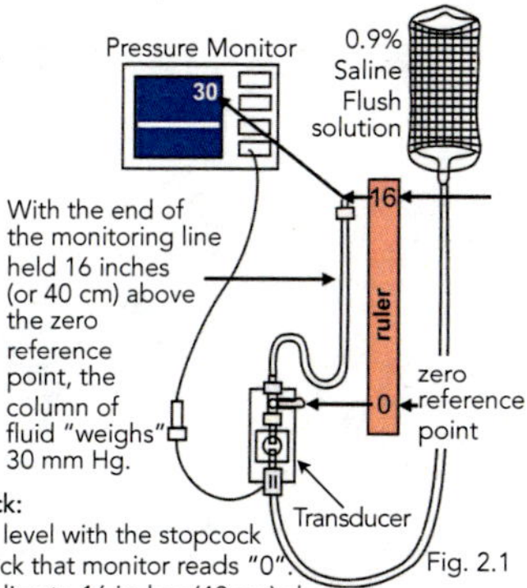

Fig. 2.1

4 **Perform Quick Transducer Check:**
Hold the end of monitoring line level with the stopcock port that was used to zero. Check that monitor reads "0".
Raise the end of the monitoring line to 16 inches (40 cm) above the zero reference point. The monitor should read "30 mm Hg."
Raise the end of the monitoring line to 32 inches (81 cm) above the zero reference point. The monitor should read "60 mm Hg."
If the monitor displays an error > 10 %, check for and correct: air bubbles in the tubing, loose connections, damaged transducer or connecting cable.
If error persists, replace the monitoring kit.

5 **Replace all vented caps with sterile dead-ender caps.**
Using bubble-free technique, connect to patient's central venous or arterial catheter. Fast flush to clear catheter of blood.

6 **Find the phlebostatic axis (PSA):**
With the patient in the supine position and HOB elevation at 0°, 30°, 45°, or 60°:
the PSA is half-way between the anterior and the posterior chest at the level of the 4th ICS.

7 **Zero the transducer to the patient's PSA:**
The zero reference point is "the air-fluid interface of the stopcock opened to air." A convenient method for zeroing is to use the stopcock closest to the patient. Turn stopcock to close the line "off" to the patient and "open" to air. Press "zero" on the monitor.

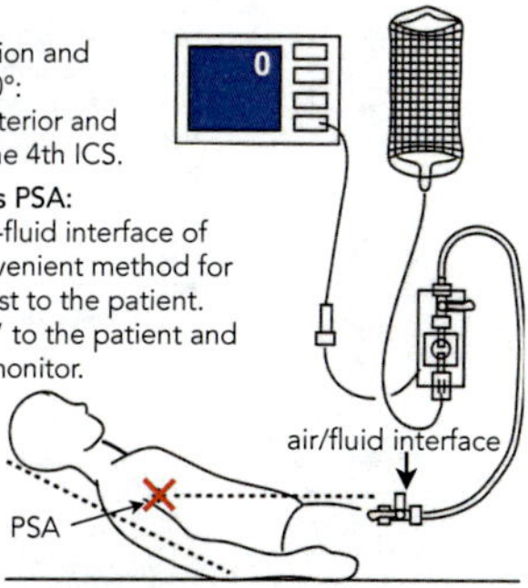

Fig. 2.2

8 **Display waveform and pressure:**
Close the zero-reference port off to air and open from transducer to the patient. Assess waveform.

9 **When to "Relevel and ReZero"**
If the position of the patient, transducer, or monitor is changed.
If there is doubt that the displayed pressure is correct.

10 If the patient is moved to a **Lateral** position (no HOB elevation), the PSA is altered. Relevel and rezero according to new landmarks:
30° right or left lateral position: The PSA is half the distance from the surface of the bed to the left sternal border.
90° right lateral position: 4th ICS at the midsternum
90° left lateral position: 4th ICS at the left sternal border)

Arterial Pressure Monitoring

Fig 2.3.a
Normal ECG with
Arterial Pressure Wave

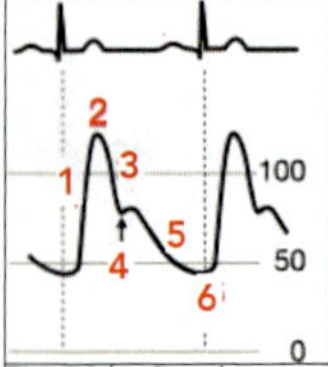

Fig 2.3.b Good
Square Wave Test

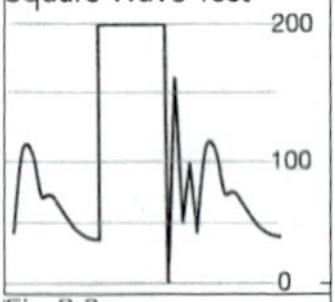

Fig 2.3.c
Overdamped

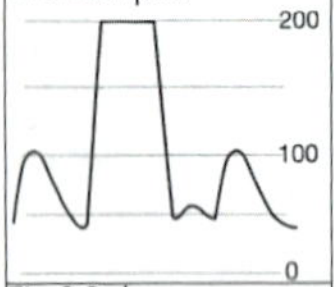

Fig 2.3.d
Underdamped

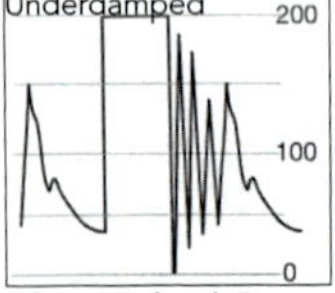

The Normal Arterial Waveform:

1 Systolic upstroke
2 Systolic peak pressure
3 Systolic decline
4 Dicrotic notch
5 Diastolic runoff
6 End-diastolic pressure

Accuracy is Improved When:

- The catheter is short and stiff, the gauge is maximum.
- A maximum of 3 foot length of pressure tubing is used between the arterial catheter and the transducer, and the tubing is completely free of air bubbles.
- 300 mm Hg pressure is constantly supplied to the catheter, infusing 3 - 5 mL/minute to maintain patency.
- The "zero stopcock" is level to the phlebostatic axis.
- When the zero stopcock is "closed to pt, opened to air," the transducer measures "0" (indicating no transducer drift has occurred since the last "zeroing" was done).
- The waveform is crisp and displays a dicrotic notch.
- Flick the pressure tubing between patient and transducer, or perform Fast Flush. Look for abrupt increase in pressure, followed by abrupt decrease, followed by 2 oscillations, and then return of a crisp pressure waveform. See Fig. 2.3.b.

Inaccuracy Occurs When:

- The Dicrotic notch is "Missing": (aka "Overdamped") Caused by conditions that impede or dissipate the transmission of the pulse to the transducer, resulting in a false low systolic pressure and false high diastolic pressure. This situation is caused by:
  1. bubbles or clot in the tubing or catheter
  2. arterial spasm due to cannulation trauma
  3. infection or plaque at the insertion site
  4. kink in or collapse of the arterial catheter (the later is often due to overly vigorous technique when obtaining blood samples).
- It has "Fling" (aka "Underdamped") Occurs when the natural frequency of the monitoring system is identical to the frequency of pressure waves being transmitted by the patient. Result is vibrations that produce spikes of overshoot and undershoot, and thus false high systolic and false low diastolic pressures.

Always Relevel, Rezero, and Flush when:

1. Accuracy of the displayed pressure is in doubt.
2. The patient's position relative to the transducer has changed.
3. The level of the transducer relative to the pressure monitor has changed.
4. The transducer set was disconnected from the monitor.

Why Arterial Lines are Dangerous:

Inaccuracies, leading to inappropriate treatment.
Accidental disconnect or removal, resulting in hemorrhage.
Compartment syndrome due to vasospasm or thrombosis distal to the catheter.
Accidental injection of medication → catastrophic ischemia of the extremity.
Air Embolism (the danger is greatest with left atrial or aortic arch monitoring, but can also result from fast flushing an arterial catheter placed at any location).
Infection, local or systemic.
Specific to radial arterial line: paralysis of the radial nerve.
Specific to femoral arterial line: retroperitoneal bleeding, bleeding into the leg.

Contraindications:

- Recent administration of fibrinolytic or anticoagulant.
- History of previous vascular surgery at the selected insertion site.
- Presence of infection, wound, or burn at the selected insertion site.
- History of peripheral vascular disease.
- Allen Test demonstrated insufficient ulnar blood flow to the hand.

Central Venous Pressure Monitoring

Description:

- A venous catheter positioned ideally in the distal innominate or proximal superior vena cava, 3 - 5 cm above the junction of the vena cava and right atrium.
- Central Venous Pressure is a direct measure of pressure in the great thoracic veins, right atrium, and right ventricle at end-diastole when the tricuspid valve is open.
- CVP is an indirect measure of volume status, and function of the left ventricle.
- Normal CVP: 0 - 6 mm Hg (0 - 8 cm H_2O)

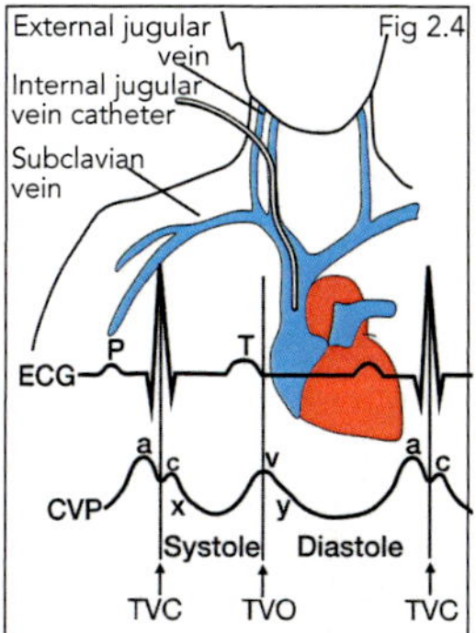

a = peak atrial contraction (follows P wave on the ECG)
TVC = tricuspid valve closes, **dicrotic notch** results.
c = RV contraction bulges the tricuspid valve into the RA
x descent = atrial pressure falls during atrial relaxation
v = atria fills, against a closed tricuspid valve
TVO = tricuspid valve opens
y descent = passive blood flow from RA to RV
a = atrial contraction with peak atrial pressure

1 mm Hg = 1.355 cm H2O
1 cm H2O = 0.738 mm Hg

Causes of decreased CVP:

1. True Hypovolemia:
   Hemorrhage or Dehydration
2. Relative Hypovolemia
   Capillary Leak Syndrome
   Vasodilation (e.g., septic shock, anaphylaxis, neurogenic shock)
   Vasodilator medications
   Third-spacing due to ↓ albumin

Causes of increased CVP:

1. Hypervolemia
2. Conditions that ↑ intrathoracic pressure:
   Hemo or Pneumothorax, PEEP, Intra-abdominal hypertension
3. Conditions that ↓ cardiac elasticity:
   Myocardial ischemia, infarction, fibrosis. Pericardial tamponade or pericarditis.
4. Tricuspid stenosis elevates the "a" wave.
5. Tricuspid regurgitation elevates "c" and "v" waves.

Dangers of the CVP catheter:

The Internal Jugular Vein is large, has a straight course, low rate of malposition, high blood flow rate, but has close proximity to the carotid artery.
Hemorrhage at the insertion site: subclavian vein injury may cause hemothorax.
Femoral vein injury may→ retroperitoneal hematoma, or bleeding into the thigh.
For both insertion and removal of a central venous catheter placed in the neck or thorax, place the patient in Trendelenberg position if possible.
Placement of the catheter tip in the right ventricle can result in ventricular irritability and dysrhythmias; perforation of the RV chamber.
Untreated hypovolemia, or fluid overload, due to error in CVP measurement.
Other complications: Embolism (air, clot, catheter, or wire), Infection, Sepsis, Thrombosis, Venous Erosion, Pneumothorax, Hydrothorax.

Avoid Measurement Error:

- Measure CVP at the end of expiration.The dicrotic notch is ideal.
- If the dicrotic notch is not visible, use the monitor to compute "mean" CVP.
- Recall the conditions in which elevated CVP does not reflect volume status: ↑ intrathoracic pressure, decreased myocardial elasticity, tricuspid disease.
- When NOT to use the monitor to record the "mean" CVP:
  1. Tricuspid stenosis: Record CVP on a calibrated paper. Ignore the large "a" wave, determine the pressure that is half-way down the systolic downslope.
  2. Tricuspid regurgitation: ignore the large "c" or "v" waves, use the "a".

A Tool to Test Fluid Responsiveness:

- A rapid infusion of 300 mL of fluid to a normovolemic, healthy adult raises the CVP about 2 - 4 mm Hg, and returns to normal in about 10 - 15 minutes.
- Rapid ↑ in CVP that does not decrease toward normal values within 10 minutes suggests a noncompliant RV, increased intravascular volume, or both.
- CVP that fails to increase in response to fluid challenge, or increases and then returns to baseline within 5 minutes, suggests hypovolemia.

Noninvasive Cardiac Output

Method 1: with Doppler Ultrasound (refer to USCOM.com.au)

Ultrasound transducer positioned at the suprasternal notch and directed toward the aortic root, determines the velocity of blood flow into the aorta (cardiac output

Ultrasound positioned at the left parasternal border 4th ICS and directed toward the pulmonic valve, determines the velocity of blood flow into the pulmonary artery.

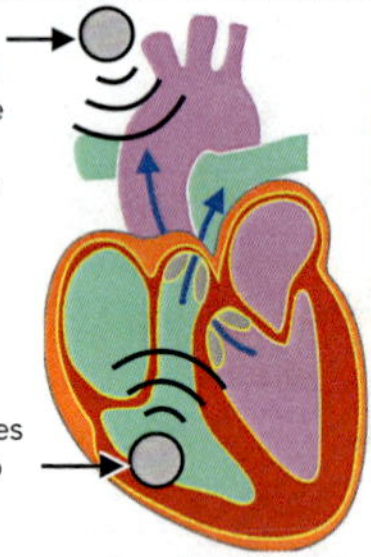

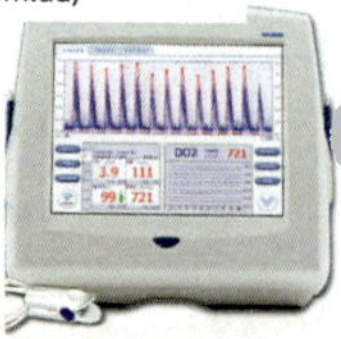

Beat-by-beat stroke volume and heart rate are recorded, cardiac output and systemic vascular resistance are calculated.

- Probe is positioned over the suprasternal notch. By bouncing high-frequency sound waves off of the red blood cells passing through the aortic valve, the velocity of blood flow (i.e., the cardiac output) is estimated.
- Probe positioned over the 3 ICS, left of the sternum estimates velocity of blood flow through the pulmonic valve.
- Trended information is displayed for all variables
- Fast, accurate, portable. Touch screen interface
- Performed by doctors, nurses, paramedics.
- No consumables are required.

inaudible, high-frequency sound waves

Method 2: with Bioimpedence (refer to Cheetah medical.com)

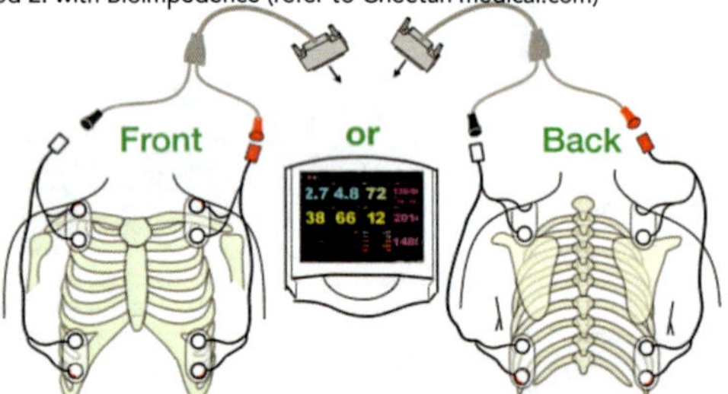

- When a low-level alternating current is applied to the upper thorax electrodes, it is propagated to the electrodes positioned on the lower thorax.
- The pulsatile blood flow in the large thoracic arteries causes the amplitude of the applied voltage to change. A time delay (called a "phase shift") occurs between the applied and the measured voltage. Research has shown that these phase shifts are tightly correlated with stroke volume (SV).
- Comparison between data collected by NICOM and data collected by Swan Ganz PAC demonstrated that the NICOM is accurate, precise, and responsive.
- Accuracy is unaffected by patient movement or by different body types.
- After 48 hours of use, NICOM sensors should be replaced with a new set.
- Re-calibration must be performed when new sensors are applied, after sensor replacement, and once daily.

The Passive leg raise (PLR) maneuver (to test Fluid Responsiveness): The patient is positioned supine with HOB elevation at 0°. Both lower extremities are raised 45°. This mobilizes about 250 mL blood from the legs to the heart. A positive PLR test (increase of ≥ 10% in SVI or CI) implies that there is sufficient cardiac reserve to pump the increased preload forward, indicates that the patient is on the ascending limb of the Starling curve, and would respond well to fluids. "It's a self-volume challenge.... it's quick, safe, and reversible." Monnet X and Teboul J-L. Passive leg raising. Inten Care Med,2008;34:659-663.

Pulmonary Artery Catheter Insertion

Indications for PA Catheterization:
1. Monitor and manage complicated acute myocardial infarction.
2. Distinguish cardiogenic from non-cardiogenic pulmonary edema.
3. Assess the hemodynamic response to fluids, blood, diuretics, vasoactive agents, and inotropes, and target predetermined hemodynamic goals.
4. Manage hemodynamic instability after cardiac surgery.
5. Assess and manage patients with vasodilatory shock.
6. Assess high-risk perioperative surgical patients.
7. Diagnose intracardiac shunts, cardiac tamponade, pulmonary embolus.

Contraindications to PA Catheterization:
1. Tricuspid or pulmonary mechanical valve, or valve endocarditis
2. Endocardial pacemaker
3. Right heart mass (thrombus or tumor)

Complications of PA Catheterization:
1. RBBB, Ventricular tachycardia, ventricular fibrillation, cardiac arrest
2. Dissection of subclavian artery or vein, tricuspid valve avulsion
3. Laceration of internal jugular vein, hematoma that compromises the airway
4. Pneumothorax (incidence is 2-4%), hemothorax, chylothorax
5. Ventricular dysrhythmia (requires treatment in < 1%), Atrial dysrhythmias
6. Thromboembolism, air embolism, pulmonary thrombosis or infarction
7. Pulmonary artery injury or rupture (mortality rate is 50%)
8. Catheter knotting (occurs in < 1%). Surgery is required for catheter removal
9. Inaccurate measurements, resulting in improper patient management
10. Endocarditis, sepsis

Supplies Needed:
1. Pressure monitoring line
2. Flush for each lumen
3. PA Catheter and Introducer sheath
4. Sterile protective catheter sleeve
5. Insertion tray
6. Drapes, gowns, gloves, masks, caps
7. Amiodarone 300 mg, Atropine 1 mg
8. ECG and BP monitoring
9. SpO_2 monitoring
10. Cardiac output monitor
11. Oximeter for SvO_2

Equipment on standby:
1. Defibrillator and Crash cart
2. Pacemaker

Insertion Procedure:
1. Have pressure monitoring line ready, leveled to patient, and monitor zeroed.
2. To the sterile field, deliver sterile insertion tray, catheter, introducer.
3. Provide Lidocaine 1% for local anesthesia, if not available in insertion tray.
4. Catheter is passed through the sterile protective sleeve.
5. Integrity of balloon is tested. All lumens may be flushed manually.
6. Integrity of thermistor is tested by momentarily connecting to CO computer.
7. If SvO_2/$ScvO_2$ catheter used, connect to Oximeter and calibrate.
8. Help connect pressure monitoring line/s and flush all lumens.
9. When the PAC is inserted to the 20-cm mark (30-cm mark if femoral route), the balloon is inflated with air (no more than a total of 1.5 mL of air). The balloon helps to flow direct the PAC.
10. Watch bedside monitor to evaluate waveforms and thus identify catheter location as it is floated. Note the right atrial & right ventricular pressures.
11. The catheter is floated into the PA and advanced until PCWP and waveform are noted. The balloon is then deflated. Confirm PA waveform.
12. During flotation, watch bedside monitor for arrhythmias, alert physician.
13. Check for PA waveform. If PCWP waveform is present, catheter is positioned too distally. Catheter must be withdrawn until PA waveform is present and the balloon requires about 1 - 1.5 mL to occlude.
14. Catheter should be secured. Insertion site is dressed.
15. Assess the patient for complications. Request postinsertion chest x-ray. Catheter tip should not be located beyond the cardiac silhouette.
16. Once catheter has warmed (in 5 - 15 minutes), check for catheter migration (appearance of PCWP waveform). Reposition catheter if necessary.
17. Never flush the catheter or inject CO thermal indicator while the catheter is in the wedged (PA occluded) position.

PA Pressures and Waveforms

Right atrial pressure

Fig. 2.6

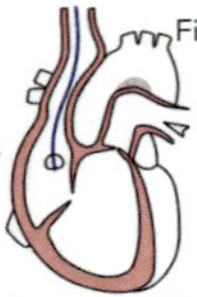

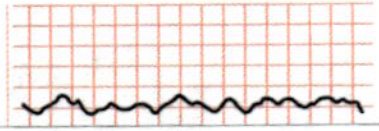

Right ventricular pressure

Fig. 2.7

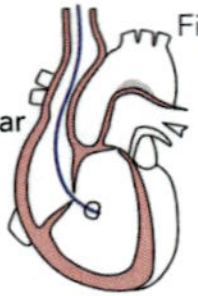

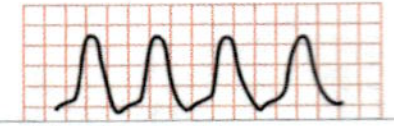

Pulmonary artery pressure

Fig. 2.8

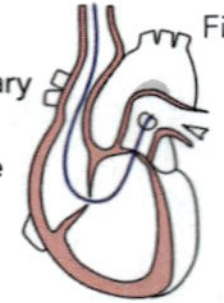

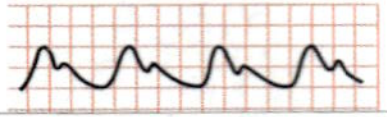

Pulmonary capillary wedge (occlusion) pressure

Fig. 2.9

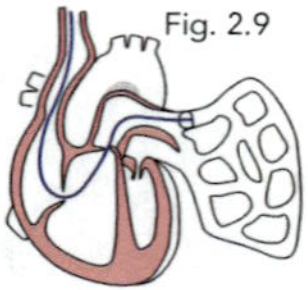

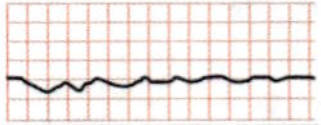

Normal Values:	RAP = 0 - 6 mm Hg (or 0 - 8 cm H20)	RVP = $\frac{15 - 25}{0 - 8}$ mm Hg	PAP = $\frac{15 - 25}{8 - 10}$ mm Hg MPAP = 10 - 20 mm Hg	PCWP = 8 - 12 mm Hg
Causes of ↓ :	Hypovolemia Venodilation	Hypovolemia Venodilation	Hypovolemia Venodilation	Hypovolemia Venodilation
Causes of ↑ :	Hypervolemia Impedance to RA emptying due to: Tricuspid stenosis RV ischemia, infarct, failure ↑ PVR (due to ↓ PaO_2, PE, COPD ARDS, pulmonary hypertension) Mitral stenosis/insufficiency Aortic stenosis LV ischemia, infarct, failure Pericardial tamponade ↑ Intrapleural pressure due to: PEEP, auto PEEP Tension pneumothorax ↑ Intra-abdominal pressure	Hypervolemia Impedence to RV emptying due to RV ischemia, infarct, failure ↑ PVR (due to ↓ PaO_2, PE, COPD ARDS, pulmonary hypertension) Mitral stenosis/insufficiency Aortic stenosis LV ischemia, infarct, failure Pericardial tamponade ↑ Intrapleural pressure due to: PEEP, auto PEEP Tension pneumothorax ↑ Intra-abdominal pressure Left-to-right intracardiac shunt	Hypervolemia Impedance to pulmonary blood flow: ↑ PVR (due to ↓ PaO_2, PE, COPD, ARDS, pulmonary hypertension) Mitral stenosis/insufficiency Aortic stenosis LV ischemia, infarct, failure Pericardial tamponade ↑ Intrapleural pressure due to: PEEP, auto PEEP Tension pneumothorax ↑ Intra-abdominal pressure Left-to-right intracardiac shunt	Hypervolemia Impedance to LA emptying: Mitral stenosis/insufficiency Aortic stenosis LV ischemia, infarct, failure Pericardial tamponade ↑ Intrapleural pressure due to: PEEP, auto PEEP Tension pneumothorax Intra-abdominal hypertension Left-to-right intracardiac shunt

Accuracy in Measuring PA Pressures

Accuracy is improved if:

1. Monitoring tubing properly flushed, bubble-free and kink-free, connections tight, properly leveled and zeroed to patient's phlebostatic axis, transducer is accurate, catheter-to-transducer tubing length is ≤ 3 ft, waveforms crisp.
2. Catheter tip is located in lung zone III (3 cm below the carina on AP CXR) (If PCWP > PAD, catheter tip is likely in zone I or II)
3. Balloon requires ≤ 1.5 mL to obtain PCWP waveform.
4. Pressures are properly measured at end-expiratory phase of the respiratory cycle. (Difficulty identifying the point on the waveform that correlates with end-expiration can be overcome by displaying the airway pressure).

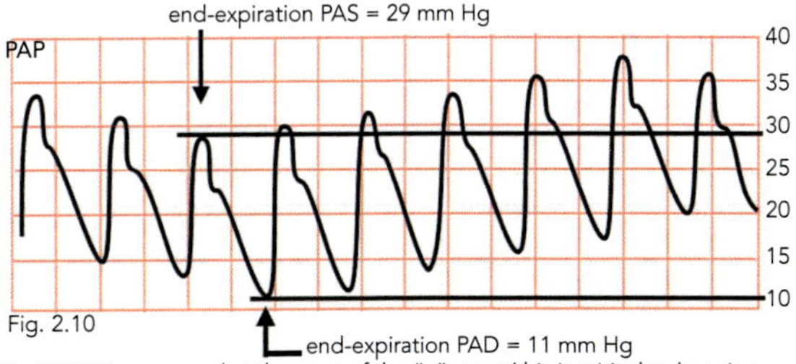

Fig. 2.10

5. PCWP is measured at the crest of the "a" wave (this is critical to keeping the "v" wave of mitral regurgitation from being averaged into the PCWP):
   "a"wave: represents atrial contraction, occurs during ventricular diastole, is found after the "p" wave of a simultaneously recorded ECG. The pressure at the crest of the "a" wave approximates LVEDP.
   "v" wave: represents atrial filling, occurs during ventricular systole, is found after the QRS of a simultaneously recorded ECG, can be significantly increased with mitral regurgitation:

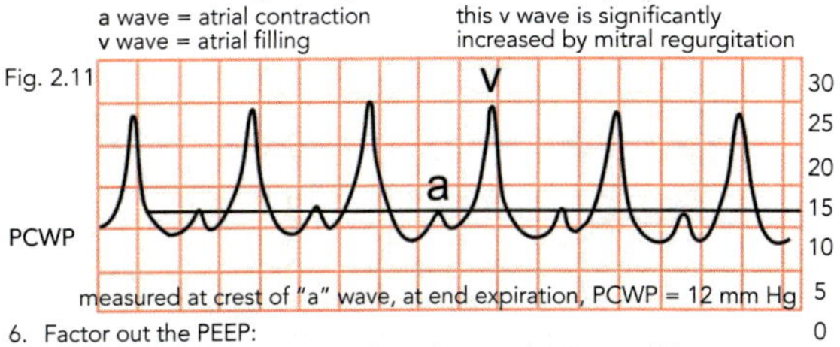

Fig. 2.11

6. Factor out the PEEP:
   Without interrupting mechanical ventilation, subtract 1/3 of the PEEP from the measured PCWP (with this formula, it is unnecessary to convert PEEP in cm H_2O to PEEP in mm Hg.). For example, while patient is receiving PEEP 18 cm H_2O, pt's PCWP is measured as 20 mm Hg. His "Actual PCWP" (the PCWP were the patient off the ventilator) is calculated:

   Actual PCWP = Measured PCWP - PEEP/3
   = 20 mm Hg - 18 /3
   = 20 - 6
   = 14 mm Hg

When PCWP is > LVEDP (and thus poorly reflects LVEDV)
Increased PVR
Decreased LV compliance
Increased intrathoracic pressure
Increased pericardial pressure
Catheter placement in Zone I or II

Desirable features in any form of monitoring
Accurate
Easy to use
Precise
Continuous
Noninvasive
Fast response time
Minimal operator time
No injury to patient

de Waal EEC, Wappler F, Buhre WF. Cardiac output monitoring. Curr Opin Anesth, 2009;22:71-77.

Cardiac Output Measurement

Intermittent Cardiac Output:

- A thermistor located on the distal end of the PAC measures the extent of temperature change after cool or iced D5W is injected into the right atrium, mixes with blood, and is delivered by blood flow to the pulmonary artery.
- The change in temperature in the PA is displayed as an inverse curve. The transit time and degree of temperature change are used to calculate the CO. The curve can be used to judge validity of the measurement.

Continuous Cardiac Output:

- CCO uses the "thermodilution" principle, but uses heat instead of cold. A 10 cm long heating filament positioned on the right ventricular section of the PA catheter emits pulses of heat which are detected by the thermistor. Thermal transit time and change in temperature are use to calculate CO.
- The CO is continuously displayed on the computer as a value averaged from the last 3 - 6 minutes and is updated every 30 - 60 seconds.
- The displayed value for CCO is not real-time. Treatment effect will not be visible in the displayed value until several minutes after treatment is given.

Need to Know:

1. Conditions that create abnormal blood flow patterns into the RA or RV (tricuspid or pulmonic regurgitation, VSD, ASD) cause unreliable results.
2. Risk factors for pulmonary artery injury/rupture include advanced age and pulmonary hypertension. To avoid injury, always confirm presence of PAP waveform (i.e., absence of PCWP waveform) before pushing the injectate.
3. Small fluctuations in CO are expected. Normally the heart adjusts its output from moment to moment according to the tissue demand for oxygen.
4. Sequential compression devices (SCDs) affect CO measurements by briefly cooling the pulmonary circulation and thus, affecting the pulmonary thermodilution curve. The SCD should be turned off during CO measurement.
5. At resting metabolic rate, normal CO = 4 - 8 LPM; CI = 2.5 - 4 L/min/m2; CI < 1.5 may be life threatening; CI < 1 is incompatible with life.

Fig. 2.12

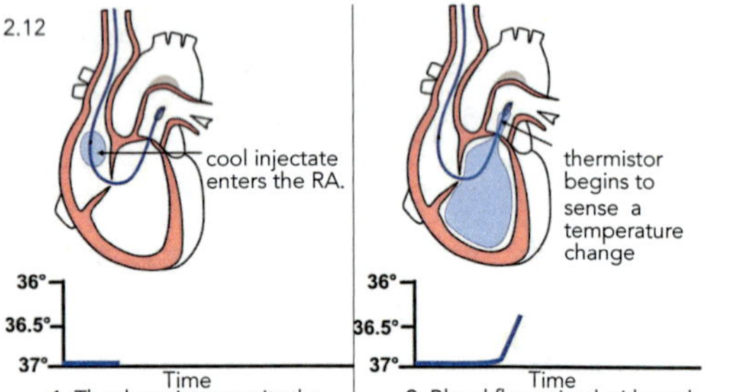

1. The thermistor awaits the change in temperature.

2. Blood flow mixed with cool injectate reaches the thermistor.

Fig. 2.13

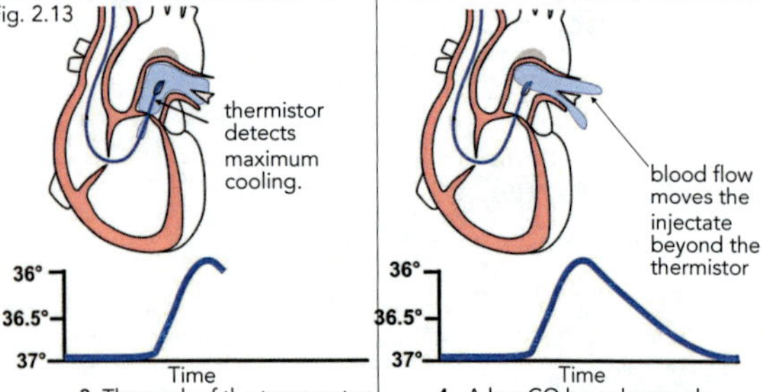

3. The peak of the temperature change occurs.

4. A low CO has a low peak, a high CO has a high peak.

Invasive CO Measurement Accuracy

Consider the cardiac output "the center of the universe" of hemodynamic assessment. CO determines blood pressure and oxygen delivery to tissue, and is used to calculate several dozen hemodynamic variables.

An accurate measurement of CO is critical to the accurate calculation of the hemodynamic profile and to the prescription of appropriate therapy.

Accuracy of the CO measurement is affected by:

Equipment preparation and operation	Respiratory influences
Injection technique	Dysrhythmias
Thermistor responsiveness	Intracardiac flow abnormalities

1. Verify presence of PA waveform. Confirm proper position of the PA catheter: PCWP that is measurable with 1 - 1.5 mL balloon inflation volume generally confirms proper PAC position.
2. Position the patient supine, with HOB 0° - 20°. If HOB is 30° or higher, the measured CO will be lower due to postural effect on venous return.
3. Assess the route for the delivery of the injectate:
   - There is serious safety hazard if there is a continuous infusion of a vasoactive or inotropic agent connected to the injectate port. To avoid rapid infusion of the agent ahead of the injectate, aspirate the agent and irrigate the line with NS. Move the agent to another infusion site.
   - Dampened RA waveform may indicate kink, clot, or sheath introducer obstruction of the RA lumen.
4. Verify that correct computation constant is entered in the CO computer.
   - Each manufacturer includes a table of computation constants on the package insert of each PA catheter. Post this table on the CO computer.
   - The constant informs the computer of the type PA catheter you are using, the size of the lumen that will be used for injection of the thermal indicator, the volume of thermal indicator, and the heat-carrying characteristics of D5W, which is the presumed choice for the thermal indicator. NS can be used, but will produce a 2% error (the measured CO will be 2% lower than the actual CO).
   - If the patient's PA catheter is changed to a different type (e.g., to a pacing PA catheter), remember to change the computation constant.
5. Room temperature injectate has been shown to produce accurate results, but iced injectate may provide more consistent results when:
   - the patient is hypothermic and the room is warm
   - the volume of the injectate must be reduced from 10 mL to 5 mL (which is sometimes necessary for fluid-restricted patients).
6. If at all possible, use an in-line temperature probe. If an external temp probe is used, accidental warming of the syringed injectate causes error.
   1° increase in syringed iced injectate causes a 2.7% error in measured CO.
   1° increase in syringed room temp injectate causes a 7.7% error.
7. Check the CO computer display to verify that the value given for PA temp is reasonable and that the PA temp is stable.
8. If the PA catheter has a separate venous infusion port, briefly suspend fluid administration through this port. Otherwise, CO may be underestimated.
9. Perform and average 3 measurements. Be certain that:
   - Injectate volume is accurately measured (a 0.5 mL error in injectate volume can cause a 10% error in CO measurement).
   - Injection is delivered smoothly and in < 4 sec for 10 mL; < 2 sec for 5 mL
   - The injection is timed to start at end-expiration of the respiratory cycle in order to minimize respiratory effect on the temp. in the pulmonary artery.
   - A delay of at least 90 seconds is allowed between measurements.
   - Thermodilution curves are smooth. Reject any CO measurement that has an irregular CO curve. Also exclude "Rogue" results.
10. Recall that abnormal flow patterns cause unreliable results. For example, tricuspid incompetence will cause an erroneously low value for CO, ventricular or atrial septal defects will cause erroneously high values for CO.
11. AFib, PAC's, PVC's, brief runs of tachycardia or bradycardia cause wide fluctuations in measured CO.

The Support of CO

CO = Stroke Volume x HR

Stroke Volume: Preload, Afterload, Contractility

Preload

The volume that fills the left ventricle (LV) at the end of diastole.

Fig. 2.14

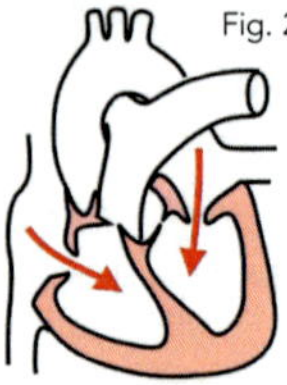

- Filling volume cannot be directly measured.
- But PCWP and LAP can be indicators of LV end diastolic pressure (LVEDP), which is a reflection of filling volume:
- PCWP < 5 mm Hg = dry
- PCWP > 15 mm Hg = wet
- Contraction strength depends in part on the degree of cardiac filling (Starling's Law)
- In patients with LV dysfunction, increased filling volume fails to elicit as much contractile force:

Fig. 2.15

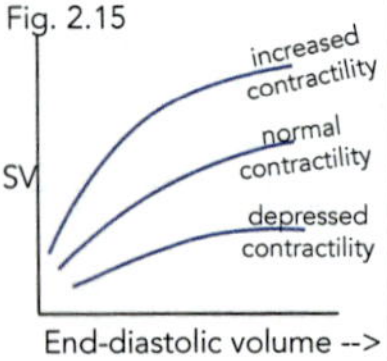

- Agents which ↓ preload:
  Diuretics (Lasix)
  Venodilators (NTG)
- IV solutions ↑ preload:
  Crystalloids (NS, RL)
  Colloids:
  - Plasma
  - Albumin
  - Plasmanate
  - Hespan
  - Dextran
  - Blood

Afterload

Wall tension generated by the LV during systole, to open the aortic valve and eject the contents.

Fig. 2.16

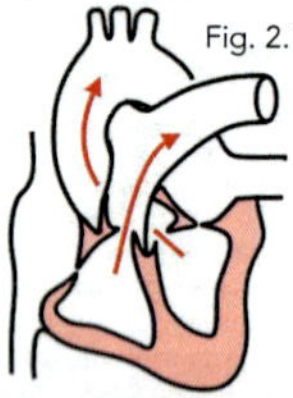

- Wall tension and heart work required to open the aortic valve cannot be directly measured.
- Once the aortic valve is open, much of the work of the heart is directed toward ejecting against the resistance of thevasculature. ↑ SVR is therefore used as a measure of afterload.

Fig. 2.17

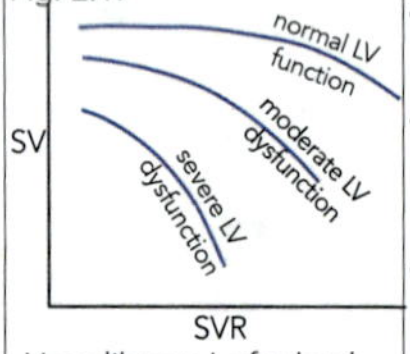

Vasodilators ↓ afterload. In LV failure, ↓ the SVR can ↑ the CO, resulting in little or no ↓ in MAP:

MAP	=	CO	x	SVR
60	=	2	x	30
60	=	3	x	20
60	=	4	x	15

- Agents that ↓ afterload (vasodilators):
  Nitroprusside
  Nitroglycerine
- Agents that ↑ afterload (vasoconstrictors)
  Norepinephrine
  Epinephrine
  Phenylephrine
  High dose Dopamine
  Vasopressin

Contractility

The inherent force of the myocardium.

- Can't be directly measured. The calculation of LVSWI is used as an estimate.
- Causes of decreased contractility:
  1. ↓ sympathetic activity
  2. Electrolyte imbalance (↓K, ↓Ca, ↓Mg)
  3. ↓ Myocardial O_2:
     ↓ Coronary perfusion pressure
     ↓ Coronary blood flow
     ↓ PaO_2/SaO_2
  4. Myocardial depressant meds such as:
     Beta-blockers
     Antidysrythmics
     CCB's
  5. Hypothermia
- No inotropes are given until volume deficit is corrected.
- Hypoxemia and electrolyte imbalan acid-base imbalance should be corrected
- Afterload reducing agent should be given with an inotrope in patients with LV failure.
- Common Inotropes:
  Dobutamine
  Dopamine
  Epinephrine
  Milrinone
  Inamrinone
  Norepinephrine
  Isoproterenol
  Calcium Chloride

Shock and The Physiologic Response

A. The purpose of the Sympathetic-Adrenal Response is to:

1. Maintain perfusion pressure:

MAP	=	CO	x	SVR*
90	=	6	x	15 (Normal)
90	=	3	x	30 (Shock)

2. Maintain O_2 delivery to tissue:

$DO_2I = CI(1.34 \times Hgb \times SaO_2) \times 10$
$= 3(1.34 \times 15 \times .99)10$
$= 600\ mL/min/m^2$

B. Receptors monitor for threats to Blood Pressure and Oxygen Delivery:

1. Aortic baroreceptors, to detect hypotension
2. Chemoreceptors, to detect acidosis (the consequence of tissue hypoxia)
3. Renal and Adrenal receptors, to detect reduced blood flow
4. Fear, pain, tissue injury, and CNS ischemia can trigger an intense response

C. The Body's Response to Shock:

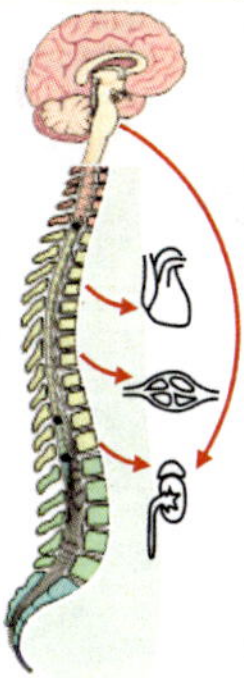

Fig. 2.18

1. Cardiovascular: release of norepinephrine and decreased vagal tone result in increased heart rate and contractility and constriction of peripheral blood vessels., which ↑ SVR and also increases venous return to the heart.
2. Hematologic: the coagulation cascade is activated, releasing chemicals (thromboxane A_2) to constrict vessels.
3. Renal: increase in renin secretion culminates in vasoconstriction of arteriolar smooth muscle.
4. Adrenal cortex: releases glucocorticoids, and increases aldosterone secretion to reabsorb sodium and water.
5. Adrenal medulla releases epinephrine to:
   - ↑ HR and contractility
   - dilate the coronary arteries
   - bronchodilate
   - ↑ sweating to dissipate heat
   - promote glycogenolysis to ↑ blood sugar

   and norepinephrine to ↑ contractility, and ↑ SVR
6. Neuroendocrine: ADH is released from the posterior pituitary gland, leading to increased renal reabsorption of water, sodium, and chloride.
7. Respiratory: increases the rate and depth of respiration to maintain oxygenation and remove CO_2 to maintain pH.

D. Classic signs of shock:

1. Cool/cold (sometimes clammy) skin
2. Weak, thready pulse
3. Slow capillary refill
4. Tachycardia
5. Increased respiratory rate
6. Decreased urinary output
7. Dilated, but reactive pupils
8. Deteriorating level of consciousness

Sympathetic control of the vasculature

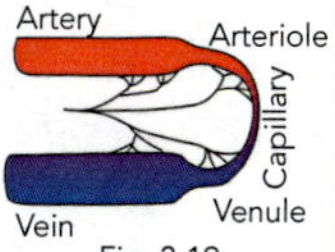

Fig. 2.19

E. Causes of ↓ BP — MAP = ↓ SVR x ↓ CO

Causes of ↓ DO_2 — DO_2 = ↓ CO x (1.34 x ↓ Hgb x ↓ SaO_2) x 10

- ↓ SVR → **Vasodilation**: Septic shock, Anaphylaxis, Neuro insult, Hypoglycemia
- ↓ CO → **Bradycardia**, **Pump failure**: CHF/AMI, Effusion/tamponade, ↓K, ↓Ca, ↓PO_2, ↓Mg, ↓pH; **Volume depletion**: Dehydration, Third Spacing, Hemorrhage, Burns
- ↓ Hgb → **Hemorrhage**, **Anemia**
- ↓ SaO_2 → **Pulmonary insufficiency**: Acute Lung Injury, Pneumothorax, Pulm. Embolism, Pulm. Edema, Atelectasis, Bronchospasm

*For simplicity, SVR is calculated in Wood units. Compare to SVR in dynes:

$$SVR = \frac{(MAP - CVP)}{CO} = \frac{(93 - 3)}{6} = 15 \text{ Wood units}$$

$$SVR = \frac{(MAP - CVP)80}{CO} = \frac{(93 - 3)80}{6} = 1200 \text{ dynes}$$

Cardiogenic Shock due to AMI

Description Decreased cardiac output and inadequate tissue perfusion that can lead to a downward spiral of ischemia, progressive myocardial dysfunction, organ failure, and death.
AMI is the most common cause. The presence of shock after AMI indicates a loss of at least 40% of functional myocardium.

CS due to AMI:
- Shock occurs in 5-8% of STEMI pts. and in 2% of NSTEMI pts.
- After infarction, average time to shock onset is 7 hours.
- 1/3 have renal dysfunction within 24 hours of shock onset.
- High grade lesions, multiple vessel involvement are common. Prognosis is worse for shock due to LV than for RV infarct.
- Without rapid revascularization, mortality rates approach 70%. Rapid revascularization (PCI, CABG) can ↓ mortality to < 40%.

Other Causes: Papillary muscle rupture, resulting in acute mitral regurgitation
Constrictive pericarditis; Pericardial tamponade
Acute Ventricular Septal Defect
Myocarditis, Cardiomyopathy

Risk factors for the development of cardiogenic shock include:
1. Preexisting myocardial disease (diabetes, previous inferior MI, triple vessel disease, pericarditis)
2. Advanced age
3. Unstable Angina, STEMI, NSTEMI, large or anterior wall AMI
4. Tachyarrhythmias, conduction abnormalities.

Pathophysiology:

Figure 2.20

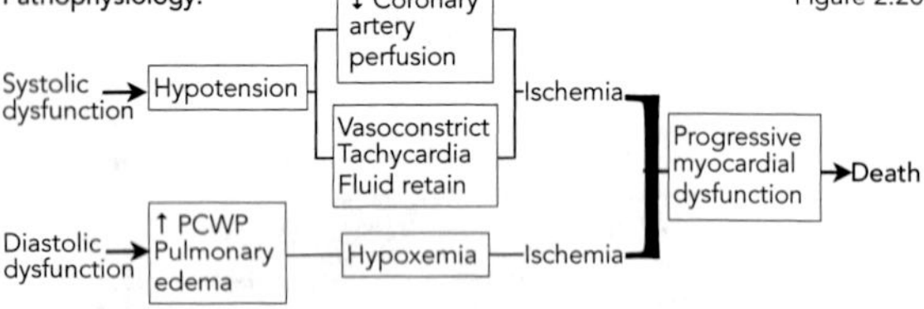

Assessment Findings:

CV: CI < 1.8 L/min/m^2, PCWP > 18 mm Hg
SBP < 90 mm Hg, MAP < 60 mm Hg
↑ HR, ↑ SVR > 1200 dynes (> 2400 dynes/m^2)
SvO_2 < 50% (unless there is septal defect)
Peripheral pulses are weak/thready, capillary refill > 2 sec
Pulse pressure may be low.
Heart sounds may be diminished; but may have S3 or S4
Large "v" wave in PCWP waveform if there is mitral regurg.

ECG: Dysrhythmias of any type, but usually SVT, VTach, Sinus bradycardia, AV block, and intraventricular conduction delays. However, 12-lead ECG may be normal.

Resp: May be dyspneic, may have audible crackles or wheezing, pulmonary edema, ↑ CVP, ↑ PAP, neck vein distention

Renal: ↓ Urinary output (< 0.5 mL/kg/hr)

Skin: Vasoconstriction produces cold/clammy skin
Poor perfusion produces ashened, mottled, extremities

Neuro: Often visibly distressed. Restless, agitated, confused, slow, anxious, impaired mental function in some, syncope.

Gi: Thirst, nausea/vomiting, decreased bowel sounds

Hibernating Myocardium:
- Severely reduced coronary blood flow produces "hibernating myocardium," areas of persistently impaired myocardial function that improve when reperfused or revascularized.
- Also, there are areas of "stunned" myocardium, which remain dysfunctional despite restoration of blood flow, but which respond to inotropic stimulation.
- Aggressive treatment hinges on the recovery of these areas.

Lab findings: Hypoxemia, metabolic acidosis, hypocapnia,
Lactic acidosis (prognosis is poor if > 4 mmol/L)
Normal BUN in early stages, then progressive $\uparrow$ in BUN and K.
Elevated Brain Natriuretic Peptide (BNP).

Treatment of Cardiogenic Shock

Initial care:	High flow O_2, IV access, monitor BP, SpO_2, ECG. Arterial pressure monitoring, CVP catheter are recommended. Hold Diuretics, Nitrates, β-blockers, ACE inhibitors, CCB's.
Fluids:	If there is no clinical evidence of volume overload, 50 mL of NS or RL may be given and repeated to maintain CVP 10 mm Hg or PCWP > 15 mm Hg (especially if infarct is right ventricular). Beware that initially an elevated PCWP may represent diastolic dysfunction rather than fluid excess. Ultrasound can be used to guide fluid management.
Support Oxygenation:	Adjust FiO_2 to maintain PaO_2 > 80 mm Hg. Intubate and ventilate if necessary + PEEP if FiO_2 > 70%. Blood may be given to keep Hgb > 7 Gms, and support DO_2. If pulmonary congestion develops, cautious use of Lasix.
Inotropes:	If hypotension is unresponsive to fluids, support SBP: If SBP 70-100, no signs of shock: Dobutamine 5-20 mcg/kg/min, but not if pt has tachyarrhythmia, or develops tachyarrhythmia. If SBP 70-100, signs of shock: Dopamine 5-10 mcg/kg/min If SBP < 70, signs of shock: Norepinephrine 0.5-30 mcg/min.
IABP:	IABP if myocardial ischemia is not quickly reversed. IABP is also a stabilizing measure prior to revascularization.
Improve Contractility:	Prevent/treat $\downarrow$ Temp, $\downarrow$ pH, $\downarrow$ K, $\downarrow$ Mg. Monitor coronary perfusion pressure, maintain > 50 mm Hg. If CO measurement is available, assess oxygen delivery: CI x 1.34 x Hgb x SaO_2 x 10. The goal is DO_2 > 400 mL/min/m^2
Manage arrhythmias:	Do not use β-blockers (myocardial depressant) for $\uparrow$ HR. Treat $\downarrow$ K and $\downarrow$ Mg, which are arrhythmogenic. Although it can cause hypotension, Morphine 2 mg IV can relieve pain, and can also $\downarrow$ sympathetic discharge, thus indirectly managing tachycardia and decreasing MVO_2.
Reduce VO_2:	Manage fever, pain, agitation, anxiety. Reduce work of breathing. Pace the nursing care to maintain $ScvO_2$ or SvO_2 > 50%.
Fibrinolytic?	When used early in the management of AMI, reduces the likelihood of subsequent development of cardiogenic shock. As the sole method of reperfusion in CS secondary to MI, has not been found to improve survival.
Hold Nitroglycerine:	Nitrates should not be given to patients with SBP < 90 mm Hg (or ≥ to 30 mm Hg below patient's baseline), or HR < 50 bpm, or HR > 100 bmp, or suspected RV infarction.
Revascularize:	Coronary angiograph/PCI is needed within 90 mins of arrival. CI or CABG is recommended for STEMI patients: who are < 75 yo, (and for suitable candidates ≥ 75 yo), and who develop shock within 36 hours of MI, and if revascularization can be done within 18 hrs of shock onset.
Good Outcome:	Cardiogenic shock patients who present 0 - 6 hours after symptom onset before undergoing PCI have the lowest mortality rate. 80% are asymptomatic 18 months later.
Pts at Risk for Poor Outcome:	Age > 75; Multiple vessel disease; Shock > 24 hours; Previous MI

Hemorrhagic Shock

Description:

- The losses from hemorrhage include not only red blood cells, but also water, electrolytes, colloid, clotting factors, platelets.
- Clotting ability is hampered by the loss of, and dilution of, clotting factors and platelets.
- Hemorrhage stimulates an inflammatory response that results in capillary leaking, which contributes to the hypovolemic state.
- The most common replacement fluid, Ringer's Lactate, may also stimulate inflammatory responses.
- Sustained decrease in perfusion pressure and oxygen delivery are primary causes of organ insult and eventual failure.
- The combination of hypothermia (due to exposure and due to cold IV solutions) + acidosis + coagulopathy constitute the self-propagating and lethal state known as the "Triad of Death."

The Threat to Cardiac Output:

1. The loss of blood volume undermines venous return to the heart, causing SV (Stroke Volume) to fall.
2. Tachycardia can compensate somewhat for the low stroke volume

	CO mL/min	=	SV mL/beat	x	HR bpm	
Normal:	6,000	=	80	x	75	
Shock:	4,000	=	40	x	100	(beware the pt
Severe shock:	3,000	=	20	x	150	who takes rate
Profound shock:	2,000	=	10	x	200	limiting meds)

The Threat to Blood Pressure

CO	x	SVR	=	MAP	
6	x	15	=	90	Normal
4	x	20	=	80	Shock
3	x	25	=	75	Severe shock
2	x	30	=	60	Profound shock

and to Oxygen Delivery to Tissue

CI	x	Hgb	x	SaO2	x	13.4	=	DO2
3	x	15	x	1.0	x	13.4	=	600
2.5	x	10	x	1.0	x	13.4	=	500
2.5	x	9	x	.98	x	13.4	=	300
2	x	8	x	.95	x	13.4	=	200

Assessment of Hemorrhagic Shock:

Neuro: In the early stages, patient may complain of being thirsty. Loud/repeated verbal stimuli may be required to arouse patient. Level of consciousness slowly decreases with severity of shock. Pupils dilate (but remain reactive) in response to sympathetic response to hypotension.

CV: Quick Assessment of Blood Pressure:

- If radial pulse is palpable, SBP is at least 80 mm Hg.
- If femoral pulse is palpable, SBP is at least 70 mm Hg.
- If carotid pulse is palpable, SBP is at least 60 mm Hg.

Signs of sympathetic-adrenal response: cold, clammy skin, tachycardia tachypnea, slow capillary refill.
HR > 130, MAP < 90, CVP < 5 represents serious shock.
Acidosis and hypothermia depress myocardial contractility

Renal: ↓ urinary output and ↓ urinary Na are early responses to ADH and Aldosterone.

Respiratory: Tachypnea is an early response to sympathetic stimulus.
↓ DO2 leads to progressive metabolic acidosis.
Hypothermia and deficit of 2,3 DPG (due to bank blood) increase the affinity of hemoglobin for oxygen, thus impairing the unloading of oxygen at the tissue level.

Temperature: Inadequately warmed IV's/blood + cold environment + open body cavities (in OR), causing progressive hypothermia, which results in coagulopathy and myocardial depression

Lab Work: Base deficit ≥ 6 mEq/L describes severe shock.
A fall in Hgb/Hct follows acute bleed by 3 - 6 hrs.
Transfusions and muscle ischemia may cause ↑ K.
Coagulopathy is revealed by prolonged PT, PTT, INR.

The American Trauma Society, Degree of Shock:

Assessment Finding:	I Mild	II Moderate	III Severe	IV Profound
Heart Rate:	< 100	100 - 120	120 - 140	> 140
Blood Pressure:	120/80	110/80	90/70	< 50 systolic
Pulse Pressure:	36	30	20	10
Skin:	normal	cool/pale	cool/pale	cold/mottled
Respiratory Rate:	14 - 20	20 - 30	30 - 40	> 35
Urinary output:	30 - 35	25 - 30	5 - 15	negligible
Level of Consciousness:	anxious	anxious	confused	lethargy-coma
Blood volume loss:	15%	20%	30%	40%
Estimate the pt's total blood volume (TBV) →	**7%** of body weight is the total blood volume (TBV). Example patient: 70 kg x .07 = 4.9 L = about 5 L			
Now estimate the amount of the patient's blood loss →	5 L TBV x 15% loss 750 mL	5 L TBV x 20% loss 1000 mL	5 L TBV x 30% loss 1500 mL	5 L TBV x 40% loss 2000 mL

The European Shock Index (SI):

In a 2013 European study of **21,853 patients,** Shock Index (SI) offered earlier identification of the extent of bleeding, than did the ATS Degrees of Shock.

Heart Rate/Systolic blood pressure = Shock Index (SI).

72/120 = 0.6	Upper limit of normal
90/100 = 0.9	Look for hidden source of bleeding
110/90 = 1.2	31% of these patients required massive transfusion
120/80 = 1.5	57% required massive transfusion. Mortality was 39.8%

Mutschler M, Nienaber U, Munzberg M, et al.The Shock Index revisited – a fast guide to transfusion requirement? CriticalCare, 2013;17:R172

The Treatment of Hemorrhagic Shock

New Strategies for Fluid Replacement and Blood Component Therapy:

- Restrict use of crystalloid. RL stimulates a greater inflammatory response, produces more capillary leaking, and dilutes red blood cells, clotting factors, and platelets, delaying the formation of stable clots. Other harmful effects, include abdominal and extremity compartment syndrome, gastrointestinal and cardiac complications,
- Earlier blood transfusion, with higher platelet-to-red cell ratios.
- FFP and platelets to minimize the development of coagulopathy.
- In patients without head injury, permissive hypotension (SBP = 80 mm Hg) allows clot formation and moderates the amount of crystalloid or colloid that is given. In head injury patients with GCS ≤ 8, maintain SBP ≥ 120 mm Hg.
- Colloid and Hypertonic Saline solutions can be beneficial in pts with head injury: less volume is required to support blood pressure, while the increased osmolarity produces less cerebral edema.

Tranexamic Acid (TXA)

- Inhibits plasminogen and plasmin (endogenous factors that dissolve clots) is recommended for patients with uncontrollable bleeding.
- In trauma patients, TXA cannot be given if it is 3 or more hours after injury.
- TXA is commonly used in cardiac surgery (it replaced aprotinin)

Norepinephrine

- May be required if there is myocardial depression (CVP > 15 mm Hg) or hypotension that persists despite fluids and blood replacement.
- MAP must be kept > 60 mm Hg in order to maintain minimal coronary artery perfusion pressure.
- Norepinephrine is started at 0.05 mcg/kg/min, increased in increments of 0.05 mcg/kg/min. Maximum Norepinephrine dose is 0.2 mcg/kg/min
- The measures above have been incorporated by many trauma centers and have resulted in improvements in mortality and morbidity.
- If Base Deficit remains unresponsive to treatment, prognosis is poor.

Severe Sepsis and Septic Shock

Patho-physiology: The Inflammatory response involves the release of chemical mediators intended to contain and disable infection at its source:

1. vasodilators increase blood flow to the area of infection.
2. activated mediators increase capillary permeability, to allow the delivery of WBC's, and antibodies to the tissue.
3. activated white blood cells engulf, disable, and destroy organisms using chemicals that lyse, dismantled, and necrose.
4. coagulation is activated to divert blood flow elsewhere.
5. if these measures succeed, fibrinolytics are released to dissolve the clots and restore capillary blood flow.

If these efforts fail to contain the infection, the host response may become exaggerated and widespread, causing injury to the circulation and eventually to every organ.

The Immune System: on Standby to Fight Infection:

Fig. 2.21a

Neutrophils
Engulf bacteria, and kill with proteolytic and lysing enzymes

Macrophages
Destroy cells that are tagged with antibodies, then kill with necrosis factor and IL-8

Mast Cells
Release histamine to ↑ capillary permeability and vasodilate,

B Lymphocytes
Become plasma cells, which secrete antibodies, which attach to known bacteria, marking it for destruction.

Artery 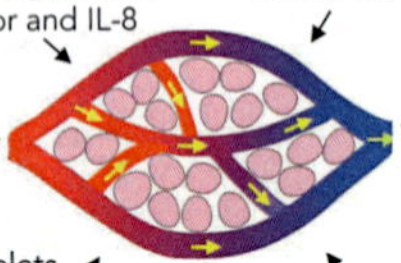 Vein

Complement
Once activated, breaks the cell membrane of the organism.

Platelets
Once activated, obstruct blood flow to contain the infection.

Oxygen Radicals
Like peroxide, can kill organisms (but also injure cells)

T Lymphocytes
Secrete cytokines, which attach to infected cells, marking them for destruction.

The Purpose of the Immune System is to contain infection, which usually begins in tissue. If infection gains access to the circulation, however, the cardiovascular consequences can contribute to organ failure and death:

Injury to the Microvasculature:

Fig. 2.21b Sepsis	Severe Sepsis Fig. 2.21c
Artery 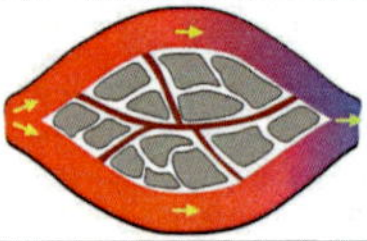 Vein	Artery 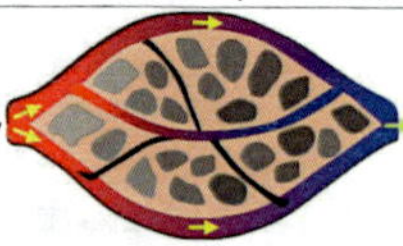 Vein
The microvasculature constricts. Peripheral shunting ensues, depriving cells of adequate amounts of oxygen. SvO_2 reflects impaired O_2 uptake. Sodium-Potassium pump failure leads to cell swelling. Blood pressure may still be acceptable.	The microvasculature is constricted or obstructed with clot. Cells become ischemic or necrotic, fail to function, and leak edema fluid. Progressive organ dysfunction or failure may be evident. Oxygenation of both arterial and venous blood is often less than normal.

"When we sense invading organisms, we are likely to turn on every defense at our disposal; we will bomb, blockade, seal off, and destroy all tissue in the area. Leukocytes become actively phagocytic, release lysosomal enzymes, turn sticky, and aggregate together in dense masses, occluding capillaries and shutting off the blood supply. It is our response to the invaders that makes the disease. Our arsenals for fighting off infection are so powerful, and involve so many defense mechanisms, we may be in as much danger from them, as we are from the invaders. We live in the midst of explosive devices; we are mined."

Lewis Thomas. The Lives of the Cell, 1974

Severe Sepsis and Septic Shock Assessment

Identify those at highest risk for the development of sepsis:

- Extremes of age (<10 and >70 yrs)
- Immunosuppression
- Major trauma, surgery, burns
- Invasive procedures
- Prolonged hospitalization
- Previous antibiotic treatment

Expect Prognosis may be poor if the patient has:

- Advanced age
- Resistant organism
- Impaired immune response
- Poor prior functional status
- Vasopressors for > 24 hours
- Sequential organ failure

Assessment	Sepsis A response to infection that produces system-wide inflammation.	Severe Sepsis Sepsis with hypoperfusion or evidence of acute organ dysfunction.
CNS	Altered mental state	Confusion, lethargy, coma
Cardio-vascular	SBP may be minimal acceptable MAP may be minimal acceptable HR > 90/min, ↓ capillary refill, Lactate > 1 mmol/L	SBP < 90, MAP < 70 mm Hg, or in adults, SBP is ↓ > 40 mm Hg. Lactate ≥ 4 mmol/L, decreased capillary refill or tissue mottling.
Immune system	Fever (> 38.3° C), or Hypothermia (core temp < 36° C) Leukocytosis (WBC > 12,000) Procalcitonin > 0.5 - 2 ng/mL (but up to 10 - 100 ng/mL) in pts with bacterial (not viral) infection. > 10% bands (immature WBC's) Increased C-reactive protein	Fever (> 38.3° C), or Hypothermia (core temp < 36° C) Leukopenia (WBC < 4000) Procalcitonin 10 - 100 ng/mL, or higher in some cases. WBC count > 12,000 or < 4,000,
Pulmonary	$PaO_2/FiO_2 < 300$ Tachypnea	$PaO_2/FiO_2 < 250$ in pts without pneumonia; < 200 in pts with pneumonia. Tachypnea.
Renal	UO < 0.5 mL/kg/hr for ≥ 2 h despite adequate fluids. Creatinine increase > 0.5 mg/dL or > 44.2 umol/L Marked edema or positive fluid balance (> 20 mL/kg over 24 hr)	UO < 0.5 mL/kg/hr for ≥ 2 h despite adequate fluids. Creatinine increase > 2 mg/dL, or > 176.8 umol/L
GI	Hypoactive bowel sounds	ileus/ absent bowel sounds
Hematology	INR > 1.5, aPTT > 60 seconds, or platelets < 100,000/uL	INR > 1.5, aPTT > 60 seconds, Platelets < 100,000/uL
Other	Hyperglycemia > 140 mg/dL, or > 7.7 mmol	Total bilirubin > 2 mg/dL or > 34 umol/L

Sepsis Treatment Goals

Words of Warning

Less than half of patients with the signs and symptoms of sepsis have a positive blood culture, and at least half have an acceptable blood pressure. Kalil A, Pinsky M. http://emedicine.medscape.com/article/168402-overview. 4/17/2015.

Treatment goals improve outcome

- Recognize sepsis early
- Give antibiotic early
- Control the source of the infection
- Early hemodynamic resuscitation
- Proper ventilatory management

Measurable Resuscitation Goals

MAP	≥	65 mm Hg (or higher if pt has hypertension history)
CVP	=	8 - 12 mm Hg (12-15 mm Hg if mechanically ventilated)
UO	≥	0.5 mL/kg/hr
$ScvO_2$	≥	65% (or $SvO_2 \geq 70\%$)
SaO_2	>	94%
Lactate	<	2.2 mmol/L

De Backer D, Biston P, Devriendt J, et al. Comparison of dopamine and norepinephrine in the treatment of shock. NEJM, 2010,363:779-789.

Pollard S, Edwin SB, Alaniz C. Vasopressor and Inotropic management of patients with septic shock. Pharmacy & Therapeutics, July 2015;40(7):438-442, 449-450.

Treatment of Severe Sepsis and Septic Shock

"Normal MAP when $ScvO_2$ is < 70% can occur when CO and SVR are adequate to maintain MAP, but Oxygen Delivery (CI x Hgb x SaO_2 x 1.34) is inadequate to meet the needs of tissue. The outcome of these patients is often worse because of delay in recognition and treatment". Kalil A, Pinsky M. http://emedicine.medscape.com/article/168402-overview. accessed 4/17/2015.

Within 3 hours of the identification of Sepsis:

1. Measure blood lactate.
2. Before giving antibiotics, obtain blood cultures, 1 drawn percutaneously and 1 from a vascular access device that has been in place > 48 hours.
3. Broad spectrum antibiotics should be given within the first hour of identifying severe sepsis or septic shock. Each hour's delay in giving antibiotics increases the risk of death by 5%.
4. For hypotension, hypoperfusion, or if lactate ≥ 4 mmol/L crystalloid 30 mL/kg are given. Fluids reverse hypotension in 50% of patients.
5. In patients who require greater amounts of fluid, albumin may be considered. The use of hetastarch should be avoided.

Within 6 hours:

6. If fluids do not improve blood pressure, vasopressors are given to maintain MAP ≥ 65 mm Hg.
7. If hypotension continues despite fluids or if initial lactate is ≥ 4 mmol/L, initiate the measurement of CVP and $ScvO_2$ (or SvO_2).

For Hypotension (MAP < 65 mm Hg)	
Norepinephrine 2 - 20 mcg/minute (max 0.19 mcg/kg/min)	The **FIRST CHOICE** vasopressor to maintain mean arterial pressure ≥ 65 mm Hg. Is considered more potent and less arrhythmogenic than Dopamine.
Epinephrine 2 - 10 mcg/minute (max 0.1 mcg/kg/min)	When norepinephrine is insufficient to maintain MAP ≥ 65 mm Hg, epinephrine should be added to or substituted for norepinephrine. But lactate level may ↑.
Vasopressin 0.03 units/minute	Should not be used as the initial pressor, but may be an alternative to norepinephrine to raise mean arterial pressure to target, or to decrease norepinephrine dose.
Dopamine 2 - 20 mcg/kg/min	An alternative to norepinephrine for select patients who have low risk for brady and/or tachyarrhythmias. **However,** 1 study found increased death rate when used to treat hypotension caused by cardiogenic shock. No longer considered effective for renal preservation.
Dobutamine 2 - 20 mcg/kg/min	May be given or added to a vasopressor in those with: 1. myocardial dysfunction (elevated cardiac filling pressures and low cardiac output), or 2. ongoing signs of hypoperfusion despite achieving adequate MAP and intravascular volume.
Phenylephrine	**Not** recommended except in circumstances where: 1. norepinephrine caused serious arrhythmias 2. cardiac output is high while blood pressure is persistently low (i.e., SVR is low) 3. other agents have failed

Steroids for Refractory Shock:

- Steroids are not recommended if fluids and pressors restore blood pressure.
- In patients with refractory shock (SBP remains < 90 mm Hg despite fluids and pressors) then intravenous hydrocortisone 200 mg per day should be given as a continuous infusion for 5 - 7 days, then tapered down and discontinued.
- ACTH stimulation test is no longer recommended.

Neuromuscular Blockade:

- Avoid Neuromuscular Blocking Agents in patients without ARDS, due to the risk of prolonged paralysis when the agent is discontinued.
- If NMBAs must be given, either intermittent bolus or continuous infusion with train-of-four monitoring of the depth of blockade should be used.
- A short course of NMBA of not greater than 48 hours may be given to those with early sepsis-related ARDS and who have a PaO_2/FIO_2 < 150 mm Hg.

Treatment of Severe Sepsis and Septic Shock (cont'd)

Source Control:

- Within the first 12 hours after diagnosis of sepsis, the source of the infection must be controlled. Techniques of least insult are recommended.

Sepsis-Induced ARDS:

- To limit aspiration risk and to prevent ventilator-associated pneumonia, septic patients who require mechanical ventilation should be maintained with HOB elevation of 30 - 45°
- A tidal volume of 6 mL/kg predicted body weight should be targeted.
- Plateau pressures should be measured. Initial upper-limit goal in a passively inflated lung (i.e., no respiratory effort by patient) should be ≤ 30 cm H_2O.
- To prevent end-expiratory alveolar collapse, positive end-expiratory pressure (PEEP) should be applied.
- In patients with moderate to severe sepsis-induced ARDS, higher rather than lower levels of PEEP should be used.
- In sepsis patients with severe refractory hypoxemia, alveolar recruitment maneuvers should be performed.
- In patients with PaO_2/FiO_2 ratio ≤ 100 mm Hg, employ prone positioning.
- Noninvasive mask ventilation should be reserved for the minority of sepsis-induced ARDS patients. Carefully weigh the benefits versus the risks.
- Do not routinely use a PAC catheter for patients with sepsis-induced ARDS.
- In patients who have sepsis-induced ARDS with no evidence of tissue hypoperfusion, fluid therapy should be conservative.
- Because of side effects (particularly tachycardia, myocardial ischemia, peripheral vasodilation), beta 2-agonists should not be used.

Sedation:

- Sedation should be minimized in mechanically ventilated sepsis patients.
- When sedating the patient, use a standardized subjective sedation scale.
- Target sedation to predetermined endpoints.

Glucose Control:

- Use a protocol for insulin infusion when two consecutive blood glucose levels exceed 180 mg/dL. Maintain BG ≤ 180 mg/dL.
- Provide a glucose source and check blood glucose every 1 - 2 hours.

Bicarbonate Therapy:

- In pts with hypoperfusion lactic acidemia with pH ≤ 7.15, bicarbonate should not be used to improve hemodynamics or reduce vasopressor requirements.

Blood Products:

- Target a hemoglobin of 7 – 9 g/dL (or higher if there is severe hypoxemia, ischemic coronary artery disease, or acute hemorrhage)
- Erythropoietin should not be used for anemic patients with severe sepsis.
- Do not use FFP to correct clotting abnormalities unless there is bleeding or there are planned invasive procedures.
- Platelets are given when platelet count is:
  < 10,000/mm^3, or
  < 20,000/mm^3 in patients with significant bleeding risk, or
  < 50,000/mm^3 in patients requiring surgery or invasive procedure.

DVT Prevention:

- Patients with severe sepsis should receive daily subcutaneous low-molecular weight heparin (LMWH). An option is subcutaneous UFH given bid or tid.
- If creatinine clearance is < 30 mL/min, dalteparin or another form of LMWH that has a low degree of renal metabolism should be used.
- Patients with severe sepsis should also be treated with intermittent pneumatic compression devices when possible.
- Septic patients who have contraindications to heparin (such as thrombocytopenia, severe coagulopathy, active bleeding, recent intracerebral hemorrhage) should not receive Heparin but rather mechanical prophylaxis, such as graduated compression stockings or intermittent compression devices
- Antithrombin therapy should not be used.

continued on next page →

Stress Ulcer Prophylaxis:

- Patients who have risk factors for bleeding should be given H_2 blocker or proton pump inhibitor to prevent prevent gastric stress ulcer.

CRRT:

- Intermittent hemodialysis and CVVH are considered equivalent.
- CVVH is better tolerated by hemodynamically unstable patients.

Nutritional Support:

- Oral or enteral feeding as tolerated is preferred over complete fasting and over the administration of only IV glucose.
- Enteral feeding is preferred over total parenteral nutrition (TPN) and should start at low dose (up to 500 calories/day) and then advanced as tolerated.

Discontinue Mechanical Ventilation:

- The septic patient recovering from ARDS should be evaluated for the discontinuation of mechanical ventilation when the patient:
  1. is arousable
  2. is hemodynamically stable without vasopressors
  3. has no new potentially serious conditions
  4. has little requirement for ventilatory and end-expiratory pressure
  5. requires an FiO_2 that can be safely given with cannula or face mask
  6. is hemodynamically stable (without vasopressor agents)
  7. has no new potentially serious conditions
  8. has low ventilatory and end-expiratory pressure requirements
- A weaning protocol should be followed and spontaneous breathing trials (SBT) should be performed regularly.
- If the SBT is successful, extubation should be considered.

Other Therapies:

- Intravenous immunoglobulins should not be given to patients with severe sepsis or septic shock.
- Intravenous selenium should not be given.
- Activated Protein C (Xigris) failed to show a survival benefit and has been withdrawn from the market.

Considerations Regarding Continuation of Life Support:

- Within 72 hours of admission to ICU, discuss the treatment plan, and as appropriate, end-of-life planning.

Dellinger RP. et al. Surviving Sepsis Campaign: Guidelines 2012. CCM, Feb 2013;41(2): 580-637.

If no evidence of infection is found:

A low procalcitonin level (< 0.5 ng/mL) or similar biomarker should be used to confirm the decision to discontinue empiric antibiotics in patients who initially appeared septic, but have no subsequent evidence of infection.

Procalcitonin level:	< 0.5 ng/mL = no infection
	2 - 10 ng/mL = severe sepsis
	> 10 ng/mL = septic shock
	up to 100 ng/mL in some patients with severe sepsis

Hemodynamics: Adult normal values

Abbrv	Parameter	Normal Value	Formula (if applicable)
HR	Heart Rate	70 - 100 bpm	
SBP	Systolic blood pressure	< 120 mm Hg	
DBP	Diastolic Blood pressure	60 - 80 mm Hg	
MAP	Mean arterial pressure	70 - 105 mm Hg	$\frac{\text{Sys} + (2 \times \text{Dias})}{3}$
CVP RAP	Central venous pressure or Right atrial pressure	2 - 6 mm Hg 2 - 8 cm H_2O	Convert cm H_2O to mm Hg mm Hg = cm H_2O /1.34
RVS	Right Ventricle Systolic	15 - 30 mm Hg	
RVD	Right Ventricle Diastolic	0 - 8 mm Hg	
PAS	Pulmonary artery systolic pressure	15 - 30 mm Hg	
PAD	Pulmonary artery diastolic pressure	8 - 15 mm Hg	
PAM	Pulmonary artery mean pressure	9 - 18 mm Hg	(PAS + 2PAD) / 3
PCWP	Pulmonary capillary wedge (occlusion) pressure	6 - 12 mm Hg	
LAP	Left atrial pressure	6 - 12 mm Hg	
CO	Cardiac output	4 - 8 LPM	
CI	Cardiac index	2.5 - 4 L/min/m^2	CO/BSA
ICP	Intracranial pressure	10 mm Hg	
CerPP	Cerebral perfusion pressure	70 - 90 mm Hg	MAP - ICP
CorPP	Coronary perfusion pressure	60 - 80 mm Hg	BP Dias - PCWP
SV	Stroke volume	60 - 100 mL/beat	$\frac{\text{CO} \times 1000}{\text{HR}}$
SVI	Stroke volume index	33 - 47 mL/beat/m^2	SV/BSA
SVR	Systemic vascular resistance (Dynes)	800 - 1200 dyne•sec/cm^5	$\frac{(\text{MAP} - \text{CVP})80}{\text{CO}}$
SVRI	Systemic vascular resistance index	1970-2390 dyne•sec/cm^5m^2	SVR x BSA
SVR	Systemic vascular resistance (Wood Units)	12 - 16 wood units	$\frac{(\text{MAP} - \text{CVP})}{\text{CO}}$
PVR	Pulmonary vascular resistance	40 - 150 dynes•sec/cm^5	$\frac{(\text{PAM} - \text{PCWP})80}{\text{CO}}$
PVRI	Pulmonary vascular resistance index	255 - 285 dyne•sec/cm^5m^2	PVR x BSA
RVEDV	Right ventricular end-diastolic volume	100 - 160 mL/beat	SV/RVEF
RVEDVI	Right ventricular end-diastolic volume index	60 - 100 mL/beat /m^2	RVEDV/BSA
RVESV	Right ventricular end-systolic volume	50 - 100 mL/beat	RVEDV - SV
RVESVI	Right ventricular end-systolic volume index	30 - 60 mL /beat/m^2	RVESV/BSA
RVEF	Right ventricular ejection fraction	40 - 60 %	RVESV/RVEDV
RVSWI	Right ventricular stroke work index	5 - 10 gm /beat/m^2	SVI(PAM - CVP).0136
LVEF	Left ventricular ejection fraction	> 75 %	SV/End Diastolic Volume
LVSWI	Left ventricular stroke work index	50 - 62 gm /beat/m^2	SVI(MAP - PCWP) x 0.0136

Edwards Labs. Quick Guide to Cardiopulmonary Care, 2010 fmed.ulaval.ca (accessed Sept 2015)
NIH National Heart Lung & Blood Institute, Normal Lab Values. Investigations Operations Manual 2014, www.lab values, fda.gov.pdf. (accessed Sept 2015).

Pulmonary Parameters: Adult Normal Values

Abbrv	Parameter	Normal Value	Formula (if applicable)
RR	Respiratory rate	10 - 20 BPM	
TV	Tidal volume	5 - 7 mL/kg	
VD	Volume of dead space	150 mL (2 mL/kg)	
VC	Vital capacity	40 - 70 mL/kg	IRV + TV + ERV
VA	Alveolar ventilation	4200 mL/min	RR(TV - VD)
MV	Minute ventilation	6000 mL/min	RR x TV
FRC	Functional residual capacity	M = 2.4 L; F = 1.9 L	ERV + RV
ERV	Expiratory reserve volume	M = 1.2 L; F = 0.93 L	
RV	Residual volume	M = 1.2 L; F = 0.93 L	FRC - ERV
IRV	Inspiratory reserve volume	M = 3 L; F = 2.3 L	
IC	Inspiratory capacity	M = 3.5 L; F = 2.7 L	IRV/TV
TLC	Total lung capacity	M = 6 L; F = 4.7 L	IRV + TV + FRC
FEV1	After maximum inspiration, volume expired in 1 second	> 10 mL/kg	
MIP	Maximum inspiratory pressure	- 50 to - 100 cm H_2O	
C	Compliance	200 mL/cm H_2O	
SC	Static compliance	100 mL/cm H_2O	$\frac{\text{Tidal Volume}}{\text{(Plateau pressure - PEEP)}}$
pH	Concentration of H^+ ions	7.35 - 7.45	
HCO_3	Bicarbonate	22 - 26 mEq/L	
$PaCO_2$	Partial pressure of arterial CO_2	35 - 45 mm Hg	
$ETCO_2$	End-tidal CO_2	35 - 45 mm Hg	
$PvCO_2$	Partial pressure of venous CO_2	40 - 50 mm Hg	
PaO_2	Partial pressure of arterial O_2	75 - 100 mm Hg	
SaO_2	Arterial oxygen saturation	95 - 100 %	
PiO_2	Partial pressure of inspired O_2	Barometric pressure - 47 cm H_2O	
FiO_2	Percentage of O_2, inspired air	21% if breathing room air	
P/F ratio	Ratio of PaO_2 to FiO_2	300 - 500 < 200 = respiratory failure	PaO_2/FiO_2
PB	Barometric pressure	760 mm at sea level	
PH_2O	Water vapor pressure	47 mm Hg	
RQ	Respiratory quotient	0.8	
PAO_2	Partial pressure of alveolar O_2	100 mm Hg at sea level	$FiO_2(PB - PH_2O)-(PaCO_2/0.8)$
$A\text{-}aDO_2$	Difference in partial pressure of alveolar O_2 and arterial O_2	< 10 mm on room air < 70 mm on 100% O_2	$PAO_2 - PaO_2$
CaO_2	O_2 content of arterial blood	16 - 22 mL O_2/dL	1.39 x Hgb x SaO_2
PvO_2	Partial pressure of venous O_2	40 mm Hg	
SvO_2	Venous oxygen saturation	60 - 80 %	
CvO_2	O_2 content of venous blood	15 mL O_2/dL	1.39 x Hgb x SvO_2
$C(a\text{-}v)O_2$	AV O_2 Difference	4 - 6 mL O_2/dL	CaO_2- CvO_2
CcO_2	O_2 content of pulmonary end-capillary blood	20.5 mL O_2/dL	
Q	Cardiac output	5 LPM	
QS/QT	Pulmonary Shunt	3 - 5 %	CcO_2- CaO_2/CcO_2 - CvO_2
DO_2I	Oxygen delivery index	500 - 600 mL/min/m^2	CI(1.39 x Hgb x SaO_2)10
VO_2I	Oxygen consumption index	120 - 160 mL/min/m^2	(SaO_2-SvO_2) x CI x Hgb x13.9
V/Q	Ventilation perfusion ratio	0.8	$\frac{\text{Ventilation LPM}}{\text{Perfusion LPM}}$
OER	Oxygen extraction rate	22 - 30 %	(CaO_2 - CvO_2)/CaO_2

Neligan P. Critical Care Medicine Tutorial: Oxygen. www.ccmtutorials.com accessed 9/11/2015

ACLS

ACLS

BLS by Healthcare Providers

Recognize: Patient is unconscious, is not breathing, or is gasping.

Activate:
- Emergency Response System
- Call for emergency equipment and another ACLS provider
- Proceed immediately to compressions

Chest Compressions:
- Check for pulse. If absent, give compressions as follows:
- Place heel of 1 hand over the back of the other hand, keeping the hands parallel to each other.
- Position over the lower half of the sternum.
- Compress to a depth of 2 inches (5 cm).
- Allow complete chest recoil after each compression.
- Compression rate is 100 - 120 compressions/minute.
- Give 30 compressions, then 2 breaths. Continue 30:2 cycles.

Airway:
- Use head tilt-chin lift; for the injured patient, use jaw-thrust.
- Placement of advanced airway must not delay CPR or defib.

1 Rescuer: No artificial airway 30:2	1 Rescuer: Yes, Artificial airway
• Give 30 compressions, at a rate of 100 - 120/min. • Depress sternum 2 inches. • Allow full chest recoil. • At end of 30 compressions, pause < 10 seconds to give 2 breaths via mouth-to-mouth or mouth-to-mask. • Focus on quality CPR. • Minimize interruptions.	• Give 30 compressions, at a rate of 100 - 120/min. • Depress sternum 2 inches. • Allow full chest recoil. • At end of 30 compressions, pause < 10 seconds to give 2 breaths via mouth-to-artificial airway. • Focus on quality CPR. • Minimize interruptions.
2 Rescuers: No artificial airway 30:2	**2 Rescuers: Yes, Artificial airway**
• First provider gives continuous compressions, at a rate of 100 - 120/min. • Depress sternum 2 inches. • Allow full chest recoil. • Every 6 seconds compressions are paused to allow second provider to give 2 breaths via mouth-to-mouth or mouth-to-mask. • Focus on quality CPR. Minimize interruptions in compressions. • Change roles q 5 cycles (≈ q 2 min).	• Continuous compressions, at a rate of 100 - 120/min. No pauses. • Depress sternum 2 inches. • Allow full chest recoil. • Every 6 seconds, second provider gives 1 breaths of 600 mL via bag-to-airway with O_2 at 5 LPM. Do **not** synch with or pause compressions. • Focus on quality CPR. Interruptions in compressions must be minimized. • Change roles q 5 cycles (≈ q 2 min).

Lone provider should not use bag/mask, but rather mouth-to-mouth or mouth-to-mask (or to ET tube if one is in place).

Resuscitation bag requirements: 1- 2 L capacity, no pressure relief valve, O_2 at 10 - 15 liters/min., and breath volume of 600 mL.

High Quality CPR
1. Chest compressions of adequate rate and depth
2. Full chest recoil allowed between compressions
3. Interruptions in chest compressions are minimized
4. Excessive ventilation is avoided

Return of Spontaneous Circulation (ROSC)
1. Pulse and blood pressure present
2. $P_{ET}CO_2$ increases abruptly (to $\geq$ 40 mm Hg)
3. Intra-arterial monitoring displays arterial pressure waves

Outcome

One study revealed that achieving ROSC was:
> 90 % among patients resuscitated for < 10 minutes
< 50 % among patients resuscitated for > 30 minutes

See last page of this chapter for summary of BLS for adult vs child vs infant.

Kleinman ME, Brennan EE, Goldberger ZD, et al. Part 5: Adult BLS and CPR Quality. 2015 AHA Guidelines Update for CPR and ECC. Circulation. November 2015;132(18) suppl 2:S414-S435.

Ventricular Fibrillation or Pulseless V Tach

"High-quality CPR and rapid defibrillation are of primary importance"

Recognize:	The patient is unresponsive, pulseless, not breathing or agonal. Start CPR, administer Oxygen. Call for AED (automatic external defibrillator).
Compression:	Press hard (at least 2 inches in depth) and fast (100 - 120/min). Allow full chest recoil. Assess quality of CPR often.
Airway and Breathing:	When a second (and trained) provider is available, bag-mask ventilation may be used, to deliver 600 mL over 1 second. CPR and defibrillation for VF should not be delayed by pulse checks or by placement of an advanced airway. End-tidal CO_2 monitor will be beneficial.
Prepare Defibrillator:	Ventricular Fib (VF) or Pulseless VTach (pVT) is identified. Continue compressions without interruption, while 2nd responder applies defib pads and charges the defibrillator.
#1 "Shock":	Continue compressions until the warning "stand clear" is given. • If biphasic defibrillator: 120 - 200 joules • If monophasic defibrillator: 360 joules If VF/pVT continues, resume CPR for 2 minutes.
#2 "Shock":	Continue compressions until the warning "stand clear" is given. • If biphasic defibrillator: 120 - 200 joules • If monophasic defibrillator: 360 joules If VF/pVT continues, resume CPR for 2 minutes. Rotate the compressor every 2 minutes. Consider advanced airway and capnography.
Epinephrine:	1 mg IV/IO (if no IV/IO: 2 - 2.5 mg in 5 - 10 mL NS per ETT). May repeat q 3 - 5 minutes. Follow IV bolus injections with 20 mL flush. If given via peripheral IV, elevate extremity for 10 - 20 seconds. If additional dose/s given, calculate total dose to avoid toxicity.
#3 "Shock":	Continue compressions until the warning "stand clear" is given. • If biphasic defibrillator: 120 - 200 joules • If monophasic defibrillator: 360 joules If VF/pVT continues, resume CPR for 2 minutes. Rotate the compressor every 2 minutes.
Amiodarone:	300 mg IV or IO; may give additional 150 mg once. May follow with infusion of 1 mg/min. Maximum total is 2.2 g over 24 hours.
Improve delivery of CPR if:	$PetCO_2 < 10$ mm Hg or Intra-arterial diastolic BP < 20 mm Hg (Some studies show that $PetCO_2 > 20$ mm Hg and DBP > 40 mm Hg offer significant survival benefit.)
Manage Reversible Causes:	Hypovolemia Hypoxia Hydrogen ion (acidosis) Hypo/hyperkalemia Hypothermia Toxins Tamponade, cardiac Tension pneumothorax Thrombosis, coronary Thrombosis, pulmonary
ROSC: Return of Spontaneous Circulation	Pulse and blood pressure are present. There is abrupt sustained increase in PO_2 (typically $\geq$ 40 mm Hg). Spontaneous arterial pressure waves are present. Proceed to Post Cardiac Arrest Care.

Ultrasound may help in detecting hypovolemia, pneumothorax, pericardial tamponade, or pulmonary embolism; but the effect on outcome during cardiac arrest is uncertain.

Link MS, Berkow LC, Kudenchuk PJ, et al. Part 7: ACLS 2015 AHA Guidelines Update for CPR and Emergency CV Care. Circulation, 2015;132(suppl 2):S444-S464.

Defibrillation with External Defibrillator

Facts:

- Every minute from the time circulation ceases to the time circulation is restored decreases the chance of survival by 7-10%.
- ≤ 3 mins from collapse to first defibrillation attempt is ideal goal.
- Padded/Adhesive electrodes can be placed in advance (allowing ECG monitoring and analysis, and faster delivery of each shock).
- Other features offer advantages for in-hospital use: audible ACLS prompts, audible and recorded analysis of EKG and CPR quality, SpO_2, exhaled CO_2, noninvasive BP, multiple-lead ECG, pacing, ST segment analysis, pressure monitoring, and audible warnings regarding cable integrity.
- One manufacturer offers a single adhesive electrode pad (placed over the heart) for both monitoring and cardioversion.

2 types: Biphasic defibrillator

- A smaller capacitor allows a lighter-weight, more portable device.
- Utilizes a two-directional flow of current. When discharged, the current flows from one electrode to the other, then reverses to flow in the opposite direction. The amount and duration of the shock is automatically adjusted based on the patient's impedance.
- Biphasic may be superior to monophasic defibrillator for: cardioversion of AFib, defibrillation of VFib in an out-of-hospital environment, and in high impedance patients (e.g., large chest, increased air in the lungs, chest hair, dry/flaky skin).

Monophasic defibrillator

- The traditional monophasic defibrillator delivers current that flows from the negative electrode to the positive electrode.
- One shock of 360 joules is recommended for VF/Pulseless VT.
- The monitoring capabilities offer many advantages.

Adult pads:

- Adult size is 8 - 12 cm (12 cm size is best).
- If patient is ≥ 8 years old, use smallest adult size.

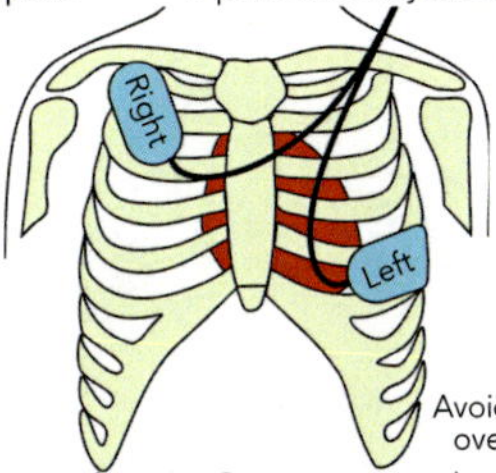

Fig. 3.4 Usual Electrode Placement
Right: Below the right clavicle.
Left: Below and lateral to the left breast.

Fig. 3.5 Path of the current

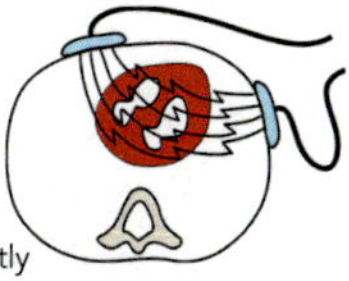

Avoid placing pads directly over implanted devices.

Procedure:

1. Remove any medication patches and wipe area clean.
2. Remove any body piercings of the torso. Remove all jewelry.
3. Apply electrode pads to patient's chest, or to chest and back.
4. Confirm VFib/Pulseless VTach.
5. Select the energy level:
   Biphasic AED: 120 j, 150 j, or 200 j
   Monophasic: 360 j
6. Announce "Charging defibrillator." Press "charge" button.
7. It may take several seconds to reach full charge.
8. If paddle electrodes used, apply firm pressure.
9. Make certain that no one is in contact with the patient, stretcher/bed, or ventilator.
10. Check that O_2 is not directed over or toward the chest.
11. Give an "all clear" warning. CPR is stopped. Press "shock."
12. Immediately resume with compressions first, then ventilation.

Safety:

- A fire hazard exists when a shock is given in the presence of O_2.
- After shocks are given to a patient with Pacemaker or ICD, the function of that device should be evaluated.

Link MS, Berkow LC, Kudenchuk PJ, et al. 2015 American Heart Association Guidelines for CPR & Emergency Cardiovascular Care. Part 7: Adult ACLS. Circulation, 2015;132(suppl2):S444-S464.

Asystole or Pulseless Electrical Activity (PEA)

Recognize:
Patient is unresponsive, pulseless, not breathing.
ECG monitor displays Asystole or PEA.
Activate Emergency Response Team.

CPR x 2 minutes, then trade roles:
- 30 Compressions at rate of 100 - 120/min.
- Depress sternum 2 inches. Allow full chest recoil.
- Pause compressions for second provider to deliver 2 breaths, using bag-to-mask attached to 5 LPM O_2
- Focus on quality CPR.
- Rotate compressor every 2 minutes.
- Minimize interruptions in compressions.

Airway and Breathing:
Consider advanced airway.
Once advanced airway in place, give 1 breath every 5 - 6 seconds (10 - 12 breaths/min), without pauses in chest compressions.

Epinephrine: 1 mg IV/IO q 3 - 5 minutes.

Rhythm √: Take < 10 seconds to check rhythm/pulse. If still Asystole or PEA,

CPR:
Resume CPR, minimize interruptions.
Repeat Epinephrine q 3 - 5 minutes.
Pacing is not recommended for Asystole or pulseless rhythm.

Monitor CPR Quality:
Improve CPR if $PetCO_2$ < 10 mm Hg or Diastolic BP < 20 mm Hg
Continuous $ScvO_2$ monitoring may be helpful.
Keep $ScvO_2$ > 50%.

Causes:
Recall H's and T's (on page 2) as possible causes of arrest.
Progressive volume loss (hemorrhage) is a common cause of Pulseless Electrical Activity.

Symptomatic Bradycardia with Pulse

Assessment: HR is < 50 bpm, or is less than expected.

Correct possible causes:
- Secure and maintain the airway.
- Assist breathing if necessary.
- Administer O_2 if hypoxemic; monitor SpO_2 if possible.
- Identify rhythm on cardiac monitor.
- Monitor blood pressure.
- Establish IV access.
- 12 Lead ECG if available, but don't delay treatment.

Immediate treatment is required if there is:
Hypotension
Sudden change in mental state
Signs of hypotension/shock
Chest discomfort or pain
Signs of acute heart failure

Atropine:
Atropine 0.5 mg IV
May repeat q 3 - 5 minutes to a total of 3 mg.
Calculate total dose of repeated meds to avoid toxicity.
(Atropine will be ineffective in cardiac transplant patients)

If Atropine ineffective:
Transcutaneous pacing
or
Dopamine: 2 - 20 mcg/kg/min infusion. Titrate to response.
or
Epinephrine: 2 - 10 mcg/min infusion. Titrate to response.

Call expert: For consultation and/or transvenous pacing.

Link MS, Berkow LC, Kudenchuk PJ, et al. Part 7: Adult Advanced Cardiovascular Life Support: 2015 AHA Guidelines Update for Cardiopulmonary Resuscitation and Emergency CV Care. Circulation, 2015;132(suppl 2):S444-S464.

Transcutaneous Pacing (TCP)

Description: The use of external electrodes to provide temporary cardiac pacing when symptomatic bradycardia persists despite meds. TCP is considered a temporary measure to be used until transvenous pacing can be accomplished.
Other names include: noninvasive pacing, external transthoracic pacing, external pacing, precordial pacing, transdermal pacing.

Other Indications:

- Mobitz Type II 2° AV Block; 3° AV Block
- New left, right, or alternating BBB or bifasicular block
- Bradycardia with symptomatic ventricular escape rhythms
- Overdrive pacing of tachycardia refractory to drug therapy
- As standby in pts with myocardial ischemia/infarction with:
  Symptomatic sinus node dysfunction
  Asymptomatic Mobitz type II 2° AV block
  Asymptomatic 3° AV block, or new BBB

Procedure:

1. Provide sedation and/or analgesia in conscious patients.
2. Clean and dry the skin. Clip, don't shave, excess hair. Avoid use of alcohol on skin.
3. Apply ECG electrodes and connect ECG cable to the pacer. Select lead I, II, or III. (Some devices provide combination pacing electrodes/ECG monitoring leads).
4. Apply the pacing electrode pads, connect to pacing device.

Anterior-Posterior offers a more direct path to and through the heart, allows a lower pacing threshold, and avoids the stimulation of large skeletal muscles.

Fig. 3.6

Anterior
the negative electrode is placed on the left anterior chest, 4th ICS, midclavicular line (ECG-lead position V4). Do not place lead over the diaphragm.

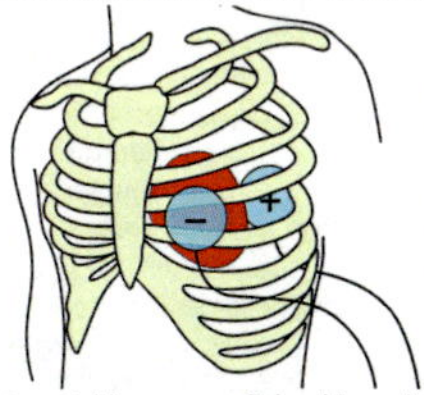

Posterior
the positive electrode is placed on the left posterior chest, beneath the scapula, lateral to the spine. Do not place directly over the spine.

Anterior-Lateral position is quickly accomplished but delivers less energy directly to the heart. Higher energy levels may be required. It also interferes with placement of defib pads if you're using "pace only" TCP equipment.

Fig. 3.7

Anterior
the negative electrode is placed below the patient's right clavicle, lateral to the sternum

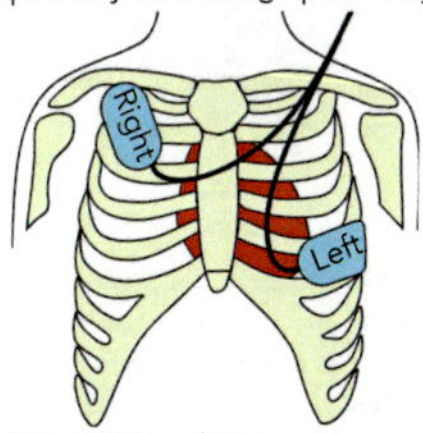

Lateral (apex)
Place positive electrode at the left 5th ICS, anterior axillary line (ECG-lead position V5).

STAT Fixed Rate Pacing:

1. Administer STAT sedative.
2. For immediate pacing, select Fixed-rate (non-demand) and set pacing rate on 60. Press "Start." Observe for skeletal muscle contraction (which occur at levels as low as 10 mA).
3. Increase the output (mA) in 10 mA increments, until there is capture (pacer spike is followed by a wide QRS and broad T).
4. For a margin of safety, set output at 2 mA above that which produces consistent capture. Often 50 - 100 mA are required.
5. Remember that muscle contraction does not mean capture. Monitor femoral (not carotid) pulse, blood pressure, skin color.
6. It is safe to touch patient during pacing.

(cont'd on next page) ➞

American Board of Anesthesia. Transcutaneous Pacing. www.open anesthesia.org. Jan 2016

Transcutaneous Pacing (cont'd)

Monitor:

1. Check that capture has resulted in:
   - Palpable pulses. Pulse oximeter or arterial line is also helpful.
   - Improved level of consciousness
   - Improved blood pressure
   - Improved skin color and temperature
2. Patients who may require greater current (mA) are those with:
   - barrel chest
   - recent thoracic surgery
   - pericardial effusion/tamponade
   - hypoxia, acidosis
3. Assess patient for sedation/analgesia requirements. 1/3 of patient's rate the pain as "severe" or "intolerable" especially if pacing is set at > 50 mA.
4. Correct possible causes of bradycardia and plan for placement of transvenous pacing leads.

DEMAND Pacing:

1. For demand pacing, adjust ECG size until pacer identifies the QRS (the pacer will place a mark on the QRS).
2. Set pacing rate at 10 - 20 beats higher than pt's heart rate.
3. Slowly increase mA until there is consistent capture. Reduce pacing rate to 60 bpm (or prescribed rate).

Trouble-Shooting:		
	No pacing of the heart: (Failed to capture)	1. Increase current (the mA). 2. Reposition electrodes, insure contact. 3. If skeletal muscle contractions are absent, check the pacer's power supply. 4. Patient may be unresponsive to pacing due to: • severe hypoxemia • prolonged arrest • severe metabolic disorder • extensive myocardial infarction • cardiac trauma
	Patient discomfort:	1. Sedative and/or analgesic may be needed. 2. Some devices have adjustable pulse width duration. Increasing the pulse width allows reduction in the mA.
	Failed to sense during demand mode:	1. Increase ECG size. 2. Change to a different lead. Try Lead I. 3. Reposition ECG leads to find a position that displays the tallest QRS possible.
	Over sensing:	1. Reduce ECG size. 2. Change to different ECG monitoring lead (Lead I may be better). 3. Reposition or replace ECG electrode/s. 4. Place ECG electrodes as far from pacing electrodes as possible.

If VFib develops:

1. Some temporary pacers have defibrillation capability. Switch from "Pacer On" to "Defib On," select energy level, press "Charge" buttons, give "all clear," press "Discharge."
2. Most temporary pacers do not have defibrillation capability. Consult the instructions provided with your transcutaneous pacer to determine if you should turn off the pacer's power.
3. Place defibrillator paddles at least 1 inch away from the pacing electrodes.

Continued Care:

1. Check pulse often. Pacing threshold may increase over time. Capture can suddenly be lost.
2. Check the skin often. Insure electrode contact with skin.
3. Consult manufacturer's recommendations for frequency of electrode replacement.
4. Plan for transvenous pacing.

ABA (American Board of Anesthesia). Transcutaneous Pacing. www.open anesthesia.org. accessed Jan 2016

Endotracheal Intubation (EI)

Facts:
- There is no difference in survival rate or neurologic outcome when ventilation is provided with bag-mask ventilation versus an endotracheal tube (ETT) or a supraglottic airway (SGA).
- During the time of Insertion, absent CPR means no perfusion, ventilation, oxygenation.
- Experienced providers may use either ETT or SGA.

Benefits: Permits delivery of high concentration of O_2, some medications, a quantifiable tidal volume, and pt-specific mode of ventilation. Maintains airway patency. Allows suction of secretions.

Indications: Unable to ventilate an unconscious pt adequately with bag/mask

Supplies:

ECG & BP monitor	ET tubes (adult size is 8 - 9.5 cm I.D.)
IV Access	Tube connector for ambu bag
O_2 supply at 15 LPM	10 cc syringe
Resus Bag & Mask	Water soluble lubricant
Suction, ET and oral	Tube stylette is inside the ET tube
SpO_2 monitor	Method of securing tube
End-tidal CO_2 monitor	Laryngoscope, back-up batteries, bulb

Intubation Procedure during CPR	
Preoxygenate:	30:2 CPR is performed with 100% O_2 at 15 LPM by bag-mask.
Prepare:	The goal is to limit the intubation attempt to < 10 seconds. Ready the supplies while compressions are being given. Some have found that 100% high-flow O_2 by nasal cannula offers an O_2-enriched environment that moderates hypoxemia.
Place:	While compressions are in progress: 1. The blade is advanced to the base of the tongue. 2. Traction is exerted on the handle of laryngoscope to lift the mandible away from the posterior oropharynx. 3. The vocal cords are visualized. 4. The ET tube is in hand. 5. Cricoid pressure should not be applied.
Pause CPR:	Compressions are stopped. The tube is advanced about 1 - 2 cm beyond the vocal cords. In adults, teeth to tube-tip distance is 19 - 23 cm.
Resume CPR:	Compressions are immediately resumed at 100 - 120/minute, **no longer** paused for ventilations, (1 breath q 6 seconds or 10 bpm)
Confirm Placement:	1. ETT stylette is removed, cuff is inflated to prevent air leak. 2. Use Resus-bag to ventilate; confirm bilateral chest expansion. 3. Confirm no breath sounds are heard over the epigastrium. 4. Confirm that breath sounds are heard over left and right anterior chest, as well as left and right midaxillary line. 5. Secure tube. Indicate tube depth with mark at the front teeth. 6. Confirm placement with exhaled CO_2 device. 7. If there is doubt, laryngoscope may be used to visualize the tube passing through the cords. If confirmed, secure tube. 8. Ventilate with 6 - 7 mL/kg (or 500 - 600 mL), 10 breaths/min. 9. Cuff pressure of 25 - 35 mm Hg is ideal. 10. Chest x-ray to confirm placement or evidence of airway injury.
Failure:	Remove tube, resume bag-mask ventilation with 100% O_2. Consider a second attempt, or consider supraglottic airway.
Complications of ET intubation:	Cuff pressure > 40 mm Hg will ↓ tracheal capillary blood flow. Injury to lips, gums, teeth, tongue, pharynx, larynx, trachea, vocal cords; avulsion of arytenoid cartilage. Hypoxemia, hypercapnea, gastric inflation. Bleeding, hematoma, infection, airway obstruction. Bronchospasm, laryngospasm, vomiting, aspiration. Intubation of esophagus, pyriform sinus. Catecholamine surge may ↑ BP, ↑ HR, or cause arrhythmia. Right mainstem bronchus intubation → Rt lung pneumothorax,

Link MS, Berkow LC, Kudenchuk PJ, et al. Part 7: Adult ACLS: 2015 AHA Guidelines Update for CPR and Emergency CV Care. Circulation, 2015;132(suppl 2):S444-S464.

Emergency Percutaneous Dilational Cricothyrotomy

Description: To provide an airway in patients in whom at least three intubation attempts have failed, or who have oral/facial/oropharyngeal/or laryngeal injuries that contraindicate oral or nasal intubation. Contraindicated in pts with expanding anterior neck hematoma, in children < 40 kg, and in patients in whom the anatomical landmarks cannot be defined (e.g., thick or obese neck).

Procedure: Size 6 Cook Melker kit. Have suction ready. The skin is prepped. The cricothyroid membrane is identified and the skin insized.

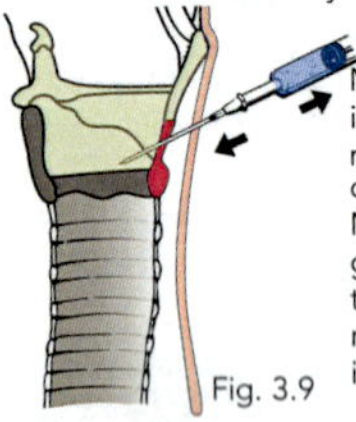

Fig. 3.9

Needle-within-catheter is inserted through cricothyroid membrane. Aspiration of air confirms placement into airway. Needle is removed and the guidewire is threaded through the catheter. The catheter is removed, leaving the guidewire in place.

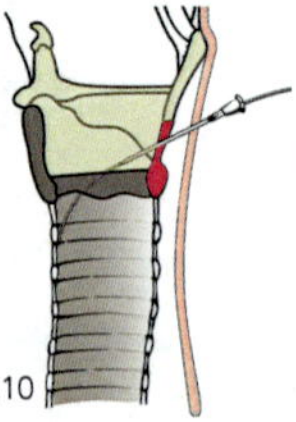

Fig. 3.10

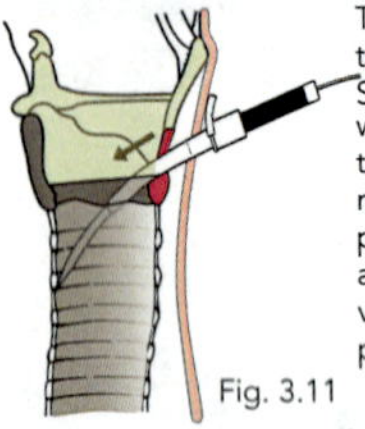

Fig. 3.11

The dilator/airway assembly is threaded over the guidewire. Support is given to the trachea while advancing the dilator through the skin. The dilator is removed, leaving the airway in place. The airway is secured and placement is verified when ventilation with ambu bag produces breath sounds.

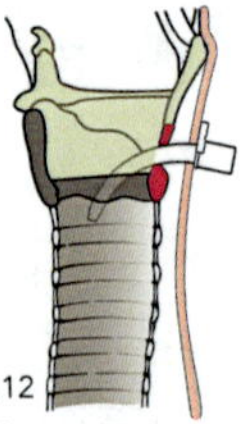

Fig. 3.12

Complications: Injury to thyroid, trachea, vocal cords, esophagus, blood supply. Pneumothorax, subcutaneous air, bleeding, hematoma, vomiting/aspiration, bronchospasm, laryngospasm.

Emergency Surgical Cricothyrotomy

Supplies:

- Scalpel with # 11 blade
- Endotracheal tube size ≥ 6.5 mm
- 2 sterile hemostats
- Tracheal hooks

Procedure: Cricothyroid membrane is identified. The skin is prepped. A 2 - 3 cm vertical skin incision is made over the membrane. A horizontal incision is made through the membrane. The patient may breathe air or cough secretions through the incision. The hemostats are used to enlarge the opening and stabilize it. The ET tube is inserted and advanced to only 1 - 2 cm above the superior border of the cuff. The hemostats are removed. Cuff is inflated. Ventilate with ambu bag. Suctioning may be required. Verify position of tube. Secure the tube.

Fig. 3.13

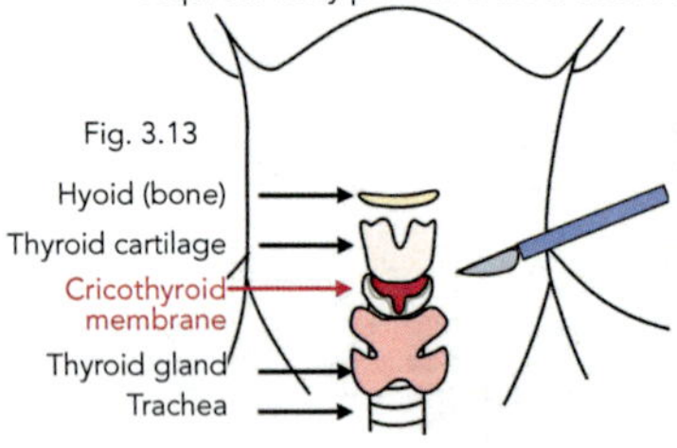

Complications:
Injury to thyroid, trachea, vocal cords, esophagus.
Bleeding
Hematoma
Bronchospasm
Airway obstruction
Subcutaneous air
Pneumothorax
Vomiting/aspiration
Infection

Post-Cardiac Arrest Care

with return of spontaneous circulation

Optimize Oxygenation and Ventilation:

- Continue bag-to-mask ventilation. Endotracheal intubation with bag-to-ET tube ventilation offers no ***immediate*** survival advantage over bag-to-facemask ventilation. Give 100% O_2, and titrate to maintain SaO_2 > 92%.
- Oropharyngeal airway may be inserted:
  only in unresponsive patients who have no cough or gag reflex, and
  only by trained caregivers
- Monitor and maintain oxygen saturation > 92%.
- Patients with episodes of apnea, shallow breathing, and poor oxygenation will require an advanced airway and mechanical ventilation.
- Following placement of an advanced airway, capnography is recommended to guide ventilatory rate and depth and avoid hypo/hyper ventilation.

Circulation:

- Hypotension (SBP < 90 mm Hg, MAP < 65 mm Hg) must be avoided during post-resuscitation care.
- Immediately intervene, with IV/IO fluid bolus, and/or vasopressor infusion.
- Target goal is MAP > 65 mm Hg (and as high as 80 mm Hg).
- 12-Lead ECG is required for the detection of cardiac ischemia.
- Immediate angiography is needed for patients with ST elevation.
- Hypoxemia, ischemia, and reperfusion injury caused by cardiac arrest may cause damage to multiple organ systems: primarily neuro, pulmonary, renal.

Neuroprotection with Hypothermia:

1. The development of hyperthermia in the first few days after cardiac arrest increases cerebral metabolic rate, and thus the oxygen required by the brain.
2. Up to 1/4 of patients who remain comatose after cardiac arrest develop seizures and/or nonconvulsive status epilepticus (NCSE). The use of intermittent or continuous EEG is critical to the identification of NCSE.
3. Therapeutic hypothermia, also know as Targeted Temperature Management (TTM) should be implemented in post-arrest patients who remain in coma.
   - The patient is cooled to 32 - 34° C (some suggest 36° C).
   - Hypothermia is maintained for at least 24 hours.
   - After 72 or more hours of normothermia, neurologic function re-evaluated. (see details on next page)
4. The earliest time to predict Neurologic Outcome can be made:
   - In patients not treated with TTM: 72 hours after cardiac arrest
   - In coma patients treated with TTM: $\geq$ 72 hours after normothermia
   - The use of sedation or paralysis may extend the time beyond 72 hours.
5. Poor Neurologic Outcome is Likely:
   - In coma patients (treated or not with TTM): absent pupillary light reflex after 72 or more hours.
   - Presence of status myoclonus (in combination with other diagnostic tests) during the first 72 hours after cardiac arrest.
   - In patients not treated with hypothermia, fever is poorly controlled or is untreated.
   - EEG:
     a. persistent absence of EEG reactivity to external stimuli at 72 hrs.
     b. intractible status epilepticus or persistent burst suppression after rewarming.

*Some report that targeting temperatures < 36° C is difficult to achieve, may elicit more complications, and probably does not offer additional benefit. A target of 36° C may be sufficient. (Nielsen N et al, for the TTM investigators. Targeted Temperature Management at 33°C versus 36°C after Cardiac Arrest. N NEJM, Dec 5, 2013;369:2197-2206)

Callaway CW, Donnino MW, Fink EL, et al.Part 8: Post-Cardiac Care. 2015 AHA Guidelines Update for CPR and ECC. Circulation. 2015;132(suppl 2):S465-S482.

Therapeutic Hypothermia after Cardiac Arrest

Description:

- Brain death is the end result for 23% of patients after in-hospital cardiac arrest and for 68% of patients after out-of-hospital cardiac arrest.
- The outcome of patients who survive cardiac arrest but have a GCS < 8 may be improved with rapid application and careful maintenance (for 12-24 hours) of therapeutic hypothermia

Immediate Care after ROSC:

- The cause of cardiac arrest and hypotension must be identified and treatment continued uninterrupted during therapeutic hypothermia.
- Epinephrine, dopamine, or norepinephrine may be required to maintain SBP ≥ 90, MAP ≥ 65.
- Seizures occur in 5 - 20 % of comatose cardiac arrest survivors.
- Once the patient is stabilized, head of bed elevation of 30° (if tolerated) is recommended to reduce the incidence of cerebral edema, aspiration, and ventilator-associated pneumonia.

The Challenges of Therapeutic Hypothermia:

- Reducing core body temp to ≤ 36° C in less 3 - 6 hours, maintaining for at least 24 hr, while simultaneously treating the cause of cardiac arrest.
- Minimizing the neurologic consequences of cardiac arrest, as well as the consequences of hypothermia, mechanical ventilation, and immobility.

Patient Selection, Temp Targets, Temp Duration:

- Adult patients (> 18 yo), who are in coma (no meaningful response to verbal commands, GCS < 8), with Return of Spontaneous Circulation (ROSC) after:
  a. in-hospital cardiac arrest: target temp 32°- 36° C maintained at least 24 hr, and outcome prediction 72 hrs or more after return of normothermia.
  b. out-of-hospital cardiac arrest: target temp 32°- 34° C maintained 12 - 24 hr
- Temp target must be achieved in less than 3 - 6 hours.

Methods of Cooling:

- Immediate methods of cooling:
  a. Cold (4° C) Sodium Chloride or Ringer's Lactate, 30 mL/kg (up to 1500 mL) is infused over 30 minutes via a peripheral or femoral catheter.
  b. Iced Normal Saline gastric lavage.
- Conventional approach: 2 cooling blankets (to 1 machine) positioned over and under the patient. A sheet is placed between the patient and each of the cooling blankets. Hypothermia unit that features hydrogel-coated pads and continuous temperature monitoring is preferred.
- Endovascular approach: An intravascular catheter with several heat-exchanging balloons, is inserted usually via the femoral artery. This is the most reliable method of achieving rapid, stable, desired body temperature. Reduces staff workload, but incurs insertion/set-up time, much higher cost.

Methods of Monitoring Temp:	Recommended	Unreliable
	Esophageal thermometer	Oral
	Bladder catheter in nonanuric patients	Axillary
	Pulmonary artery catheter, if one is in place	Tympanic
	Endovascular device, if one is in place	Rectal

Three Phases: (Arterial line and Central Venous Catheter are recommended).

1. FAST Induction Phase:
   - The goal: reduce body temp rapidly, in order to minimize short-term events (shivering, hypovolemia, electrolyte imbalance, hyperglycemia) and without overshooting the target temperature.
   - Sedatives are given in low dose boluses (hypothermia significantly reduces drug clearance). Paralytic agent may be given for shivering.
   - Cooling causes intracellular shifts of potassium, magnesium, calcium, and phosphate, resulting in low serum levels of these electrolytes.
   - Glucose goal: 110 - 150 mg/dL using intensive insulin therapy.
   - Induction may be faster in older patients, because of their lower rate of metabolism, ↓ vascular responsiveness, and often a lower lean body mass.

Callaway CW, Donnino MW, Fink EL, et al. Part 8: Post-Cardiac Arrest Care. 2015 AHA Guidelines Update for CPR and ECC. Virc, 2015;132(suppl2):S465-482.
Nielsen N, Wettersley J, Cronberg T, et al. Targeted Temperature Management at 33°C versus 36°C after Cardiac Arrest. NEJM 2013;369:2197-2206.

Therapeutic Hypothermia after Cardiac Arrest (cont'd)

2. **MAINTENANCE** Phase (maintain at least 24 hours):
   - When core temp is < 33.5°C the patient tends to become more stable, fluid shifts abate, shivering diminishes/ceases. The NMBA (which masks the adequacy of sedation as well as seizure activity) is discontinued.
   - Temp is tightly controlled, allow only minor fluctuations of 0.2°- 0.5° C.
   - Sedatives are given in low dose as a continuous infusion.
   - Attention shifts toward the prevention of long-term side effects such as pneumonia, wound infections, and decubiti.
   - Achieve end-tidal CO_2 = 35 - 40 mm Hg, $PaCO_2$ = 35 - 45 mm Hg.
   - SpO_2 forehead sensors are more accurate in the setting of hypothermia. O_2 is titrated to achieve $SpO_2 \geq 94\%$.
   - Vital signs every 30 minutes during induction, every hour once the temperature goal has been met, and every hour during rewarming.
   - Since peripheral nerve conduction is slowed by cooling, peripheral nerve stimulation may not be a reliable method for monitoring blockade. The neurologic exam is generally limited to pupil reaction to light.
   - Capillary glucose values can be falsely decreased by cold-induced vasoconstriction.
3. **SLOW** Rewarming Phase: (has been described as the most difficult phase):
   - Stop all Potassium supplements 8 hours prior to rewarming.
   - Strive for a rewarming rate of 0.5 degrees/hr (range of 0.2° - 0.5° C/hr). Too-rapid rewarming can erase any achieved neuroprotective benefits.
   - Continue sedation, analgesia. Avoid neuromuscular blockade since seizures are likely. Manage the same as seizures of any other etiology.
   - Carefully monitor and manage fluid and electrolyte imbalance.
   - Once normothermia is achieved (37° C), the sedation dose can be decreased by 50%, and then slowly titrated down until off.

Lab: CBC, PT, PTT, INR, blood sugar, chemistry (Na, Cl, K, Mg, P, Ca), and arterial blood gases every 6-8 hours until the patient is again normothermic.

Complications	
↑ blood pressure, ↑ CVP, ↓↑ heart rate, ↓ CO	Vasoconstriction causes slight increase in BP; Reduced tissue oxygen demand prompts a slower HR, lower cardiac output, and ↑ $ScvO_2$.
EKG changes: ↓ HR, ↑ PR interval, ↑ QT interval, widened QRS.	Risk for severe arrhythmias begins when core temperature decreases to < 30° C and is significant when < 28° C. Initial arrhythmia is usually atrial fibrillation; VF is a possibility.
↓ PCO_2 and alkalosis	CO_2 production is slower. Ventilator rates and volume must be lower than routine settings.
Electrolyte disorders (K, Mg, P, Ca)	Intracellular shift may cause ↓ K during Phase 1 and 2. Extracellular shift may cause hyperkalemia during Phase 3 (rewarming). Rewarm slowly. Keep electrolyte levels in the high normal range.
Coagulopathy	Platelet count and function are impaired during hypothermia. Platelets may be given before an invasive procedure.
Shivering (is the most significant impediment to achieving target temperature)	Shivering causes rewarming and must be controlled with analgesia (meperidine or quick-acting opiates), and/or sedation (propofol or benzodiazepines). Minimize the use of short-acting paralytic agents. Usually shivering abates when temp is < 33.5° C.
Glycemic Control	Insulin requirement may increase during the cooling phase, and decrease during rewarming. Target BG of 144 - 180 mg/dL (8 - 10 mmol/L)
Vasoconstriction, immobilization, and immune suppression	These multiple risk factors should focus attention on the prevention of decubitus, wound infections, and ventilator associated pneumonia (VAP).
Decreased drug clearance	Bolus doses, infusion rates may require adjustment.

Neurologic outcome cannot be determined until 72 hr after phase 3 is complete.

Gessner P, Target temperature within 3 hours. AACN AdvCritCare, 2012;23(3):245-257.

Unstable Tachycardia, HR ≥ 150 bpm
Synchronized Electrical Cardioversion (SEC)

Description:
- Synchronized cardioversion is timed to discharge on the R wave, thus avoiding the vulnerable refractory period, during which a shock could cause ventricular fibrillation.
- The energy level for SEC is less than that used for defibrillation.

The Unstable Patient is identified by:
- Hypotension
- Acute change in mental status
- Signs of shock
- Ischemic chest pain/discomfort
- Signs of acute heart failure

Immediate Interventions
- Maintain airway
- Assist Breathing if needed
- Apply O_2 if patient is hypoxemic
- Analyze ECG, identify rhythm
- Monitor blood pressure and SpO_2

Indications for Urgent SEC*:
- Unstable SVT due to reentry
- Unstable Atrial Fibrillation
- Unstable Atrial Flutter
- Unstable Atrial Tachycardia
- Unstable Monomorphic V Tach (with pulses)

DO NOT use SEC for:
- Junctional Tachycardia
- Pulseless Ventricular Tachycardia
- Ventricular Fibrillation (VF)
- Torsades de pointes (irregular rate makes synchronization impossible). Defibrillation is required.

* For regular rhythm narrow complex, Adenosine may be considered.

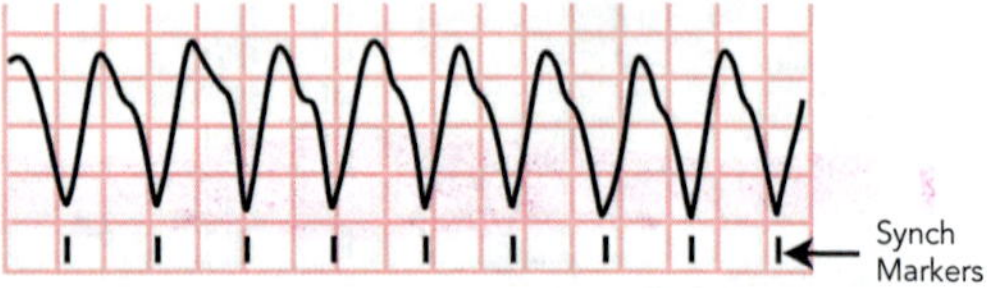

Fig. 3.8

Select the energy level according to the duration and regularity of the QRS:

QRS duration (seconds) is	And the rhythm is	And the arrhythmia is identified as	Biphasic dose (joules) is:	Monophasic dose (joules) is:
< 0.12	Regular:	SVT, or A Flutter	50 - 100 j	200 j
	Irregular:	A Fib	120 - 200 j	200 j
≥ 0.12	Regular:	Monomorphic VT	100 j	100 j
	Irregular:	Torsades des pointes	unsynchronized defibrillation	

Remove piercings of the torso. Remove jewelry. Consider sedation.

Cardioversion Procedure:
1. Give proper warning, then press and hold the "shock" button/s until the R wave is sensed by the cardioverter and shock is delivered.
2. If cardioversion fails, confirm (or reset, if needed) synch mode and try again.
3. When the QRS is wide, the cardioverter may be unable to identify (and thus unable to synchronize to) the QRS. Synch markers will be absent. Assume Ventricular Tach and proceed to unsynchronized cardioversion.

Complications:
1. Failure of the cardioverter to detect the R wave.
2. Cardioversion attempt results in ventricular tachycardia, ventricular fibrillation, or asystole.
3. Myocardial dysfunction, especially with repeated shocks and higher energy.

Link MS, Berkow LC, Kudenchuk PJ, et al. Part 7: Adult ACLS: 2015 AHA Guidelines Update for CPR and Emergency CV Care. Circulation, 2015;132(suppl 2):S444-S464.
Hazinski MF, Shuster M, Donnino MW, et al. 2015 Handbook of Emergency Cardiovascular Care for Healthcare Providers. American Heart Association, November 2015.
Zoll.com. Cardioversion. (accessed 1/31/2016)

Atrial Fibrillation

Consequences of AFib:

- Formation of intra-atrial clots → 5 fold risk of stroke
- Adverse effect on contractility → 3-fold risk of heart failure
- Decreased cardiac filling and cardiac output → poor perfusion, hypotension
- Sympathetic nervous system activation → hypertension

Signs and Symptoms of AFib:

- There may be no symptoms. Symptoms usually occur at HR ≥ 150.
- Any or all of the following: irregular pulse, fatigue, dyspnea, palpitations, syncope, hypertension or hypotension, heart failure.
- Bradycardia, Tachycardia, or Normal (although irregular) rate.

Medications for AFib:

AFib meds, for stable pt
The following meds are used for HFpEF* and with caution in those with COPD or history of mild congestive heart failure:
Beta blocker, Diltiazem, or Verapamil. That failing, then: Amiodarone

AFib meds, for pt with cardiac hx
If the patient has LV Dysfunction, or has history of Heart Failure, then the following meds:
Beta blocker (with caution), Digoxin. That failing, then: Amiodarone

*HFpEF = Heart Failure with preserved Ejection Fraction

AFib in Patients with Acute Coronary Syndrome (ACS):[1]

- AFib occurs in 10 - 21% of patients with ACS; the incidence increases with age and with the extent of myocardial ischemia.
- For new-onset AF patients with hemodynamic compromise, heart failure, intractable Ischemia, or inadequate rate control: Prepare for Urgent Synchronized Electrical Cardioversion (SEC).[1] (See previous page for details.)
- Initiating anticoagulation should not delay cardioversion.
- For those without heart failure and without hemodynamic instability:
  1. don't delay administration of anticoagulant (Heparin)
  2. intravenous beta blockers are recommended (if there are no contra-indications, namely HF, hemodynamic instability, or bronchospasm) in order to slow a rapid ventricular response to AFib.
- For patients with ACS and AF, a score has been proposed to emphasize which patients require anticoagulant therapy.[2] If the score is 2 or greater, and contraindications are absent, warfarin is recommended.

Anticoagulant Therapy absent in some pts
A review [2] of antithrombotic therapy in high-risk AFib patients before admission for stroke revealed that: • 29% of patients were **not** receiving antithrombotic therapy. • Only about one quarter of the 39% receiving warfarin achieved therapeutic INR (international normalized ratio). • 31% were prescribed anti-platelet therapy.

CHA_2DA_2-VASc	score
CHF	1
Hypertension	1
Age ≥ 75 yo	2
Diabetes mellitus	1
Stroke/TIA	2
Vascular disease	1
Age 65 - 74	1
Sex (Gender)	1
Maximum Score =	9

Anticoagulants are required, when CHA_2DA_2-VASc score is > 2:

Prevention of thromboembolism[1]

- Antithrombotic agents: Heparin, warfarin, direct thrombin inhibitor, factor Xa inhibitor, and/or anti-platelet agent (aspirin and clopidogrel) are prescribed.
- Platelet inhibitors: are less effective than warfarin, but better tolerated by some patients, while also offering a lower risk of intracerebral hemorrhage.

1. January CT, Wann LS, Alpert JS, et al. 2014 AHA/ACC/HRS Guideline for the Management of Patients With Atrial Fibrillation. JACC, 2014;64(21):2246-2280.
2. Lane DA, Lip GYH. Use of the CHA_2DS_2-VASc Score to Aid Decision Making for Thromboprophylaxis in Nonvalvular Atrial Fibrillation. Circ, 2012;126:860-865. accessed 2/21/16.

Stable Tachycardia

Initial Management	Since the patient is stable, there is time to:
• Continuous ECG. • Provide oxygen if needed. • Establish IV access. • Identify/treat reversible causes (see "Look for Possible Causes" listed below)	• Obtain a 12-lead ECG • Evaluate the rhythm • Measure QRS duration, determine if QRS < 0.12 or ≥ 0.12 seconds • Measure the length of the QT interval • Consider treatment options • Decide if treatment risk exceeds benefit • Seek expert consultation
If QRS is < 0.12 seconds:	**If QRS is ≥ 0.12 seconds:**
12 lead ECG, if available Vagal maneuvers (which is effective in 25% of patients) Adenosine (if rhythm is regular) Beta-blocker, or Calcium Channel Blocker may be considered. May consider expert consultation	12 lead ECG, if available Adenosine is considered, only if the QRS is regular and monomorphic Antiarrhythmic infusion may be considered May consider expert consultation

Medications for Stable Tachycardia	
Adenosine	6 mg rapid (1 - 3 seconds) IV push, followed by NS flush; if the rate fails to convert, may follow with a second dose of 12 mg.
Amiodarone	150 mg IV over 10 minutes. May be repeated as needed if VTach recurs. Maintenance infusion is 1 mg/min for the first 6 hours.
Procainamide	Avoid use in patients with prolonged QT or CHF. 20 - 50 mg/min may be given until: The arrhythmia is suppressed Hypotension ensues QRS duration increases > 50%, or The maximum dose of 17 mg/kg has been given. Maintenance dose: 1 - 4 mg/min
Sotalol	Avoid use in patients with prolonged QT. 1.5 mg/kg (or 100 mg) over 5 minutes.

Look for Possible Causes	
Hypovolemia	Toxins
Hypoxia	Tamponade, cardiac
Hydrogen ion (acidosis)	Tension Pneumothorax
Hypo/Hyperkalemia	Thrombosis, coronary
Hyperthermia	Thrombosis, pulmonary

Link MS, Berkow LC, Kudenchuk PJ, et al. Part 7: Adult ACLS: 2015 AHA Guidelines Update for CPR and Emergency CV Care. Circulation, 2015;132(suppl 2):S444-S464.
Hazinski MF, Shuster M, Donnino MW, et al. 2015 Handbook of Emergency Cardiovascular Care for Healthcare Providers. American Heart Association, November 2015.

Acute Ischemic Stroke

Facts:
Stroke is the leading cause of adult disability.
87% of strokes are ischemic (10% of strokes are hemorrhagic).
25% of patients deteriorate during the first 24 hours.
19% have ↑ BP at stroke onset; 80% have ↑ BP within 24 hours.

Risk Factors for Stroke:
Atrial fib 17x (A Fib increases the risk for stroke 17 times)

Previous CVA,TIA 10x	Smoking 2x	Advanced age
Hypertension 6x	Prosthetic heart valve	Black race
Heart disease 2x - 6x	Family history	Male
Diabetes 2x - 4x	Hypercoagulopathy	
Carotid bruit 3x	Sickle cell anemia	

Signs and Symptoms of Stroke:
Sudden weakness or numbness of the face, arm, or leg, especially if only one side of the body is affected.
Confusion, trouble speaking or understanding.
Trouble seeing with one or both eyes.
Trouble walking, dizziness, loss of balance or coordination.
Severe headache with no known cause.

Stroke Mimics:
Recognize conditions that initially mimic stroke: postictal state, syncope, hypoglycemia, complex migraine, arrhythmias.

The Cincinnati Prehospital Stroke Scale

If any 1 of these 3 signs is abnormal, the probability of a stroke is 72%.

Test	Method of Testing	Normal Response	Abnormal
Facial Droop	have pt smile or show teeth	both sides of face move equally	one side of face does not move as well
Arm drift	with eyes closed, pt can hold arms out straight for 10 seconds	both arms move the same or not at all	one arm does not move or one arm drifts down.
Speech	ask pt to repeat a statement	Pt uses correct words with no slurring	slurs, uses the wrong words, or can't speak

Kothari RU, Pancioli A, Liu T, et al. Cincinnati Prehospital Stroke Scale. Ann of Emerg Med 1999 33(4):373-8.

NIH Stroke Scale (score "0" if normal in any category)

Assessment		Score
Motor, of each limb at 90° if sitting 45° if lying	Limb held 90°/45° drifts in < 10 seconds. Can't attain or maintain 90°/45° position. No effort against gravity No movement	1 2 3 4
Limb ataxia	Ataxia in 1 limb Ataxia in 2 limbs	1 2
Sensory*	Mild sensory loss Severe sensory loss	1 2
Language	Mild aphasia Severe aphasia Global aphasia/mute	1 2 3
Articulation	Mild slurring Severe slurring	1 2
Extinction/ Inattention to Sensory* stimulus	Unaware of bilateral stimuli to 1 of the senses Unaware of bilateral stimuli to 2 senses	1 2

Assessment		Score
LOC	Drowsy Obtunded Coma	1 2 3
Orientation to two questions	Answers one Answers neither	1 2
Response to 2 commands	Performs one Performs none	1 2
Gaze	Partial gaze palsy Complete palsy	1 2
Visual fields	Partial hemianopia Complete Bilateral	1 2 3
Facial movement	Minor paralysis Partial paralysis Total paralysis	1 2 3

*The 5 senses: taste, smell, hearing, vision, touch, and position sense

Powers WJ, Derdeyn C, Biller J, et al. 2015 AHA/ASA Focused update of the 2013 Guidelines for the early management of patients with acute ischemic stroke. Stroke, 2015;46:3020-3035.
Jauch EC, Saver JL, Adams HP, et al. Guidelines for the early management of patients with acute ischemic stroke: summary. AHA/ASA. Stroke. 2013;44:870 - 947.

Acute Ischemic Stroke

➔ ED arrival		
	STAT	ABC's if needed. Activate Stroke Team.
	O2	If needed, to maintain $SpO_2 > 94\%$.
	IV access	for immediate treatment of elevated BP, or for hypotension, or for possible administration of r-tPA.
	BG	The only lab result that must be known before r-tPA may be given. Blood Glucose must = 80 - 110 mg/dL. Other required lab: CBC, coagulation studies.
	BP	Immediate treatment of BP > 185/110
➔ < 10 mins	ECG	Check Bedside Monitor for AFib or AMI, as possible cause of embolic stroke. Order 12-lead ECG.
	Stroke onset	Identify "the last time the patient was observed to be normal." If that time was before the pt retired for the night, the pt's time "asleep" must be included.
	History	Patient's past medical history
➔ < 25 mins	Neuro Assess	Neuro Assessment (NIH Scoring System is preferred. See previous page) Remember Stroke Mimics: postictal state, systemic infection, brain tumor, hypoglycemia, hyponatremia.
	CT	Non-contrast head CT in most cases, to screen for intracranial hemorrhage. If no ICH, evaluate for r-tPA
	Temp	Fever worsens neurologic outcome. Keep T ≤ 37.5° C. Use Tylenol. ASA cannot be given 24 hrs before or after r-tPA
	BP	To be eligible for r-tPA: Systolic must be ≤ 185 mm Hg Diastolic must be ≤ 110 mm Hg
➔ < 45 mins	r-tPA	Assess for contraindications (see next page) Pt should receive r-tPA even if endovascular procedure (stent retrieval of the clot) is being considered.
➔ < 60 mins	r-tPA	This is the maximum "door-to-needle time," from door of the ED to the administration of r-tPA in the pt who: 1. is < 6 hrs since last observed to be normal, and 2. has no contraindications. No anticoagulants or antiplatelets for 24 hr after r-tPA. Activase dose: 0.9 mg/kg (maximum total dose is 90 mg)
	CXR	should not delay initiation of r-tPA
➔ ASAP	ECG-12	for AFib or AMI, but should not delay initiation of r-tPA
	Troponin	for AMI, but should not delay initiation of r-tPA

< 3 hours	from ED admit to Critical Care:
↓↑ Blood pressure:	NS 75-100 mL/hr to maintain normovolemia. Hypovolemic patients may require NS boluses, given carefully to avoid volume excess. Urgently manage hypertension (see next page).
Oxygen and Ventilation:	Ischemic brain injury is compounded by hypoxia and acidosis. Risk for aspiration or upper airway obstruction is high. Maintain PaO_2 80 - 100 mm Hg, $SaO_2 \geq 94\%$, $PaCO_2$ 35 mm Hg, pH 7.3 - 7.5
Glycemic control:	Hyperglycemia can be a marker of severe stroke. Insulin is given if BG > 185 mg/dL (> 7.8 mmol/L). Hypoglycemia must be treated urgently.
Temp:	Fever worsens neurologic outcome. Keep T ≤ 37.5° C.
If ICP increases:	Osmotherapy (mannitol or glycerol) and/or corticosteroids for malignant cerebral edema have not proven beneficial. Ventricular drain may be needed for acute hydrocephalus. Surgical decompression can be life-saving in select patients.
ASA:	If the patient is ineligible for r-tPA and hemorrhage is absent, ASA 325 mg is recommended early (within 24 - 48 hours of stroke onset).
Seizures:	Occur in 2 - 23% of patients, usually within 24 hours of stroke.

Activase for Acute Ischemic Stroke

Intravenous recombinant tissue plasminogen activator, Activase (aka r-tPA) dissolves clots (fibrinolysis).

- Benefits are substantial when given within 3 hours of symptom onset.
- Benefits are moderate when given within 3 - 6 hours of symptom onset.

Is the AIS Patient **Eligible for Fibrinolysis?**

- Diagnosis is ischemic stroke with measurable neurologic deficit.
- Time from symptom onset to initiating r-tPA is < 6 hrs.
- SBP is < 185 mm Hg and DBP is < 110 mm Hg.

↑ BP Treatment:	If the patient IS NOT eligible for r-tPA:
If SBP > 220 or If DBP >120	Control of BP is urgent in patients with acute ischemic stroke. The goal is to lower BP by 15 - 25% during the first 24 hrs. Labetalol 10-20 mg IV over 1-2 min. Dose may be repeated or doubled every 10 mins to a maximum of 300 mg.
↑ BP Treatment:	**If the patient IS eligible for r-tPA, but BP is elevated:**
If SBP > 180 or If DBP > 105	To limit the bleeding risk, BP must be controlled to < 185/110 Labetalol 10 - 20 mg over 1 - 2 mins. May repeat x 1. or Nicardipine 5 mg/hr, titrate up by 2.5 mg/hr q 5 - 15 mins, max of 15 mg/hr. When desired BP achieved, ↓ to 3 mg/h or Other agents (hydralazine, enalaprilat) If BP remains > 180/105, r-tPA cannot be given.

Absolute Contraindications to r-tPA (Activase.com, Dec 2015):
Do not administer Activase to treat acute ischemic stroke in the following situations in which the risk of bleeding is greater than the potential benefit:

- Current intracranial hemorrhage
- Subarachnoid hemorrhage
- Active internal bleeding
- Recent (within 3 months) intracranial or intraspinal surgery, or serious head trauma
- Presence of intracranial conditions that may increase the risk of bleeding (e.g., some neoplasms, arteriovenous malformations, or aneurysms)
- Bleeding diathesis platelet count < 100,000/mm^3, or on anticoagulant with INR > 1.7 or prothrombin time (PT) > 15 seconds.
- Current severe uncontrolled hypertension (SBP > 185 or DBP > 110 mm Hg)

Relative Contraindications to r-tPA (Activase.com, Dec 2015)
Risks of bleeding with Activase therapy for all approved indications are increased and should be weighed against the anticipated benefits in pts with:

- Recent major surgery or procedure, (e.g., coronary artery bypass graft, obstetrical delivery, organ biopsy, puncture of noncompressible vessels)
- Cerebrovascular disease
- Recent intracranial hemorrhage
- Recent gastrointestinal or genitourinary bleeding
- Recent trauma
- Hypertension: systolic BP > 175 mm Hg or diastolic BP > 110 mm Hg
- High likelihood of left heart thrombus, e.g., mitral stenosis with atrial fibrillation
- Acute pericarditis
- Subacute bacterial endocarditis
- Hemostatic defects including those due to severe hepatic or renal disease
- Significant hepatic dysfunction
- Pregnancy
- Diabetic hemorrhagic retinopathy, or other hemorrhagic ophthalmic conditions
- Septic thrombophlebitis or occluded AV cannula at seriously infected site
- Advanced age
- Patients currently receiving anticoagulants (e.g., warfarin sodium)
- Any other condition in which bleeding constitutes a significant hazard or would be particularly difficult to manage because of its location.

*Powers WJ, Derdeyn CP, Biller J, et al. 2015 AHA/ASA Focused Update of the 2013 Guidelines for the Early Management of Patients With Acute Ischemic Stroke Stroke, 2015;46:3020 - 3035.
Hazinski MF, et al. Adult suspected stroke. 2015 Handbook of Emergency CV Care:19-22.

Acute Ischemic Stroke (continued)

During and after rtPA:	
r-tPA Dose:	0.9 mg/kg (not to exceed 90 mg total) given as follows: 10% of total dose given as IV bolus over 1 minute, then the remaining 90% infused over 60 minutes. (see Activase.com)
Caution:	To limit the risk for bleeding, BP must be controlled. From the start of rtPA, monitor BP q 15 mins x 2 hours then q 30 mins x 6 hours, then q 1 hour x 16 hours.
If SBP >180 or If DBP > 105:	Labetalol 10 mg IV, follow with infusion 2 - 8 mg/min. or Nicardipine 5 mg/hr continuous IV, titrating up by 2.5 mg/hr q 5-15 mins if needed, to maximum of 15 mg/hr. If BP not controlled or diastolic BP > 140, Nipride is considered

Intracranial hemorrhage is the major complication of r-tPA; occurs in 5% of pts.

1. No ASA or antiplatelet agent may be given 24 hour prior to r-tPA, and for 24 hrs after, until CT shows no hemorrhage.
2. If signs of intracranial bleeding (severe HA, acute ↑ BP, nausea/vomiting), r-tPA must be discontinued immediately, followed by urgent CT. Treatment for cerebral edema or intracranial hemorrhage may follow.
3. For signs of internal bleeding, get urgent abdominal or chest CT, lab test for Hgb/Hct, PT/PTT; may need to T & C for 4 units PRBC, 4 - 6 units cryo or FFP.

Removal of Cerebral Thrombus with a Stent Retriever*	
Description:	• r-tPA should still be given to eligible patients. • Endovascular therapy requires the patient to be at an experienced stroke center with rapid access to cerebral angiography and qualified neuro interventionalists. • A Stent Retriever is a tiny wire mesh tube that once deployed, expands and entraps a thrombus. • The thrombus is removed by pulling back the deployed stent into the guide catheter, where the struts of the stent engage the thrombotic material. • The stent is slowly retrieved while the microcatheter is continuously aspirated. • The stent may be applied repeatedly until all of the thrombus is removed. The average number of passes is 3. • The most common sites for cerebral thrombectomy include ICA Internal carotid artery MCA Middle cerebral artery • Stent Retrieval should be achieved within 6 hrs of stroke onset and can be performed after r-tPA is given. • Studies support Class I, Level of Evidence A (the highest) recommendation, but only for a carefully defined patient.
Patient Criteria for use of Stent Retriever:	1. Prestroke mRS score 0 to 1, 2. Acute ischemic stroke receiving r-tPA within 4.5 hr of onset. 3. Occlusion of the ICA or proximal MCA 4. Age ≥18 years, 5. NIHSS score of ≥6, (National Institutes of Health Stroke Scale 6. ASPECTS of ≥6 (Alberta Stroke Program Early CT Score) 7. Treatment can be initiated (via groin puncture) within 6 hours of symptom onset.

Acute Stroke Patients Are At Risk for:	
Hypertensive crisis Aspiration pneumonia Upper airway obstruction Hypoventilation Another stroke	Hypoxic secondary brain injury Deep vein thrombosis Urinary tract infection Neurogenic pulmonary edema

*Excellent Video on Stent Retriever: Burathoki S. Endovascular Treatment of AS. youtube.com.

BLS by Healthcare Providers, AHA 2015

Actions	Adult or Adolescent	Child (1 yo to puberty)	Infant (< 1 yo)
Recognize:	Unconscious, no breathing (or is gasping)	Unconscious, no breathing (or is gasping)	Unconscious, no breathing (or is gasping)
Check pulse in < 10 seconds:	Check for carotid pulse. Activate Emergency Response System	Check carotid or femoral pulse. Activate Emergency Response System	Check brachial pulse. If HR < 60, activate Emergency Response
Compression: Site	Heel of 1 hand, on the lower half of the sternum. Other hand placed on the back of the first hand, keeping hands parallel,	Heel of 1 hand, or 2 hands as for adults, on the lower half of the sternum	2 fingers at midsternum, just below nipple line. If 2nd rescuer, both hands encircle the chest, compress below nipple line.
Depth	At least 2 inches (5 cm) allow complete chest recoil	at least 1/3 of the AP diameter of chest, about 2 inches (5 cm)	at least 1/3 of the AP diameter of chest, 1.5 inches (4 cm)
Rate	30 initial compressions at 100 - 120/min	30 initial compressions at 100 - 120/min	30 initial compressions at 100 - 120/min
Airway:	head tilt-chin lift, or jaw-thrust for the injured patient.	head tilt-chin lift (for both injured and uninjured)	head tilt-chin lift (for both injured and uninjured)
Compress/ventilate ratio	30:2 if 1 or 2 rescuers	30:2 if single rescuer 15:2 if two rescuers (HCP)	30:2 if single rescuer 15:2 if two rescuers (HCP)
If no artificial airway:	After 30 compressions, give 2 breaths.	1 every 3 - 5 seconds (12 - 20 breaths/minute)	1 every 3 - 5 seconds (12 - 20 breaths/minute)
If artificial airway:	1 breath every 6 seconds (10 bpm) with continuous (no pause) in compressions.	1 breath every 6 seconds (10 bpm) with continuous (no pause) in compressions.	1 breath every 6 seconds (10 bpm) with continuous (no pause) in compressions.
Self-inflating Bag:	1 - 2 L capacity, no pressure relief valve, attach O_2 at 10 - 15 LPM, give 600 mL breaths	400 - 500 mL capacity bag, attach O_2 at 10 LPM, volume according to patient size	400 - 500 mL capacity bag, attach O_2 at 10 LPM, volume according to patient size
Defibrillation x 1 for VFib or VTach, then resume CPR immediately for 2 minutes	AED: 120 - 200 J Monophasic: 360 J	initial dose of 2 J/kg subsequent dose: 4 J/kg, up to 10 J/kg, or the adult maximum dose. If AED, use of pedi attenuator is ideal.	initial dose of 2 J/kg Manual defibrillator is preferred. If AED, use of pedi attenuator is ideal.
√ pulse every 2 minutes, and change roles	If you can't detect pulse in < 10 seconds, resume CPR. Recheck q 2 min	If you can't detect pulse in < 10 seconds, resume CPR. Recheck q 2 min	If you can't detect pulse in < 10 seconds, resume CPR. Recheck q 2 min

Hazinski MF, Shuster M, Donnino MW, et al. 2015 Handbook of ECC for Healthcare Providers. American Heart Association, November, 2015.

Notes

Stat Meds

Quick CV Drips

Medication	Mix	Concentration (per mL)	Dose (See details on the pages that follow and in "Med Facts" chptr)
Amiodarone (Cordarone)	900 mg 500 mL D5W in glass	1.8 mg	Bolus: 150 mg /100 mL D5W over 10 mins. Then infuse 1 mg/min for 6 hrs, then 0.5 mg/min for 18 hrs.
Diltiazem (Cardizem)	125 mg Diltiazem 25 mL Diltiazem +100 mL D5W or NS	1 mg	Bolus: 0.25 mg/kg. If needed in 15 mins, 0.35 mg/kg over 2 min. Infuse: 5 - 15 mg/hr
Dobutamine (Dobutrex)	250 mg 250 mL D5W or NS	1,000 mcg	Infuse: 2 - 20 mcg/kg/min (up to 40 mcg/kg/min have been used).
Dopamine (Inotropin)	400 mg 250 mL D5W or NS	1,600 mcg	Infuse: 2 - 20 mcg/kg/min Higher doses vasoconstrict.
Epinephrine (Adrenalin)	1 mg 250 mL D5W or NS	4 mcg	IVP: 0.1 - 1 mg. Start infusion at 1 mcg/min, range is 2-10 mcg/min (or 0.05 - 0.1 mcg/kg/min).
Esmolol (Brevibloc)	2.5 g 250 mL D5W, NS, RL	10,000 mcg	500 mcg/kg/min x 1 min, then 50 mcg/kg/min x 5 mins, range is 50 - 200 mcg/kg/min (300 max).
Fenoldopam (Corlopam)	10 mg 250 mL D5W or NS	40 mcg	Give no IV bolus. Start infusion at 0.1 - 0.3 mcg/kg/min. Dose range is 0.025 - 0.5 mcg/kg/min
Furosemide (Lasix)	100 mg 100 mL D5W, NS, RL	1 mg	IVP: 0.1 mg/kg slowly, then Infuse: 2 - 10 mg/hr (0.1 mg/kg/hr) (maximum total is 600 mg/day).
Isoproterenol (Isuprel)	2 mg 250 mL D5W	8 mcg	Start infusion at 2 mcg/kg/min. Dose range is 2 - 20 mcg/min
Labetalol (Normodyne, Trandate)	400 mg Labetalol 80 mL Labetalol + 120 mL D5W, NS, RL	2 mg	IVP: 20 mg over 2 minutes, may repeat q 10 mins to total 300 mg. Infuse: 0.5 - 2 mg/min
Lidocaine (Xylocaine)	2 g 500 mL D5W	4 mg	Bolus: 0.5 - 0.75 mg/kg Infuse: 1 - 4 mg/min
Milrinone (Primacor)	40 mg 200 mL D5W or NS	200 mcg	Load: 50 mcg/kg over 10 minutes Infuse: 0.375 - 0.75 mcg/kg/min
Nesiritide (Natrecor)	1.5 mg 250 mL D5W or NS	6 mcg	Draw loading dose of 2 mcg/kg from mix, give over 60 seconds. Infuse: 0.01 mcg/kg/min
Nicardipine (Cardene)	25 mg 250 mL D5W or NS	0.1 mg	Start at 5 mg/hr, then ↑ by 2.5 mg/hr q 15 min to 15 mg/hr max.
Nitroglycerin	50 mg 250 mL D5W in glass (nonabsorbing tubing)	200 mcg	Load: 12.5 - 25 mcg. Start infusion at 5 mcg/min, ↑ by 5 mcg/min q 5-10 mins (max is 200 mcg/min)
Nitroprusside (Nipride)	50 mg 250 mL D5W only (protect from light)	200 mcg	Begin with 0.1 mcg/kg/min. Adjust by 0.5 - 1 mcg/kg/min q 5-15 mins Dose range is 0.1-10 mcg/kg/min.
Norepinephrine (Levophed)	4 mg 250 mL D5W	16 mcg	Start 0.5 mcg/min. Dose range is 2 - 12 mcg/min but higher doses have been used.
Phenylephrine (Neosynephrine)	20 mg 250 mL D5W or NS	80 mcg	Infuse: 100 - 180 mcg/min initially, then 40 - 60 mcg/min.
Procainamide (Pronestyl)	1 g 250 mL D5W	4 mg	Use mix to IV Load: 20 mg/min to effect, or to max of 17 mg/kg. Then Infuse 1 - 4 mg/min
Prostaglandin (Flolan)	500,000 ng 100 mL Flolan diluent	5,000 ng	Infusion started at 2 ng/kg/min. Average dose is 2 - 16 ng/kg/min
Vasopressin (Pitressin)	20 units 250 mL D5W or NS	0.08 units	Septic shock: 0.02 - 0.1 units/min

Other Quick Drips

Medication	Mix	Concentration (per mL)	Dose (See details on the following pages and in the chapters "Med Facts" and "Drip Tables")
Aminocarproic acid (Amicar)	5 g / 250 mL D5W or NS	0.02 gram	5 g/hr (250 mL/hr) for first hour, then 1 g/hr (50 mL/hr) for 8 hrs (max of 30 g/24 hr)
Aminophylline (lower dose for pt on theophylline)	500 mg / 500 mL D5W or NS	1 mg	IV load: 2.5 - 6 mg/kg given in 100 mL D5W no faster than 25 mg/min Infuse: 0.25 - 0.75 mg/kg/hr
Atracurium (Tracrium)	50 mg / 100 mL D5W or NS	0.5 mg	Bolus: 0.4 - 0.5 mg/kg Infuse: 5 - 15 mcg/kg/min
Cisatracurium (Nimbex)	40 mg / 100 mL D5W or NS	0.4 mg	IVP: 0.1 - 0.2 mg/kg. Continuous infusion range is 0.5-10 mcg/kg/min
Dexmedetomidine (Precedex)	200 mcg / 50 mL NS	4 mcg	Load: 1 mcg/kg/min over 10 mins. Infuse: 0.2 - 0.7 mcg/kg/hr < 24 hr.
Doxacurium (Nuromax)	10 mg / 100 mL D5W or NS	0.1 mg	IVP: 0.025 - 0.05 mg/kg Infuse: 0.3 - 0.5 mcg/kg/min
Fentanyl (Sublimase)	1 mg / 100 mL D5W or NS	10 mcg	IVP: 25 - 100 mcg q 1 hr. Infuse 25-200 mcg/hr (or 0.5-2 mcg/kg/hr)
Glucagon	10 mg / 100 mL D5W or NS	0.1 mg	*for severe hypoglycemia:* IVP: 0.5 - 1 mg, Infuse: 1 - 5 mg/hr
Haloperidol (Haldol)	50 mg / 50 mL D5W or NS	1 mg	IVP: 2.5 mg q 20 mins until sedated Infuse: 3 - 10 mg/hr (or 0.01 - 0.15 mg/kg/hr)
Heparin	12,500 units / 250 mL D5W or NS	50 units	50 - 80 units/kg loading dose, then Infuse: 12 - 18 units/kg/hr
Hydromorphone (Dilaudid)	40 mg / 200 mL D5W or NS	0.2 mg	IVP: 0.5 - 2 mg (10 mcg/kg) slowly. Infuse: 7 - 15 mcg/kg/hr
Insulin	125 units / 250 mL NS	0.5 units	Start infusion at 0.1 units/kg/hr or about 5 - 10 units/hr
Levosimendan (Simdax)	35 mg / 500 mL D5W	50 mcg	IVP: 6 - 12 mcg/kg over 10 minutes Infuse: 0.05 to 0.2 mcg/kg/min
Lorazepam (Ativan)	10 mg / 100 mL D5W or NS (in glass)	0.1 mg	IVP: the smaller of 0.044 mg/kg or 2 mg total; Infuse: 0.5 - 2 mg/hr (or 0.01 - 0.1 mg/kg/hr).
Magnesium Sulfate	4 g / 100 mL D5W or NS	0.04 gram	*Cardiac arrest due to Torsades or ↓ Mg* 1-2 g in 10 mL D5W over 5-20 mins *Torsades with pulse or AMI with ↓ Mg:* 1-2 g in 75 mL D5W over 30-60 min Infuse: 0.5 - 1 g/hr
Midazolam (Versed)	50 mg / 250 mL D5W or NS 100 mg / 200 mL D5W or NS	0.2 mg 0.5 mg	IVP: 1 mg over 2 mins, may repeat in 2 mins, titrating to effect. To maintain sedation: infuse 1 - 7 mg/hr
Morphine	20 mg / 100 mL D5W or NS	0.2 mg	IVP: 1-5 mg (diluted) over 3-5 mins. Infuse: 1 - 5 mg/hr
Naloxone (Narcan)	5 mg / 250 mL D5W or NS	0.02 mg	IVP: 0.1 - 2 mg for opiate overdose. Infuse: 0.4 mg/hr
Octreotide (Sandostatin)	500 mcg / 250 mL NS	2 mcg	IVP for GI bleeding: 25 - 50 mcg Infuse: 25 - 50 mcg/hr
Pentobarbital (Nembutal)	1000 mg / 250 mL D5W or NS	4 mg	For pento coma, load 2 - 10 mg/kg over 1 - 2 hrs, then 0.5 - 3 mg/kg/hr
Potassium	10 mEq / 100 mL D5W or NS 200 mEq / 1000 mL	0.1 mEq 0.2 mEq	**WARNING: CONCENTRATED!** **Give through Central line only!** Infuse: no faster than 10 mEq/hr Monitor ECG.
Propofol (Diprivan)	500 mg / 50 mL emulsion	10 mg	Start infusion with 5 mcg/kg/min Infuse: 5 - 50 mcg/kg/min
Vecuronium (Norcuron)	20 mg / 100 mL D5W or NS	200 mcg	IVP pre intubation: 80 - 100 mcg/kg Infuse: 0.8 - 1.2 mcg/kg/min

Medication	Description	Prep and Dose	Adverse Effects	Contraindications
Adenosine (Adenocard) (given by physician only in some institutions)	An endogenous nucleoside that slows conduction through the AV node. For treatment of stable narrow-complex Paroxysmal Supraventricular Tachycardia (PSVT), as well as PSVT with WPW. Does not convert AFib, AFlutter, or VT. Extremely short half-life (< 10 seconds).	Prep: 3 mg/mL in 2 mL vial & 4 mL syringe IVP: Use injection site closest to the heart, 6 mg rapidly over 1 - 2 seconds, follow with 20 mL NS flush. Record rhythm. If no response in 1 - 2 mins, may give 12 mg. May repeat this 12 mg dose in 1 - 2 minutes if needed.	Transient AVB or brief period of asystole (< 15 sec) is common. PAC's, PVC's, bradycardia, sinus tachycardia, shortness of breath, wheezing, dyspnea, facial flush, HA, ↓↑ BP, VFib, nausea, chest pain, palpitations, dizziness.	2° or 3° AVB Sick sinus syndrome WPW with wide QRS Ventricular Tach Bronchospasm Asthma or Bronchitis Bradycardia
Aminocaproic acid (Amicar, EACA)	Antifibrinolytic that inhibits plasminogen activator substance and plasmin. Used to control bleeding in states of hyperfibrinolysis (postoperative heart surgery, portocaval shunt, abruptio placentae, carcinoma). Used to prevent rebleeding in aneurysmal subarachnoid hemorrhage (see PI for dosage)	Prep: 250 mg/mL in 20 mL vial (5 g total) Mix: <u>5 g</u> / 250 mL NS, D5W, or RL — Concentration = 0.02 g/mL To control active bleeding: Load: 5 g (250 mL/hr) during first hour Infuse: 1 g (50 mL/hr) for 8 hrs until bleeding controlled (max of 30 g/24h).	Rapid administration may cause ↓ BP, ↓ HR, dysrhythmias. Confusion, seizures, dizziness. Nausea, cramps, diarrhea. Myopathy, muscle weakness, Potential for thrombosis (rare). Overdose can cause renal failure.	Any evidence of intravascular clotting
Aminophylline	A xanthine bronchodilator that directly relaxes smooth muscle of the bronchial airways and pulmonary blood vessels. For treatment of acute bronchial asthma and for bronchospasm associated with chronic bronchitis and emphysema. Also used for status asthmaticus. Has respiratory, cardiac, cerebral stimulant effects. Therapeutic theophylline level is 10 - 15 μg/mL (or 10 - 15 mg/L) and < 10 μg/mL in patients > 60 years old.	Prep: 250 mg as 25 mg/mL in 10 mL syringe 500 mg as 25 mg/mL in 20 mL syringe. Load: Usually given over 30 minutes. *<u>For pt currently receiving theophylline:</u>* 2.5 mg/kg given in 100 mL D5W. *<u>For pt not already receiving theophylline:</u>* 5 - 6 mg/kg given in 100 mL D5W give no faster than 25 mg/min. Mix: <u>500 mg</u> / 500 mL D5W or NS — Concentration = 1 mg/mL Infuse: 0.25 mg - 0.75 mg/kg/hr	Rarely occur when serum theophylline levels < 20 μg/mL. If > 20: N/V, anorexia, diarrhea, irritability, restlessness, tremor, insomnia, headache. If > 35: Tachycardia, palpitations, extrasystoles, arrhythmias, hypotension, seizures, respiratory arrest. Reduce dose in patients with heart failure, liver disease, or cor pulmonale.	Allergy to xanthine Active peptic ulcer Seizure disorder Caution in patients with coronary artery disease, hypoxemia, or hypertension. Severe renal or hepatic impairment.

Medication	Description	Prep and Dose	Adverse Effects	Contraindications
Amiodarone (Cordarone)	An antiarrhythmic with effects on Na,K, Ca channels. Slows AV conduction. Prolongs refractoriness, has vasodilatory and negative chronotropic effects. For prevention and treatment of recurrent VFib and monomorphic VTach. For stable, narrow complex tachycardia. An alternative for rate control in AFib when beta blocker is contraindicated.	Prep: 50 mg/mL in 3 mL amp, and 900 mg in 18 mL vial. IVP: cardiac arrest: 300 mg in 30 mL NS. Then, if needed, may give 150 mg over 3 - 5 min Load: 150 mg in 100 D5W over 10 minutes Mix: 900 mg / 500 mL D5W in glass. Concentration. = 1.8 mg/mL Don't use if cloudy/discolored Infuse: 1 mg/min (33 mL/hr) x 6 hrs, then: 0.5 mg/min (17 mL/hr) x 18 hrs. If VTach recurs, repeat loading dose. Maximum total daily dose is 2 g.	Hypotension in 16% of patients (related to rate of infusion), Bradycardia (occurs in 5%), AVB, New onset VTach /VFib, asystole, Torsades de Pointes, Anaphylaxis, Cardiogenic shock, Heart Failure, Elevated liver enzymes, ↓ K, ↓ Mg, Nausea, Hepatic injury, Pulmonary fibrosis.	Iodine allergy. Cardiogenic shock, Marked sinus brady, 2° or 3° AVB. Due to negative inotropic effect, use with caution in LV dysfunction. Correct ↓ K, ↓ Mg before giving.
Argatroban	A direct inhibitor of thrombin, interfering with fibrin formation, activation of factors V, VIII, XIII, protein C, and platelets. For the prevention and treatment of thrombosis in patients with Heparin Induced Thrombocytopenia (HIT). For PCI patients who have or are at risk for HIT.	Prep: 100 mg/mL in 2.5 mL vial IVP: NA Mix: 250 mg / 250 mL D5W or NS (invert to mix x 2 minutes) Concentration = 1 mg/mL Infuse: For prevention/treatment of thrombosis in adults with HIT: 2 *mcg*/kg/min (if pt has hepatic insufficiency, then 0.5 *mcg*/kg/min.) For HIT patient undergoing PCI: IVP: 350 *mcg*/kg over 3 - 5 mins, then Infuse: 25 *mcg*/kg/min, adjusting according to ACT.	Bleeding, Hypotension, Allergic reaction: fever, cough, dyspnea, rash, vasodilation, chest pain, back pain. Patients with hepatic insufficiency should receive a lower dose.	Bleeding tendency or overt bleeding. Hypersensitivity. Extreme caution in postoperative pts.
Atenolol (Tenormin)	β1 selective adrenoreceptor blocker for treatment of hypertension (lowers Sys and Dias BP by 15 - 20%), SVT and chronic angina. In hemodynamically stable AMI patients, limits infarct size, reduces incidence of dysrhythmias, and reduces mortality rate.	Prep: 0.5 mg/mL in 10 mL amp IVP: 5 mg (diluted in NS or D5W) over 5 minutes (at rate of 1 mg/min) may repeat in 10 minutes. PO: 50 mg po q 12 hrs x 6-9 days after AMI.	Pronounced fatigue and/or cold extremities in 10 - 20% of pts. Dizziness, ↓ HR, ↓ BP, conduction defects. Caution in pts with bronchospastic disease. Caution: B-blocker may prohibit compensatory tachycardia in pts with low BG or hypovolemia.	2° and 3° AVB, Symptomatic heart failure, Cardiogenic shock, Pulmonary edema, Sinus bradycardia.

Medication	Description	Prep and Dose	Adverse Effects	Contraindications
Atropine	Anticholinergic used as preop med to reduce pulmonary secretions. Enhances SA node automaticity and AV node conduction, reverses cholinergic mediated decreases in HR, SVR, BP. Drug of choice to treat symptomatic bradycardia. May benefit asystole and PEA. Antidote to insecticide poisoning.	Prep: 0.1 mg/mL, 0.4 mg/mL, 0.6 mg/mL, 0.8 mg/mL, and 1 mg/mL IVP: *for bradycardia:* 0.5 mg, repeat if needed every 3 - 5 minutes, not to exceed total dose of 0.04 mg/kg (3 mg total) *for asystole/PEA:* Atropine is no longer recommended in the ACC/AHA ACLS guidelines for Asystole/PEA.	Tachycardia (may exacerbate myocardial ischemia and could induce VTach/VFib), arrhythmia, ↓ pulmonary secretions, dry mouth, blurred vision, dilated pupils, tremor, disorientation, N/V, urinary retention. Physostigmine is the antidote to Atropine.	Obstructive GI disease Paralytic ileus Glaucoma Obstructive renal disease Mobitz Type II block (could cause paradoxical bradycardia). Unlikely to be effective for hypothermic bradycardia.
Bivalirudin (Angiomax)	Direct thrombin inhibitor, to: • reduce risk of acute ischemia in those undergoing PCI • reduce the incidence of HIT in patients undergoing PCI • replace heparin in patients with HIT undergoing cardiac surgery. • Intended for use with Aspirin. • After termination of infusion, coagulation returns to normal in 1 - 2 hrs. Incidence of bleeding is less than that of Heparin.	Prep: 250 mg/vial, reconstitute with 5 mL SWFI Mix: 250 mg/50 mL D5W or NS = 5 mg/mL *or* 250 mg/500 mL = 0.5 mg/mL IVP: *For Percutaneous Coronary Intervention:* Infuse: 0.75 mg/kg, followed by 1.75 mg/kg per hr for the duration of PCI, and/or for 4 hours post PCI, IVP: *For HIT patients undergoing PCI* Infuse: 0.75 mg/kg, followed by 1.75 mg/kg per hr for the duration of the procedure. Infusion may be continued for up to 4 hours, after which a rate of 0.2 mg/kg/hr can be used for up to 20 more hours, if needed.	Back pain, nausea, headache. Anaphylactic shock, death. Hemorrhage can occur at any site. Investigate any decrease in hemoglobin or in blood pressure. ***Reduced doses for PCI patients:* For PCI pts with CrCl < 30 mL: same bolus dose of 0.75 mg/kg, but reduce infusion to 1 mg/kg/hr. For PCI pts being treated with hemodialysis, reduce infusion to 0.25 mg/kg/hr.	Allergy to Bivalirudin. Preexisting bleeding disorders of any origin.
Bumetanide (Bumex)	A sulfonamide loop diuretic for edema caused by heart failure, hepatic or renal disease, or edema unresponsive to other diuretics, or if sensitive to other diuretics. 1 mg Bumex = 40 mg Lasix.	Prep: 0.25 mg/mL in 2, 4, 10 mL vials IVP: 1 mg over 1 - 2 minutes, may repeat q 2 - 3 hrs not to exceed max of 10 mg/24 hr. Mix: 5 mg / 100 D5W, NS Concentration = 0.05 mg/mL Protect from light Infuse: 0.5 - 2 mg/hr	↑ Blood glucose, ↑ BUN, ↓ K, ↓ Na, ↓ Cl, ↓ Ca and tetany. ↓ BP, dizziness, headache, Encephalopathy in pts with hepatic disease, Dehydration, Ototoxicity, Muscle cramps.	Allergy to sulfonamides. Anuria. Discontinue if there is marked increase in BUN or Creatinine. Electrolyte depletion. Hepatic coma.

Medication	Description	Prep and Dose	Adverse Effects	Contraindications
Buprenorphine (Buprenex)	A synthetic opioid agonist-antagonist. 0.3 mg Buprenex = 10 mg of morphine in analgesic and respiratory depressant effect. For moderate to severe pain.	Prep: 0.3 mg/mL in 1 mL amp or vial. IVP: 0.3 mg over 2 mins, q 6-8 hrs Mix: 1.5 mg / 250 mL D5W, D5NS, NS, or RL Concentration = 6 mcg/mL Infuse: 25 - 250 mcg/hr	Sedation, CNS depression, N/V, dizziness, ↓ HR, ↑↓ BP, respiratory depression, HA. May ↑ ICP, use with caution in patients with head injury. Naloxone may not reverse respiratory depression caused by Buprenex.	Allergy to Buprenex. Caution in elderly, or those with respiratory depression. Fatal respiratory depression if taken with benzodiazepine or CNS depressants. Can cause withdrawal in narcotic addicted patients.
Calcium Chloride 1 g has 273 mg of elemental calcium	To enhance myocardial contractility. To treat ↓ Ca, ↑ K, ↑ Mg, or toxicity with calcium channel blockers. Used after cardiac surgery when epinephrine fails to ↑ cardiac output Although both CaCl and Calcium Gluconate are supplied as 100 mg/mL, CaCl has 3 times the amount of calcium than Calcium Gluconate.	Prep: 1 g in 10 mL vial = 100 mg/mL IVP: *Hypocalcemic Tetany:* 1000 mg undiluted given slowly (1 mL/min) into a central vein. *Symptomatic Hypocalcemia:* 500 mg over 10 minutes, then 1000 mg over the next 6 - 12 hours, while measuring Ca levels q 4-6 hrs and correcting Mg, K, and pH. *CCB toxicity:* 500 - 1000 mg over 10 mins. *PEA/asystole:* No longer recommended in the ACLS guidelines for Asystole/PEA	Nausea, flushing, peripheral vasodilation, hypotension, arrhythmias. Extravasation can result in severe tissue injury. If given too fast, vasomotor collapse, cardiac arrest. Precipitates in alkaline solution. Central line recommended.	Hypercalcemia. Cardiac resuscitation in the presence of VFib, Asystole, or Pulseless Electrical Activity. Caution in patients on digoxin. Can cause digoxin toxicity and/or arrhythmias.
Calcium Gluconate 1 g has 93 mg of elemental calcium	Being less concentrated, Calcium Gluconate is less irritating to the veins than is Calcium Chloride. To avoid confusion and insure patient safety, hospitals are encouraged to stock Calcium Chloride **or** Calcium Gluconate **but not both.**	Prep: 1 g in 10 mL vial = 100 mg/mL IVP: *Hypocalcemic Tetany:* 1000 mg followed by 4 g daily by continuous IV until Ca level is normal *Symptomatic Hypocalcemia:* (0.5 x kg x 24)/93 mg = Ca Gluconate to add to 500 - 1000 mL D5W or NS, infuse at 0.3 - 2 mg/kg/hr, while monitoring Calcium. *Calcium Channel Blocker Toxicity*: 30 mL of 10% calcium gluconate IV over 10 - 15 min. May repeat every 15 - 20 minutes for a total of 3 doses Then check ionized Ca level.	See Calcium Chloride,	See Calcium Chloride contraindications listed above.

Medication	Description	Prep and Dose	Adverse Effects	Contraindications
Clevidipine butyrate (Cleviprex)	A calcium channel blocker for treatment of increased BP. Reduces mean arterial blood pressure by decreasing systemic vascular resistance. Does not affect venous capacity, cardiac filling pressure, or preload. Metabolism is rapid (terminal half-life is about 15 mins) and independent of the liver and kidneys. Dose adjustment for patients with renal or hepatic dysfunction is not necessary.	Prep: Pre-mixed, ready-to-use 50 mL & 100 mL vials, milky lipid emulsion, can be given via central or peripheral line. Should not be given into same line as other meds; but can piggyback to D5W, NS, D5NS, D5RL, LR. Protection from light not required. IVP: NA Infuse: Start at 1 - 2 mg/hr A 1 - 2 mg/hour increase will generally produce a 2 - 4 mm Hg decrease in systolic blood pressure. The desired effect usually occurs at doses of 4 - 6 mg/hour. Max dose is 16 mg/hr (but some patients have required up to 32 mg/hr)	Most common adverse reactions (> 2%) are headache, nausea, vomiting. Hypotension and reflex tachycardia may occur with rapid upward titration. Can produce negative inotropic effects and exacerbate heart failure. Provides no protection against the effects of abrupt beta-blocker withdrawal.	Allergies to soybeans, soy products, eggs, or egg products. Defective lipid metabolism such as pathologic hyper-lipemia, lipoid nephrosis, or acute pancreatitis with hyperlipidemia. Patients with severe aortic stenosis.
Demadex (Torsemide)	A diuretic of the sulfonylurea class that ↑ excretion of Na, Cl, and water. For treatment of edema associated with heart failure, renal failure, hepatic disease. Also used for treatment of hypertension.	Prep: 10 mg/mL in 2 mL amp or 5 mL vial IVP: 5 - 20 mg over more than 2 minutes Mix: 50 mg / 500 mL D5W, NS Concentration = 0.1 mg/mL Infuse: 3 mg/hr	HA, dizziness, N/V, nervousness, weakness, ototoxicity, hypotension, electrolyte imbalance, hypokalemia may induce arrhythmias.	Anuria, Allergy to sulfa, Lactation, Caution in those with liver failure (change in fluid and electrolytes can precipitate hepatic coma)
Desmo-pressin (DDAVP)	Synthetic analogue of ADH. Replace-ment for neurogenic causes of Diabetes Insipidus. Also maintains hemostasis in hemophilia A and in patients with von Willebrand's disease. Off label use: bleeding following cardiac surgery.	Prep: 4 mcg/mL in 1 mL amp and 10 mL vial. IVP: For Diabetes Insipidus: 1 - 4 mcg qd For bleeding: 0.3 mcg/kg, diluted in 50 mL NS given over 15 - 30 mins.	↑↓ BP, tachycardia, HA, nausea, abd cramps (which dissipate when dose is reduced), hyponatremia, water intoxication.	Correct fluid and electrolyte imbalance before giving DDAVP. Caution in patients with CAD or hypertension, may cause tachycardia.

Medication	Description	Prep and Dose	Adverse Effects	Contraindications
Dexmedetomidine (Precedex)	An alpha-2 adrenergic receptor agonist, with sedative, analgesic, sympatholytic, and hypnotic effects. For sedation of initially intubated, ventilated ICU pts. Does not cause respiratory depression, can be given during weaning from mechanical ventilation and after extubation. Reduces the requirement for morphine. Maintains arousable state.	Prep: 100 *mcg*/mL in a 2 mL clear glass vial IVP: Never give undiluted Mix: $\frac{200 \text{ mcg}}{50 \text{ mL NS}}$ Concentration = 4 mcg/mL Load: 1 mcg/kg over 10 minutes, then Infuse: 0.2 - 0.7 *mcg*/kg/hr, not to be given for longer than 24 hrs. Reduce dose in patients with impaired hepatic or renal function.	Bradycardia and hypotension (may be more pronounced in patients with hypovolemia, diabetes, or hypertension). Effects enhanced when given with other sedatives, hypnotics, or opioids. Does not cause respiratory depression.	Caution in patients who depend on sympathetic tone (e.g., bradycardia, LV dysfunction, AVB). Correct hypovolemia before giving Precedex. Caution in patients who are receiving other vasodilators or negative chronotropic agents.
Digoxin (Lanoxin)	A cardiac glycoside that increases contractility, slows the heart rate, and slows conduction through the AV node. May be used to control ventricular response in symptomatic AFib, AFlutter, and PSVT (but Diltiazem and β-blockers are preferred for this purpose). Used for heart failure, although ACE inhibitors are first choice. No longer considered an emergency drug.	Prep: 0.25 mg/mL (250 *mcg*/mL) in 2 mL amp IVP: Digitalize: 0.5 mg, then 0.25 mg in 6 hr then 0.25 mg in 6 hr, then maintenance at 0.125 - 0.375 mg/day Give IV dose over 5 minutes. ↓ dose for patients with renal failure. Signs of Toxicity: Confusion, fatigue, weakness, N/V, anorexia, abdominal pain, diarrhea, ↓ ST segment, prolonged PR, bigeminy, HA, blurred or yellow vision, halos around objects	Almost every arrhythmia - PVC, bigeminal or trigeminal pattern, bradycardia, VTach, VFib, AVB, PSVT, AV Dissociation. Anorexia, N/V, psychosis, visual disturbances, mesenteric or myocardial ischemia. Toxicity can be precipitated by ↓ K, ↓ Mg, ↑ Ca. Keep Dig level 0.5 - 2 ng/mL. Toxic level is > 2.5 ng/mL.	Hypersensitivity. Aortic stenosis, AV Block, Sinus node disease. VFib. Electrical cardioversion of pt with digoxin toxicity can lead to fatal ventricular dysrhythmia. In patients with WPW, digoxin could cause very rapid ventricular response.
Digoxin Immune Fab (Digibind)	For the treatment of Digoxin or Digitoxin toxicity with: life-threatening arrhythmia, shock, heart failure, hyperkalemia, or digoxin level >10 - 15 ng/mL. Average dose is 10 vials (400 mg). 20 vials (800 mg) have been given.	Prep: 40 mg/vial. Reconstitute each vial with 4 mL sterile water to equal 10 mg/mL. Infuse over 30 minutes. Dose is the *number of vials* needed: For OD: $\frac{\text{Total mg ingested}}{0.5}$ For Dig Toxicity: $\text{Dose} = \frac{\text{serum digoxin in ng/mL)(wt in kg)}}{100}$	Allergic reaction, anaphylaxis (rare). Heart failure in patients dependent on the inotropic support. Recurrent AFib. May cause serious drop in serum Potassium. Dig levels will be meaningless for 7 days after Digibind use.	Hypersensitivity. Should perform skin test if patient previously exposed to Digibind. Other causes of Digoxin toxicity should be corrected.

Medication	Description	Prep and Dose	Adverse Effects	Contraindications
Diltiazem (Cardizem)	Calcium channel blocker with potent negative chronotropic and mild negative inotropic effects. Slows AV node conduction. For acute AFib and AFlutter, in the absence of WPW or short PR. For PSVT (prevents atrial reentry). A coronary vasodilator to treat angina and a peripheral vasodilator for treatment of hypertension.	Prep: 5 mg/mL in 5, 10, & 25 mL vials. IVP: 0.25 mg/kg (15 - 20 mg) over 2 mins. if inadequate response, wait 15 mins, then 0.35 mg/kg over 2 minutes. Mix: 125 mg / 25 mL Diltiazem + 100 D5W, NS Concentration = 1 mg/mL Infuse: 5 - 15 mg/hr Titrate to HR Dose limit is 15 mg/hr. Infuse no longer than 24 hours.	Hypotension, flushing, HA, 2° or 3° AVB, bradycardia, asystole, VTach, VFib, left ventricular failure, dyspnea. peripheral edema, chest pain, nausea, vomiting, dry mouth, constipation, anorexia, angina, nervousness, insomnia, injection site reaction. Rare cases of hepatic injury.	WPW (Diltiazem can cause life-threatening ↑ HR and ↓ BP), short PR, SSS (can cause asystole), 2° and 3° AVB, VTach, Severe heart failure, ↓ BP, Cardiogenic shock, SBP < 90 mm Hg. Should not be given within a few hrs of IV beta blocker.
Dobutamine (Dobutrex)	Synthetic catecholamine with direct inotropic effect due to beta receptor stimulation, and with mild chrontropic and vasodilatory effects. Improves cardiac output by improving stroke volume. For short term treatment of depressed contractility in the absence of shock. Half-life is only 2 minutes.	Prep 250 mg in 20 mL vial (12.5 mg/mL) IVP: NA Mix #1: 250 mg / 250 mL D5W, NS Concentration = 1 mg/mL Mix #2: 500 mg / 250 mL D5W, NS, D5NS, RL (Incompatible with alkaline solutions; OK if solution is pink) Concentration = 2 mg/mL Infuse: 0.5 - 1 mcg/kg/min to start, then ↑ by 2 mcg/kg/min q 15 mins as needed. 2 - 20 mcg/kg/min is usual dose range.	Dose related tachycardia can cause myocardial ischemia, PVC's, and ↑ infarct size. ↑ ventricular response to AFib, palpitations, chest pain, ↑ or ↓ BP (may be precipitous) Headache, nausea, tremor, ↓ K, dyspnea, Tissue necrosis if dobutamine infiltrates.	Hypersensitivity (possibly due to sulfite). Idiopathic hypertropic subaortic stenosis, Tachycardia, Ventricular dysrhythmia. Correct hypovolemia before giving. Use with extreme caution after AMI.
Dopamine (Intropin)	Catecholamine precursor of norepinephrine and epinephrine with inotropic, chronotropic, and vasoactive effects. For shock due to heart failure, cardiac surgery, and for hypotension unresponsive to fluids. No longer recommended for acute oliguric renal failure. Treatment of Atropine-resistant bradycardia.	Prep: 40 mg/mL in 5 mL; 80 mg/mL in 5 mL. IVP: NA Mix #1: 200 mg / 250 mL D5W, NS,D5NS, RL Concentration = 800 mcg/mL Mix #2: 400 mg / 250 mL D5W, NS, D5NS, RL Concentration =1600 mcg/mL Dopamine is inactivated in alkaline solution. Infuse: 2 - 20 mcg/kg/min	At low dose, may ↓ BP. High doses ↑ HR and ↑ SVR. Tachycardia, ↑ MVO_2, PVC's, Myocardial ischemia, Atrial and ventricular arrhythmias, Renal ischemia at high dose, HA, dyspnea, N/V, Peripheral vasoconstriction, that may progress to necrosis.	Sensitivity to sulfites. Tachycardia, ↑ BP, Pheochromocytoma, Ventricular dysrhythmias, MAO inhibitors (can cause hypertensive crisis). Correct hypovolemia before giving Dopamine.

Medication	Description	Prep and Dose	Adverse Effects	Contraindications
Enalapril Vasotec	Angiotensin converting enzyme inhibitor (ACEI) decreases the formation of angiotensin II, to decrease vasopressor activity and decrease aldosterone secretion. For treatment of heart failure, hypertension, AMI.	Prep: 1.25 mg/mL in 1 mL and 2 mL vials. IVP: *For hypertension:* 1.25 mg (1 mL) over 5 mins may repeat in 1 hr, then 1.25 mg q 6 hr. *For pts with renal impairment or are on diuretics:* 0.625 mg (0.5 mL) over 5 minutes, may repeat in 1 hr, then 1.25 mg q 6 hr.	Cough, dizziness, headache. Hypotension which can cause renal failure, MI, cardiac arrest. Hyperkalemia, Angioedema (rare but life-threatening), hepatic necrosis/failure, Abd. pain, N/V, chest pain.	Hypersensitivity, aortic stenosis, hyperkalemia, hypotension, oliguria, renal failure, history of angioedema. Pregnancy (can harm or cause death of fetus)
Epinephrine 1:1,000 (Adrenalin)	Potent catecholamine with both α- and β- adrenergic agonist effect. Increases HR, BP, SVR, cerebral & coronary blood flow, myocardial O_2 demand, contractility, and automaticity. For PEA, asystole, bradycardia, or VTach or VFib unresponsive to defibrillation. Also for severe hypotension, anaphylactic shock, bronchospasm.	Prep: 1 mg/mL in 1 mL amp IVP: *For cardiac arrest:* 1 mg q 3 - 5 mins (dilute each 1 mg in 10 mL NS, or use 1:10,000 where 0.1 mg/mL = 1 mg/10 mL) *For anaphylactic reaction:* 0.1 - 0.25 mg *For profound bradycardia:* 0.5 mg ET: 2 - 2.5 mg diluted in 10 mL NS Mix: 1 mg / 250 mL D5W, NS — Concentration = 4 mcg/mL (Discard if fluid brown) Incompatible with alkaline solutions Infuse: 0.04 - 0.1 mcg/kg/min (or 1 - 10 mcg/min)	↑ BP, HA, N/V, tremors, anxiety, sweating, ↑ MVO_2, myocardial ischemia, pulmonary edema, dyspnea, tachycardia, ventricular arrhythmias, stroke, renal ischemia. Dose > 20 μg/min can result in hypertension. Tissue necrosis if infiltrates.	Cardiogenic or hemorrhagic shock, cerebral vascular disease, aortic aneurysm, narrow angle glaucoma, cardiac dilation, coronary insufficiency, α blocker overdose (giving Epi can cause irreversible ↓ in BP).
Esmolol (Brevibloc)	β-1 selective adrenergic receptor blocking agent for treatment of noncompensatory sinus tach, SVT, hypertension, and to control heart rate in AFib and AFlutter. Very short half life (10 minutes).	Prep: 100 mg in 10 mL vial (10 mg/mL) and 100 mg in 5 mL (20 mg/mL) IVP: 500 mcg/kg over 1 minute. Premix: 2.5 g/250 mL = 10,000 mcg/mL or 2 g/100 mL = 20,000 mcg/mL Infuse: 50 mcg/kg/min for 5 mins. To titrate: Increase by 50 mcg/kg/min q 5-10 mins. Repeat loading dose when infusion dose is increased. Dose range is 50-200 mcg/kg/min May continue infusion up to 48 hrs. Do not abruptly discontinue; taper down.	Hypotension (in 20-50% of pts) diaphoresis, pallor, flushing, bradycardia, heart block, heart failure, sudden cardiac death. Dizziness, confusion, HA, N/V, fever, bronchospasm, infusion site reaction, peripheral ischemia, increase in digoxin level.	Sinus bradycardia, 2° or 3° AVB, cardiogenic shock, heart failure, pulmonary edema. Caution in patients with reactive airway disease.

Emergency Meds

Medication	Description	Prep and Dose	Adverse Effects	Contraindications
Etomidate (Amidate)	Hypnotic without analgesic activity, with rapid onset (within 1 minute) and short duration (usually 3 - 5 minutes). For induction of anesthesia, and for rapid sequence intubation.	Prep: 2 mg/mL in 10 & 20 mg single dose vial IVP: 0.2 - 0.6 mg/kg, with usual dose of 0.3 mg/kg, injected over a period of 30 to 60 seconds.	Transient venous pain at site of injection, transient skeletal muscle movements, hyper or hypoventilation, transient apnea, laryngospasm, ↑↓ BP, ↑↓ HR, arrhythmias.	Pts with hypersensitivity to etomidate. Due to its suppression of cortisol and aldosterone, not intended for prolonged use.
Fenoldopam (Corlopam)	Rapid acting vasodilator with selective D1-Dopamine receptor effect. For emergency treatment of hypertension. Potential use in heart failure. Has short term effects (half life = 5 minutes) Fewer toxicities than Nipride.	Prep: 10 mg/mL in 1 mL, 2 mL, 4 mL ampuls IVP: Give no IV bolus. Mix: 10 mg / 250 mL NS, D5W. Concentration = 40 mcg/mL Infuse: 0.1 - 0.3 mcg/kg/min initially. Adjust by 0.05 - 0.1 mcg/kg/min q 15 mins. Dose range is 0.025 - 0.5 mcg/kg/min.	↑ HR if dose > 0.1 mcg/kg/min. Headache, flushing, N/V, ↓ K. Hypotension, MI, heart failure. Use with caution in patients with cerebral hemorrhage, angina, infarction, cirrhosis, glaucoma.	Sulfite sensitivity. Caution in glaucoma, may ↑ intraocular pressure. Avoid use with β-blockers.
Fentanyl (Sublimase)	Potent narcotic analgesic, rapid onset (peak effect IV in 6-7 min.) Equagesic doses: Fentanyl 100 mcg Morphine 10 mg Hydromorphone 1.5 mg Demerol 75 mg	Prep: 0.05 mg/mL (50 mcg/mL) IVP: 25 -100 mcg (or 0.5 - 2 mcg/kg) given slowly (over several mins) q 1 - 2 hrs Mix: 1 mg / 100 mL D5W, NS Concentration = 10 mcg/mL Infuse: 25 - 100 mcg/hr (0.5 - 2 mcg/kg/hr) Prolonged infusion -> accumulation in tissues -> extended effect after dc'd.	Respiratory depression is dose-related and may last longer than the analgesic effect. Muscle rigidity: ventilating pt may be impossible if dose is high or is given too rapidly. If given with tranquilizer: ↓ BP, ↓ HR Other: N/V, Torsades de pointes, bronchoconstriction.	Known intolerance to the drug or to other opioids. Caution in head injury and ↑ ICP - may obscure assessment and/or depress respiration. If high dose (> 10 mcg/kg), mechanical ventilation will be required.
Flumazenil (Mazicon Romazicon)	Benzodiazepine receptor antagonist for reversal of sedative effect of benzo-diazepine and benzodiazepine overdose. Monitor for residual benzodiazepine effect, and repeat dose/s if needed. Has no effect in absence of benzodiazepine.	Prep: 0.1 mg/mL in 5 mL and 10 mL vial. IVP: *to reverse Benzodiazepine*: 0.2 mg over 15 seconds, repeat with 0.2 mg q 60 sec for 4 more doses or to total of 1 mg *For Benzodiazepine overdose*: 0.2 mg over 30 seconds; if no response after 30 secs, 0.3 mg over 30 seconds. May give 0.5 mg q 60 secs to total of 3 mg.	Nausea, vomiting, headache, emotional lability, agitation, dizziness, confusion, seizures. Resedation - monitor pt. for 2 hr. Withdrawal or seizures in patients who are physically dependent on benzodiazepine or have history of drug dependency	Allergy to this medication or to benzodiazepines. Patients who take benzodiazepines for life-threatening illness (control of epilepticus, ↑ ICP). Cyclic antidepressant OD. Seizure-prone individuals.

Emergency Meds

Medication	Description	Prep and Dose	Adverse Effects	Contraindications
Fosphenytoin	Anticonvulsant for immediate and short term management of generalized convulsive status epilepticus (GCSE) and for prevention and treatment of seizures during neurosurgery. More compatible with intravenous solutions than Phenytoin and is better tolerated at the infusion site.	Prep: 50 mg PE/mL (PE = phenytoin units) in 2 mL and 10 mL vials. IM: Unlike Phenytoin, may be given IM. IVP: for GCSE: 10 - 20 mg PE/kg at rate of at least 100 mg PE/min, but no faster than 150 mg PE/min. (to avoid ↓ BP) Maintenance: 4 - 6 mg PE/kg/day, in a single daily dose, or divided as bid or tid. Keep plasma phenytoin level 10-20 mcg/mL. Toxic signs begin at > 20 mcg/mL.	Can cause severe cardiovascular depression - use with caution in elderly patients or those with ↓ BP or ↓ CO. Can cause V Fib, ↓ HR, AVB, coma, cardiac/respiratory arrest, dizziness, HA, paresthesia, slurred speech, somnolence, tremor, numbness, itch, rash, Hepatic injury, ↓ WBC, ↑ blood glucose.	Allergy to phenytoin. Sinus bradycardia SA block 2° or 3° AV block Stokes-Adams syndrome.
Furosemide (Lasix)	Potent, rapid acting diuretic (inhibits the reabsorption of Na, K, H_2O) used in the treatment of hypertensive crisis, nephrotic syndrome, ascites, pulmonary edema in the absence of shock. Emergency treatment of ↑ ICP. Onset: about 5 minutes Duration of effect: about 2 hours	Prep: 10 mg/mL in 2, 4, 10 mL amps and vials IVP: 20 - 40 mg (up to 0.5 - 1 mg/kg) given slowly (over 2 minutes). Load: preceding infusion: 0.1 mg/kg Mix: 100 mg / 100 mL D5W, NS Concentration = 1 mg/mL Infuse: 2 - 10 mg/hr (up to 20 mg/hr), or 0.1 mg/kg/hr (which may be doubled) (> 600 mg/day can cause ototoxicity)	Dehydration, hypotension. ↓ Na, ↓ K, ↓ Ca, ↓ Mg Hyperosmolality Metabolic alkalosis Ototoxicity with high doses or too rapid administration. ↓ BP, Cardiac arrest.	Allergy to sulfonamides. Hypovolemia Hepatic coma Electrolyte imbalance Anuria.
Glucagon	For emergency treatment of severe hypoglycemia, manifested by unconsciousness or seizures (since glucagon ↑ blood sugar by accelerating liver glycogenolysis, it is ineffective in starvation). Treatment of beta-blocker OD. Bypasses β_1-adrenergic receptors to directly activate cyclic AMP to ↑ HR and ↑ BP.	Prep: 1 mg powder (available in emergency kit) IVP: *Dose for severe hypoglycemia:* pt wt < 44 lbs: 0.5 mg pt wt ≥ 44 lbs: 1 mg Mix: 10 mg / 100 mL D5W, NS Concentration = 0.1 mg/mL Infuse: 1 - 3 mg/hr For: *b-blocker or CCB toxicity:* 5 - 10 mg IVP over 1-5 mins, follow with infusion of the "response dose" per hour.	May induce nausea and vomiting, especially if dose > 1 mg is given rapidly. Stimulates release of catecholamine which can cause sudden increase in blood pressure and heart rate. Rebound hypoglycemia (must ensure carbohydrate intake).	Pheochromocytoma Hypersensitivity (signs of allergy include tachycardia, hypotension, respiratory distress, urticaria).

Emergency Meds

Medication	Description	Prep and Dose	Adverse Effects	Contraindications
Haloperidol (Haldol)	A neuroleptic (major tranquilizer). An antipsychotic. Has been used for delirium, but this is being intensely questioned. Blocks the effects of Dopamine and Epinephrine (if ↓ BP occurs, manage with Neosynephrine or Norepinephrine).	Prep: 5 mg/mL in 1 mL amp & 10 mL vial IVP: 2.5 mg q 20 mins until sedated. (or 0.01 - 0.15 mg/kg) Mix: 50 mg / 50 mL D5W, NS Concentration = 1 mg/mL Infuse: 3 - 10 mg/hr (or 0.01 - 0.15 mg/kg/hr)	Extrapyramidal symptoms (tremors, rigidity, muscle spasms, extreme restlessness, increased muscle activity), Layngospasm, ↓ BP, ↑↓ HR, Dysrhythmias, prolonged QT, Increased risk for Torsades de pointes.	Toxic CNS depression, coma from any cause, Parkinsonism, Caution in patients with CV disease. Caution if seizure disorder: Haldol may lower seizure threshold.
Heparin Unfraction-ated (UFH)	Inhibits clotting by binding to Antithrombin III, to neutralize Thrombin and activated factors IX, X, XI, XII. Existing clot is not lysed. Used to prevent and treat deep vein thrombosis, pulmonary embolism, coronary thrombosis, and thrombosis of intravascular devices	Prep: 1000,2500,5000,7500,10000,20000 units/mL IVP: IVP: 50 - 80 units/kg (5,000 units total maximum) Mix: 10,000 units / 250 mL D5W, NS Concentration = 40 units/mL 12,500 units / 250 mL D5W, NS Concentration = 50 units/mL 25,000 units / 250 mL D5W, NS Concentration = 100 units/mL Infuse: 12 - 18 units/kg/hr (400 - 1600 units/hr)	Hemorrhage at any site. Dose to keep aPTT 1.5 - 2 x control. If bleeding occurs, Protamine sulfate 1 mg will neutralize 100 units of heparin. Thrombocytopenia (if platelet count < 100,000, stop Heparin, and assess for Heparin Induced Thrombocytopenia).	History of HIT Bleeding diathesis, Severe thrombocytopenia Recent hemorrhagic stroke, surgery, GI bleed, hematuria, or internal bleeding. Caution in severe hypertension.
Hydro-morphone (Dilaudid)	A hydrogenated ketone of morphine, an opioid analgesic for moderate to severe pain.	Prep: 10 mg/mL in 1 & 5 mL amp & 50 mL vial IVP: 0.5 - 2 mg (10 µg/kg) q 1 - 2 hr given over at least 2 - 3 minutes Mix: 40 mg / 200 mL D5W, NS Concentration = 200 mcg/mL Infuse: 7 - 15 mcg/kg/hr	Too rapid IVP → ↑ side effects. Nausea, vomiting, constipation. Sedation, respiratory depression, Bronchospasm, depressed cough, apnea, ↓ BP, fainting, shock, cardiac arrest.	Hypersensitivity Respiratory depression. Status asthmaticus, apnea. May ↑ ICP in head injury. May aggravate convulsive disorder.
Ibutilide Fumarate (Corvert)	Antiarrhythmic that slows sinus rate and AV conduction. For rapid conversion of recent onset AFib or AFlutter. Effects occur within 30 - 90 minutes.	Prep: 0.1 mg/mL in 10 mL vial Dose: If < 60 kg weight: 0.01 mg/kg If ≥ 60 kg weight: 1 mg (10 mL vial) Dilute dose to total volume of 50 mL with D5W or NS and give over 10 mins.	Polymorphic Ventricular Tach. Bradycardia, BBB, PVC's, tachycardia, ↑↓ BP, heart failure, Headache, nausea.	Torsades de pointes or pts with QT_C > 440 msec. Do not give with class Ia or III antiarryhthmics. Correct ↓ K, ↓ Mg first.

Emergency Meds

Medication	Description	Prep and Dose	Adverse Effects	Contraindications
Inamrinone	Discontinued by Bedford Labs, May 2011	No alternative source is available		
Isoproterenol 1:5,000 (Isuprel)	β-1 & 2 adrenergic receptor activity (inotrope, chronotrope, broncho-dilator). For refractory bradycardia, refractory Torsades de pointes, β-blocker poisoning, Bradycardia in heart transplant patients, Bronchospasm.	Prep: 0.2 mg/mL in 1 & 5 mL amps. IVP: 20 - 60 mcg 0.2 mg in 9 mL NS = 20 mcg/mL Mix: 2 mg / 250 mL D5W (don't use if brown or pink) Concentration = 8 mcg/mL Infuse: start at 2 mcg/min, may ↑ to 10 mcg/min, dose range is 2 - 20 mcg/min.	Myocardial ischemia, PVC's, vasodilation that ↓ BP and ↓ coronary perfusion pressure, tachycardia, arrhythmias, ↑ MVO2, ↑ BP, pulmonary edema, tremors, HA, ↓ K, cardiac arrest.	Tachycardia, ventricular arrhythmias, angina, AMI, ↓ K, heart block due to digoxin toxicity. No longer recommended in the setting of cardiac arrest.
Labetalol (Normodyne, Trandate)	Beta adrenergic receptor blocking agent that decreases SVR without markedly affecting cardiac output, renal hemodynamics, or cerebral blood flow. Used for severe hypertension.	Prep: 5 mg/mL in 20 mL & 40 mL vials. IVP: 20 mg over 2 mins. To achieve desired BP, may repeat or give double dose q 10 mins, not to exceed a total of 300 mg or give initial bolus then start infusion. Mix: 400 mg / 80 mL Labetalol + 120 mL D5W, NS, RL, D5NS Concentration = 2 mg/mL Infuse: 0.5 - 2 mg/min.	Hypotension (keep pt supine during and 3 hr after infusion), myocardial depression, dizziness, somnolence, nausea, hepatic injury, ventricular dysrhythmias, bradycardia, AVB, syncope, dyspnea, wheezing, fatigue.	Asthma, COPD, Overt heart failure, Pulmonary edema, 2° or 3° AVB, Bradycardia, Hypotension, Cardiogenic shock.
Levosimendan (Simdax)	A calcium sensitizer for the short-term treatment of acutely decompensated severe chronic heart failure (ADHF) when conventional therapy is insufficient. Improves myocardial blood flow. Due to vasodilatory effects, severe hypovolemia should be corrected prior to infusion of this medication.	Prep: 2.5 mg/mL in 5 & 10 mL vials IVP: 6 - 12 mcg/kg over 10 minutes Mix: 25 mg / 500 mL D5W Concentration = 50 mcg/mL Use solution ASAP. Storage and in-use time must never exceed 24 hrs. Infuse: 0.05 - 0.2 mcg/kg/min Response seen within 5 minutes. Peak effect within 10 - 30 minutes	May decrease the serum K+ The most frequent adverse events are ventricular tachycardia, atrial fibrillation, hypotension, heart failure, myocardial ischemia, extrasystoles, tachycardia, nausea/vomiting headache.	Allergy to Simdax. Severe hypotension and tachycardia. Any obstruction to ventricular filling or outflow. Severe renal or hepatic impairment.

Emergency Meds

Medication	Description	Prep and Dose	Adverse Effects	Contraindications
(Lidocaine) Xylocaine	An antiarrhythmia agent, for stable VTach in patients with preserved left ventricular function. Can be used for stable polymorphic ventricular tachycardia Does not affect contractility, blood pressure, or absolute refractory period. Ineffective against atrial arrhythmias.	Prep: 100 mg/5 mL in syringe; 1 gram in 50 mL; Premixed 4 mg/mL in 250 or 500 mL bag. IVP: Stable VT, PVC's: 0.5 - 0.75 mg/kg. Mix: 2 g / 500 mL D5W Concentration = 4 mg/mL Infuse: 1 - 4 mg/min. Titrate in increments of 1 mg/min. ↓ dose 50% in elderly pts, and those with liver, kidney, or left ventricular dysfunction. After 24 hr of infusion, ↓ rate by one-half.	Myocardial depression, ↓ BP, aggravation of arrhythmia, AVB, respiratory depression/arrest, bradycardia, CV collapse. Infusion > 24 hr increases risk for toxicity (signs are CNS depression or irritability which progresses to seizure). Measure Lidocaine level at 12 hrs, then q 24 h. (> 9 mcg/mL is toxic).	SA, AV, IV heart block, Bradycardia. WPW. Caution in patients with conduction disturbance, low CO, heart failure, hepatic disease. Avoid using Lidocaine to manage reperfusion PVC's following fibrinolytic therapy.
Lorazepam (Ativan)	A benzodiazepine with antianxiety, sedative, and anticonvulsant effects. Indicated for the treatment of status epilepticus. To reduce anxiety and recall prior to surgery or during mechanical ventilation.	Prep: 2 mg/mL & 4 mg/mL, in amp or vial IVP: For sedation: the smaller of 0.044 mg/kg or 2 mg total, diluted in equal amount of NS, given over 5 mins. IVP for GCSE: 4 mg given slowly (2 mg/min) Mix: 10 mg / 100 mL D5W, NS (in glass) Concentration = 0.1 mg/mL Infuse: 0.5 - 2 mg/hr (or 0.01 - 0.1 mg/kg/hr)	Hypotension, paradoxical agitation, dizziness, weakness, confusion. Can cause respiratory depression, airway obstruction, and/or hypoxic cardiac arrest. Caution in elderly patients or those with limited pulmonary reserve.	Sensitivity to benzodiazepines. Glaucoma, Sleep apnea syndrome. Patients with severe respiratory insufficiency will require mechanical ventilation.
Magnesium Sulfate	Replacement therapy for ↓ Mg. (Hypomagnesemia can precipitate refractory ventricular tachycardia, ventricular fibrillation, pump inefficiency, sudden cardiac death.) For polymorphic VTach (Torsades de pointes) and for life-threatening arrhythmias due to digoxin toxicity. Also to prevent and control seizures in severe toxemia of pregnancy.	Prep: 10% = 0.1 g/mL = 0.8 mEq/mL 20% = 0.2 g/mL = 1.6 mEq/mL 50% = 0.5 g/mL = 4 mEq/mL Load: Cardiac arrest due to Torsades or ↓ Mg: 1 - 2 g in 10 mL D5W over 5 - 20 mins. Torsades with pulse or AMI with ↓ Mg: 1 - 2 g in 50-100 mL D5W over 30 - 60 min. Mix: 4 g / 100 mL D5W, NS Concentration = 0.04 g/mL or 0.32 mEq/mL Infuse: 0.5 - 1 g/hr (or 4 - 8 mEq/hr)	Mg intoxication (especially in patients with renal dysfunction) manifested by flushing, ↓ BP, paralysis, respiratory paralysis, circulatory collapse. CNS depression. 10% Calcium Gluconate IV is used to reverse the effects of Mg toxicity.	Hypermagnesemia Heart block Renal dysfunction Respiratory depression Caution in pts receiving neuromuscular blockade. Caution in digitalized pt - if Calcium is used to treat Mg toxicity, heart block can occur.

Emergency Meds

Medication	Description	Prep and Dose	Adverse Effects	Contraindications
Mannitol (Osmitrol)	A sugar alcohol osmotic diuretic. Used to promote diuresis in acute phase of renal failure, severe trauma or surgery, as well as promote excretion of toxic substances. Used to reduce acute increases in intracranial pressure.	Prep: 20% = 0.2 g/mL in 250 mL bag = 50 g 25% = 0.25 g/mL in 50 mL = 12.5 g Infuse: for ATN: 0.2 g//kg or 12.5 g over 3 - 5 minutes for ↑ ICP: 1 - 2 g/kg over 30 minutes, then 0.25 - 0.5 g/kg q 4 - 6 hr. Effect on ICP in 15 minutes; lasts 4 hr.	Headache, tremor, dizziness, convulsions, N/V, ↑↓ BP, fluid and electrolyte imbalance, hypernatremia, acidosis, circulatory overload, pulmonary congestion, rebound increase in ICP.	Anuria, Shock, Severe dehydration, Intracranial bleeding Pulmonary edema Serum osmolality > 320 mOsm (normal = 278-298).
Metaraminol Bitartrate (Aramine)	Potent α adrenergic stimulator (vasoconstrictor) for hypotension due to ↓ SVR. For ↓ BP due to CNS injury, spinal anesthesia, or allergic reaction. Give via central line.	Prep: 10 mg/mL in 10 mL vial IVP: 0.5 - 5 mg (0.05 - 0.5 mL) over 1 min Mix: 100 mg / 250 mL D5W, NS, RL Concentration = 0.4 mg/mL Infuse: titrate to achieve desired BP.	Arrhythmias, angina, ↑ MVO_2, hypertension, pulmonary edema, cardiac arrest, stroke. Infusion site thrombosis, tissue necrosis if infiltrates.	Allergy to sulfites. Halothane or Cyclopropane anesthesia. Effects are potentiated by MAO inhibitors and tricyclics.
Methyl-prednisolone (Medrol, Depo-medrol, Solu-medrol)	Intermediate-acting synthetic adrenal corticosteroid used as an anti-inflammatory agent in acute and chronic inflammatory diseases, severe allergic responses (asthma), and acute spinal cord injury (SCI). Low dose steroid is also recommended for severe sepsis in pts with adrenal insufficiency or septic shock refractory to pressors.	Prep: 40 mg/mL & 80 mg/mL in 1 mL vial. IVP: *Inflammation:* 10 - 250 mg q 6 h *Acute SCI within 3 hrs*: 30 mg/kg in 50 mL D5W over 30 min, then 5.4 mg/kg at 10 mL/hr x 23 hr. *Acute SCI within 3-8 hrs:* same doses, but continue infusion for 47 hr. *Asthma:* 1 - 2 mg/kg IV over 5 mins, q 6 hr x 24 hrs, then 1 - 2 mg/d in 3 divided doses.	Headache, insomnia, confusion, psychosis, CHF, edema, nausea, vomiting, muscle weakness/wasting, delayed wound healing, Osteoporosis, aseptic bone necrosis, fractures.	Systemic fungal infection, Use caution in pts with: Cushing's syndrome GI ulceration Hypertension Diabetes Psychoses
Metoprolol (Lopressor)	Selective β1 receptor blocking agent. Reduces heart rate, contractility, and cardiac output. Prolongs AV node conduction, suppresses renin secretion. To treat SVT, angina, hypertension, AFib/AFlutter, and to reduce mortality in stable AMI.	Prep: 1 mg/mL in 5 mL vials. IVP: 5 mg over 2 - 5 minutes, may repeat q 15 mins to total maximum of 15 mg.	Hypotension, myocardial depression, heart failure. Bradycardia, AVB. Hypoglycemia Bronchospasm Caution in patients with hepatic dysfunction.	Bradycardia, AMI with HR < 45 bpm, 2° and 3° AVB, SBP < 100 mm Hg Moderate to severe heart failure. Bronchospastic disease.

Emergency Meds

Medication	Description	Prep and Dose	Adverse Effects	Contraindications
Midazolam (Versed)	A short-acting benzodiazepine. Central nervous system depressant used for sedation, anxiolysis, and amnesia, and as an adjunct in the management of mechanically ventilated patients. Three to four times more potent per milligram as diazepam. Used as an anesthetic induction agent, and prior to and during diagnostic procedures.	Prep: 1 mg/mL in 2, 5, 10 mL vials. 5 mg/mL in 1, 2, 5, 10 mL vials. IVP: 1 mg over 2 mins, wait at least 2 mins, repeat to titrate to adequate sedation. Maximum single dose is 2.5 mg. Total dose > 4 mg is seldom needed. Mix: 50 mg / 250 mL D5W or NS; Concentration = 0.2 mg/mL Infuse: 1 - 7 mg/hour (or 0.02 - 0.1 mg/kg/hr) (1 - 10 mg/hr is often described). Decrease infusion dose 10 - 15% q 2 - 3 hr to find the minimum effective infusion dose. Reduce dose if narcotic also given.	Fluctuations in BP, HR. Decreased respiratory rate and tidal volume in 23% of patients. Apnea in 15%, have back-up ventilatory support available. Can cause hypoventilation, airway obstruction, cardiac arrest if given too fast. Reduce dose for elderly, debilitated, and those who have received narcotic or other CNS depressant.	Hypersensitivity to benzodiazepines. Acute narrow angle glaucoma. Not intended for intrathecal or epidural administration. Shock, coma, or ETOH intoxication.
Milrinone (Primacor)	Inotropic/vasodilator agent that inhibits phosphodiesterease in in cardiac and vascular smooth muscle. Used for short-term (infuse < 48 hrs) treatment of acute decompensated heart failure (to increase CO and decrease SVR, without increasing HR or MVO_2).	Prep: 1 mg/mL in 10 mL, 20 mL, 50 mL vials. IVP: 50 mcg/kg over 10 minutes, then Mix: 40 mg; Concentration = 200 mcg/mL 40 mL Milrinone + 160 mL D5W or NS (premixes are: 200 mcg/mL. 400 mcg/mL) Infuse: 0.375 - 0.75 mcg/kg/min For renal failure, reduce dose to 0.2 - 0.33 mcg/kg/min	Ventricular irritability, PVC's, VTach, VFib, supraventricular tachycardia, angina, hypotension, sudden death, Infusion for longer than 48 hr increases arrhythmia risk. Headache, Hypokalemia.	Hypersensitivity. Correct hypokalemia and hypovolemia before giving Milrinone. Severe obstructive aortic or pulmonic valve disease. Acute phase AMI.
Morphine	An opioid analgesic. Its vasodilatory effects reduce SVR, increase venous capacity, and reduce myocardial O_2 demand in the emergency treatment of ischemic chest pain and pulmonary edema. When given IV, maximum effect occurs within 20 minutes.	Prep: 5 mg/mL, 10 mg/mL in 1 mL amp IVP: 1 - 5 mg in 10 mL NS over 3 - 5 min. *dose in AMI:* 2 - 4 mg over 1 - 5 min q 5 - 30 min, may increase to 2 - 8 mg q 5 - 15 mins Mix: 20 mg / 100 mL D5W, NS; Concentration = 0.2 mg/mL Infuse: 1 - 5 mg/hr (or 0.05 - 0.1 mg/kg/hr) (1 - 10 mg/hr is often described)	Respiratory depression, (Naloxone 0.1 - 0.2 mg IV may be used as antidote). Hypotension (especially in hypovolemic patients). Bradycardia, dizziness, N/V, confusion, delirium, insomnia. constipation with prolonged use.	↓ BP, CNS depression, respiratory insufficiency, bronchospasm, asthma, Head injury, ↑ ICP, seizures. Suspected surgical abdomen. Within 14 d of treatment with MAO inhibitor.

Medication	Description	Prep and Dose	Adverse Effects	Contraindications
Naloxone (Narcan)	Opiate antagonist that is free of morphine-like effects when given in the absence of narcotic. Used for narcotic overdose and to reverse respiratory depression, sedation, or hypotension in patients who have received narcotics.	Prep: 0.02 mg/mL in 2 mL amp 0.4 mg/mL in 1 mL amp. 1 mg/mL 2 mL amp and 10 mL vial. IVP: *Opiate OD in addict*: start at 0.05 mg *Opiate OD in nonaddicted pt*: 0.4 - 2 mg may be repeated q 2-3 minutes to total of 10 mg. *Opiate depression*: 0.1 - 0.2 mg, may be repeated q 2 - 3 minutes to 3 total doses Mix: 5 mg / 250 mL D5W or NS Concentration = 0.02 mg/mL (20 mcg/mL) Infuse: 0.4 mg/hr	↑↓ BP, tremors, agitation, ↑ pain due to analgesia reversal. Hyperventilation, dyspnea, pulmonary edema, arrhythmias, VTach, VFib, cardiac arrest. May precipitate opiate withdrawal syndrome (reduce dose and give slowly to patients with addiction). Too rapid reversal can cause catecholamine surge, nausea, vomiting, sweating, tachycardia.	Allergy to Naloxone Respiratory depression due to nonopiod drugs.
Nesiritide (Natrecor)	B-type natriuretic peptide (BNP) for acutely decompensated CHF pts who have dyspnea at rest or with minimal activity. Not to be used as primary treatment of cardiogenic shock or in pts with SBP < 90 mm Hg Dilates veins and arteries, producing 5 mm Hg ↓ in PCWP within 15 mins.	Prep: 1.5 mg vial, reconstitute with 5 mL removed from 250 mL bag D5W or NS Mix: 1.5 mg / 250 mL Concentration = 6 mcg/mL Discard mixture after 24 hours IVP: 2 mcg/kg (taken from the infusion mix) given over 60 seconds. Infuse: 0.01 mcg/kg/min (0.03 mcg/kg/min max.)	Dose related hypotension (in 4% of patients, lasting about 2 hours), especially when combined with other meds that decrease BP (e.g., NTG, ACEI's). VTach, PVC's, bradycardia, angina, dizziness, nausea, headache, anxiety.	Allergy to Nesiritide Cardiogenic shock SBP < 90 mm Hg Hypovolemia Valve stenosis Constrictive pericarditis
Nicardipine (Cardene)	A calcium channel inhibitor with potent vasodilatory effect on systemic, coronary, cerebral, and renal vasculature. Little or no negative inotropic effect. For short-term treatment of hypertension. Used as pretreatment prior to PTCA to protect against ischemia.	Prep: 2.5 mg/mL in 10 mL amp IVP: NA Mix: 25 mg / 250 mL D5W or NS, not in RL or NaHCO3 Concentration = 0.1 mg/mL (also premixed 20 mg/200 mL) Infuse: 5 mg/hr (50 mL/hr). If needed, titrate by ↑ in increments of 2.5 mg/hr (25 mg/hr) q 15 min to max of 15 mg/hr (150 mL/hr). ↓ dose in patients with hepatic disease.	Irritation of peripheral infusion site (rotate IV site q 12 hrs). HA in 14% of pts, hypotension, N/V, dizzy, flushing, sweating, tachycardia, PVC's, palpitations. Does not protect against dangers of abrupt beta-blocker withdrawal.	Allergy to Nicardipine Advanced aortic stenosis Because of negative inotropic effect, caution in patients with HF or significant LV dysfunction. Caution in patients receiving beta-blocker.

Medication	Description	Prep and Dose	Adverse Effects	Contraindications
Nimodipine (Nimotop)	A cerebro-selective calcium channel blocker used to improve neurologic outcome by reducing the incidence and severity of ischemic deficits resulting from vasospasm following recent subarachnoid hemorrhage (SAH) due to ruptured intracranial aneurysm.	Prep: 30 mg/capsule PO: Start within 96 hrs of SAH. 60 mg q 4 h for 21 d. If pt can't swallow, extract contents of the capsule, then give via NG tube. NG tube should then be irrigated with 30 mL NS. FDA issued Black-Box warning against giving this preparation intravenously.	Hypotension, especially if other calcium channel blockers are given or if dose of Nimodipine is increased. Bradycardia, Nausea, Headache, Flushing. If patient has impaired hepatic function, reduce dose.	Caution if patient is hypotensive. Caution in patients with heart failure or abnormal AV node conduction.
Nitro-glycerin (Nitro-bid) (Tridil)	Dilates peripheral/coronary vasculature by relaxing vascular smooth muscle. Initial treatment of angina in suspected ischemic pain. In heart failure to ↓ preload, ↓ afterload, ↓ pulmonary congestion. In postop cardiac surgery pts, to ↑ coronary perfusion and control BP. Preferred over Nipride in patients with CAD.	Prep: 5 mg/mL in 1, 5, & 10 mL vials. IVP: May give 12.5 - 25 mcg bolus Mix: 25 mg / 250 mL D5W or NS in glass, nonabsorbent tubing — Concentration = 100 mcg/mL or 50 mg / 250 mL D5W or NS in glass, nonabsorbent tubing — Concentration = 200 mcg/mL Infuse: Start at 5 mcg/min, then ↑ by 5 mcg/min (if needed) q 5 - 10 mins, to 10 - 20 mcg/min (max dose is 200 mcg/min). If topical or po doses started, ↓ infusion to < 20 mcg/min.	Hypovolemia, hypotension (↓ in PCWP precedes the fall in BP), bradycardia (all of which can exacerbate myocardial ischemia). Fainting if patient sits up. Reflex tachycardia, HA (in 50%), N/V, flushing, 15% are resistant to its antihypertensive effects. Tolerance develops over 1 - 2 d. May cause heparin resistance.	Allergy to nitrates. Hypovolemia, ↑ or ↓ HR, hypotension, glaucoma, constrictive pericarditis RV infarction, ↑ intracranial pressure, head injury, cerebral hemorrhage, aortic stenosis, severe anemia, Phosphodiesterease inhibitors.
Nitro-prusside (Nipride)	Potent peripheral vasodilator. Its effect is almost immediate and ends when infusion is stopped. For refractory hypertension. For afterload reduction in patients with heart failure and pulmonary edema. To reduce blood pressure in pts with aortic dissection or VSD. To promote forward blood flow in mitral or aortic regurgitation.	Prep: 25 mg/mL in 2 mL vial IVP: NA Mix: 50 mg / 250 mL D5W, shield from light, faint brown tint is OK. Discard if highly colored or > 24 hrs old. — Concentration = 200 mcg/mL Infuse: Begin 0.1 mcg/kg/min. Titrate q 5 - 10 min in increments of 0.5 - 1 mcg/kg/min. Maximum allowable dose: 10 mcg/kg/min for no longer than 10 minutes. Reduce dose in elderly, and in renal failure.	Can cause precipitous ↓ in BP. Hypotension may require fluids. Reflex tachycardia, N/V, myocardial ischemia, diaphoresis, pulmonary shunting, ↓ PaO_2. When thiocyanate level is > 12 mg/dL, look for signs of toxicity: ↓ BP confusion, hyperreflexia, tinnitus, blurred vision, HA, vomiting, seizures.	Hypovolemia Aortic stenosis Hypotension Poor cerebral circulation Renal failure (due to risk of cyanide toxicity) Head injury (Nipride may increase intracranial pressure).

Medication	Description	Prep and Dose	Adverse Effects	Contraindications
Norepi-nephrine (Levophed)	Potent alpha-1 (vasoconstriction) and beta-1 agonist. (inotropic effect and coronary artery vasodilation). Vasocontrictive effects are used to treat hypotension due to low SVR (due to anesthesia, septic shock). Avoided in ischemic heart disease due to ↑ in MVO_2, SVR, and HR.	Prep: 1 mg/mL in 4 mL amp. IVP: NA Mix: 4 mg / 250 mL D5W, not NS — Concentration = 16 mcg/mL (Don't use if solution turns pink or brown) Infuse: 0.05 - 0.5 mcg/kg/min (or 2-12 mcg/min, starting at 0.5 mcg/min; doses up to 30 mcg/min have been given). Expect great individual differences in dose required.	Excessively high BP, tachycardia, peripheral vasoconstriction that progresses to tissue ischemia. Anxiety, HA, Dizzy, Dysrhythmias, Myocardial ischemia, Dyspnea, ↓ renal/mesenteric blood flow, Tissue infiltration can cause tissue necrosis. Dose should be decreased in patients with hyperthyroidism.	Allergy to sulfite. Ischemic heart disease, hypovolemia, mesenteric or peripheral thrombosis. Cyclopropane and halothane anesthesia may cause VTach, VF. Extreme caution in those taking MAO inhibitors, tricyclic antidepressants.
Octreotide (Sandostatin	Given subcutaneously in the treatment of diarrhea related to AIDS or chemotherapy and to reduce output of GI fistulae. Off label: given to control bleeding esophageal varices until endoscopic treatment can be accomplished.	Prep: 50 mcg/mL, 100 mcg/mL, 500 mcg/mL in 1 mL amp. Also 200 mcg/mL and 1,000 mcg/mL in 5 mL vial. IVP: 50 - 100 mcg over 3 minutes Mix: 500 mcg / 250 mL D5W, NS — Concentration = 2 mcg/mL Infuse: 25 - 50 mcg/hr	Alters glucagon/insulin balance, resulting in ↓↑ blood glucose. Hypothyroidism, bradycardia, N/V, diarrhea, abdominal pain, inhibits gallbladder motility.	Allergy to the drug.
Pento-barbital (Nembutal)	Short-acting barbiturate used as a sedative, hypnotic, anticonvulsant. Used as a third line drug for refractory status epilepticus. Off label: used to reduce cerebral O_2 demand and to treat refractory increased intracranial pressure. Reduces ICP probably by reducing cerebral blood flow: in patients who do not respond to pentobarbital, mortality rate > 80%.	Prep: 50 mg/mL (is highly alkaline and incompatible with most other meds) IVP: *Pentobarbital coma for ↑ ICP*: 2 - 10 mg/kg over 1-2 hr (some give 30 mg/kg over 2 hours) Give no faster than 50 mg/min. *Status Epilepticus*: 2 - 5 mg/kg over 1-2 hr Mix: 1000 mg / 250 mL NS, RL — Concentration = 4 mg/mL Infuse: 0.5 - 3 mg/kg/hr. Titrate until blood levels = 2 - 4 mcg/mL. DC slowly, to avoid lethal rebound in ICP.	Paradoxical excitement. If given too fast, can cause respiratory depression, apnea, laryngospasm, hypotension. Injection site pain. Pain perception is unimpaired. Provide analgesia if needed. Blood levels: 0.5 - 3 mcg/mL: sedated 10 - 15 mcg/mL: coma 15 - 40 mcg/mL: may be lethal (shock and circulatory collapse).	Allergy to barbiturates Porphyria Hepatic coma Caution in patients with hepatic dysfunction Alcohol intoxication

Medication	Description	Prep and Dose	Adverse Effects	Contraindications
Pheno-barbital (Luminal)	3rd line anticonvulsant for GCSE given after Lorazepam and Phenytoin. Intubation and ventilation are required. May take 15 minutes to attain peak levels in brain.	Prep: 60 mg/mL and 130 mg/mL vials IVP: for GCSE: 10-20 mg/kg IV at 50-60 mg/min May give additional 5 - 10 mg/kg at 20 minute intervals. Max total dose 1 - 2 g.	Depression of respiration, level of consciousness, and blood pressure. Agitation, confusion. Bradycardia, N/V, HA. Many drug incompatibilities.	Sensitivity to barbiturates Porphyria
Phenyl-ephrine (Neo-Synephrine)	Synthetic, α-receptor stimulant, with potent vasoconstrictive effects and almost completely lacking of chronotropic and inotropic action. For treatment of the vasodilated state, (e.g., anaphylaxis, or the result of spinal or regional anesthesia).	Prep: 10 mg/mL in 1 mL vial. IVP: NA Mix $\frac{20\ mg}{250\ mL\ D5W\ or\ NS}$ Concentration = 80 mcg/mL (don't use if solution is brown) Infuse: 100 - 180 mcg/min to start, then 40 - 60 mcg/min (maintenance rate)	Myocardial ischemia, reflex bradycardia, peripheral and visceral vasoconstriction, HA, ↑↑BP and ↓ CO. Caution in pts with AV Block, CAD, ASVD. Potentiated by oxytocin and MAOI's. Necrosis if infiltrates.	Hypertension Halothane anesthesia Ventricular Tachycardia Severe peripheral vascular disease Caution in patients with bradycardia
Phenytoin (Diphenyl-hydantoin) (Dilantin)	An anticonvulsion agent sometimes used as second line of treatment for status epilepticus. Off label: Phenytoin prolongs the refractory period and suppresses ventricular automaticity. Used in the treatment of ventricular arrhythmias and prolonged QT.	Prep: 50 mg/mL in 2 mL and 5 mL amp. Highly alkaline. Should not be given IM. Is incompatible with most drugs. Do not give into other running IV's. IVP: *For seizures*: 10 - 20 mg/kg Then 100 mg IV q 6 - 8 hr. Do not give faster than 50 mg/min. Therapeutic level = 10 - 20 µg/mL	Hypotension (especially with rapid administration), AVB, arrhythmias, CV collapse, bradycardia, pulmonary fibrosis, exfoliative/purpuric dermatitis, liver damage or necrosis, abrupt withdrawal may cause seizures.	Hypersensitivity to hydantoins. SA block Sinus bradycardia 2° & 3° AV block Stokes-Adams syndrome Caution in pts with renal or hepatic dysfunction, asthma, or heart failure.
Potassium Chloride	To prevent or treat potassium deficiency. Hypokalemia is most often due to: diuretics, vomiting, diarrhea, NG suctioning, corticosteroids, metabolic acidosis, dialysis, hemodilution.	Prep: 2 mEq/mL in 10 and 20 mL vials Never IV push undiluted K. **Always** dilute. Mix: Rapid replacement: (central line) $\frac{10\ -\ 40\ mEq}{100\ mL\ D5W}$ Slow replacement: (may use peripheral line) $\frac{20\ -\ 40\ mEq}{1000\ mL\ D5W}$ Infuse: 10 - 20 mEq/hr (Never > 40 mEq/hr)	If given peripherally, pain/ irritation of IV site and peripheral vein. Signs of toxicity (when K > 5.5 mEq/L): confusion, irritability, flaccid paralysis, respiratory distress, ↓ BP, arrhythmias, widened QRS, prolonged QT, V Fib.	Renal failure Hemolytic reaction Dehydration Caution if urinary output < 30 mL/hr.

Medication	Description	Prep and Dose	Adverse Effects	Contraindications
Procain-amide (Pronestyl)	A Group 1A cardiac antiarrhythmic drug. Increases the refractory period of the atria, and reduces impulse conduction velocity in the atria, His-Purkinje fibers, and ventricular muscle. For the treatment of sustained life-threatening ventricular tachycardia. Because of serious side effects, the use of Pronestyl with lesser arrhythmias is not recommended.	Prep: 100 mg/mL in 10 mL; 500 mg/mL in 2 mL. Mix: 1 g / 250 mL D5W Concentration = 4 mg/mL Load: 20 mg/min for up to 25-30 mins, until: 1. Arrhythmia is suppressed 2. Hypotension develops 3. QRS widens > 50% 4. PR or QT interval lengthen > 50% 5. total of 17 mg/kg is given (if renal or cardiac dysfunction, 12 mg/kg total) Infuse: 1 - 4 mg/min	Hypotension, especially if given too fast. Widening of QRS, lengthening of PR and QT, heart block and cardiac arrest. PVC's, VTach, VFib, Asystole. Keep blood level 4 - 10 µg/mL. Risk of toxicity if patient has renal failure, high dose, or infusion for > 24 hrs. Prolonged use may lead to lupus-erythematosus-like syndrome.	Allergy to sulfite Complete heart block Prolonged QT interval 2° AVB or hemiblock Torsades de pointes Caution in patients with: AMI, CHF, digitalis toxicity, hypokalemia.
Propofol (Diprivan)	A rapid-acting sedative hypnotic for the induction or maintenance of anesthesia. In intubated and mechanically ventilated ICU patients for sedation and control of stress responses. Also used to control ICP patients with severe head injury. Avoid abrupt discontinuation, which can result in anxiety and agitation. Expect awakening to be slower in pts on long term administration.	Prep: 10 mg/mL in 20 mL, 50 mL, 100 mL glass infusion vials. Premade mixes all have concentration of 10 mg/mL Mix: 200 mg / 20 mL D5W; 500 mg / 50 mL D5W; 1000 mg / 100 mL D5W Strict aseptic technique during handling. Discard vial and tubing after 12 hours. Infuse: Start infusion at 5 mcg/kg/min., then ↑ by 5-10 mcg/kg/min over 5-10 minutes to desired level of sedation. (IVP bolus 10-20 mcg may be given). Dose range is 5 - 50 mcg/kg/min.	↓ BP in 26% of patients (avoid rapid rate changes). Respiratory depression, acidosis, hypoxia, apnea, airway/ventilatory support required. Must adjust dose down to light level of sedation during weaning from mechanical ventilation. Bradycardia, decreased CO, Respiratory acidosis during weaning. Green urine.	Allergy to soybean oil, eggs, glycerol. Strict aseptic technique must always be maintained during handling. Can support growth of micro-organisms. Discard if contamination is suspected.
Propranolol (Inderal)	Non-selective beta-adrenergic receptor blocking agent, which ↓ HR, contractility, BP, and MVO_2. For supraventricular arrhymias (PAT, noncompensatory sinus tach, PAC's, AFib/Flutter). For angina before or after AMI.	Prep: 1 mg/mL in 1 mL amp. IVP: 1 - 3 mg given no faster than 1 mg/min. May repeat q 5 mins to total dose of 0.1 mg/kg Mix: 25 mg / 250 mL D5W or NS Concentration = 0.1 mg/mL Infuse: 1 - 3 mg/hr	Bronchoconstriction/spasm, Hypotension, CHF, Dizziness, weakness, fatigue. N/V, abd pain, constipation. Effects potentiated by calcium channel blockers.	Cardiogenic shock Sinus bradycardia 2° & 3° AVB, reactive airway disease, heart failure, compensatory sinus tachycardia.

Medication	Description	Prep and Dose	Adverse Effects	Contraindications
Prostaglandin Epoprostenol (Flolan)	A potent pulmonary and systemic vasodilator for long term treatment of pulmonary hypertension and pulmonary hypertension associated with scleroderma. Also inhibits platelet aggregation.	Prep: Freeze-dried powder 0.5 mg (500,000 ng) Use only Flolan diluent. IVP: NA Mix: 500,000 ng / 100 mL Flolan Diluent — Concen. = 5,000 ng/mL (mix is incompatible with everything; stable x 8 h) Infuse: 2 ng/kg/min. ↑ in increments of 2 ng/kg/min q 15 mins. Initially, dose range is 2 - 16 ng/kg/min.	↓ BP, ↓ HR, chest pain. Reflex tachycardia at higher doses. N/V, flushing, dizziness, HA, anxiety, dyspnea, abdominal pain. Abrupt withdrawal can result in rebound pulmonary hypertension. Side effects ↑ if > 8.5 ng/kg/min. Increased risk for bleeding.	Hypersensitivity Left ventricular systolic dysfunction Pulmonary edema during dosing
Sodium Bicarbonate (NaHCO3)	The most widely used buffering agent, for treatment of persistent metabolic acidosis due to prolonged low-flow state, diabetic ketoacidosis lactic acidosis, hyperkalemia.	Prep: 1 mEq/mL in 50 mL syringe IVP: 1 mEq/kg, or calculated mEq dose = 0.5 x wt(kg) x (desired HCO3 - measured HCO3) Mix: 150 mEq / 250 mL D5W, NS — Concen. = 0.6 mEq/mL Infuse: 0.5 - 1 mEq/kg/hr	Iatrogenic alkalosis Hyperosmolality Left shift of O2/Hgb curve can compromise release of O2 to tissues.	Alkalosis Respiratory acidosis Initial stages of cardiac arrest Pulmonary edema
Tranexamic acid (Cyklokapron)	An antifibrinolytic agent that inhibits plasminogen activation and plasmin. 10 times more potent in vitro than aminocaproic acid. For patients with hemophilia to reduce or prevent hemorrhage. OFF LABEL: To reduce blood loss and transfusion requirement in orthotopic liver transplantation and in pts undergoing cardiac surgery with cardiopulmonary bypass. Effects are similar to aprotonin. An antagonist to tPA.	Prep: 100 mg/mL in 5 mL and 10 mL ampuls IVP: 10 - 40 mg/kg, followed by infusion Mix: 1000 mg / 250 mL D5W or NS — Concen. = 4 mg/mL Infuse: 1 - 5 mg/kg/hour Reduce dose in patients with reduced Creatinine Clearance.	Nausea, diarrhea. Cerebral edema and infarction in patients with subarachnoid (SAH) or intracranial hemorrhage. However, the American Heart Association states that a "reasonable " treatment approach to SAH is a short course of an antifibrinolytic agent plus early aneurysm treatment, followed by prevention of hypovolemia and cerebral vasospasm.	Patients with acquired defective color vision Patients with sub-arachnoid hemorrhage (anecdotal experience indicates that cerebral edema and cerebral infarction may occur). Patients with active intravascular clotting

Medication	Description	Prep and Dose	Adverse Effects	Contraindications
Valproate Sodium (Depacon)	Intravenous anticonvulsant for patients who take oral Valproate but who are temporarily unable to take the oral form. OFF LABEL: anticonvulsant alternative for status epilepticus	Prep: 100 mg/mL in 5 mL single dose vial. Use: As IV replacement for oral administration of Valproate in seizure patients. Mix: 20 mg/kg / 200 mL D5W, NS, or RL — Concen. = depends on the mg/kg mix. Infuse: over 60 mins, no faster than 20 mg/min. Maximum daily dose of 60 mg/kg/day. Therapeutic blood level:50-100 mcg/mL (lower for seniors) OFF LABEL for Status Epilepticus: 100 mg IV push q 5 minutes.	Hepatic toxicity and failure, which can be fatal. Incidence is highest in children < 2 yrs. Life threatening pancreatitis. Injury to fetus (neural tube defects). In the elderly, somnolence, decreased intake, weight loss. In patients receiving the drug to prevent major seizures, should not be discontinued abruptly because of the danger of precipitating status epilepticus.	Hepatic dysfunction/disease Urea cycle disorders. To prevent seizures in patients with acute head trauma. Can cause thrombocytopenia or inhibit platelet aggregation. Platelet counts, bleeding time, and coagulation studies should be determined before and during therapy.
Vasopressin (Pitressin)	Synthetic analog of the posterior pituitary hormone, ADH (anti-diuretic hormone), which increases reabsorption of water by the renal tubules and causes constriction in all parts of the vascular bed. Treatment of diabetes insipidus. May be used as an alternative to epinephrine for vasodilatory shock. In the potential organ donor (following brain death) may be used to support BP. Also used to treat acute, massive GI bleeding.	Prep: 20 units/mL and 200 units/10 mL vial SC/IM *For Diabetes Insipidus:* 5 - 10 units SC or IM 2-4 times/day Septic shock or support of Organ Donor: Mix #1: 20 units / Infuse: 250 mL D5W or NS — Concen. = 0.08 unit/mL 0.02 - 0.1 units/min (via central line) Mix #2: OFF LABEL for variceal bleeding: Infuse: 200 units / 250 mL D5W or NS — Concen. = 0.8 units/mL 0.2 - 0.4 units/min (via central line)	Allergy, anaphylaxis, tremor, sweating, N/V, angina, hypertension, cardiac arrest, heart block, myocardial infarction, decreased cardiac output, decreased coronary artery blood flow, mesenteric ischemia, gastric infarction, ishcemic colitis, peripheral ischemia, dilutional hyponatremia, intestinal cramps, broncho-constriction. Concurrent use of high dose Norepinephrine may exaggerate the adverse effects of vasopressin.	Hypersensitivity Caution in ischemic heart disease and vascular disease Chronic nephritis with nitrogen retention Caution in any condition in which rapid volume expansion could be detrimental (e.g., CHF). Vasoconstrictive effects can cause multiple organ ischemia when plasma levels exceed 100 pg/mL (normal = 20 - 30 pg/mL).

Medication	Description	Prep and Dose	Adverse Effects	Contraindications
Vecuronium (Norcuron)	A nondepolarizing blocking agent (NMBA) of intermediate duration, competes for cholinergic receptors at the motor end plate. Used to facilitate endotracheal intubation, provide skeletal muscle relaxation during surgery or during mechanical ventilation. Effects may be reversed with neostigmine, edrophonium, or pyridostigmine.	Prep: 10 mg powder, reconstitute in SWFI IVP: For intubation: 80 - 100 mcg/kg (0.08 - 0.1 mg/kg), allow 2 - 3 mins for drug effect before ET intubation. Mix: Mix in D5W, NS, RL. 10 mg/100 mL = 100 mcg/mL, or 20 mg/100 mL = 200 mcg/mL, or 100 mg/250 mL = 400 mcg/mL Infuse: 0.8 - 1.2 mcg/kg/min, adjust to lowest possible dose to maintain a 2 twitch response to peripheral nerve stimulator. If no response is elicited, hold infusion until response returns.	Respiratory insufficiency, apnea. Long term use may result in prolonged muscle weakness and in muscle atrophy. Has no effect on consciousness, therefore, analgesia and/or sedation must be provided. Allergic reaction may cause ↓ BP, ↑ HR, bronchospasm.	Hypersensitivity It is mandatory that artificial airway, mechanical ventilation, and reversal agent be available. Caution in patients with myasthenia gravis, small doses of Vecuronium may have profound effects.
Verapamil (Calan, Isoptin)	Calcium channel blocker. Has negative chronotropic and negative inotropic effects, but has fewer side effects and contra-indications than propranolol. Dilates peripheral and coronary arteries, used for angina and ↑ BP. Decreases and slows SA and AV node conduction, inhibits reentry. After Adenosine, may be used to terminate PSVT (*only* if narrow complex, with adequate BP, and preserved LV function). May be used for rate control in Multifocal Atrial Tachycardia, Atrial Fib, Atrial Flutter,	Prep: 2.5 mg/mL in 2 mL and 4 mL amp. IVP: 2.5 - 5 mg over at least 2 minutes. If response is inadequate, may give 5 mg every 15 minutes, to a total maximum of 30 mg. Mix: 50 mg / 20 mL Verap + 180 mL D5W — Concen. = 0.25 mg/mL or 100 mg / 40 mL Verap + 160 mL D5W — Concen. = 0.5 mg/mL Infuse: 5 - 10 mg/hr (or 0.1 - 2.5 mcg/kg/min)	May cause decreased myocardial contractility, vasodilation, flushing, hypotension, tachycardia, syncope, bradycardia, AV Block, asystole, heart failure, edema, rash, dizziness, HA, fatigue, depression, nausea, sleep disturbance, palpitations. Constipation (in 5 - 10% of patients).	SSS, 2° or 3° AVB PSVT with wide QRS Hypotension, cardiogenic shock, severe heart failure, left ventricular dysfunction, VTach, AFib/Flutter with WPW (could result in VT/VF), Aortic stenosis Use with extreme caution in patients receiving beta-blockers.

Adrenergic Receptors

Receptor	Location	Physiologic Response
α1 alpha 1	Blood vessels Heart	Vasoconstriction Positive inotrope (↑ contractility) Negative chronotropic (↓ heart rate)
α2 alpha 2	CNS	Vasodilation, ↓ BP, ↓ HR by limiting norepinephrine release and inhibiting sympathetic activity.
β1 beta 1	Heart	Positive inotrope (↑ contractility) Positive chronotrope (↑ heart rate) Increased automaticity Increased rate of conduction
β2 beta 2	Blood vessels and Coronary arteries Bronchioles, GI tract, Uterus Other	Vasodilation Bronchodilation, relaxation of GI and uterine smooth muscle. Glycogenolysis, Calorigenesis. Drives K intracellularly -> ↓ K. ↑ Renin release -> vasoconstriction.
DA 1 dopaminergic 1	Blood vessels	Vasodilation of renal, cerebral, coronary, mesenteric, skeletal muscle, and skin. Promotes renal excretion of Na by inhibiting aldosterone.
DA 2 dopaminergic 2	Blood vessels	Vasodilation by inhibiting release of norepinephrine. Stimulates vomiting. Inhibits prolactin release.

α and β Stimulants	Dose	α	β1	β2	DA	Arrhythmia potential
Dobutamine (Dobutrex)	2 - 30 mcg/kg/min	+	+++	++	0	++
Dopamine (Intropin)	1 - 2 mcg/kg/min 2 - 10 mcg/kg/min > 10 mcg/kg/min	+ ++ +++	+ ++ +++	0 + ++	+++ +++ +++	+ ++ +++
Epinephrine	0.5 - 1 mg IVP 1 - 20 mcg/min infusion	+ ++	++ ++	+ +	0 0	+++ +++
Isoproterenol (Isuprel)	2 -10 mcg/min	0	+++	+++	0	+++
Metaraminol (Aramine)	1 mcg/min	+++	+	0	0	++
Norepinephrine (Levophed)	low dose high dose	++ +++	+ ++	0 0	0 0	++ ++
Phenylephrine (Neo-synephrine)	20 - 200 mcg/min	+++	0	0	0	+

Phosphodiesterase Inhibitors	Dose	α	β1	β2	DA	Arrhythmia potential
Inamrinone (Inocor)	2 - 15 mcg/kg/min	0	0	0	0	++
Milrinone (Primacor)	0.375-0.75 mcg/kg/min	0	0	0	0	++

α and β Blockers	Trade name		Blocks	
Phentolamine	(Regitine)	α		
Esmolol	(Brevibloc)		β1	
Metoprolol	(Lopressor)		β1	
Propranolol	(Inderal)		β1	β2
Labetalol	(Normodyne)	α	β1	β2

Med Facts

Med Facts

ACE Inhibitors (ACEI)

(Angiotensin Converting Enzyme Inhibitors)

Action: Inhibits the enzyme that converts angiotensin I to angiotensin II. Angiotensin II is a potent vasoconstrictor, stimulates the secretion of aldosterone, and breaks down bradykinin (a vasodilator kinin).
Reduces vascular resistance, improves LV function.
Venodilation benefits heart failure patients by ↓ venous return.
Reduces myocardial oxygen demand, thereby improving CO.
Has indirect antiarrhythmic effect by relieving heart failure, increasing serum potassium, and decreasing norepinephrine levels.

Uses:

- A first line of therapy for hypertension.
- Essential to treatment of heart failure (↓ LV systolic function)
- Given within the first 24 hours following AMI
- Patients with LVEF < 35% following CABG

Adverse effects:

- Cough (may require discontinuation of the drug)
- Dizziness, headache, fatigue, vertigo, insomnia, photosensitivity
- Abdominal pain, nausea/vomiting, cramps, disturbance in taste
- Palpitations, atrial fibrillation, bradycardia
- Paresthesia, somnolence, weakness
- Hypotension (may rarely cause renal failure)
- Hyperkalemia, hepatic necrosis/failure
- Angioedema (rare but life-threatening)

ACEI's:

Benazepril (Lotensin)	Moexipril (Univasc)
Captopril (Capoten)	Perindopril (Aceon)
Enalapril (Vasotec)	Quinapril (Accupril)
Fosinopril (Monopril)	Ramipril (Altace)
Lisinopril (Prinivil, Zestril)	Trandolapril (Mavik)

Contra-indications:

Sensitivity to ACEI's	Clinically relevant renal failure
Aortic stenosis	Hypotension (SBP < 100 mm Hg)
Hyperkalemia	Bilateral renal artery thrombosis
Pregnancy	History of angioedema

Angiotensin II Receptor Blockers (ARB's)

Action:

- Blocks the binding of angiotensin I to Angiotensin II receptors in smooth muscle of the heart and blood vessels.
- Unlike ACEI's, ARB'S have no effect on bradykinin.

Uses:

- Hypertension, LV hypertrophy, Heart Failure, AMI.
- To decrease the risk of kidney failure in patients who have both Type 2 diabetes and hypertension.
- Primarily used in patients who do not tolerate ACEI's.
- Are more consistent in blocking the effects of Angiotensin II.
- There is ongoing research on when to give ACEI vs ARB.

Adverse effects:

- Hyperkalemia, abdominal pain, nausea, vomiting, diarrhea
  Fainting, dizziness, lightheadedness, palpitations, headache
- Shortness of breath, difficulty swallowing
- Much lower incidence of cough, compared to ACEI
- Swelling of head, face, neck. Skin rash.
- Flu-like syndrome, joint or muscle pain or weakness
- Maintaining hydration is important to preventing side effects
- Individuals who take an ARB and spend time in the heat are more likely to experience side effects.
- Much more expensive than ACEI's.

ARBs:

Candesartan (Atacand)	Olmesartan (Benicar)	Losartan (Cozaar)
Eprosartan (Teveten)	Telmisartan (Micardis)	
Irbesartan (Avapro)	Valsartan (Diovan)	

Contra-indications:

Sensitivity to ACEI's or ARB's	Angioedema	Liver disease
Aortic or mitral stenosis	Kidney disease	Pregnancy
Hypotension (SBP < 100 mm Hg)	Hyperkalemia	

Analgesia, Intravenous

Facts: Studies showed that pain is under-managed in more than 50% of mechanically ventilated patients and in 20% of paralyzed patients. However, 50% of patients given analgesics/sedatives are over medicated Health professionals are strongly urged to be give effective pain control.

Unrelieved pain:

- May cause inadequate sleep, exhaustion, disorientation.
- Evokes the stress response: tachycardia, increased myocardial O2 demand, hypercoagulability, immunosuppression, catabolism.
- Splinting and hypoventilation may lead to pulmonary dysfunction.
- It's easier to prevent escalating pain, than to manage out-of-control pain.
- The most common reasons given for withholding analgesia are:
- Concern for respiratory depression, hypotension, addiction.
- Hepatic and/or renal dysfunction may reduce drug clearance.
- The maximum dose of an opioid is limited only by the adverse effects.

Adverse Effects of Opioids:

- Respiratory depression, prolonged time on ventilator.
- Reduced intestinal motility, constipation, gastric distention, nausea/vomiting
- Hypotension due to histamine release; bradycardia mediated by the vagus.
- Allergic reaction, histamine release, hypotension, bronchospasm.
- Agitation, hallucinations, and increased ICP in head injury patients.
- Opioid-dependent patients may require very large doses.
- Naloxone given to opioid addict may cause acute withdrawal syndrome.
- High dose opioid may cause muscle rigidity, can interfere with ventilation.
- More than 1 week of high-dose opioid may lead to physiologic dependence.
- Rapid withdrawal may precipitate symptoms (agitation, tachypnea, delirium, sweating, hypertension). Opioid infusion dose should not be decreased faster than 25% each day. Methadone can decrease withdrawal effects.

Recommendations:

1. Proper titration requires regular, objective assessment of pain and dosing according to an established protocol.
2. Assess the level of pain with a numeric scale (score 1 - 10).
3. In patient who cannot communicate, assess pain by observing movement, facial expression, posturing, HR, BP, RR.
4. Set analgesia goals and a pain-management plan for each patient.
5. Opioids should be given along with sedatives, with opioids given first.
6. Reduce the dose in the elderly and in those with renal dysfunction.
7. Recommended IV opioids are morphine, hydromorphone, fentanyl.
8. Slowing the rate of IV push injections may reduce adverse reactions.
9. Those on continuous infusion opioid who need more opioid should receive intravenous bolus dose rather than an increase in the infusion rate.
10. For rapid onset in acutely distressed patients, use fentanyl.
11. For patients with hemodynamic instability or allergy to morphine, fentanyl or hydromorphone are used. Hydromorphone is 3 times more potent than Morphine and induces less histamine release.
12. Most NSAIDS are avoided due to adverse effects (GI bleeding, platelet inhibition, renal insufficiency).
13. Oral, transdermal, or IM route should not be used in unstable patients.
14. Because of the risk of renal failure, GI bleeding, or postoperative bleeding, limit Ketorolac to a maximum of five days.

Analgesic	Intermittent IV dose	Constant Infusion
Morphine	0.01 - 0.15 mg/kg q 1 - 2 hr	0.07 - 0.5 mg/kg/hr
Fentanyl	0.35 - 1.5 mcg/kg q 0.5 - 1 hr	0.7 - 10 mcg/kg/hr
Hydromorphone	10 - 30 mcg/kg q 1 - 2 hr	7 - 15 mcg/kg/hr
Ketorolac	30 mg q 6 hr, or 15 mg q 6 hr if age > 65 years, wt < 50 kg, or renal insufficiency	Not applicable
Remifentanil	is ultra-short-acting	0.15 - 1 mcg/kg/min
Demerol or Codeine	not recommended	not recommended

Beta Blockers

Description: Beta Blockers block the effects of catecholamines (epinephrine and norepinephrine) at the beta-adrenergic receptors, in order to decrease heart rate, contractility, and/or vascular resistance, and ultimately to decrease myocardial oxygen demand.

Indications:
- Hypertension
- Unstable angina
- Stable heart failure
- Non-ST elevation myocardial infarction
- Supraventricular tachycardia (A Fib, PSVT)
- Aortic dissection (to ↓ BP and thus stall bleeding)

Contra-indications:
Asthma, reactive airways
HR < 60, SBP < 100
2° or 3° AV block
Sick sinus syndrome
PR > 0.23 seconds
NYHA Class IV LV failure
Unstable Class III LV failure
Cardiogenic shock
Prinzmetal's variant angina
Kidney or liver disease
Severe peripheral vascular disease

	Target	Action	When Beta Blockade is indicated (or not)
β1	Cardiac contractility	↓ contractility	To decrease MvO_2 in Unstable Angina, Non-ST elevation myocardial infarction
	Conduction though the AV node (which affects heart rate)	↓ heart rate	Supraventricular tachycardia (A Fib, PSVT) Prevention of AFib during cardiac surgery
β2	Vascular and bronchial smooth muscle	Vasodilation, Broncho-constriction	Unfortunately, β2 beta-blockers are contraindicated in those with bronchospastic disease.
α1	Hypertension	Vasodilation	Hypertension (calcium channel blocker is preferred, but a beta-blocker also helps). Aortic dissection (to ↓ BP/prevent bleed) Stable heart failure (to decrease afterload) Migraine headache, anxiety disorder.

Oral preparations of Beta-blockers:

Generic name	Trade name	Blockade of	Initial dose per day (mg)	Maximum dose per day (mg)
Atenolol	Tenormin	β1	12.5 - 50	100
Betaxolol	Kerlone	β1	5	20
Bisoprolol	Zebeta	β1	2.5 - 10	20
Metoprolol	Lopressor	β1	100 - 200	400
Nebivolol	Bystolic	β1	5	40
Nadolol	Corgard	β1, β2	40	240
Pindolol	Visken	β1, β2	20	60
Propranolol	Inderal	β1, β2	120 - 240	320 - 640
Sotalol	Betapace	β1, β2	160	320
Timolol	Blocadren	β1, β2	20	60
Carvedilol	Coreg	α1, β1, β2	6.25	50
Labetolol	Normodyne	α1, β1, β2	400 - 800	2400
Propafanone	Rythmol	α1, β1, β2	450	900

See the "Stat Meds" chapter for details on the injectable beta-blockers.

Adverse Effects:
Hypotension
Myocardial depression
Heart block
Severe bradycardia
Drowsy, weak, fainting
Memory loss, depression
Bronchospasm, wheeze, SOB
Pallor, flushing, diaphoresis
Fatigue, HA, N/V, diarrhea
Hepatic injury
Sensitivity to cold
↓ Sex drive, Erectile dysfunction

Calcium Channel Blockers

Description Calcium channel blockers inhibit the inward current of calcium into cardiac and vascular smooth muscle, resulting in:

- ↓ Heart rate
- ↓ Contractility
- Vasodilation of peripheral arteries
- Vasodilation of coronary arteries
- ↓ AV conduction and ↑ duration of AV node refractory period

Indications: Calcium channel blockers inhibit the inward current of calcium into cardiac and vascular smooth muscle, resulting in:

- ↓ Heart rate
- ↓ Contractility
- Vasodilation of peripheral arteries
- Vasodilation of coronary arteries
- ↓ AV conduction and ↑ duration of AV node refractory period

Two Types:

1. Dihydropyridines (amlodipine, felodipine, nicardipine, nifedipine) - peripheral vasodilation but no affect on HR or contractility. Used for hypertension, but not arrhythmias.
2. Nondihydropyridines (diltiazem, verapamil) - decreased HR and conduction through SA and AV nodes, coronary artery vasodilation, and negative inotropic effect. For atrial arrhythmias and angina.

	Generic name:	Brand name	Generic name:	Brand name
Calcium Channel Blockers:	Nicardipine	Cardene	Amlodipine	Norvasc, Lotrel
	Nifedipine	Procardia, Adalat	Bepridil	Vascor
	Nimodipine	Nimotop	Diltiazem	Cardizem
	Nisoldipine	Sular	Felodipine	Lexxel, Plendil
	Verapamil	Calan, Isoptin	Flunarizine	Sibelium
			Isradipine	DynaCirc

See "Stat Meds" chapter for details on Diltiazem, Nicardipine, Nimodipine

Adverse Effects:

- Flushing, headache, pedal edema, N/V, constipation
- ↓ SVR can cause ↓ BP, dizziness, weakness, lightheadedness
- Bradycardia, AV blocks, asystole, especially if patient also on Digoxin or β–blockers
- Tachycardia, palpitation, dyspnea
- Muscle, back, joint pain
- Depression. Parkinson-like symptoms
- In severe LV failure, can lead to hemodynamic compromise, myocardial ischemia, infarction, renal failure.

Contra-indications:

- Due to negative inotropic effects, all CCB's are contra-indicated in patients with LV failure or aortic stenosis.
- Because CCB's inhibit the action potential of the AV node, some CCB's (Verapamil and Diltiazem) are contraindicated in patients with 2° or 3° AVB, WPW, SSS.
- Because of the negative inotropic effects of both CCB's and β-blockers, concomitant administration should be avoided.

Calcium Channel Blocker Toxicity (signs may occur suddenly):

Signs of CCB Toxicity	Treatment
Hypotension and ↓ CO due to heart failure.	Dobutamine 2 - 20 mcg/kg/min Calcium Chloride 1 - 4 g, Glucagon 5 - 15 mg IV
Hypotension due to ↓ SVR	Dopamine > 10 mcg/kg/min or Epinephrine, Norepinephrine, Neosynephrine
Bradycardia or High-degree AV block	Atropine 0.5 - 1 mg q 2 - 3 mins up to a total of 3 mg If no response, Isoproterenol 2 - 10 mcg/min or transcutaneous pacing may be used.
↓ Level of consciousness	O_2, check blood glucose.

Clotting and Lysing

(the "a" that appears after the name of a clotting factor indicates that the factor has been activated")

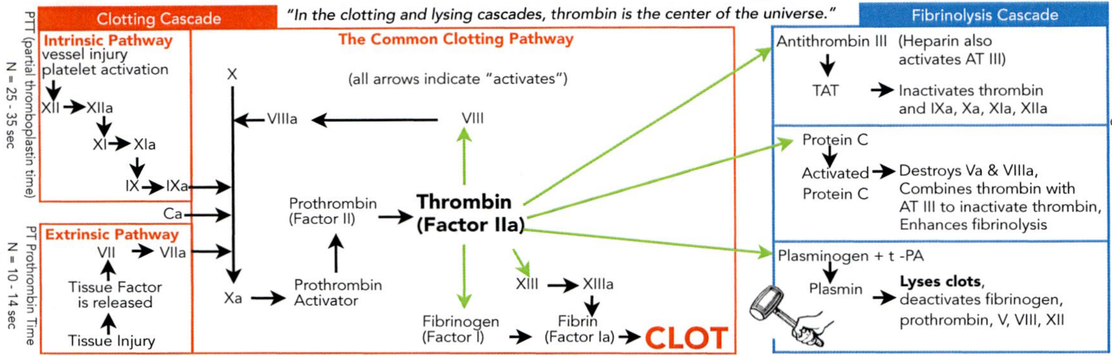

Antiplatelets	Name	Brand
Aspirin (ASA)	Aspirin	
Thieno-pyridines	Ticlopidine Clopidogrel Prasugrel Ticagrelor	Ticlid Plavix Effient Brilinta
GP IIb/IIIa platelet inhibitor	Abciximab Eptifibatide Tirofiban	Reopro Integrilin Aggrastat

VKA	Brand
Warfarin	Coumadin

Vitamin K Antagonist (VKA) inhibits Factors II, VII, IX, X

Details on the anticoagulants are on the next 10 pages.

Anti-thrombin		Brand
Heparin	Heparin (UFH)	
LMWH	Dalteparin Enoxaparin Fondaparinux	Fragmin Lovenox Arixtra
Direct Thrombin Inhibitors	Lepirudin Bivalirudin Argatroban Antithrombin III Dabigatran	Refludan Angiomax Argatroban Thrombate Pradaxa

Fibrinolytics	Brand
Alteplase	Activase
Reteplase	Retavase
Streptokinase	Streptase
Tenecteplase	TNKase
Urokinase	Abbokinase

if needed for bleeding

Coagulants	Brand
Tranexamic acid	Cyclopron
Aminocaproic acid	Amicar
Factor VIIa	Novoseven

Clot Inhibitor: Heparin, Unfractionated (UFH)

Description:

- Heparin acts at multiple sites in the normal coagulation system.
- Low dose Heparin binds to antithrombin III to inactivate Factor Xa, and thus inhibit the conversion of prothrombin to thrombin.
- The heparin-AT III complex also inactivates activated factors IX, XI, XII
- Higher dose Heparin can inhibit further coagulation by inactivating thrombin, thus preventing the conversion of fibrinogen to fibrin.
- Heparin also prevents the formation of a stable fibrin clot by inhibiting the activation of the fibrin stabilizing factor.
- Heparin has no fibrinolytic action and therefore will not lyse existing clots.

The Problems with Heparin:

- Requires careful lab monitoring and frequent dose adjustment.
- 3% of patients develop HIT (Heparin Induced Thrombocytopenia).
- Some of these develop life-threatening thrombosis (see next page).
- 5 - 10% develop significant bleed (risk is greatest on day 3).
- Age > 60 is a significant risk factor for bleeding.
- There is over a 3-fold increase in bleeding risk in patients receiving
- 25 units/kg/hr compared to patients receiving 15 units/kg/hr.
- Hypersensitivity reactions include chills, hives, asthma, N/V, ↓ BP.
- In the future, direct thrombin inhibitors and/or low-molecular-weight heparin may be preferred to unfractionated heparin.

Contra-indications to Heparin:			
	Known allergy to Heparin	Recent GI bleed	Hematuria
	Uncontrolled hypertension	Recent major surgery	Recent stroke
	Active bleeding in last 72 hr	Severe liver disease	Head trauma
	Recent intracranial surgery	Recent eye surgery	History of HIT
	Spinal or epidural catheter	Thrombocytopenia	

Dosing:

Deep Subcutaneous	Initial dose	Maintenance Dose
	333 units/kg	250 units/kg q 12 h
Intermittent intravenous	IVP Loading dose	Maintenance Dose
	10,000 units, undiluted or diluted in 50 - 100 mL NS	5,000 - 10,000 units q 4 - 6 hr undiluted or diluted
Continuous infusion	IVP Loading dose	Infusion Dose
	5,000 units	1,000 units/h

Normal aPTT is 20 - 35 seconds. Therapeutic range is 1.5 - 2 times normal.
Check aPTT q 4 - 6 hr and adjust dose accordingly.
Weight based dosing achieves shorter time to therapeutic aPTT.
Bleeding risk is lower with continuous infusion than with intermittent dosing.
Must reduce dose in patients with renal insufficiency, particular the elderly, the diabetic, or the patient with other causes of bleeding.

Heparin Infusions: (see "Drip Tables" chapter for dosing tables)

Heparin Mixes	Concentration
10,000 units / 250 mL D5W or NS	= 40 units/mL
12,500 units / 250 mL D5W or NS	= 50 units/mL
25,000 units / 250 mL D5W or NS	= 100 units/mL

Invert container at least 6 times to ensure adequate mixing.

Effects are Potentiated by:				
	Aspirin	Indomethacin	High dose penicillin	Clopidogrel
	Ibuprofen	Dipyridamile	GP IIb/IIIa inhibitors	Fibrinolytics

Antidote: Protamine sulfate 1 mg neutralizes 100 units UFH.
Protamine is given as 50 mg very slowly, over at least 10 minutes.

Heparin Flush Solutions for vascular catheters are:

- no more effective than 9% NaCL alone for maintaining patency of venous IV catheters in peripheral veins when blood is not aspirated into the device.
- more effective than 0.9% NaCL alone in maintaining patency of arterial and venous catheters used to obtain blood specimens.

Clot Inhibitor: Heparin, Low Molecular Weight (LMWH)

Description: LMWH is produced by fractionating heparin into molecules that are 1/3 the size. LMWH inhibits activated clotting factor X (designated as "Xa"), to prevent the conversion of prothrombin to thrombin in the common clotting pathway.

Advantages over UFH:

1. More predictable anti-thrombotic response and longer half-life over UFH permits once/day or twice/day dosing.
2. Does not affect aPTT (lab monitoring not required, although plasma Anti-Xa level may be done).
3. Less effect on platelet function and vascular permeability, results in fewer hemorrhagic events.
4. Less risk of HIT (Heparin Induced Thrombocytopenia)
5. Not neutralized by heparin-binding proteins, so there is a lower incidence of "heparin resistance."

Disadvantages: More expensive than UFH. Can't neutralize with Protamine.

Indications for LMWH:

- Prevention of DVT/VTE in patients at risk.
- Treatment of DVT and nonmassive PE except for patients with severe renal failure (creatinine clearance < 30 mL/minute). Treatment of pt with massive PE, and those with severe renal failure are treated with UFH).
- In UA/NSTEMI, with aspirin and other therapy, to reduce the risk of acute cardiac ischemic events (death and/or myocardial infarction).

LMWH	Prevent DVT/PE	Treat DVT or acute non-massive PE	Prevent Thrombosis in: UA, NSTEMI, or STEMI
Dalteparin (Fragmin)	2500 - 5000 units SC q day. If CrCl < 30 mL/min ↓ dose by 50%	200 units/kg SC q d in 1 or 2 divided doses for at least 5 days.	UA/NSTEMI: 120 units/kg SC q 12h usually for 5 - 8 d AFIB lasting > 48 hrs and prior to electrical cardioversion: 200 units/kg
Enoxaparin (Lovenox)	30 - 40 mg SC q 12 h for 7 - 10 days (longer for knee or hip replacement). If Cr Cl < 30 mL/min, i frequency to q 24 h	1 mg/kg SC q 12 hr or 1.5 mg/kg q 24 hr. for 7 days. Daily dose should not exceed 180 mg	UA/NSTEMI: 1 mg/kg SC q 12 h, for 2 - 8 days. ACUTE STEMI, adjunct to thombolysis: Pt < 75 yrs: 30 mg IVP then 1 mg/kg SC q 12h Pt ≥ 75 yrs: no IVP. Dose is 0.75 mg/kg SC q 12 hr
Fonda-parinux (Arixtra)	2.5 mg SC q d in pts who weigh ≥ 50 kg starting 8 - 12 hours after surgery, for 5 - 9 days, or 10 - 11 days after hip or knee surgery.	Pt wt < 50 kg: 5 mg SC q d. Pt wt = 50 - 100 kg: 7.5 mg SC q d Pt wt > 100 kg: 10 mg SC q d until INR ≥ 2 for 24 hrs	NSTEMI + delayed PCI: 2.5 mg IVP, then SC q d up to 9 days + additional dose prior to PCI. STEMI + no PCI: 2.5 mg IVP, then SC q d up to 9 d. STEMI + primary PCI: not recommended

Contra-indications:

1. Heparin Induced Thrombocytopenia (HIT)
2. Major bleeding
3. Thrombocytopenia
4. Sensitivity to pork or heparin

Adverse Effects: Spinal hematoma in pts with epidural catheter or spinal puncture Thrombocytopenia (HIT), Anemia, Fever, Bleeding or pain at the injection site, Nausea. To reduce adverse effects:

- Avoid use of NSAIDS, platelet inhibitors, other anticoagulants during treatment with LWMH.
- Avoid traumatic and/or repeat spinal puncture.
- Stop LWMH 24 hrs prior to surgery, (last dose reduced by 1/2), then resume 24 hrs postop, when hemostasis achieved.
- Monitor anti Xa level 4 hours after dosing.

Warfarin: Warfarin is started on day 1 of LMWH, adjust to achieve INR = 2. Stop LMWH after 4-5 days of combined therapy when INR = 2.5

Heparin Induced Thrombocytopenia (HIT)

Description:
- A sudden fall in platelet count usually occurring 5 - 10 days from the start of or exposure to heparin therapy, reaching a ≥ 50% platelet count decline between days 7 - 12, even if Heparin has already been discontinued.
- In 30% of pts, the platelet counts falls immediately ("Rapid Onset HIT) in response to heparin administration, indicating previous exposure to Heparin (in the last 100 days) and the presence of already-circulating HIT antibodies.
- 38 - 76% develop venous or arterial thrombosis. In some patients, thrombosis occurs before the platelet count falls, or even after Heparin has been halted.
- Thrombosis causes loss of limb in 20% and death in 30 - 50%.

Risk factors: (">" indicates "more so than")
- Use of Bovine UFH > porcine UFH > low-molecular-weight heparin [LMWH]
- The type of heparin-exposed patient (postsurgery > medical > pregnancy)
- Recent heparin exposure (within past 100 days) or Heparin duration > 4 days
- Patient gender (female > male)

Pathophysiology:
- Heparin binds to platelet factor 4 to form an antigen on the platelet surface.
- 1 - 5% of patients develop IgG antibody to the antigen. The antibody activates
- and aggregates the platelets and promotes thrombin generation. Clots form.
- The reticuloendothelial system removes the activated platelets, i platelet count.
- The platelet-rich white fibrin clots can cause multi-organ thrombosis.
- Antibody disappears within 2 - 3 months of stopping heparin.

Diagnosis:
- Heparin injection sites may exhibit lesions.
- Platelets < 100,000 or a 30 - 50% decline from baseline.
- Positive platelet aggregation test (50 - 80% sensitive).
- ELISA assay detection of the HIT antibody (> 90% sensitive).
- Rarely, acute anaphylaxis (e.g., fever/chills, tachycardia)
- Rarely, hypertension, dyspnea, cardiac arrest after IV heparin bolus.
- Evidence of single or multi-organ thrombosis.

Treatment: STOP ALL FORMS OF HEPARIN, Start Non-Heparin Treatment!
- If the patient is on warfarin, STOP IMMEDIATELY, give Vit K 5-10 mg IV.
- If the patient is not receiving warfarin, DO NOT GIVE warfarin (until later). Warfarin suppresses Protein C, a natural anticoagulant, and if given in the absence of an antithrombin agent, can cause limb gangrene.
  Once antithrombin is given, however, and platelets begin to recover, warfarin is started, 5 mg/day, to overlap the antithrombin for a minimum of 4 - 5 days, to a target INR. One of the 3 following antithrombins is given:
  1. Argatroban (Novastan)
     - For prevention and treatment of HIT: 2 mcg/kg/min IV x 6 days.
     - Dose reduced to 0.5 - 1.2 mcg/kg/min. in pts with hepatic insufficiency.
     - Resolution of thrombocytopenia usually by day 3 in 53% of treated pts.
     - For patients with HIT undergoing PCI: 350 mcg/kg over 3 - 5 minutes, then 25 mcg/kg/min, adjusting dose to keep ACT > 300 seconds.
     - May be continued after PCI, but at much lower dose of 2 mcg/kg/min.
  2. Bivalirudin (Angiomax)
     - Reduces risk for HIT patients undergoing PCI: IVP 0.75 mg/kg, then
     - 1.75 mg/kg/hr during PCI. If ACT < 225 seconds, may give additional IVP dose of 0.3 mg/kg. May continue after PCI with 0.2 mg/kg/hr.
     - Success also reported in HIT pts undergoing cardiac or vascular surgery.
  3. Lepirudin (Refludan) Discontinued by Bayer HealthCare on 5/31/2012.
- Platelet monitoring q 4 hrs.
  No IM injections. Provide protective skin care. Provide pain management. For strongly suspected or confirmed HIT, ultrasound of the lower-limbs.

Clot Inhibitor: GP IIb/IIIa Receptor

Description: Glycoprotein IIb/IIIa receptor antagonists bind with glycoprotein IIb/IIIa receptors on the surface of activated platelets, thereby preventing platelet aggregation and thrombus formation.

Indications: Reduce the incidence of cardiac ischemic events (including infarction, death, need for revascularization procedures) in
Non-W-wave Myocardial Infarction
High risk Unstable Angina
Angioplasty

IV Heparin: Must be given concomitantly with GP receptor antagonists during PCI, titrated to keep the activated clotting time (ACT) 200 - 300 seconds and/or the aPTT at 2 times control (50 - 70 sec).

Contra-indications:
Active or recent clinically significant bleeding in last 30 days
Recent (within 6 weeks) GI or GU bleeding
Relevant trauma or major surgery within 6 weeks
History of stroke within last 30 days, or stroke with significant neuro deficit, or any history of hemorrhagic stroke
Clotting disturbance (INR > 1.5, aPTT > 1.2 times control, platelet count < 100,000/mm^3)
Major trauma or surgery in the last 6 weeks
Intracranial neoplasm, AV malformation, aneurysm, hemorrhage
Malignant hypertension
Severe liver failure
History, symptoms, findings suggestive of aortic dissection
Hemorrhagic retinopathy
History of vasculitis
Acute pericarditis
Use of IV Dextran before PCI, or intent to use during PCI
Hypersensitivity to this or other murine proteins
Thrombolytic therapy, due to bleeding risk

Risk Factors for bleeding:
Body weight < 75 kg
Prolonged procedure (> 70 mins)
Repeat or unsuccessful procedures
Age > 65 yrs
PCI within 12 hrs of AMI
Heparin and ASA

Bleeding Precautions:
1. To decrease the incidence of bleeding, some physicians give IV boluses, but not continuous infusion of GP Antagonist.
2. Give careful attention to all potential bleeding sites: vascular access sites, wounds, pulmonary, GI, GU, retroperitoneal space, intracranial.
3. Minimize arterial and venous punctures, IM injections, use of urinary, nasotracheal and nasogastric tubes, and frequent measurements of BP with automatic BP cuff.
4. Avoid use of non-compressible sites (e.g., subclavian).
5. If bleeding occurs, discontinue GP IIb/IIIa and Heparin immediately.
6. While vascular femoral sheath in place, keep pt at bedrest with HOB ≤ 30° and affected limb kept straight.
7. Discontinue heparin after completion and remove sheath within 6 hours if aPTT ≤ 50 seconds or ACT ≤ 175 seconds. Apply pressure for at least 30 mins. Maintain at bedrest for 6-8 hrs following sheath removal or end of GP 11b/IIIa or four hours following end of Heparin, whichever is later.

Adverse Effects: Thrombocytopenia in 1 - 5% of patients who receive GP IIb/IIIa. If platelet count decreases to < 100,000, discontinue the infusion of GP receptor antagonist and discontinue Heparin.
If platelet count < 50,000, platelets may be given.
The most common bleeding site is the arterial access for PCI. Other adverse effects: hypotension, nausea, vomiting, dizziness, bradycardia, extremity pain, pelvic pain.

Details on each GP IIb/IIIa receptor antagonists are summarized on the next page →

Clot Inhibitor: GP IIb/IIIa Receptor Antagonists

Agent	Preparation	Indications and Dosage	Administration info	Caution
Abciximab (Reopro)	10 mg/5 mL = 2 mg/mL Infusion Mix: 10 mg / 250 mL D5W, NS =40 mcg/mL	1. <u>Prior to PCI to prevent ischemic complications</u> Bolus: 0.25 mg/kg IV over at least 1 min (too rapid injection is linked to hypotension) given 10-60 minutes prior to PCI, then Infuse: 0.125 mcg/kg/min (max of 10 mcg/min) for 12 hours. 2. <u>Unstable angina or NSTEMI not responding to conventional therapy and PCI planned within 24 hours</u> Bolus: same as above. Infuse: 10 mcg/min (15 mL/hr) for 18 - 24 hr, ending 1 hr after PCI.	When started 18-24 hr before PCI, keep aPTT 60 - 85 sec. During PCI, ACT 200-300 seconds After PCI, keep aPTT 55 - 75 sec. Don't shake vial. Do not use if vial contains opaque particles. Filter through a 0.2 or 5 mcm filter. Use separate IV line.	Risk of bleeding & ↓ BP. Risk of thrombocytopenia: If < 100,000 or ↓ 25% of baseline, check platelets, stop Reopro. If ↓ to 60,000, discontinue heparin and ASA. If < 50,000, give platelets. Eli Lilly PI dated 11/2013
Eptifibatide (Integrilin)	For bolus dose: 20 mg/10 mL = 2 mg/mL For infusion: 75 mg /100 mL = 0.75 mg/mL and 200 mg/100 mL = 2 mg/mL	1. <u>Prior to PCI to prevent ischemic complications:</u> Bolus: 180 mcg/kg IVP over 1-2 mins immediately prior to PCI, then start infusion immediately after the bolus, then repeat the bolus in 10 minutes. Infuse: 2 mcg/kg/min until hospital discharge or up to 18-24 hr. If renal insufficiency, reduce infusion dose by 50%. 2. <u>Acute Coronary Syndrome (UA, NSTEMI), both in patients who are managed medically and those undergoing PCI:</u> Bolus: 180 mcg/kg IVP over 1-2 mins (no repeat bolus), then Infuse: 2 mcg/kg/min until hospital discharge, CABG, or up to 72 hours, unless goes to PCI, then infuse 18 - 24 hrs. If renal insufficiency, bolus does is the same, but infusion dose is reduced by 50%.	Bolus should be withdrawn from the 10 mL vial. Infusion should be administered undiluted directly from the 100 mL vial, which has been spiked with a vented set. Give with: ASA 160-325 mg. For PCI, give Heparin to achieve ACT 200 - 300 seconds. Heparin after PCI is strongly discouraged. Refrigerate. Protect from light. No filtration is needed. NSTEMI pts should also receive Clopidogrel 300 mg prior to PCI.	Risk of bleeding & ↓ BP. No dose adjustments needed for elderly or female, but dose adjustment is necessary for Cr Cl < 50 mL/min or serum Cr > 2 mg/dL. If platelets ↓ to < 100,000, stop Heparin and Integrilin. Avoid in patients treated with hemodialysis. Merck PI dated 4/2014
Tirofiban (Aggrastat)	Premixed: 5 mg/100 mL = 50 mcg/mL and 12.5 mg/250 mL = 50 mcg/mL	For <u>Non ST Elevation Acute Coronary Syndrome (NSTEMI):</u> If managed medically or by PCI: Bolus: 25 mcg/kg over 5 minutes (no dose adjustment in bolus dose for patients with renal insufficiency). > 90% inhibition of platelets occurs within 10 minutes. Infuse: If normal renal function: 0.15 mcg/kg/min up to 18 hrs If CrCl is $\leq$ 60 mL/min: 0.075 mcg/kg/min up to 18 hrs. Given in combination with heparin or bivalirudin.	Protect from light during storage. May give into same line as heparin, atropine, dobutamine, potassium, epinephrine, furosemide, NTG. When infusion stopped, platelet function returns to normal in 4 hr. Discard solution after 24 h.	Platelet aggregation is inhibited > 90% within 30 minutes of loading dose. May cause thrombocytopenia Monitor platelets and H/H. Half-life is about 2 hours. Aggrastat PI dated 4/2015

Clot Inhibitor: Warfarin (Coumadin)

Description: Inhibitor of Vitamin K-dependent clotting factors (II, VII, IX, X). The peak effect may not occur until 36 - 72 hrs after it is given, the dose is difficult to titrate, effects last 2 - 5 days.

Uses: Prevention and treatment of thromboembolic events of DVT, PE, AFib > 48 hr., myocardial infarction, heart valve replacement.

Contra-indications:
- Recent stroke
- Active internal bleeding
- Recent or planned neurosurgery
- Recent or planned eye surgery
- Severe systemic hypertension
- Renal or hepatic insufficiency
- Thrombocytopenia
- Pregnancy
- Hypercoagulable state
- Intracranial tumor
- Recent major surgery
- Recent GI bleed
- Hematuria
- Pericarditis
- Spinal puncture
- Malignant hypertension

In patients with HIT, giving warfarin in the absence of an anti-thrombin can result in limb ischemia and gangrene.

Heparin to Warfarin: If the pt is on heparin, it should be continued for the first 5 - 7 d of oral warfarin therapy. Dose must increase prothrombin time (PT) to 1.5 - 2.5 times control (normal PT is 11 - 14 seconds).

Dose: 5 mg/day for first 2 days, then 2 - 5 mg/day according to INR. Stop Warfarin 4 days before surgery.

If the INR is	And there is no evidence of bleeding
2.0 - 3.0:	INR is therapeutic for DVT, or AFib, or MI
2.5 - 3.5:	INR is therapeutic for mechanical heart valve
4 - 10:	Hold warfarin, check INR frequently,
> 10:	Oral vitamin K should be given.

If there is major bleeding at any dose:
May give intravenous vitamin K 10 mg slowly.
Reverse bleeding rapidly with 4-factor prothrombin complex (contains Factors II, VII, IX, X) given as 500 - 1500 IU.

Warfarin effects are potentiated by		Effects are diminished by:
Amiodarone	Dipyridamole	Alcohol
Allopurinol	Ethacrynic acid	Antacids
Anabolic steroids	Ibuprofen	Barbiturates
Antibiotics	Indomethacin	Corticosteroids
Aspirin	Naproxen	Estrogen
Celphalosporin	Sulfonamides	Haloperidol
Chloramphenicol	Thyroxine	Penicillin
Chloral hydrate		Thiazide diuretics

Adverse effects: 5 - 10% have significant bleed (intracerebral, GI, retroperitoneal). Nausea, vomiting, diarrhea, hepatitis, jaundice, leukopenia, alopecia. Rarely, skin and soft tissue necrosis, leading to pain, "purple toe" syndrome, and sometimes gangrene, amputation, death. Believed to be caused by severe depletion of protein C and failure to reduce thrombin generation. Usually occurs on days 3-8 of warfarin therapy.

Advise Patient:

1.

Avoid foods high in Vitamin K		
Cauliflower	Kale	Spinach
Brussel sprouts	Chick peas	Broccoli
Turnip greens	Green tea	Liver

Avoid foods medium high in Vit. K	
Coffee	Cheddar cheese
Rolled oats	Chicken liver
Cabbage, Lettuce, Asparagus	

2. Report adverse effects:
   - Severe nosebleed
   - Severe headache
   - Black/bloody stools
   - Blood in the urine
   - Coughing up blood
   - Blue or purple toes
   - Vomiting blood
   - Any unexpected bleeding
3. Have INR checked q 4 - 6 weeks.
4. Don't take other meds/supplements without consulting physician.
5. Don't stop taking warfarin without consulting physician.

Clot Busters — aka Fibrinolysis, aka Thrombolysis

Description:

- Tissue plasminogen activator is a natural substance present in vascular endothelial cells. When exposed to a clot, tPA catalyzes the conversion of plasminogen to plasmin. Plasmin is the major enzyme responsible for clot breakdown (fibrinolysis).
- Fibrinolytics are used to dissolve clots in 4 life-threatening ischemic conditions: STEMI (ST Elevation Myocardial Infarction), Acute Pulmonary Embolism, Acute Ischemic Stroke, Peripheral Arterial Thrombosis.
- Fibrinolytics can cause life-threatening bleeding. It is imperative that the contraindications be identified before administration.

Absolute Contraindications:

- Any prior Intracerebral Hemorrhage
- Known structural cerebral vascular lesion (eg, AV malformation)
- Known malignant intracranial neoplasm (primary or metastatic)
- Ischemic stroke within 3 months EXCEPT acute ischemic stroke within 4.5 hr.
- Suspected aortic dissection
- Active bleeding or bleeding diathesis (excluding menses)
- Significant closed-head or facial trauma within 3 months
- Intracranial or intraspinal surgery within 2 months
- Severe uncontrolled hypertension (unresponsive to emergency therapy)
- For streptokinase, prior treatment within the previous 6 months

Relative Contraindications

- History of chronic, severe, poorly controlled hypertension
- Significant hypertension (SBP >180 mm Hg or DBP >110 mm Hg)
- History of prior ischemic stroke >3 months prior √ 2015
- Known intracranial pathology not covered in absolute contraindications
- Traumatic or prolonged (>10 min) CPR
- Major surgery in the previous 3 weeks
- Recent (within 2 to 4 weeks) internal bleeding
- Noncompressible vascular punctures
- Oral anticoagulant therapy
- Active peptic ulcer
- Pregnancy
- Dementia

About 5 percent of patients will have some problem with bleeding. One out of five who bleed will have a serious episode of bleeding.

Anticoagulant Therapy?

Anticoagulants such as Heparin, Antithrombins, or Antiplatelets are given as adjuncts for STEMI patients treated with fibrinolytic, but are contraindicated in Acute Ischemic Stroke both during and 24 hours after Fibrinolysis.

Post Infusion Care:

1. Invasive procedure (e.g., PCI or CABG) should not be performed within the first 2 to 3 hours after administration of fibrinolytic therapy.
2. Monitor for signs of bleeding (intracranial, GI, GU, vascular access site)
   HR, BP: q 15 mins x 2 hours after starting fibrinolytic, then
   q 30 minutes x 6 hours, then q 1 hour x 24 hours.
   GCS: If neurologic status declines during or after fibrinolytic, presume ICH. Discontinue fibrinolytic, antiplatelet, and anticoagulant. Stat CT.
   GI/GU: Check for blood in urine, stool, gastric drainage.
3. Usually 2 peripheral lines, one exclusively for fibrinolytic.
4. Avoid central venous access placement, arterial punctures, and the insertion
5. of a nasogastric tube or urinary catheter.
6. Place NIBP cuff on arm without IV's, arterial line, or wounds.
7. Insert IV catheter/Hep-lock for venous blood samples.
8. Avoid IM injections during and for 24 hrs after.
9. If ABG drawn or IV catheter removed, compress site for 30 minutes.

If Serious Bleeding Occurs:

Immediately discontinue fibrinolytic and anticoagulants.

- Aminocaproic acid (Amicar) may be given for life-threatenting bleeding. Amicar 5 g/250 mL over 1 hr, then 1 g/hr (i.e. 50 mL/hr) x 8 hrs.
- Fresh frozen plasma, cryoprecipitate, or both may also be given.

Clot buster: Alteplase (Activase)

Effects: t-PA binds to fibrin in a thrombus and converts the entrapped plasminogen to plasmin. This initiates local fibrinolysis. Alteplase is identical to native tPA.

Indications:
- ST Segment Elevation Myocardial Infarction (STEMI) with symptom onset within the previous 12 hrs, and PCI cannot be completed within 120 mins of first medical contact and the patient has no contraindications (AHA/ACC 2013).
- Acute Ischemic Stroke
- Pulmonary Embolism with hemodynamic compromise
- Arterial Occlusion

Prep: Reconstitute 100 mg vial with 100 mL SWFI without preservatives (use no other diluent) to concentration of 1 mg/mL. Do not agitate the contents. Use within 8 hrs.

Side Effects: In addition to general side effects of fibrinolytics, there may be allergic reaction, hypotension, arrhythmias.

STEMI dose
- Bolus 15 mg, then follow with: Infusion of 0.75 mg/kg (maximum of 50 mg) for 30 minutes,
- Then 0.5 mg/kg (maximum of 35 mg) over the next 60 mins.
- Total dose not to exceed 100 mg
- Also, Heparin 60 U/kg bolus for a maximum of 4,000 U, then 12 U/kg/hr (1,000 U/h maximum) adjust to keep APTT of 50 - 70 seconds, and continued for 48 hours.
- 73% - 84% patency rate in 90 mins

Acute Ischemic Stroke
- 0.9 mg/kg (not to exceed 90 mg total dose) infused over 60 minutes with 10% of the total dose administered as an initial intravenous bolus over 1 minute.
- No Heparin or ASA within 24 hours of alteplase administration

Pulmonary embolism
- Prior to giving alteplase, unfractionated heparin should be started at full dose. Some suspend Heparin during Alteplase infusion, then restart restart the Heparin when aPTT or thrombin time return to twice normal or less.
- Alteplase is given as 100 mg IV over 2 hours (i.e., 50 mL/hr).

Arterial thrombosis
- 0.05 - 0.1 mg/kg/hr for 1 - 8 hours.
- 0.02 mg/kg per hour over 1 – 7 hours may also be effective.

Clot buster: Tenecteplase (TNKase)

Effects: Tenecteplase is a modified form of human tissue plasminogen activator (tPA) that binds to fibrin and converts plasminogen to plasmin, which degrades fibrin clot.

Indication: Acute ST-Elevation Myocardial Infarction:

Prep: TwinPak kit. Reconstitute by directing 10 mL sterile water for injection without preservative (use no other diluent) into the powder. Gently swirl, don't shake.
50 mg/10 mL = 5 mg/mL, Precipitates in D5W, so flush line with NS. Discard unused TNKase after 8 hours.

Dose for STEMI:

85% patency in 90 minutes

Patient weight	IV bolus total dose
< 60 kg	30 mg
60 – 69 kg	35 mg
70 – 79 kg	40 mg
80 – 89 kg	45 mg
≥ 90 kg.	50 mg

Also Heparin: 60 U/kg bolus for a maximum of 4,000 U, followed by 12 U/kg/h (1,000 U/h maximum) adjusted to maintain an APTT of 50 to 70 seconds, and given for 48 h

Side effects: Bleeding, rare allergic reactions, arrhythmias, heart failure, cardiac arrest, embolism, N/V, hypotension, fever.

Clot Buster: Reteplase (Retavase)

Retavase is on longterm backorder as of 12/16/2015. ashp.org

Effects:	A recombinant plasminogen activator that generates plasmin, which degrades the fibrin matrix of the thrombus.
Indications:	For ST Segment Elevation Myocardial Infarction (STEMI), to improve ventricular function, reduce the incidence of heart failure and cardiogenic shock, and reduce mortality. (Not approved for Acute Ischemic Stroke)
Prep:	Supplied in a kit with two vials of 10 units each for double bolus injection. Reconstitute each vial by using dispensing pens to inject 10 mL SWFI into vial. Do not use any other diluent. Gently roll, do _not_ shake. Should be used immediately.
Dose for STEMI:	Two 10-unit IV injections each over 2 minutes, 30 minutes apart. Inject into dedicated IV line of D5W or NS. Sterile normal saline flush before and after each bolus.
Also Heparin:	60 U/kg bolus for a maximum of 4,000 U, followed by 12 U/kg/hr (1,000 U/hr maximum) adjusted to maintain an APTT of 50 to 70 seconds, and given for 48 h
Dose for PE:	Not FDA approved for PE. Clinical trials are in progress.
Side Effects:	In addition to general side effects of fibrinolytics, there may be rare allergic reaction, arrhythmias, heart failure, venous thrombosis, vomiting, hypotension, fever.

Clot buster: Streptokinase (Streptase)

Availability:	Streptokinase is highly antigenic and therefore no longer marketed in the US or the UK. However, it is available/affordable worldwide, thus important to pts with limited access to cardiac catheterization
Effects:	Acts with plasminogen to produce an "activator complex" that converts plasminogen to the proteolytic enzyme plasmin, which degrades fibrin clots.
Prep:	Slowly direct diluent at the side of the vial rather than into the drug powder. Roll and tilt the vial gently to reconstitute. Avoid shaking. The reconstituted solution can be filtered through a 0.8 mcm or larger pore size filter. Must be used within 8 hours following reconstitution if stored at 2 - 8°C (36 - 46°F)
STEMI dose:	1.5 million units IV given over 30 – 60 minutes
PE dose:	250,000 IU over 30 minutes IV, then 100,000 IU for 24 - 72 hours 60% to 68% patency in 90 minutes
Heparin for STEMI and PE pts:	UFH by IV bolus plus continuous infusion, target aPTT 50-75 sec; or Subcutaneous UFH q 12 hr x 48 hours are recommended. Heparin is not given to PE patients until the aPTT has decreased to less than twice the normal control value.
Bleeding risk:	ACCP recommends that in STEMI patients, streptokinase not be used with any GP IIb/IIIb inhibitor.
Side effects:	Bleeding. Highly antigenic, Allergic reaction occurs in 10%, and is therefore absolutely contraindicated within 6 months of previous exposure. Back pain, Arrhythmia, Hypotension, Pulmonary embolism Because of antibodies to Streptase, may be ineffective if given 5 days - 12 months after prior Streptokinase administration.

Citation: The Pharmaceutical Journal, 19 July 2014, Vol 293, No 7819, online | DOI: 10.1211/PJ.2014.20065679

The clot buster rivalry of the 1990s came to an abrupt end when studies showed that primary percutaneous coronary intervention (PCI) yielded better results than any of the pharmacological options.

Delirium

Definition:	A change in mental status that is characterized by inattention, disorganized thinking, disturbed perception, confusion, altered level of consciousness, and sometimes hallucinations. Develops over a short time. Fluctuates during the day.
Facts:	Develops in up to 80% of patients in the ICU. Causes distress for both family and caregivers. Often increases the use of sedatives and restraints. Increases cost, length of stay, and mortality rate.

Delirium Subtypes	Description	% of delirium pts
Hyperactive	Agitation, fidgeting, or combativeness	1.6%
Hypoactive	Lethargy, quiet (delirium is often unsuspected)	43.5%
Mixed	Fluctuation between hyper- and hypo-active	54.9%

Patho-physiology:	Thought to be related to imbalances in the neurotransmitters that modulate the control of cognitive function, behavior, and mood (dopamine, y-aminobutyric acid, acetylcholine, catecholamine, serotonin, endorphin). Inflammation may also play a role.

Risk Factors		Precipitating Factors
Age > 70 years	Renal insufficiency	Hypoxia, Hypotension,
History depression, stroke,	Recent ETOH abuse	Electrolyte imbalance
dementia, or epilepsy	Liver disease	Acute infection
Psychoactive meds	History of heart failure	Sleep deprivation
Sodium imbalance	Presence of gastric, urinary,	Withdrawal syndrome
Hypo or hyperglycemia	rectal, or vascular catheter.	Metabolic disturbances
Hypo or hyperthyroidism	Physical restraints	Isolation, Noise
Hypo or Hyper thermia	Malnutrition	Alarms, Fear
Intracranial pathology	Voicelessness due to ETT	Benzodiazepine,
Elevated Creatinine	Visual/hearing impairment	Opioid, or Haldol

Medications that may precipitate delirium:

anticonvulsants	antipsychotics	hypnotics	ranitidine
antidepressants	benzodiazepines	narcotics	sedatives
antiemetics	cimetidine	nifedipine	
antihistamines	digoxin	prednisone	

Confusion Assessment Method for ICU (CAM-ICU):

The following is a summary of the assessment:

1. Recent change in mental status or fluctuation in mental status.
2. Inattention (insufficient attention to succeed in simple tests).
3. Disorganized thinking (cannot correctly answer at least 3 of 4 questions, cannot complete simple commands).
4. Altered level of consciousness (patient is anything other than alert)

Management of Delirium:

- Although antipsychotic medications (Haldol), benzodiazepines, and opioids have been recommended for delirium, recent studies indicate that these medications may actually cause and/or intensify the delirious state.
- Reorient to reality and reassure (do this often).
- Assess and address the patient's risk factors.
- Assess and attend to pain.
- Employ the patient's eye glasses, hearing aid, magnifying lenses.
- Minimize unnecessary noise, lights, and other stimuli.
- Inform, explain, and reassure, but keep it short and simple.
- Find ways to give the patient some control of his/her care.
- Listen to and acknowledge the patient's fears.
- Encourage mobilization.
- Involve and inform the family on ways they can help.
- Consider using relaxation techniques.

Epidural Analgesia

Description: An opiate, sometimes combined with a local anesthetic, given through a catheter placed in the space above the dura (which covers the spinal cord) and the vertebra.
Administration of epidural analgesia produces reversible blockade of opioid receptors in the spinal cord, while leaving sensory and motor intact, sympathetic function unchanged, and without affecting consciousness. Catheter is usually left in place 48 - 72 hrs.

Benefits: Provides longer-lasting pain relief with lower narcotic dose. (5 mg morphine lasts 6 - 24 hrs, vs 3 - 4 hrs if given systemically)
Decreases the incidence of pulmonary complications: reduces need for and time on mechanical ventilation, reduces need for tracheostomy, reduces ICU length of stay.
May decrease the stress response following surgery or trauma.
Contributes to earlier mobilization and ambulation.
After abdominal surgery, GI motility recovers earlier.

Contrandications: Absolute
Infection at proposed catheter site Systemic infection (risks meningitis) Acute, symptomatic hypovolemia ↑ ICP (risk of brainstem herniation) Allergy to local anesthetic or opioids

Contrandications: Relative
Neurologic disorder such as multiple sclerosis, which could cloud the assessment of sensory/motor function Spine deformity (e.g., scoliosis) Previous back surgery Coagulopathy (spinal hematoma risk)

Adverse Effects:

- Pruritis (moderate to severe) in up to 44% of patients given morphine, and in 11% of patients given hydromorphone.
- Nausea, vomiting, urinary retention.
- Blocking sympathetic nerve fibers may cause bradycardia and hypotension (due to vasodilation).
- Side effects related to opioids (hydromorphone has the least side-effects).
- Respiratory depression and SpO_2 < 90% occurs in 25% of pts given morphine.
- Spinal or epidural hematoma can cause paralysis, which can be permanent:
  1. Risk factors: hemostatic disorder, vertebral column abnormalities, traumatic needle or catheter insertion, insertion in presence of high level of anticoagulation, use of continuous epidural catheters, older age, catheter removal in presence of anticoagulant effect.
  2. Monitor/report symptoms and signs of spinal cord compression: progression of lower-extremity numbness or weakness, bowel or bladder dysfunction, and new onset of back pain.
- Local anesthetic toxicity - dizzy, agitation, seizures, ↓ BP.
- Inadvertant subdural migration of catheter resulting in opioid overdose.
- Intravenous migration of the catheter can result in inadequate analgesia.

Catheter insertion:

1. Catheter insertion site is usually between vertebrae T 6-7 or L 2-3.
2. After catheter insertion, physician will check placement:
   a. The catheter is aspirated and will be removed if:
      - > 1 mL of clear fluid that tests positive for glucose: the catheter is intrathecal (under the dura, between dura and spinal cord).
      - Bloody fluid obtained (epidural vein is injured)

   b. Physician may inject a local anesthetic that contains epinephrine (1.5 % Lidocaine + epinephrine 1:200,000).
      - If HR and BP increase, catheter is in epidural vein.
      - If there is loss of sensory or motor function in the lower extremities and BP falls for 1 - 5 mins, catheter is intrathecal (between the arachnoid and the pia).
3. The catheter is covered with sterile occlusive dressing and secured.
4. Application of a 0.22 micron in-line filter is recommended.
5. Clearly mark the dressing, tubing, pump as EPIDURAL to avoid confusion with parenteral agents. Some use yellow color-coded tubing.

Epidural Analgesia (cont'd)

Facts on Epidural Administration:

- The epidural space contains fatty tissue, which functions as a "depot" for the opioids and local anesthetic. The slow diffusion of medication from the depot, across the meninges to the spinal cord produces a longer duration of action.
- Water soluble opioids (Morphine, Hydromorphone) diffuse more slowly, have a slower onset, a longer duration, and affect a wider area than do fat-soluble opioids (Fentanyl, Demerol).
- Local anesthetics are combined with opioid to produce a synergistic effect.
- Common anesthetics infused with opioid: Bupivacaine (Marcaine 0.125%) (most often used, long duration, good safety profile). Also Ropivacaine (Naropin) 0.05 - 0.2%, Lidocaine (Xylocaine 1%). All must be preservative-free.

Epidural opioid (must be preservative-free)	Intermittent epidural dose	Time to peak effect	Duration of effect	Continuous epidural dose
Morphine (Duramorph)	2 - 6 mg	30 - 60 min	12 - 24 hr	0.2 - 0.3 mg/hr
Hydromorphone	0.5 - 1.5 mg	15 - 30 min	6 - 18 hr	0.05 - 0.4 mg/hr
Fentanyl (Sublimase)	25 - 100 mcg	5 - 15 min	2 - 3 hr	0.5 - 1 mcg/kg/hr (50 - 100 mcg/hr)

Safety Measures:

1. Only preservative-free medications may be infused into the epidural space.
2. Medications intended for intravenous use, if given epidurally, can be fatal.
3. Maintain venous access during epidural analgesia, to use for fluids (hypotension is common), narcotic antagonist, antiemetic, or antihistamine.
4. Do not use alcohol or any other neurotoxic agent on the epidural catheter or on the infusion tubing.
5. Do not give IV opioids or CNS depressant while epidural is used.
6. Do not initiate or change anticoagulation therapy. Those patients receiving anticoagulant (Heparin, LMWH, antiplatelet med, NSAID) are at greater risk for spinal hematoma.

Assessment is Critical:

- Monitor BP, heart rate, pain level, sedation level, respiratory rate and depth, SpO2, sensory/motor every 2 - 4 hours, according to hospital policy.
- Monitor frequently for signs and symptoms of neurological impairment. Epidural analgesics do not cause sensory loss, motor weakness, or back pain. However, inadvertent subdural infusion can result in spinal cord compromise, nerve impingement, or neurologic dysfunction/toxicity. Report numbness, tingling, ↓ motor in lower extremities, low back pain. Prompt management can prevent permanent paralysis.
- Prompt recognition of opiate excess allows prompt intervention/support.
- If sedation score is low and respiratory rate is < 8, presume opiate excess and stop epidural infusion. Naloxone 100 mcg IV over 1 minute may be repeated
  q 3 - 5 minutes until symptoms have been reversed. Half life of Naloxone is 55 minutes, so a repeat dose may be needed later.
- Administration of sedatives may potentiate the effects of epidural opioids.
- If pain relief is inadequate, increase the bolus dose and/or infusion rate:
  - 25 % for mild improvement in analgesia
  - 50 % for moderate improvement
  - 75 % for pronounced improvement

Assess Catheter and insertion site:

1. Assess catheter insertion site q 8 hours for infection, bleeding, hematoma,
2. CSF leak, blood in catheter. Report to physician any abnormal findings.
3. Do not reinforce or change dressing (can obscure drainage, may dislodge catheter). Dressing will be removed with catheter in 48 - 72 hours.
4. Determine the status of coagulation before catheter removal.
5. Clear or bloody fluid on dressing may indicate catheter break, CSF leak, or injury to epidural vein. Notify physician and stop the administration of epidural meds.

Insulin and Glycemic Control: SCCM Guidelines*

Description:

- In critically ill patients, the acute stress response is a well-known cause of hyperglycemia (BG > 150 mg/dL).
- The adverse effects of hyperglycemia include:
  1. Increased vascular permeability
  2. Endothelial dysfunction, capillary occlusion
  3. Fluid, Electrolyte, and Acid-Bases disturbance
  4. Immune dysfunction, higher incidence of infection
  5. Catabolism
- But treatment hypoglycemia carries serious complications:
  1. BG < 70 mg/dL leads to increased mortality. A brief episode of BG < 40 mg/dL is even worse.
  2. In patients with brain injury, severe hypoglycemia
  3. (< 100 mg/dL) can produce or compound focal neurologic deficits, encephalopathy, seizures or status epilepticus, permanent cognitive dysfunction, and death)

Recommended measures:

- BG ≥ 150 mg/dL should trigger initiation of insulin therapy.
- Insulin therapy should be titrated to keep BG < 150 mg/dL.
- Insulin therapy should absolutely maintain BG < 180 mg/dL.
- Monitor BG every 1 - 2 hrs for pts receiving insulin infusion.
- Point of Care testing is recommended to speed BG results.
- Blood sample should be arterial or venous.
- Fingerstick is the "source of last resort."
- When a BG sample is drawn from a multilumen catheter being infused with IV fluid, care must be taken to avoid contaminating the sample with any infused IV fluid.

The Insulin Infusion:

Prepare a 1 unit/mL continuous infusion.
Prime new tubing immediately prior to starting the infusion (polyvinyl chloride and polyolefin plastics adsorb insulin).
Use new tubing each time a new bag is hung.

Beware Hypoglycemia:

- Hypoglycemia is defined as:
  - BG ≤100 mg/dL must be avoided in pts with brain injury
  - BG ≤ 70 mg/dL in all other patients
- Insulin" is in the top five "high-risk" medications that account for 1/3 of all major drug-related injuries.
- One study found that 33% of errors causing death within 48 hours involved insulin.

Risk Factors for Hypoglycemia:

- Insulin therapy
- Patients with diabetes, renal failure, mechanical ventilation, female gender, greater severity of illness, longer ICU stays
- Interruption of caloric intake without insulin adjustment
- Sepsis with the use of vasoactive infusions
- CRRT using HCO_3-based replacement fluid

Treatment of Hypoglycemia:

- Stop insulin infusion immediately and administer 10 - 20 g of hypertonic (50%) dextrose.
- Repeat the BG in 15 minutes, with further dextrose administration as needed to achieve BG ≥ 70 mg/dL (beware that rapid administration of dextrose in repeated doses has been linked to cardiac arrest and hyperkalemia)
- Repeat BG q 15 minutes until stable, then q 1 hr
- In patients with stable BG, testing may be changed to q 4 hr.

Insulin, IV or SQ?

- IV insulin is preferred for patients with type 1 diabetes mellitus, hemodynamically unstable pts with hyperglycemia, and changing clinical status, such as hypothermia, edema, frequent interruption of dextrose intake.
- SQ insulin may be adequate to maintain BG < 180 mg/dL in patients who are stable and have low insulin requirements.
- Delay transition to SQ insulin until there are no planned interruptions of nutrition for procedures, until peripheral edema has resolved, and until vasopressors are off.

Jacobi J, Bircher N, Krinsley J, et al. Guidelines for insulin infusion for hyperglycemia in critically ill patients. CritCareMed, 2012;40(12):3251-3276.

Neuromuscular Blockade

Normal Muscle Contraction:	1. The neuron releases acetylcholine, which binds with the receptors of the motor end-plate, changing its permeability. 2. The permeability change causes depolarization, which releases Calcium. Increased Ca in the cytoplasm causes bridging of actin-myosin proteins and muscle contraction. 3. Acetylcholinesterase then destroys acetylcholine, freeing the receptors of the motor end-plate for new stimuli.

Fig. 5.1

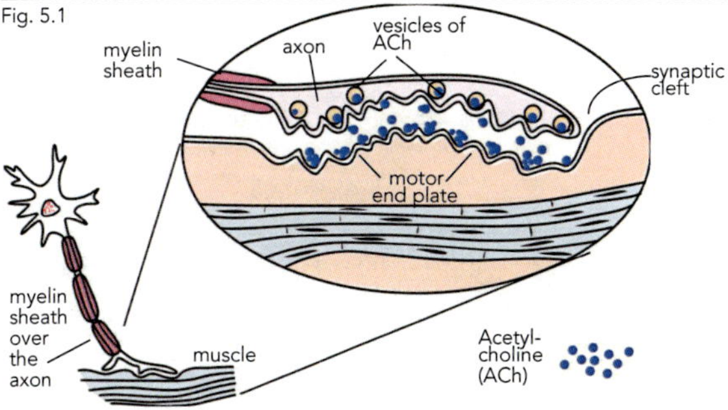

2 Types of Blocking Agents:	Depolarizing - binds to the receptors of the motor end-plate causing depolarization, which prevents subsequent activation. Nondepolarizing - binds to (but does not activate) acetylcholine receptors, thus blocking ACh from depolarizing the muscle.
Indications:	1. Produce apnea to facilitate intubation 2. Produce apnea to facilitate mechanical ventilation 3. Produce paralysis for treatment of refractory seizures/tetanus 4. Decrease tissue O2 demands during therapeutic hypothermia following cardiac arrest 5. Decrease tissue O2 demands during critically elevated ICP.
Prior to Administration:	NMB's cause paralysis, apnea, with NO effect on consciousness. Before NMBA is given, the pt <u>must</u> be sedated and intubated. For those patients who have pain, analgesics such as morphine or fentanyl must be given prior to giving a NMBA. Sedatives such as lorazepam (Ativan), must be given (usually by continuous drip) prior to giving NMBA. All appropriate alarms must be set. Position patient carefully.
Dosage:	There is wide variability in dosage requirements for individual patients and these requirements may change over time. Reduce the dosage for these patients: 1. the elderly 2. those with hepatic or renal dysfunction 3. those with conditions or factors which increase the sensitivity to NMB's (see next page)
Administration:	If rapid onset needed, give full loading dose. If rapid onset not needed, give 1/4 - 1/2 the loading dose. Slower IV push rate ↓ histamine release with certain agents. Muscles stop moving in the following order: 1. Eyes, face, neck 2. Extremities, abdomen, chest 3. Glottis, diaphragm
Effective dose:	The goal, using "train of four" testing with a peripheral nerve stimulator, is a score of 1 or 2 (see next topic). If intermittent NMBA is given, test 15 mins after each dose. If continuous NMBA infusion is used, test q 4 hr.

continued on next page →

Neuromuscular Blocking Agents (cont'd)

Factors that ↑ the effect of NMBAs:	Neuromuscular diseases Hepatic or renal disease Inhaled anesthetics ↓ body temp ↓ Na ↓ K, ↓ Ca, ↓ Mg ↓ pH Barbiturates Sedatives Aminoglycosides Antibiotics Ca Channel blockers Lithium Lidocaine Procainamide Nitroglycerin Quinidine Diuretics Beta blockers
Factors that ↓ the effect of NMBAs:	Prolonged immobilization Burns, Massive trauma Upper motor neuron lesions Lower motor neuron lesions Demyelinating lesions Epinephrine, Norepinephrine Ranitidine (Zantac) Aminophylline Theophylline Corticosteroids Phenytoin, Fosphenytoin Furosemide ↑ pH ↑ K ↑ Ca
Drugs that reverse NMBs:	Acetylcholinesterase inhibitor + Anticholinergic agent: 1. Neostigmine 0.05 mg/kg + Atropine 1 mg for each 1 mg Neostigmine given, or 2. Neostigmine 0.05 mg/kg + Glycopyrrolate 0.2 mg for each 1 mg Neostigmine given. Acetycholinesterase inhibitors should not be given to reverse NMB until some spontaneous motor movement is seen.
Care:	Reposition patient carefully/regularly, or use turning bed. The eyes must be protected with artificial tears ointment. Prevent exposure to heat or cold. Assess clinically with Train-of-Four to maintain 1 - 2 twitches. Assess the level of sedation. Sedation is inadequate if: 1. HR increases when patient is stimulated 2. BP changes when patient is stimulated 3. SaO_2 falls during routine care 4. Patient is diaphoretic Give eye care and DVT prophylaxis. When NMB is discontinued, may need to give more sedative.
Before extubation:	The patient must have: • Equal responses in the 1st and 4th "train-of-four" • Adequate tidal volume • Peak inspiratory pressure < - 25 cm H_2O • Sustained 5 second head-lift, and 5 second hand grip • Sustained response to 5 second, 50 Hz tetanus.
Complications:	• Anxiety, pain, panic if paralyzed without sedation or analgesia • Ventilator disconnect or airway mishap • Autonomic and CV effects (↑ HR, ↓ BP) • Development of deep vein thrombosis • Generalized deconditioning • Peripheral nerve injury • Corneal abrasion, conjunctivitis • Prolonged muscle weakness • Prolonged paralysis: Occurs in 5-10% of patients who have been given NMBA > 24 h. The risk is increased when given concurrently with corticosteroids. • AQMS (paresis and myonecrosis + abnormal EMG) can be a devastating complication, and is linked to administration of NMBA with corticosteroid, or use of steroid based NMBA. • Myositis Ossificans - ossification in connective tissue or muscle, ligaments, tendons, fascia, joint capsule

Neuromuscular Blocking Agents (NMBA)

	NMBA	IV Push intubate dose	Duration of action, minutes	Time to recovery, minutes	Intermittent IVP dose for maintenance	Mix for continuous infusion	Concentration of the infusion	Continuous infusion dose	Metabolism	Adverse Effects
Short-Acting	Mivacurium (Mivacron) (not in the US)	150 - 200 mcg/kg	10 - 20	15 - 30	100 mcg/kg q 15 mins	50 mg / 100 mL D5W premixed	0.5 mg/mL	6 - 7 mcg/kg/min	plasma cholinesterase	16% have flushing of face, neck, chest. Few major side effects except at ↑ doses: ↓ BP, arrhythmias, bronchospasm
	Succinly-choline (Anectine) (Quelicin)	0.6 mg/kg	< 10	4-6	0.04 - 0.07 mg/kg q 5 - 10 mins	500 mg / 250 mL D5W, NS, or D5NS	2 mg/mL	0.5 - 10 mg/min	plasma cholinesterase	The only approved depolarizing agent. Arrhythmias, ↑↓ BP, prolonged paralysis with continued used, Increased introcular pressure. Malignant hyperthermia.
Intermediate-Acting	Vecuronium (Norcuron)	0.08 - 0.1 mg/kg	20 - 35	45-65	0.01 - 0.015 mg/kg q 25 - 45 mins	20 mg / 100 mL D5W, NS, or D5NS	0.2 mg/mL	0.8 - 1.2 mcg/kg/min	30% renal 50% biliary	Minimal histamine release, minimal vagal blockade, Minimal CV side effects, Long term use may result in prolonged weakness
	Atracurium (Tracrium)	0.4 - 0.5 mg/kg	20 - 35	60	80 - 100 mcg/kg q 25-45 mins	50 mg / 100 mL D5W, NS, or D5NS	0.5 mg/mL	2 - 15 mcg/kg/min	Independent of renal and hepatic function	↓ BP, dyspnea, wheezing, laryngospasm. Slow administration minimizes histamine release. No vagal blockade. Fewer reports of prolonged paralysis.
	Rocuronium (Zemuron)	0.6 - 1.2 mg/kg	20 - 30	60	0.1 - 0.2 mg/kg	50 mg / 100 mL D5W or LR	0.5 mg/mL	10 - 12 mcg/kg/min	Primariy hepatic 33% renal	Occur in < 1% of pts. Tachycardia, ↑↓ BP, N/V, bronchospasm, rash, itch, wheezing. Less histamine release than Atracurium.
Long-Acting	Cisatracurium (Nimbex)	0.1 - 0.2 mg/kg	45 - 60	90	0.03 mg/kg q 20-30 mins	40 mg / 100 mL D5W, NS, or D5NS	0.4 mg/mL	3 mcg/kg/min (range is 0.5 - 10 mcg/kg/min)	organ independent Hoffman elimination	Minimal histamine release. Minimal, if any, cardiovascular effects. Can be used in hemodynamically unstable patients. Cumulative paralysis is rare.
	Pancuronium (Pavulon)	0.06 - 0.1 mg/kg	60 - 100	120 - 180	0.01 - 0.02 mg/kg q 1-3 hr	10 mg / 100 mL	0.1 mg/mL	1 - 2 mcg/kg/min	60-90% renal 15-40% hepatic	No histamine release, but > 90% develop ↑ HR > 10 bpm due to vagal blockade. Avoid use in renal or hepatic disease.
	Doxacurium (Nuromax)	50 - 80 mcg/kg	60 - 160	120 - 180	5 - 10 mcg/kg q 30-45 mins	NA	NA	NA	60-90% renal	Most potent NMBA available. May have prolonged weakness after dc'd. Flushing, wheezing, bronchospasm, ↓ BP, VFib.

* Doses listed in this table are the doses prescribed for "prolonged surgical procedures with anesthesia."

Peripheral Nerve Stimulator (PNS)

Train of Four (TOF) Monitoring

Purpose: To determine the effective dose for neuromuscular blockade.

Description of the PNS: Delivers 4 electrical stimuli at 0.5 seconds apart, with an output of 20 - 80 milliamps, to stimulate the ulnar nerve. (See alternate monitoring sites on next page)
Normally, 4 thumb adductions occur. These twitches become weaker and successively disappear as the dose of NMB is ↑

	4	twitches	Little or no neuromuscular blockade
	3	twitches	30% blockade.
desired level:	2	twitches	50% blockade; some spontaneous movement and some reflexes may be preserved
	1	twitch	70% blockade; no spontaneous movement or reflexes. 1 or two twitches is the desired level.
	0	twitches	> 90% blockade; blockade is excessive.

Set-up:

1. Explain to patient that PNS can be uncomfortable and that sedatives and analgesics are necessary.
2. Locate the site of placement for the electrodes:
   a. the negative (black) terminal: on the ulnar nerve, 1 - 2 cm proximal to the skin crease at the wrist.
   b. the positive (red) terminal: on the ulnar nerve, 3 - 5 cm behind the first electrode.
3. Prep site by shaving if necessary and cleaning skin with alcohol. Apply pediatric-sized electrodes.

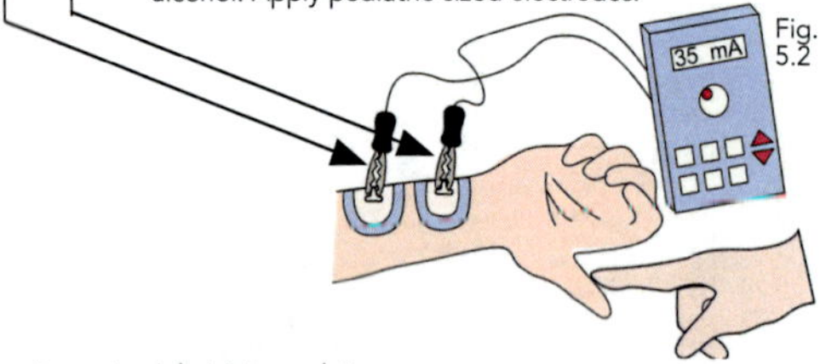

Fig. 5.2

Determine the initial threshold:

1. Administer sedative.
2. Place your fingertips on the patient's thumb. With output set at lowest level, press TOF, palpate single thumb twitch.
3. If none occurs, increase mA, and try again. Continue until a single twitch occurs (usually occurs at 5 - 10 mA). Allow at least 10 seconds of rest between each stimulus discharge.
4. If more than 15 mA is required, reposition the electrodes.

Determine the supra-maximal threshold:

1. Multiply the initial threshold by 3 (e.g., 5 mA x 3 = 15 mA).
2. Starting at the initial threshold, increase mA and press "TOF". Read the digital display and note the mA discharged. Increase the mA and press "TOF" until you reach the mA level that is 3 times initial threshold.
3. Place your fingertips on the patient's thumb. Press "TOF" and palpate 4 thumb twitches.

Achieve best NMB dose:

1. Administer loading dose of neuromuscular blocking agent.
2. Perform TOF. Adjust dose to achieve 2 twitches.
3. Recheck TOF q 15 - 30 minutes until steady state achieved, then assess TOF every 1 - 4 hours, unless conditions alter the effects of the NMB.
4. Continue sedative administration with NMB.

Discontinue:

1. Discontinue the blocking agent, assess TOF q 30 - 60 minutes for equal strength of all 4 thumb twitches.
2. Physician may order anticholinesterase inhibitor (edrophonium, neostigmine) with an anticholinergic (Atropine) to reverse any residual NMB effect.

Peripheral Nerve Stimulator (PNS)

Alternative Monitoring Sites:

Nerve	Electrode Placement	Response
Ulnar	Between the elbow and wrist	Thumb adduction
Facial	2 cm from the outer canthus of the eye, proximal to the tragus of the ear	Eye twitch and facial movement
Posterior Tibial	Behind the medial malleolus in the groove adjacent to the Achilles tendon	Flexion of the great toe
Peroneal	Lateral to the neck of the fibula and posterior to the lateral malleolus	Dorsiflexion of the foot

Before Neuromuscular Blocking Agent is given:

Problem	Possible Causes	Interventions
Unable to elicit thumb adduction TOF = 0	Peripheral edema Obesity, thick skin Cold extremity	Reposition electrodes Make sure electrodes are close Attempt alternative wrist
	PNS not working Electrodes not conducting	Check battery Replace electrodes Use pedi size electrodes Shave and clean the skin
	Output (mA) set too low	Output should be 3 times the initial threshold.
High level mA required to evoke initial threshold	Peripheral edema Obesity, thick skin Cold extremity Electrodes not conducting	Reposition electrodes Make sure electrodes are close Attempt alternative wrist Change electrodes Use pedi-sized electrodes Shave and clean the skin
Fingers twitch, but thumb does not	Nerve is understimulated, or Median nerve is being stimulated	Increase the mA Reposition electrodes

After Neuromuscular Blocking Agent is given:

Problem	Possible Causes	Interventions
TOF = 0 Patient is not moving	NMB dose too high. Drugs or conditions have potentiated the NMB effect TOF test done too soon after the last test.	Reduce or turn off the NMB. Retest TOF q 15 mins until desired level achieved, then restart NMB. Wait 30 seconds between tests.
TOF = 0 Patient is moving	TOF test done too soon after the last test.	Wait 30 seconds between tests.
	Other muscles are less sensitive to NMB than is the thumb.	May need to increase the NMB dose, discuss with physician.
TOF = 4 Patient is moving	Drugs or conditions have antagonized the effect of NMBA	Give repeat loading dose and increase drip rate of NMBA.
TOF = 4 Patient is not moving	False positive TOF test due to direct stimulus of muscle instead of nerve.	Reposition electrodes.
	Output (mA) is set too high, overstimulating the nerve.	Check that output is 3 times the initial threshold.

Sedation

Sedation in the ICU:

1. The use of pharmacologic agents, usually in intubated patients, to induce a state of relaxation or sleep. Indications include:
   - Control anxiety, agitation, delirium
   - Decrease VO_2 (due to agitation, work of breathing, posturing)
   - Abolish asynchrony with mechanical ventilation
   - Ensure patient comfort, ensure patient safety
   - Eliminate awareness/recall during therapeutic paralysis
   - Reduce awareness and recall during pain management
2. 85% of ICU patients receive IV sedation for anxiety, pain, or agitation.
3. Studies have shown that a nurse-directed sedation protocol using a sedation assessment scale can reduce the amount of sedative given. The result is ↓ duration of mechanical ventilation and decreased ICU and hospital LOS.
4. Administering the proper level of sedation requires:
   - Sedating only after providing analgesia and treating reversible physiologic causes of agitation
   - Establishing the sedation goal for each patient
   - Using a protocol for monitoring and adjusting sedative dosage
   - Using bolus rather than continuous infusion
   - Conducting daily "wake-up" sedative withdrawal, to allow patient reassessment and reduction/titration of the dose
   - Adjusting for factors that influence drug effectiveness

Over and Undersedation (one study found 54% of ICU pts receiving sedation were over sedated, 15% were undersedated, 30% were appropriately sedated).

	Oversedation	Undersedation
Risk factors:	Renal or hepatic insufficiency Obesity Prolonged sedative use (particularly Midazolam)	History of alcohol/drug abuse Low albumin levels Concomitant use of NMBA
Adverse effects:	↓ respiratory drive Prolonged mechanical ventilation Ventilator associated pneumonia Increased ICU length of stay CV instability ↑ Neurodiagnostic testing	↑ anxiety -> ↑ catecholamines Restlessness, self harm Ventilator asynchrony Hypoxia, ↑ O_2 demand by tissues Hemodynamic instability Unnecessary use of NMBA

Two often-used Sedation Assessment Scales (SAS):

Modified Ramsay Sedation Assessment Scale	
1	Anxious, Agitated, Restless
2	Cooperative, Oriented, Tranquil, Accepts mechanical ventilation
3	Responds to commands only
4	Asleep, has brisk response to light glabellar* tap or loud noise
5	Asleep, has sluggish response to a light glabellar tap or loud noise
6	Asleep, has no response to light glabellar tap or loud noise

* the glabella is the smooth area of frontal bone between the eyebrows; above the root of the nose; the lower forehead.

Richmond Agitation Sedation Scale (RASS)		
+4	Combative	Overtly combative, violent, immediate danger to staff
+3	Very agitated	Pulls or removes tube(s) or catheter(s); aggressive
+2	Agitated	Frequent non-purposeful movement, fights ventilator
+1	Restless	Anxious but movements not aggressive, vigorous
0	Alert	Awake, calm, aware of surroundings
-1	Drowsy	Not fully alert, but has sustained awakening (eyes-opening/eye contact) to voice (≥ 10 seconds)
-2	Light sedation	Briefly awakens with eye contact to voice (< 10 secs)
-3	Moderate sedation	Movement or eye opening to voice (but no eye contact)
-4	Deep sedation	Movement or eye opening only to physical stimulation.
-5	Unarousable	No response to voice or physical stimulation

Agitation Causes:	Pain and/or Anxiety	Excessive stimulation	Shortness of breath
	Perceived threat	Sleep deprivation	Constant noise
	Cannot communicate	Immobility or restraint	Sudden noise

Recommended Meds (SCCM Sedation Guidelines)	
Analgesia:	If hemodynamically stable: Morphine 2 - 5 mg IVP q 5 - 15 mins. until pain relieved. If hemodynamically unstable: Fentanyl 25 - 100 mcg IVP q 5 - 15 mins until pain relieved or Hydromorphone 0.25 - 0.75 mg IVP q 5 - 15 mins until relieved.
Sedation:	If acute agitation, use rapid onset benzodiazepine: Midazolam 2 - 5 mg IVP q 5-15 mins until sedated. If ongoing agitation: Lorazepam 1 - 4 mg q 10-20 mins until sedated, then q 2 - 6 hr or Propofol 5 mcg/kg/min, titrate q 5 mins to achieve goal.
(See "Stat Meds" chapter for details on the above medications)	

Reversal Agents: Benzodiazipine antagonist: Flumazenil 3 - 45 mcg/kg
Opiate antagonist: Naloxone 3 - 30 mcg/kg
Opiate antagonist: Nalmefene 0.5 - 1 mg

A Better Sedative: Dexmedetomidine (Precedex) 1 mcg/kg over 10 mins, followed by 0.4 mcg/kg/hr infusion, then 0.2 - 0.7 mcg/kg/hr, titrated to effect.

As an alpha $_2$ agonist, Precedex does not depress respiration.
Can be used during weaning from mechanical ventilation, and before, during, and after extubation. Also has analgesic effects.
Because of its short 6-minute half-life, no reversal agent is needed.

Sedative Withdrawal:

1. If patient has been on high dose sedative > 1 week, withdraw slowly (20% dose reduction each day) and do not give reversal agents.
2. Signs and symptoms of opioid withdrawal: sweating, lacrimation, rhinorrhea, tachycardia, vomiting, diarrhea, fever, tachypnea, anxiety, restlessness, irritability, muscle aching and cramps, ↑ BP.
3. Signs of benzodiazepine withdrawal: dysphoria, tremor, HA, nausea, sweating, fatigue, anxiety, agitation, ↑ sensitivity to light and sound, muscle cramps, sleep disturbance, delirium, seizures.

Procedural Sedation

Definition: The use of pharmacologic agents in unintubated patients to induce a relaxed state for a diagnostic or surgical procedure.
The goal is a minimal ↓ in level of consciousness in which the pt:

- Retains protective reflexes (cough, swallow, gag),
- Is able to maintain his/her airway, and
- Responds appropriately to verbal commands.

Prior to the Procedure:

Baseline assessment: Level of consciousness, airway and respiratory status, vital signs, ECG, SpO_2, pulses and circulatory status. NPO at least 4 hrs prior to procedure. Emergency meds and equipment available.

During the Procedure:

One nurse to monitor patient, another to assist physician.
Vital signs q 5 - 15 minutes; LOC q 5 - 15 minutes

- If ↓ resp rate, ↓ SpO_2, or ↑ pCO_2 or the patient does not respond to stimuli: Perform chin lift, head tilt, jaw thrust, ambu ventilate with supplemental O_2, reverse with Naloxone and/or Flumazenil.
- If BP ↓ by 20 - 30%, but SpO_2 OK: Lie patient flat, start O_2, give fluids (NS) unless contraindicated. May need Dopamine.
- If patient has preexisting hypertension (SBP > 140, DBP > 90): Start with benzodiazepine. If BP stays ↑, may need to cancel procedure. If BP initially good, but ↑ during procedure, may need analgesic for pain, diuretic for fluid excess, or β-blockade for catecholamine excess.

Seizures Meds for Status Epilepticus (SE)

		IV Loading dose	IV Push Rate	Maintenance	Warning	Therapeutic Level
First 30 minutes	**Line 1: Rapid acting** - Rapidly enter the brain and control seizures until peak brain concentrations of longer acting meds are reached.					
	Lorazepam (Ativan)	4 mg IV, may repeat 2 mg q 10 mins, not to exceed a total of 0.1 mg/kg	Slower than 2 mg/min.	None	Lorazepam is favored because of quick onset and long half-life. Benzodiazepines can cause respiratory depression, ↓ BP	
	Diazepam (Valium)	5 - 10 mg (0.15 mg/kg) q 15 mins. Max is 30 mg/8 hrs.	Slower than 5 mg/min.		Follow Benzodiazepine with Phenytoin	
Next 30-60 minutes	**Line 2: Long acting** - Peak brain concentrations are not achieved for up to 1 hour after IV injection.					
	Fosphenytoin (Cerebyx) or	15 - 20 mg PE/kg May give total dose of 30 mg PE/kg.	75 PE/min. at first, then up to 150 mg/min. Too fast can cause cardiac arrest.	4 - 6 mg PE/kg/24 hr	Fosphenytoin poses less risk for vein irritation than Phenytoin. Both can cause cardiac depression. ↓ BP occurs in 28 - 50%. Monitor for ↓ BP, ↓ HR	
	Phenytoin	18 - 20 mg/kg given directly into vein or into tubing with NS. May give total of 30 mg/kg	25 mg/min at first, then up to 50 mg/min (can cause hypotension and arrhythmia)	NA	Contraindicated in sinus bradycardia, SA block, 2° and 3° AV block. Has slow onset, so give Benzodiazepine first.	10 - 20 mcg/mL
	Midazolam (Versed)	0.2 mg/kg	Over 2 - 3 mins, may be repeated in 10 - 15 mins	0.1 - 0.4 mg/kg/hr	Intubation and pressor support and ECG monitoring are necessary.	
2nd hour of treatment	**Line 3: Refractory SE** (does not respond to Line 1 and 2 meds) occurs in 31 - 44% of all SE patients.					
	Propofol (Diprivan)	1 - 2 mg/kg	10 mg/min. Rapid bolus causes hypotension	0.1 - 0.2 mg/kg/min (100-200 mcg/kg/min)	Intubation and ventilation required. ECG monitoring. Manage hypotension.	
	Phenobarbital (Luminal)	10 - 20 mg/kg. In 20 mins, may give additional 5 mg/**kg** if needed.	No faster than 75 mg/min.	NA	Slow onset, may need 15 mins for effect. Requires intubation and respiratory and/or hemodynamic support.	15 - 40 mcg/mL
	Pentobarbital (Nembutal)	3 mg/kg	over 1 **hour**	1 - 3 mg/kg/hr	Hypotension may limit dose. Requires intubation and respiratory support, ECG monitoring, EEG, neuro consult.	3 - 4.5 mg/dL
	Valproic acid (Depacon)	15 - 30 mg/kg	No faster than 6 mg/kg/min	500 mg tid	Box warning: Toxic to the liver and pancreas Increases phenobarb and phenytoin levels Contraindicated in thrombocytopenia.	80 - 120 mcg/mL

Drip Tables

Drip Tables

Infusion Formulas

$$\text{mg/mL} = \frac{\text{mg of med}}{\text{mL of solution}}$$

$$\text{mg/hr} = \frac{\text{mg of med}}{\text{mL of solution}} \times \text{infusion rate (mL/hr)}$$

$$\text{mg/min} = \left[\frac{\text{mg of med}}{\text{mL of solution}} \times \text{infusion rate (mL/hr)}\right] / 60$$

$$\text{mg/kg/min} = \left[\frac{\text{mg of med}}{\text{mL of solution}} \times \text{infusion rate (mL/hr)}\right] / 60 / \text{kg}$$

$$\text{mcg/mL} = \frac{\text{mg of med} \times 1000}{\text{mL of solution}}$$

$$\text{mcg/hr} = \frac{\text{mg of med} \times 1000}{\text{mL of solution}} \times \text{infusion rate (mL/hr)}$$

$$\text{mcg/min} = \left[\frac{\text{mg of med} \times 1000}{\text{mL of solution}} \times \text{infusion rate (mL/hr)}\right] / 60$$

$$\text{mcg/kg/min} = \left[\frac{\text{mg of med} \times 1000}{\text{mL of solution}} \times \text{infusion rate (mL/hr)}\right] / 60 / \text{kg}$$

$$\text{Rate in gtts/min} = \frac{\text{volume to be given}}{\text{hrs to be given}} \times \text{\# of gtts/ml of IV set} / 60$$

$$\text{Rate in mL/hr} = \frac{\text{mcg/kg/min to be given} \times 60 \times \text{pt weight in kg}}{\text{drip concentration in mcg/mL}}$$

$$\text{Rate in mL/hr} = \frac{\text{mg/kg/min to be given} \times 60 \times \text{pt weight in kg}}{\text{drip concentration in mg/mL}}$$

When calculating a weight-based dose, do you use the patient's actual weight?
Here is 1 recommendation:
- If dialysis pt, use dry weight.
- If pt weighs > 200 lbs, use Ideal body weight, by gender:
  F: 45 + (2.3 × inches over 5 feet)
  M: 50 + (2.3 × inches over 5 feet)
- Everyone else: use the patient's actual weight.

NOREPINEPHRINE (Levophed)

IV load: None

Mix: $\frac{\text{4 mg}}{\text{250 mL D5W}}$

Concen: **16 mcg/mL**

Infuse: 2 - 12 mcg/min

Infusion rate mL/hr	Dose mcg/min
4	1
8	2
11	3
15	4
19	5

Table 6.1

Using the Infusion Tables:

1. The grid tables (e.g., Dopamine), offer the dose computed in mcg/kg/min. Some meds will have more than 1 table, for situations requiring a different concentration. Before using any one particular table, be sure you select the table with the concentration that matches the infusion you are giving your patient.
2. The vertical tables (e.g., Heparin, Lidocaine) are computed in either mg/hr, mg/min, mcg/min, or units/hr. Some meds, like Heparin, have several tables, each with a different concentration.
3. The areas shaded in blue are the doses that are outside the recommended dose range for that medication.

If you are using a drip concentration that is half of or twice that of the table you find in this chapter, you may halve or double the values accordingly.
For example: Suppose you have a mixture of Norepinephrine that is:

$\frac{\text{2 mg}}{\text{250 mL D5W}}$

The concentration of your drip would be 8 mcg/mL instead of the 16 mcg/mL in this table. Therefore, using this Norepinephrine table, if the infusion pump rate is set on 15 mL/hr, then your patient would receive half of the 4 mcg/min in this table, which would be 2 mcg/min. Not an ideal work-around, but it will do in a pinch.

AMIODARONE
(Cordarone)

IV load: 150 mg in 100 mL D5W over 10 mins.

Mix: 900 mg / 500 mL D5W

Concen: **1.8** mg/mL

Infuse: 1 mg/min x 6 hrs, then 0.5 mg/min x 18 hrs

Infusion rate mL/hr	Dose mg/min
5	0.2
10	0.3
13	0.4
16	0.5
20	0.6
23	0.7
25	0.8
28	0.8
30	0.9
33	1
40	1.2

Table 6.2

DEXMEDETOMIDINE
(Precedex)

Loading Dose Table

IV load: 1 mcg/kg over 10 min (use the mix to give the loading dose)

Mix: 200 mcg / 50 mL NS

Concen: **4** mcg/mL

To give a loading dose of 1 mcg/kg over 10 minutes:

Pt wt (kg)	Volume (mL) to give over 10 minutes
40	10
45	11.3
50	12.5
55	13.8
60	15
65	16.3
70	17.5
75	18.8
80	20
85	21.3
90	22.5
95	23.8
100	25.0
105	26.3
110	27.5

Table 6.3a

DILTIAZEM
(Cardizem)

IV load: 0.25 mg/kg over 2 mins.

Mix: 125 mg / 25 mL Diltiazem + 100 mL D5W, NS

Concen: **1** mg/mL

Infuse: 5 - 15 mg/hr

Infusion rate mL/hr	Dose mg/hr
4	4
5	5
6	6
7	7
8	8
9	9
10	10
11	11
12	12
13	13
14	14
15	15
20	20
25	25

Table 6.4

Table 6.3b

DEXMEDETOMIDINE (Precedex)

Continuous Infusion Table (using the mix in table 6.3a)

Use this table for find the infusion rate to give a dose between **0.2-0.7 mcg/kg/hr**

Patient weight (kg) is:

dose (mcg/kg/hr)	50	55	60	65	70	75	80	85	90	95	100	105	110	115	120
	Infusion rate (mL/hr):														
0.2	3	3	3	3	4	4	4	4	5	5	5	5	6	6	6
0.3	4	4	5	5	5	6	6	6	7	7	8	8	8	9	9
0.4	5	6	6	7	7	8	8	9	9	10	10	11	11	12	12
0.5	6	7	8	8	9	9	10	11	11	12	13	13	14	14	15
0.6	8	8	9	10	11	11	12	13	14	14	15	16	17	17	18
0.7	9	10	11	11	12	13	14	15	16	17	18	18	19	20	21

(Shaded) Doses outside the therapeutic range.

DOBUTAMINE

(Dobutrex)

IV loading dose: None

Mixture: 250 mg Nipride
250 mL D5W, NS D5NS, or RL

Concentration: 1000 mcg/mL

Infusion dose: 2 - 20 mcg/kg/min

(mcg/kg/min = Infusion rate x concentration/60/pt wt)

Table 6.5

Infusion rate (mL/hr)	Patient weight (kg) 35	40	45	50	55	60	65	70	75	80	85	90	95	100	105	110	115	120	125	130
	Dose (mcg/kg/min)																			
3	1.4	1.3	1.1	1.0	0.9	0.8	0.8	0.7	0.7	0.6	0.6	0.6	0.5	0.5	0.5	0.5	0.4	0.4	0.4	0.4
4	1.9	1.7	1.5	1.3	1.2	1.1	1.0	1.0	0.9	0.8	0.8	0.7	0.7	0.7	0.6	0.6	0.6	0.6	0.5	0.5
5	2.4	2.1	1.9	1.7	1.5	1.4	1.3	1.2	1.1	1.0	1.0	0.9	0.9	0.8	0.8	0.8	0.7	0.7	0.7	0.6
6	2.9	2.5	2.2	2.0	1.8	1.7	1.5	1.4	1.3	1.3	1.2	1.1	1.1	1.0	1.0	0.9	0.9	0.8	0.8	0.8
7	3.3	2.9	2.6	2.3	2.1	1.9	1.8	1.7	1.6	1.5	1.4	1.3	1.2	1.2	1.1	1.1	1.0	1.0	0.9	0.9
8	3.8	3.3	3.0	2.7	2.4	2.2	2.1	1.9	1.8	1.7	1.6	1.5	1.4	1.3	1.3	1.2	1.2	1.1	1.1	1.0
9	4.3	3.8	3.3	3.0	2.7	2.5	2.3	2.1	2.0	1.9	1.8	1.7	1.6	1.5	1.4	1.4	1.3	1.3	1.2	1.2
10	4.8	4.2	3.7	3.3	3.0	2.8	2.6	2.4	2.2	2.1	2.0	1.9	1.8	1.7	1.6	1.5	1.4	1.4	1.3	1.3
15	7.1	6.3	5.6	5.0	4.5	4.2	3.8	3.6	3.3	3.1	2.9	2.8	2.6	2.5	2.4	2.3	2.2	2.1	2.0	1.9
20	9.5	8.3	7.4	6.7	6.1	5.6	5.1	4.8	4.4	4.2	3.9	3.7	3.5	3.3	3.2	3.0	2.9	2.8	2.7	2.6
25	11.9	10.4	9.3	8.3	7.6	6.9	6.4	6.0	5.6	5.2	4.9	4.6	4.4	4.2	4.0	3.8	3.6	3.5	3.3	3.2
30	14.3	12.5	11.1	10.0	9.1	8.3	7.7	7.1	6.7	6.3	5.9	5.6	5.3	5.0	4.8	4.5	4.3	4.2	4.0	3.8
35	16.7	14.6	13.0	11.7	10.6	9.7	9.0	8.3	7.8	7.3	6.9	6.5	6.1	5.8	5.6	5.3	5.1	4.9	4.7	4.5
40	19.0	16.7	14.8	13.3	12.1	11.1	10.3	9.5	8.9	8.3	7.8	7.4	7.0	6.7	6.3	6.1	5.8	5.6	5.3	5.1
45	21.4	18.8	16.7	15.0	13.6	12.5	11.5	10.7	10.0	9.4	8.8	8.3	7.9	7.5	7.1	6.8	6.5	6.3	6.0	5.8
50	23.8	20.8	18.5	16.7	15.2	13.9	12.8	11.9	11.1	10.4	9.8	9.3	8.8	8.3	7.9	7.6	7.2	6.9	6.7	6.4
55	26.2	22.9	20.4	18.3	16.7	15.3	14.1	13.1	12.2	11.5	10.8	10.2	9.6	9.2	8.7	8.3	8.0	7.6	7.3	7.1
60	28.6	25.0	22.2	20.0	18.2	16.7	15.4	14.3	13.3	12.5	11.8	11.1	10.5	10.0	9.5	9.1	8.7	8.3	8.0	7.7
65	31.0	27.1	24.1	21.7	19.7	18.1	16.7	15.5	14.4	13.5	12.7	12.0	11.4	10.8	10.3	9.8	9.4	9.0	8.7	8.3
70	33.3	29.2	25.9	23.3	21.2	19.4	17.9	16.7	15.6	14.6	13.7	13.0	12.3	11.7	11.1	10.6	10.1	9.7	9.3	9.0

DOBUTAMINE
(Intropin)

IV loading dose: **None**

Mixture: 500 mg Dobutamine
250 mL D5W, NS D5NS, or RL

Concentration: **2000** mcg/mL

Infusion dose: 2 - 20 mcg/kg/min

mcg/kg/min = Infusion rate x concentration/60/pt wt

Table 6.6

Infusion rate (mL/hr)	Patient weight (kg) 35	40	45	50	55	60	65	70	75	80	85	90	95	100	105	110	115	120	125	130
	Dose (mcg/kg/min)																			
3	2.9	2.5	2.2	2.0	1.8	1.7	1.5	1.4	1.3	1.3	1.2	1.1	1.1	1.0	1.0	0.9	0.9	0.8	0.8	0.8
4	3.8	3.3	3.0	2.7	2.4	2.2	2.1	1.9	1.8	1.7	1.6	1.5	1.4	1.3	1.3	1.2	1.2	1.1	1.1	1.0
5	4.8	4.2	3.7	3.3	3.0	2.8	2.6	2.4	2.2	2.1	2.0	1.9	1.8	1.7	1.6	1.5	1.4	1.4	1.3	1.3
6	5.7	5.0	4.4	4.0	3.6	3.3	3.1	2.9	2.7	2.5	2.4	2.2	2.1	2.0	1.9	1.8	1.7	1.7	1.6	1.5
7	6.7	5.8	5.2	4.7	4.2	3.9	3.6	3.3	3.1	2.9	2.7	2.6	2.5	2.3	2.2	2.1	2.0	1.9	1.9	1.8
8	7.6	6.7	5.9	5.3	4.8	4.4	4.1	3.8	3.6	3.3	3.1	3.0	2.8	2.7	2.5	2.4	2.3	2.2	2.1	2.1
9	8.6	7.5	6.7	6.0	5.5	5.0	4.6	4.3	4.0	3.8	3.5	3.3	3.2	3.0	2.9	2.7	2.6	2.5	2.4	2.3
10	9.5	8.3	7.4	6.7	6.1	5.6	5.1	4.8	4.4	4.2	3.9	3.7	3.5	3.3	3.2	3.0	2.9	2.8	2.7	2.6
15	14.3	12.5	11.1	10.0	9.1	8.3	7.7	7.1	6.7	6.3	5.9	5.6	5.3	5.0	4.8	4.5	4.3	4.2	4.0	3.8
20	19.0	16.7	14.8	13.3	12.1	11.1	10.3	9.5	8.9	8.3	7.8	7.4	7.0	6.7	6.3	6.1	5.8	5.6	5.3	5.1
25	23.8	20.8	18.5	16.7	15.2	13.9	12.8	11.9	11.1	10.4	9.8	9.3	8.8	8.3	7.9	7.6	7.2	6.9	6.7	6.4
30	28.6	25.0	22.2	20.0	18.2	16.7	15.4	14.3	13.3	12.5	11.8	11.1	10.5	10.0	9.5	9.1	8.7	8.3	8.0	7.7
35	33.3	29.2	25.9	23.3	21.2	19.4	17.9	16.7	15.6	14.6	13.7	13.0	12.3	11.7	11.1	10.6	10.1	9.7	9.3	9.0
40	38.1	33.3	29.6	26.7	24.2	22.2	20.5	19.0	17.8	16.7	15.7	14.8	14.0	13.3	12.7	12.1	11.6	11.1	10.7	10.3
45	42.9	37.5	33.3	30.0	27.3	25.0	23.1	21.4	20.0	18.8	17.6	16.7	15.8	15.0	14.3	13.6	13.0	12.5	12.0	11.5
50	47.6	41.7	37.0	33.3	30.3	27.8	25.6	23.8	22.2	20.8	19.6	18.5	17.5	16.7	15.9	15.2	14.5	13.9	13.3	12.8
55	52.4	45.8	40.7	36.7	33.3	30.6	28.2	26.2	24.4	22.9	21.6	20.4	19.3	18.3	17.5	16.7	15.9	15.3	14.7	14.1
60	57.1	50.0	44.4	40.0	36.4	33.3	30.8	28.6	26.7	25.0	23.5	22.2	21.1	20.0	19.0	18.2	17.4	16.7	16.0	15.4
65	61.9	54.2	48.1	43.3	39.4	36.1	33.3	31.0	28.9	27.1	25.5	24.1	22.8	21.7	20.6	19.7	18.8	18.1	17.3	16.7
70	66.7	58.3	51.9	46.7	42.4	38.9	35.9	33.3	31.1	29.2	27.5	25.9	24.6	23.3	22.2	21.2	20.3	19.4	18.7	17.9

DOPAMINE
(Intropin)

Mixture: <u>200 mg Dopamine</u>
250 mL D5W, NS, or D5NS

Concentration: **800** mcg/mL

Infusion dose: 2 - 20 mcg/kg/min

IV loading dose: **None**

mcg/kg/min = Infusion rate x concentration/60/pt wt

Table 6.7

Infusion rate (mL/hr)	35	40	45	50	55	60	65	70	75	80	85	90	95	100	105	110	115	120	125	130
	Patient weight (kg)																			
	Dose (mcg/kg/min)																			
3	1.1	1.0	0.9	0.8	0.7	0.7	0.6	0.6	0.5	0.5	0.5	0.4	0.4	0.4	0.4	0.4	0.3	0.3	0.3	0.3
4	1.5	1.3	1.2	1.1	1.0	0.9	0.8	0.8	0.7	0.7	0.6	0.6	0.6	0.5	0.5	0.5	0.5	0.4	0.4	0.4
5	1.9	1.7	1.5	1.3	1.2	1.1	1.0	1.0	0.9	0.8	0.8	0.7	0.7	0.7	0.6	0.6	0.6	0.6	0.5	0.5
6	2.3	2.0	1.8	1.6	1.5	1.3	1.2	1.1	1.1	1.0	0.9	0.9	0.8	0.8	0.8	0.7	0.7	0.7	0.6	0.6
7	2.7	2.3	2.1	1.9	1.7	1.6	1.4	1.3	1.2	1.2	1.1	1.0	1.0	0.9	0.9	0.8	0.8	0.8	0.7	0.7
8	3.0	2.7	2.4	2.1	1.9	1.8	1.6	1.5	1.4	1.3	1.3	1.2	1.1	1.1	1.0	1.0	0.9	0.9	0.9	0.8
9	3.4	3.0	2.7	2.4	2.2	2.0	1.8	1.7	1.6	1.5	1.4	1.3	1.3	1.2	1.1	1.1	1.0	1.0	1.0	0.9
10	3.8	3.3	3.0	2.7	2.4	2.2	2.1	1.9	1.8	1.7	1.6	1.5	1.4	1.3	1.3	1.2	1.2	1.1	1.1	1.0
15	5.7	5.0	4.4	4.0	3.6	3.3	3.1	2.9	2.7	2.5	2.4	2.2	2.1	2.0	1.9	1.8	1.7	1.7	1.6	1.5
20	7.6	6.7	5.9	5.3	4.8	4.4	4.1	3.8	3.6	3.3	3.1	3.0	2.8	2.7	2.5	2.4	2.3	2.2	2.1	2.1
25	9.5	8.3	7.4	6.7	6.1	5.6	5.1	4.8	4.4	4.2	3.9	3.7	3.5	3.3	3.2	3.0	2.9	2.8	2.7	2.6
30	11.4	10.0	8.9	8.0	7.3	6.7	6.2	5.7	5.3	5.0	4.7	4.4	4.2	4.0	3.8	3.6	3.5	3.3	3.2	3.1
35	13.3	11.7	10.4	9.3	8.5	7.8	7.2	6.7	6.2	5.8	5.5	5.2	4.9	4.7	4.4	4.2	4.1	3.9	3.7	3.6
40	15.2	13.3	11.9	10.7	9.7	8.9	8.2	7.6	7.1	6.7	6.3	5.9	5.6	5.3	5.1	4.8	4.6	4.4	4.3	4.1
45	17.1	15.0	13.3	12.0	10.9	10.0	9.2	8.6	8.0	7.5	7.1	6.7	6.3	6.0	5.7	5.5	5.2	5.0	4.8	4.6
50	19.0	16.7	14.8	13.3	12.1	11.1	10.3	9.5	8.9	8.3	7.8	7.4	7.0	6.7	6.3	6.1	5.8	5.6	5.3	5.1
55	21.0	18.3	16.3	14.7	13.3	12.2	11.3	10.5	9.8	9.2	8.6	8.1	7.7	7.3	7.0	6.7	6.4	6.1	5.9	5.6
60	22.9	20.0	17.8	16.0	14.5	13.3	12.3	11.4	10.7	10.0	9.4	8.9	8.4	8.0	7.6	7.3	7.0	6.7	6.4	6.2
65	24.8	21.7	19.3	17.3	15.8	14.4	13.3	12.4	11.6	10.8	10.2	9.6	9.1	8.7	8.3	7.9	7.5	7.2	6.9	6.7
70	26.7	23.3	20.7	18.7	17.0	15.6	14.4	13.3	12.4	11.7	11.0	10.4	9.8	9.3	8.9	8.5	8.1	7.8	7.5	7.2

DOPAMINE
(Intropin)

IV loading dose: **None**

Mixture: 400 mg Dopamine / 250 mL D5W, NS, or D5NS

Concentration: **1600** mcg/mL

Infusion dose: 2 - 20 mcg/kg/min

mcg/kg/min = Infusion rate x concentration/60/pt wt

Table 6.8

Infusion rate (mL/hr)	35	40	45	50	55	60	65	70	75	80	85	90	95	100	105	110	115	120	125	130
	Patient weight (kg)																			
	Dose (mcg/kg/min)																			
3	2.3	2.0	1.8	1.6	1.5	1.3	1.2	1.1	1.1	1.0	0.9	0.9	0.8	0.8	0.8	0.7	0.7	0.7	0.6	0.6
4	3.0	2.7	2.4	2.1	1.9	1.8	1.6	1.5	1.4	1.3	1.3	1.2	1.1	1.1	1.0	1.0	0.9	0.9	0.9	0.8
5	3.8	3.3	3.0	2.7	2.4	2.2	2.1	1.9	1.8	1.7	1.6	1.5	1.4	1.3	1.3	1.2	1.2	1.1	1.1	1.0
6	4.6	4.0	3.6	3.2	2.9	2.7	2.5	2.3	2.1	2.0	1.9	1.8	1.7	1.6	1.5	1.5	1.4	1.3	1.3	1.2
7	5.3	4.7	4.1	3.7	3.4	3.1	2.9	2.7	2.5	2.3	2.2	2.1	2.0	1.9	1.8	1.7	1.6	1.6	1.5	1.4
8	6.1	5.3	4.7	4.3	3.9	3.6	3.3	3.0	2.8	2.7	2.5	2.4	2.2	2.1	2.0	1.9	1.9	1.8	1.7	1.6
9	6.9	6.0	5.3	4.8	4.4	4.0	3.7	3.4	3.2	3.0	2.8	2.7	2.5	2.4	2.3	2.2	2.1	2.0	1.9	1.8
10	7.6	6.7	5.9	5.3	4.8	4.4	4.1	3.8	3.6	3.3	3.1	3.0	2.8	2.7	2.5	2.4	2.3	2.2	2.1	2.1
15	11.4	10.0	8.9	8.0	7.3	6.7	6.2	5.7	5.3	5.0	4.7	4.4	4.2	4.0	3.8	3.6	3.5	3.3	3.2	3.1
20	15.2	13.3	11.9	10.7	9.7	8.9	8.2	7.6	7.1	6.7	6.3	5.9	5.6	5.3	5.1	4.8	4.6	4.4	4.3	4.1
25	19.0	16.7	14.8	13.3	12.1	11.1	10.3	9.5	8.9	8.3	7.8	7.4	7.0	6.7	6.3	6.1	5.8	5.6	5.3	5.1
30	22.9	20.0	17.8	16.0	14.5	13.3	12.3	11.4	10.7	10.0	9.4	8.9	8.4	8.0	7.6	7.3	7.0	6.7	6.4	6.2
35	26.7	23.3	20.7	18.7	17.0	15.6	14.4	13.3	12.4	11.7	11.0	10.4	9.8	9.3	8.9	8.5	8.1	7.8	7.5	7.2
40	30.5	26.7	23.7	21.3	19.4	17.8	16.4	15.2	14.2	13.3	12.5	11.9	11.2	10.7	10.2	9.7	9.3	8.9	8.5	8.2
45	34.3	30.0	26.7	24.0	21.8	20.0	18.5	17.1	16.0	15.0	14.1	13.3	12.6	12.0	11.4	10.9	10.4	10.0	9.6	9.2
50	38.1	33.3	29.6	26.7	24.2	22.2	20.5	19.0	17.8	16.7	15.7	14.8	14.0	13.3	12.7	12.1	11.6	11.1	10.7	10.3
55	41.9	36.7	32.6	29.3	26.7	24.4	22.6	21.0	19.6	18.3	17.3	16.3	15.4	14.7	14.0	13.3	12.8	12.2	11.7	11.3
60	45.7	40.0	35.6	32.0	29.1	26.7	24.6	22.9	21.3	20.0	18.8	17.8	16.8	16.0	15.2	14.5	13.9	13.3	12.8	12.3
65	49.5	43.3	38.5	34.7	31.5	28.9	26.7	24.8	23.1	21.7	20.4	19.3	18.2	17.3	16.5	15.8	15.1	14.4	13.9	13.3
70	53.3	46.7	41.5	37.3	33.9	31.1	28.7	26.7	24.9	23.3	22.0	20.7	19.6	18.7	17.8	17.0	16.2	15.6	14.9	14.4

EPINEPHRINE
(Adrenalin)

Mixture: 4 mg Epinephrine
250 mL D5W, NS, D5NS, or RL

Concentration: 16 mcg/mL

Infusion dose: 0.05 - 0.1 mcg/kg/min

IV loading dose: 0.1 - 1 mg

mcg/kg/min = Infusion rate x concentration/60/pt wt.

Table 6.9

Infusion rate (mL/hr)	Patient weight (kg)																			
	35	40	45	50	55	60	65	70	75	80	85	90	95	100	105	110	115	120	125	130
	Dose (mcg/kg/min)																			
4	0.03	0.03	0.02	0.02	0.02	0.02	0.02	0.02	0.01	0.01	0.01	0.01	0.01	0.01	0.01	0.01	0.01	0.01	0.01	0.01
5	0.04	0.03	0.03	0.03	0.02	0.02	0.02	0.02	0.02	0.02	0.02	0.01	0.01	0.01	0.01	0.01	0.01	0.01	0.01	0.01
6	0.05	0.04	0.04	0.03	0.03	0.03	0.02	0.02	0.02	0.02	0.02	0.02	0.02	0.02	0.02	0.01	0.01	0.01	0.01	0.01
7	0.05	0.05	0.04	0.04	0.03	0.03	0.03	0.03	0.02	0.02	0.02	0.02	0.02	0.02	0.02	0.02	0.02	0.02	0.01	0.01
8	0.06	0.05	0.05	0.04	0.04	0.04	0.03	0.03	0.03	0.03	0.03	0.02	0.02	0.02	0.02	0.02	0.02	0.02	0.02	0.02
9	0.07	0.06	0.05	0.05	0.04	0.04	0.04	0.03	0.03	0.03	0.03	0.03	0.03	0.02	0.02	0.02	0.02	0.02	0.02	0.02
10	0.08	0.07	0.06	0.05	0.05	0.04	0.04	0.04	0.04	0.03	0.03	0.03	0.03	0.03	0.03	0.02	0.02	0.02	0.02	0.02
11	0.08	0.07	0.07	0.06	0.05	0.05	0.05	0.04	0.04	0.04	0.03	0.03	0.03	0.03	0.03	0.03	0.03	0.02	0.02	0.02
12	0.09	0.08	0.07	0.06	0.06	0.05	0.05	0.05	0.04	0.04	0.04	0.04	0.03	0.03	0.03	0.03	0.03	0.03	0.03	0.02
13	0.10	0.09	0.08	0.07	0.06	0.06	0.05	0.05	0.05	0.04	0.04	0.04	0.04	0.03	0.03	0.03	0.03	0.03	0.03	0.03
14	0.11	0.09	0.08	0.07	0.07	0.06	0.06	0.05	0.05	0.05	0.04	0.04	0.04	0.04	0.04	0.03	0.03	0.03	0.03	0.03
15	0.11	0.10	0.09	0.08	0.07	0.07	0.06	0.06	0.05	0.05	0.05	0.04	0.04	0.04	0.04	0.04	0.03	0.03	0.03	0.03
16	0.12	0.11	0.09	0.09	0.08	0.07	0.07	0.06	0.06	0.05	0.05	0.05	0.04	0.04	0.04	0.04	0.04	0.04	0.03	0.03
17	0.13	0.11	0.10	0.09	0.08	0.08	0.07	0.06	0.06	0.06	0.05	0.05	0.05	0.05	0.04	0.04	0.04	0.04	0.04	0.03
18	0.14	0.12	0.11	0.10	0.09	0.08	0.07	0.07	0.06	0.06	0.06	0.05	0.05	0.05	0.05	0.04	0.04	0.04	0.04	0.04
19	0.14	0.13	0.11	0.10	0.09	0.08	0.08	0.07	0.07	0.06	0.06	0.06	0.05	0.05	0.05	0.05	0.04	0.04	0.04	0.04
20	0.15	0.13	0.12	0.11	0.10	0.09	0.08	0.08	0.07	0.07	0.06	0.06	0.06	0.05	0.05	0.05	0.05	0.04	0.04	0.04
21	0.16	0.14	0.12	0.11	0.10	0.09	0.09	0.08	0.07	0.07	0.07	0.06	0.06	0.06	0.05	0.05	0.05	0.05	0.04	0.04
22	0.17	0.15	0.13	0.12	0.11	0.10	0.09	0.08	0.08	0.07	0.07	0.07	0.06	0.06	0.06	0.05	0.05	0.05	0.05	0.05
23	0.18	0.15	0.14	0.12	0.11	0.10	0.09	0.09	0.08	0.08	0.07	0.07	0.06	0.06	0.06	0.06	0.05	0.05	0.05	0.05

EPINEPHRINE

IV load: 0.1 - 1 mg

Mix: 1 mg / 250 mL D5W

Concen: 4 mcg/mL

Infuse: 2 - 10 mcg/min

Infusion rate mL/hr	Dose mcg/min
15	1
30	2
45	3
60	4
75	5
90	6
105	7
120	8
135	9
150	10
165	11
180	12

Table 6.10

EPINEPHRINE

IV load: 0.1 - 1 mg

Mix: 2 mg / 250 mL D5W

Concen: 8 mcg/mL

Infuse: 2 - 10 mcg/

Infusion rate mL/hr	Dose mcg/min
6	0.8
8	1.1
15	2.0
23	3.1
30	4.0
38	5.1
45	6.0
53	7.1
60	8.0
68	9.1
75	10.0
80	10.7
85	11.3
90	12.0
95	12.7
100	13.3

Table 6.11

EPINEPHRINE

IV load: 0.1 - 1 mg

Mix: 4 mg / 250 mL D5W

Concen: 16 mcg/mL

Infuse: 2 - 10 mcg/min

Infusion rate mL/hr	Dose mcg/min
6	1.6
8	2.1
10	2.7
12	3.2
14	3.7
16	4.3
18	4.8
20	5.3
22	5.9
24	6.4
26	6.9
28	7.5
30	8.0
32	8.5
34	9.1
36	9.6
38	10.1
40	10.7
42	11.2
44	11.7
46	12.3
48	12.8
50	13.3

Table 6.12

FENTANYL
(Sublimase)

IV load: 25 - 100 mcg (0.5 - 2 mcg/kg)

Mix: 1 mg / 100 ML D5W

Concen: 10 mcg/mL

Infuse: 25 - 200 mcg/hr

Infusion rate mL/hr	Dose mcg/hr
2	20
3	30
4	40
5	50
6	60
7	70
8	80
9	90
10	100
15	150
20	200
25	250
30	300

Table 6.13

Doses outside the therapeutic range.

ESMOLOL
Brevibloc

A fib

IV Loading dose:
Use the mix to give
500 mcg/kg x 1 min.,
then 50 mcg/kg/min x 5 mins.

Mixture: 2.5 g Esmolol
250 mL D5W, NS, 1/2 NS, or RL

Concentration: **10,000** mcg/mL (10 mg/mL)

Infusion dose: 50 - 200 mcg/kg/min

mcg/kg/min = Infusion rate x concentration/60/pt wt

Table 6.14

Infusion rate (mL/hr)	Patient weight (kg) 35	40	45	50	55	60	65	70	75	80	85	90	95	100	105	110	115	120	125	130
	Dose (mcg/kg/min)																			
5	24	21	19	17	15	14	13	12	11	10	10	9	9	8	8	8	7	7	7	6
10	48	42	37	33	30	28	26	24	22	21	20	19	18	17	16	15	14	14	13	13
15	71	63	56	50	45	42	38	36	33	31	29	28	26	25	24	23	22	21	20	19
20	95	83	74	67	61	56	51	48	44	42	39	37	35	33	32	30	29	28	27	26
25	119	104	93	83	76	69	64	60	56	52	49	46	44	42	40	38	36	35	33	32
30	143	125	111	100	91	83	77	71	67	63	59	56	53	50	48	45	43	42	40	38
35	167	146	130	117	106	97	90	83	78	73	69	65	61	58	56	53	51	49	47	45
40	190	167	148	133	121	111	103	95	89	83	78	74	70	67	63	61	58	56	53	51
45	214	188	167	150	136	125	115	107	100	94	88	83	79	75	71	68	65	63	60	58
50	238	208	185	167	152	139	128	119	111	104	98	93	88	83	79	76	72	69	67	64
55	262	229	204	183	167	153	141	131	122	115	108	102	96	92	87	83	80	76	73	71
60	286	250	222	200	182	167	154	143	133	125	118	111	105	100	95	91	87	83	80	77
65	310	271	241	217	197	181	167	155	144	135	127	120	114	108	103	98	94	90	87	83
70	333	292	259	233	212	194	179	167	156	146	137	130	123	117	111	106	101	97	93	90
75	357	313	278	250	227	208	192	179	167	156	147	139	132	125	119	114	109	104	100	96
80	381	333	296	267	242	222	205	190	178	167	157	148	140	133	127	121	116	111	107	103
85	405	354	315	283	258	236	218	202	189	177	167	157	149	142	135	129	123	118	113	109
90	429	375	333	300	273	250	231	214	200	188	176	167	158	150	143	136	130	125	120	115
95	452	396	352	317	288	264	244	226	211	198	186	176	167	158	151	144	138	132	127	122
100	476	417	370	333	303	278	256	238	222	208	196	185	175	167	159	152	145	139	133	128

HEPARIN

IV load: 50 - 80 units/kg

Mix: 10,000 units / 250 mL D_5W

Concen: 40 units/mL

Infuse: 400-1600 units/hr

Infusion rate mL/hr	Dose units/hr
8 (shaded)	320
10	400
11	440
12	480
13	520
14	560
15	600
16	640
17	680
18	720
19	760
20	800
22	880
24	960
25	1000
26	1040
28	1120
30	1200
32	1280
34	1360
36	1440
38	1520
40	1600
42 (shaded)	1680
44 (shaded)	1760

Table 6.15

HEPARIN

IV load: 50 - 80 units/kg

Mix: 12,500 units / 250 mL D_5W

Concen: 50 units/mL

Infuse: 400-1600 units/hr

Infusion rate mL/hr	Dose units/hr
7 (shaded)	350
8	400
9	450
10	500
11	550
12	600
13	650
14	700
15	750
16	800
17	850
18	900
19	950
20	1000
22	1100
24	1200
26	1300
28	1400
30	1500
32	1600
34 (shaded)	1700
36 (shaded)	1800
38 (shaded)	1900
40 (shaded)	2000

Table 6.16

HEPARIN

IV load: 50 - 80 units/kg

Mix: 25,000 units / 250 mL D_5W

Concen: 100 units/mL

Infuse: 400-1600 units/hr

Infusion rate mL/hr	Dose units/hr
3 (shaded)	300
4	400
5	500
6	600
7	700
8	800
9	900
10	1000
11	1100
12	1200
13	1300
14	1400
15	1500
16	1600
18 (shaded)	1800
20 (shaded)	2000

Table 6.17

Shaded: Doses outside the therapeutic range.

INAMRINONE
(Inocor)

Mixture: <u>500 mg Inamrinone</u>
100 mL Inamrinone +
100 mL NS or 1/2 NS

Concentration: 2,500 mcg/mL

IV Push dose: 0.75 mg/kg over 5 mins

Infusion dose: 5 - 10 mcg/kg/min

mcg/kg/min = Infusion rate x concentration/60/pt wt.

Table 6.18

Dose (mcg/kg/min)

Infusion rate (mL/hr)	Patient weight (kg) 35	40	45	50	55	60	65	70	75	80	85	90	95	100	105	110	115	120	125	130
4	4.8	4.2	3.7	3.3	3.0	2.8	2.6	2.4	2.2	2.1	2.0	1.9	1.8	1.7	1.6	1.5	1.4	1.4	1.3	1.3
5	6.0	5.2	4.6	4.2	3.8	3.5	3.2	3.0	2.8	2.6	2.5	2.3	2.2	2.1	2.0	1.9	1.8	1.7	1.7	1.6
6	7.1	6.3	5.6	5.0	4.5	4.2	3.8	3.6	3.3	3.1	2.9	2.8	2.6	2.5	2.4	2.3	2.2	2.1	2.0	1.9
7	8.3	7.3	6.5	5.8	5.3	4.9	4.5	4.2	3.9	3.6	3.4	3.2	3.1	2.9	2.8	2.7	2.5	2.4	2.3	2.2
8	9.5	8.3	7.4	6.7	6.1	5.6	5.1	4.8	4.4	4.2	3.9	3.7	3.5	3.3	3.2	3.0	2.9	2.8	2.7	2.6
9	10.7	9.4	8.3	7.5	6.8	6.3	5.8	5.4	5.0	4.7	4.4	4.2	3.9	3.8	3.6	3.4	3.3	3.1	3.0	2.9
10	11.9	10.4	9.3	8.3	7.6	6.9	6.4	6.0	5.6	5.2	4.9	4.6	4.4	4.2	4.0	3.8	3.6	3.5	3.3	3.2
11	13.1	11.5	10.2	9.2	8.3	7.6	7.1	6.5	6.1	5.7	5.4	5.1	4.8	4.6	4.4	4.2	4.0	3.8	3.7	3.5
12	14.3	12.5	11.1	10.0	9.1	8.3	7.7	7.1	6.7	6.3	5.9	5.6	5.3	5.0	4.8	4.5	4.3	4.2	4.0	3.8
13	15.5	13.5	12.0	10.8	9.8	9.0	8.3	7.7	7.2	6.8	6.4	6.0	5.7	5.4	5.2	4.9	4.7	4.5	4.3	4.2
14	16.7	14.6	13.0	11.7	10.6	9.7	9.0	8.3	7.8	7.3	6.9	6.5	6.1	5.8	5.6	5.3	5.1	4.9	4.7	4.5
15	17.9	15.6	13.9	12.5	11.4	10.4	9.6	8.9	8.3	7.8	7.4	6.9	6.6	6.3	6.0	5.7	5.4	5.2	5.0	4.8
16	19.0	16.7	14.8	13.3	12.1	11.1	10.3	9.5	8.9	8.3	7.8	7.4	7.0	6.7	6.3	6.1	5.8	5.6	5.3	5.1
18	21.4	18.8	16.7	15.0	13.6	12.5	11.5	10.7	10.0	9.4	8.8	8.3	7.9	7.5	7.1	6.8	6.5	6.3	6.0	5.8
20	23.8	20.8	18.5	16.7	15.2	13.9	12.8	11.9	11.1	10.4	9.8	9.3	8.8	8.3	7.9	7.6	7.2	6.9	6.7	6.4
22	26.2	22.9	20.4	18.3	16.7	15.3	14.1	13.1	12.2	11.5	10.8	10.2	9.6	9.2	8.7	8.3	8.0	7.6	7.3	7.1
24	28.6	25.0	22.2	20.0	18.2	16.7	15.4	14.3	13.3	12.5	11.8	11.1	10.5	10.0	9.5	9.1	8.7	8.3	8.0	7.7
26	31.0	27.1	24.1	21.7	19.7	18.1	16.7	15.5	14.4	13.5	12.7	12.0	11.4	10.8	10.3	9.8	9.4	9.0	8.7	8.3
28	33.3	29.2	25.9	23.3	21.2	19.4	17.9	16.7	15.6	14.6	13.7	13.0	12.3	11.7	11.1	10.6	10.1	9.7	9.3	9.0
30	35.7	31.3	27.8	25.0	22.7	20.8	19.2	17.9	16.7	15.6	14.7	13.9	13.2	12.5	11.9	11.4	10.9	10.4	10.0	9.6

LABETALOL
(Normodyne, Trandate)

IV load: 20 mg over 2 minutes

Mix: 400 mg / 80 mL Labetalol + 120 mL D5W

Concen: **2** mg/mL

Infuse: 0.5 - 2 mg/min

Infusion rate mL/hr	Dose mg/min
14	0.47
15	0.5
18	0.6
21	0.7
24	0.8
27	0.9
30	1
36	1.2
42	1.4
48	1.6
54	1.8
60	2

Table 6.19

LIDOCAINE

IV load: 0.5 - 1.5 mg/kg

Mix: 2 g / 500 mL D5W

Concen: **4** mg/mL

Infuse: 1 - 4 mg/min

Infusion rate mL/hr	Dose mg/min
10	0.7
15	1
20	1.3
25	1.7
30	2
35	2.3
40	2.7
45	3
50	3.3
55	3.7
60	4
65	4.3

Table 6.20

LORAZEPAM
(Ativan)

IV load: 0.44 mg/kg (or 2 mg total), dilute in equal amount of NS give over 5 mi

Mix: 10 mg / 100 mL D5W in glass

Concen: **0.1** mg/mL

Infuse: 0.5 - 2 mg/hr

Infusion rate mL/hr	Dose mg/hr
4	0.4
5	0.5
6	0.6
7	0.7
8	0.8
9	0.9
10	1
12	1.2
14	1.4
16	1.6
18	1.8
20	2
22	2.2
24	2.4
26	2.6
28	2.8
30	3
32	3.2
34	3.4
36	3.6
38	3.8
40	4

Table 6.22

Doses outside the therapeutic range.

1

MIDAZOLAM
(Versed)

IV load: 1 mg over 2 mins. repeat as needed q 2 - 5 mins, maxium total dose is 5 mg

Mix: 50 mg / 250 mL D5W or NS

Concen: **0.2** mg/mL

Infuse: 1 - 7 mg/hr (1 - 10 mg/hr is also often described)

Infusion rate mL/hr	Dose mg/hr
5	1
10	2
15	3
20	4
25	5
30	6
35	7
40	8
45	9
50	10

Table 6.23

2

MIDAZOLAM
(Versed)

IV load: 1 mg over 2 mins. repeat as needed q 2 - 5 mins, maxium total dose is 5 mg

Mix: 100 mg / 250 mL D5W or NS

Concen: **0.5** mg/mL

Infuse: 1 - 7 mg/hr (1 - 10 mg/hr is also often described)

Infusion rate mL/hr	Dose mg/hr
2	1
4	2
6	3
8	4
10	5
12	6
14	7
16	8
18	9
20	10

Table 6.24

MORPHINE

IV load: 1 - 5 mg

Mix: 20 mg / 100 mL D5W or NS

Concen: **0.2** mg/mL

Infuse: 1 - 5 mg/hr (1 - 10 mg/hr is also often described)

Infusion rate mL/hr	Dose mg/hr
2	0.4
3	0.6
4	0.8
5	1
6	1.2
7	1.4
8	1.6
9	1.8
10	2
12	2.4
14	2.8
15	3
16	3.2
18	3.6
20	4
22	4.4
24	4.8
25	5
30	6
35	7
40	8
45	9
50	10

Table 6.25

Doses outside the therapeutic range.

MILRINONE
(Primacor)

Mixture: 40 mg Milrinone / 200 mL D5W

Concentration: 200 mcg/mL

IV Push dose:
50 mcg/kg over 10 minutes

Infusion dose: 0.375 - 0.75 mcg/kg/min

mcg/kg/min = infusion rate x concentration/60/pt wt

Table 6.26

Dose (mcg/kg/min)

Infusion rate (mL/hr) \ Patient weight (kg)	35	40	45	50	55	60	65	70	75	80	85	90	95	100	105	110	115	120	125	130
4	0.38	0.33	0.30	0.27	0.24	0.22	0.21	0.19	0.18	0.17	0.16	0.15	0.14	0.13	0.13	0.12	0.12	0.11	0.11	0.10
5	0.48	0.42	0.37	0.33	0.30	0.28	0.26	0.24	0.22	0.21	0.20	0.19	0.18	0.17	0.16	0.15	0.14	0.14	0.13	0.13
6	0.57	0.50	0.44	0.40	0.36	0.33	0.31	0.29	0.27	0.25	0.24	0.22	0.21	0.20	0.19	0.18	0.17	0.17	0.16	0.15
7	0.67	0.58	0.52	0.47	0.42	0.39	0.36	0.33	0.31	0.29	0.27	0.26	0.25	0.23	0.22	0.21	0.20	0.19	0.19	0.18
8	0.76	0.67	0.59	0.53	0.48	0.44	0.41	0.38	0.36	0.33	0.31	0.30	0.28	0.27	0.25	0.24	0.23	0.22	0.21	0.21
9	0.86	0.75	0.67	0.60	0.55	0.50	0.46	0.43	0.40	0.38	0.35	0.33	0.32	0.30	0.29	0.27	0.26	0.25	0.24	0.23
10	0.95	0.83	0.74	0.67	0.61	0.56	0.51	0.48	0.44	0.42	0.39	0.37	0.35	0.33	0.32	0.30	0.29	0.28	0.27	0.26
11	1.05	0.92	0.81	0.73	0.67	0.61	0.56	0.52	0.49	0.46	0.43	0.41	0.39	0.37	0.35	0.33	0.32	0.31	0.29	0.28
12	1.14	1.00	0.89	0.80	0.73	0.67	0.62	0.57	0.53	0.50	0.47	0.44	0.42	0.40	0.38	0.36	0.35	0.33	0.32	0.31
13	1.24	1.08	0.96	0.87	0.79	0.72	0.67	0.62	0.58	0.54	0.51	0.48	0.46	0.43	0.41	0.39	0.38	0.36	0.35	0.33
14	1.33	1.17	1.04	0.93	0.85	0.78	0.72	0.67	0.62	0.58	0.55	0.52	0.49	0.47	0.44	0.42	0.41	0.39	0.37	0.36
15	1.43	1.25	1.11	1.00	0.91	0.83	0.77	0.71	0.67	0.63	0.59	0.56	0.53	0.50	0.48	0.45	0.43	0.42	0.40	0.38
16	1.52	1.33	1.19	1.07	0.97	0.89	0.82	0.76	0.71	0.67	0.63	0.59	0.56	0.53	0.51	0.48	0.46	0.44	0.43	0.41
17	1.62	1.42	1.26	1.13	1.03	0.94	0.87	0.81	0.76	0.71	0.67	0.63	0.60	0.57	0.54	0.52	0.49	0.47	0.45	0.44
18	1.71	1.50	1.33	1.20	1.09	1.00	0.92	0.86	0.80	0.75	0.71	0.67	0.63	0.60	0.57	0.55	0.52	0.50	0.48	0.46
19	1.81	1.58	1.41	1.27	1.15	1.06	0.97	0.90	0.84	0.79	0.75	0.70	0.67	0.63	0.60	0.58	0.55	0.53	0.51	0.49
20	1.90	1.67	1.48	1.33	1.21	1.11	1.03	0.95	0.89	0.83	0.78	0.74	0.70	0.67	0.63	0.61	0.58	0.56	0.53	0.51
21	2.00	1.75	1.56	1.40	1.27	1.17	1.08	1.00	0.93	0.88	0.82	0.78	0.74	0.70	0.67	0.64	0.61	0.58	0.56	0.54
22	2.10	1.83	1.63	1.47	1.33	1.22	1.13	1.05	0.98	0.92	0.86	0.81	0.77	0.73	0.70	0.67	0.64	0.61	0.59	0.56
23	2.19	1.92	1.70	1.53	1.39	1.28	1.18	1.10	1.02	0.96	0.90	0.85	0.81	0.77	0.73	0.70	0.67	0.64	0.61	0.59

NESIRITIDE
(Natrecor)

Mix: 1.5 mg / 250 mL D5W, NS

Concen: 6 mcg/mL

Load: 2 mcg/kg over 60 seconds

Infuse: 0.01 mcg/kg/min

Pt wt (kg)	Infusion rate (mL/hr) to give 0.01 mcg/kg/min
40	4
45	4.5
50	5
55	5.5
60	6
65	6.5
70	7
75	7.5
80	8
85	8.5
90	9
95	9.5
100	10
105	10.5
110	11
115	11.5
120	12
125	12.5
130	13
135	13.5
140	14
145	14.5
150	15

Table 6.27

NITROGLYCERIN

IV load: 12.5 - 25 mcg

Mix: 25 mg / 250 mL D5W

Concen: 100 mcg/mL

Infuse: 5 - 20 mcg/min (200 mcg/min max)

Infusion rate mL/hr	Dose mcg/min
3	5
5	8
6	10
9	15
12	20
15	25
18	30
21	35
24	40
30	50
36	60
42	70
48	80
54	90
60	100
66	110
72	120
78	130
84	140
90	150
96	160
105	175
114	190
120	200

Table 6.29

NITROGLYCERIN

IV load: 12.5 - 25 mcg

Mix: 50 mg / 250 mL D5W

Concen: 200 mcg/mL

Infuse: 5 - 20 mcg/min (200 mcg/min max)

Infusion rate mL/hr	Dose mcg/min
1	3.3
2	6.7
3	10
6	20
7	23
9	30
12	40
15	50
18	60
21	70
24	80
27	90
30	100
33	110
36	120
39	130
42	140
45	150
48	160
54	180
60	200
66	220
72	240
78	260

Table 6.30

Table 6.28

NICARDIPINE
(Cardene)

is on page 18.

Doses outside the therapeutic range. (shaded)

NITROPRUSSIDE
(Nipride)

IV loading dose: None

Mixture: 50 mg Nipride
250 mL D5W

Concentration: 200 mcg/mL

Infusion dose: 0.5 - 5 mcg/kg/min
(maximum of 8 mcg/kg/min for no more than 10 mins)

mcg/kg/min = Infusion rate x concentration/60/pt wt

Table 6.31

Infusion rate (mL/hr)	Patient weight (kg) 35	40	45	50	55	60	65	70	75	80	85	90	95	100	105	110	115	120	125	130
	Dose (mcg/kg/min)																			
5	0.5	0.4	0.4	0.3	0.3	0.3	0.3	0.2	0.2	0.2	0.2	0.2	0.2	0.2	0.2	0.2	0.1	0.1	0.1	0.1
10	1.0	0.8	0.7	0.7	0.6	0.6	0.5	0.5	0.4	0.4	0.4	0.4	0.4	0.3	0.3	0.3	0.3	0.3	0.3	0.3
15	1.4	1.3	1.1	1.0	0.9	0.8	0.8	0.7	0.7	0.6	0.6	0.6	0.5	0.5	0.5	0.5	0.4	0.4	0.4	0.4
20	1.9	1.7	1.5	1.3	1.2	1.1	1.0	1.0	0.9	0.8	0.8	0.7	0.7	0.7	0.6	0.6	0.6	0.6	0.5	0.5
25	2.4	2.1	1.9	1.7	1.5	1.4	1.3	1.2	1.1	1.0	1.0	0.9	0.9	0.8	0.8	0.8	0.7	0.7	0.7	0.6
30	2.9	2.5	2.2	2.0	1.8	1.7	1.5	1.4	1.3	1.3	1.2	1.1	1.1	1.0	1.0	0.9	0.9	0.8	0.8	0.8
35	3.3	2.9	2.6	2.3	2.1	1.9	1.8	1.7	1.6	1.5	1.4	1.3	1.2	1.2	1.1	1.1	1.0	1.0	0.9	0.9
40	3.8	3.3	3.0	2.7	2.4	2.2	2.1	1.9	1.8	1.7	1.6	1.5	1.4	1.3	1.3	1.2	1.2	1.1	1.1	1.0
45	4.3	3.8	3.3	3.0	2.7	2.5	2.3	2.1	2.0	1.9	1.8	1.7	1.6	1.5	1.4	1.4	1.3	1.3	1.2	1.2
50	4.8	4.2	3.7	3.3	3.0	2.8	2.6	2.4	2.2	2.1	2.0	1.9	1.8	1.7	1.6	1.5	1.4	1.4	1.3	1.3
55	5.2	4.6	4.1	3.7	3.3	3.1	2.8	2.6	2.4	2.3	2.2	2.0	1.9	1.8	1.7	1.7	1.6	1.5	1.5	1.4
60	5.7	5.0	4.4	4.0	3.6	3.3	3.1	2.9	2.7	2.5	2.4	2.2	2.1	2.0	1.9	1.8	1.7	1.7	1.6	1.5
65	6.2	5.4	4.8	4.3	3.9	3.6	3.3	3.1	2.9	2.7	2.5	2.4	2.3	2.2	2.1	2.0	1.9	1.8	1.7	1.7
70	6.7	5.8	5.2	4.7	4.2	3.9	3.6	3.3	3.1	2.9	2.7	2.6	2.5	2.3	2.2	2.1	2.0	1.9	1.9	1.8
75	7.1	6.3	5.6	5.0	4.5	4.2	3.8	3.6	3.3	3.1	2.9	2.8	2.6	2.5	2.4	2.3	2.2	2.1	2.0	1.9
80	7.6	6.7	5.9	5.3	4.8	4.4	4.1	3.8	3.6	3.3	3.1	3.0	2.8	2.7	2.5	2.4	2.3	2.2	2.1	2.1
85	8.1	7.1	6.3	5.7	5.2	4.7	4.4	4.0	3.8	3.5	3.3	3.1	3.0	2.8	2.7	2.6	2.5	2.4	2.3	2.2
90	8.6	7.5	6.7	6.0	5.5	5.0	4.6	4.3	4.0	3.8	3.5	3.3	3.2	3.0	2.9	2.7	2.6	2.5	2.4	2.3
95	9.0	7.9	7.0	6.3	5.8	5.3	4.9	4.5	4.2	4.0	3.7	3.5	3.3	3.2	3.0	2.9	2.8	2.6	2.5	2.4
100	9.5	8.3	7.4	6.7	6.1	5.6	5.1	4.8	4.4	4.2	3.9	3.7	3.5	3.3	3.2	3.0	2.9	2.8	2.7	2.6

NITROPRUSSIDE
(Nipride)

Mixture: 100 mg Nipride / 250 mL D5W

Concentration: 400 mcg/mL

Infusion dose: 0.5 - 5 mcg/kg/min (maximum of 8 mcg/kg/min for no more than 10 mins)

IV loading dose: None

mcg/kg/min = Infusion rate x concentration/60/pt wt

Table 6.32

Infusion rate (mL/hr)	Patient weight (kg) 35	40	45	50	55	60	65	70	75	80	85	90	95	100	105	110	115	120	125	130
	Dose (mcg/kg/min)																			
5	1.0	0.8	0.7	0.7	0.6	0.6	0.5	0.5	0.4	0.4	0.4	0.4	0.4	0.3	0.3	0.3	0.3	0.3	0.3	0.3
10	1.9	1.7	1.5	1.3	1.2	1.1	1.0	1.0	0.9	0.8	0.8	0.7	0.7	0.7	0.6	0.6	0.6	0.6	0.5	0.5
15	2.9	2.5	2.2	2.0	1.8	1.7	1.5	1.4	1.3	1.3	1.2	1.1	1.1	1.0	1.0	0.9	0.9	0.8	0.8	0.8
20	3.8	3.3	3.0	2.7	2.4	2.2	2.1	1.9	1.8	1.7	1.6	1.5	1.4	1.3	1.3	1.2	1.2	1.1	1.1	1.0
25	4.8	4.2	3.7	3.3	3.0	2.8	2.6	2.4	2.2	2.1	2.0	1.9	1.8	1.7	1.6	1.5	1.4	1.4	1.3	1.3
30	5.7	5.0	4.4	4.0	3.6	3.3	3.1	2.9	2.7	2.5	2.4	2.2	2.1	2.0	1.9	1.8	1.7	1.7	1.6	1.5
35	6.7	5.8	5.2	4.7	4.2	3.9	3.6	3.3	3.1	2.9	2.7	2.6	2.5	2.3	2.2	2.1	2.0	1.9	1.9	1.8
40	7.6	6.7	5.9	5.3	4.8	4.4	4.1	3.8	3.6	3.3	3.1	3.0	2.8	2.7	2.5	2.4	2.3	2.2	2.1	2.1
45	8.6	7.5	6.7	6.0	5.5	5.0	4.6	4.3	4.0	3.8	3.5	3.3	3.2	3.0	2.9	2.7	2.6	2.5	2.4	2.3
50	9.5	8.3	7.4	6.7	6.1	5.6	5.1	4.8	4.4	4.2	3.9	3.7	3.5	3.3	3.2	3.0	2.9	2.8	2.7	2.6
55	10.5	9.2	8.1	7.3	6.7	6.1	5.6	5.2	4.9	4.6	4.3	4.1	3.9	3.7	3.5	3.3	3.2	3.1	2.9	2.8
60	11.4	10.0	8.9	8.0	7.3	6.7	6.2	5.7	5.3	5.0	4.7	4.4	4.2	4.0	3.8	3.6	3.5	3.3	3.2	3.1
65	12.4	10.8	9.6	8.7	7.9	7.2	6.7	6.2	5.8	5.4	5.1	4.8	4.6	4.3	4.1	3.9	3.8	3.6	3.5	3.3
70	13.3	11.7	10.4	9.3	8.5	7.8	7.2	6.7	6.2	5.8	5.5	5.2	4.9	4.7	4.4	4.2	4.1	3.9	3.7	3.6
75	14.3	12.5	11.1	10.0	9.1	8.3	7.7	7.1	6.7	6.3	5.9	5.6	5.3	5.0	4.8	4.5	4.3	4.2	4.0	3.8
80	15.2	13.3	11.9	10.7	9.7	8.9	8.2	7.6	7.1	6.7	6.3	5.9	5.6	5.3	5.1	4.8	4.6	4.4	4.3	4.1
85	16.2	14.2	12.6	11.3	10.3	9.4	8.7	8.1	7.6	7.1	6.7	6.3	6.0	5.7	5.4	5.2	4.9	4.7	4.5	4.4
90	17.1	15.0	13.3	12.0	10.9	10.0	9.2	8.6	8.0	7.5	7.1	6.7	6.3	6.0	5.7	5.5	5.2	5.0	4.8	4.6
100	19.0	16.7	14.8	13.3	12.1	11.1	10.3	9.5	8.9	8.3	7.8	7.4	7.0	6.7	6.3	6.1	5.8	5.6	5.3	5.1
110	21.0	18.3	16.3	14.7	13.3	12.2	11.3	10.5	9.8	9.2	8.6	8.1	7.7	7.3	7.0	6.7	6.4	6.1	5.9	5.6

NICARDIPINE
(Cardene)

IV load: None

Mix: 25 mg / 250 mL D5W or NS

Concen: 0.1 mg/mL

Infuse: 5 - 15 mg/hr

Infusion rate mL/hr	Dose mg/hr
25	2.5
50	5
60	6
70	7
80	8
90	9
100	10
110	11
120	12
130	13
140	14
150	15
160	16
170	17
180	18
190	19
200	20

Table 6.28

NOREPINEPHRINE
(Levophed)

IV load: None

Mix: 4 mg / 250 mL D5W

Concen: 16 mcg/mL

Infuse: 2 - 12 mcg/min (doses up to 30 mcg/min have been used)

Infusion rate mL/hr	Dose mcg/min
4	1
8	2
11	3
15	4
19	5
22	6
26	7
30	8
34	9
38	10
41	11
45	12
49	13
53	14
56	15
60	16
64	17
68	18
71	19
75	20
80	21
85	23
90	24
95	25
100	27
105	28
110	29
115	31

Table 6.33

See Norepinephrine mcg/kg/min tables on next two pages

PHENYLEPHRINE
(Neosynephrine)

Mix: 20 mg / 250 mL D5W, NS

Concen: 80 mcg/mL

Infuse: 100-180 mcg/min to start, then 40 - 60 mcg/min

Infusion rate mL/hr	Dose mcg/min
28	37
30	40
32	43
34	45
36	48
38	51
40	53
42	56
44	59
46	61
48	64
50	67
55	73
65	87
75	100
85	113
95	127
105	140
115	153
125	167
135	180
145	193

Table 6.37

Shaded: Doses outside the therapeutic range.

NOREPINEPHRINE
(Levophed)

Mixture:	8 mg Norepinephrine 250 mL D5W
Concentration:	32 mcg/mL
Infusion dose:	0.05 - 0.5 mcg/kg/min
(in septic shock:	0.5 - 1.5 mcg/kg/min has been used)

IV loading dose: None

mcg/kg/min = Infusion rate x concentration/60/pt wt.

Table 6.34

Dose (mcg/kg/min)

Infusion rate (mL/hr)	Patient weight (kg) 35	40	45	50	55	60	65	70	75	80	85	90	95	100	105	110	115	120	125	130
5	0.08	0.07	0.06	0.05	0.05	0.04	0.04	0.04	0.04	0.03	0.03	0.03	0.03	0.03	0.03	0.02	0.02	0.02	0.02	0.02
10	0.15	0.13	0.12	0.11	0.10	0.09	0.08	0.08	0.07	0.07	0.06	0.06	0.06	0.05	0.05	0.05	0.05	0.04	0.04	0.04
15	0.23	0.20	0.18	0.16	0.15	0.13	0.12	0.11	0.11	0.10	0.09	0.09	0.08	0.08	0.08	0.07	0.07	0.07	0.06	0.06
20	0.30	0.27	0.24	0.21	0.19	0.18	0.16	0.15	0.14	0.13	0.13	0.12	0.11	0.11	0.10	0.10	0.09	0.09	0.09	0.08
25	0.38	0.33	0.30	0.27	0.24	0.22	0.21	0.19	0.18	0.17	0.16	0.15	0.14	0.13	0.13	0.12	0.12	0.11	0.11	0.10
30	0.46	0.40	0.36	0.32	0.29	0.27	0.25	0.23	0.21	0.20	0.19	0.18	0.17	0.16	0.15	0.15	0.14	0.13	0.13	0.12
35	0.53	0.47	0.41	0.37	0.34	0.31	0.29	0.27	0.25	0.23	0.22	0.21	0.20	0.19	0.18	0.17	0.16	0.16	0.15	0.14
40	0.61	0.53	0.47	0.43	0.39	0.36	0.33	0.30	0.28	0.27	0.25	0.24	0.22	0.21	0.20	0.19	0.19	0.18	0.17	0.16
45	0.69	0.60	0.53	0.48	0.44	0.40	0.37	0.34	0.32	0.30	0.28	0.27	0.25	0.24	0.23	0.22	0.21	0.20	0.19	0.18
50	0.76	0.67	0.59	0.53	0.48	0.44	0.41	0.38	0.36	0.33	0.31	0.30	0.28	0.27	0.25	0.24	0.23	0.22	0.21	0.21
55	0.84	0.73	0.65	0.59	0.53	0.49	0.45	0.42	0.39	0.37	0.35	0.33	0.31	0.29	0.28	0.27	0.26	0.24	0.23	0.23
60	0.91	0.80	0.71	0.64	0.58	0.53	0.49	0.46	0.43	0.40	0.38	0.36	0.34	0.32	0.30	0.29	0.28	0.27	0.26	0.25
65	0.99	0.87	0.77	0.69	0.63	0.58	0.53	0.50	0.46	0.43	0.41	0.39	0.36	0.35	0.33	0.32	0.30	0.29	0.28	0.27
70	1.07	0.93	0.83	0.75	0.68	0.62	0.57	0.53	0.50	0.47	0.44	0.41	0.39	0.37	0.36	0.34	0.32	0.31	0.30	0.29
75	1.14	1.00	0.89	0.80	0.73	0.67	0.62	0.57	0.53	0.50	0.47	0.44	0.42	0.40	0.38	0.36	0.35	0.33	0.32	0.31
80	1.22	1.07	0.95	0.85	0.78	0.71	0.66	0.61	0.57	0.53	0.50	0.47	0.45	0.43	0.41	0.39	0.37	0.36	0.34	0.33
85	1.30	1.13	1.01	0.91	0.82	0.76	0.70	0.65	0.60	0.57	0.53	0.50	0.48	0.45	0.43	0.41	0.39	0.38	0.36	0.35
90	1.37	1.20	1.07	0.96	0.87	0.80	0.74	0.69	0.64	0.60	0.56	0.53	0.51	0.48	0.46	0.44	0.42	0.40	0.38	0.37
95	1.45	1.27	1.13	1.01	0.92	0.84	0.78	0.72	0.68	0.63	0.60	0.56	0.53	0.51	0.48	0.46	0.44	0.42	0.41	0.39
100	1.52	1.33	1.19	1.07	0.97	0.89	0.82	0.76	0.71	0.67	0.63	0.59	0.56	0.53	0.51	0.48	0.46	0.44	0.43	0.41

NOREPINEPHRINE
(Levophed)

This table is calculated for a concentrated mix that may be required for some patients with severe shock.

IV loading dose: None

Mixture: 16 mg Norepinephrine / 250 mL D5W

Concentration: **64** mcg/mL

Infusion dose: 0.05 - 0.5 mcg/kg/min

Profound Shock: 0.5 - 1.5 mcg/kg/min

mcg/kg/min = infusion rate x concentration/60/pt wt

Table 6.35

Dose (mcg/kg/min)

Infusion rate (mL/hr)	Patient weight (kg) 35	40	45	50	55	60	65	70	75	80	85	90	95	100	105	110	115	120	125	130
5	0.15	0.13	0.12	0.11	0.10	0.09	0.08	0.08	0.07	0.07	0.06	0.06	0.06	0.05	0.05	0.05	0.05	0.04	0.04	0.04
10	0.30	0.27	0.24	0.21	0.19	0.18	0.16	0.15	0.14	0.13	0.13	0.12	0.11	0.11	0.10	0.10	0.09	0.09	0.09	0.08
15	0.46	0.40	0.36	0.32	0.29	0.27	0.25	0.23	0.21	0.20	0.19	0.18	0.17	0.16	0.15	0.15	0.14	0.13	0.13	0.12
20	0.61	0.53	0.47	0.43	0.39	0.36	0.33	0.30	0.28	0.27	0.25	0.24	0.22	0.21	0.20	0.19	0.19	0.18	0.17	0.16
25	0.76	0.67	0.59	0.53	0.48	0.44	0.41	0.38	0.36	0.33	0.31	0.30	0.28	0.27	0.25	0.24	0.23	0.22	0.21	0.21
30	0.91	0.80	0.71	0.64	0.58	0.53	0.49	0.46	0.43	0.40	0.38	0.36	0.34	0.32	0.30	0.29	0.28	0.27	0.26	0.25
35	1.07	0.93	0.83	0.75	0.68	0.62	0.57	0.53	0.50	0.47	0.44	0.41	0.39	0.37	0.36	0.34	0.32	0.31	0.30	0.29
40	1.22	1.07	0.95	0.85	0.78	0.71	0.66	0.61	0.57	0.53	0.50	0.47	0.45	0.43	0.41	0.39	0.37	0.36	0.34	0.33
45	1.37	1.20	1.07	0.96	0.87	0.80	0.74	0.69	0.64	0.60	0.56	0.53	0.51	0.48	0.46	0.44	0.42	0.40	0.38	0.37
50	1.52	1.33	1.19	1.07	0.97	0.89	0.82	0.76	0.71	0.67	0.63	0.59	0.56	0.53	0.51	0.48	0.46	0.44	0.43	0.41
55	1.68	1.47	1.30	1.17	1.07	0.98	0.90	0.84	0.78	0.73	0.69	0.65	0.62	0.59	0.56	0.53	0.51	0.49	0.47	0.45
60	1.83	1.60	1.42	1.28	1.16	1.07	0.98	0.91	0.85	0.80	0.75	0.71	0.67	0.64	0.61	0.58	0.56	0.53	0.51	0.49
65	1.98	1.73	1.54	1.39	1.26	1.16	1.07	0.99	0.92	0.87	0.82	0.77	0.73	0.69	0.66	0.63	0.60	0.58	0.55	0.53
70	2.13	1.87	1.66	1.49	1.36	1.24	1.15	1.07	1.00	0.93	0.88	0.83	0.79	0.75	0.71	0.68	0.65	0.62	0.60	0.57
75	2.29	2.00	1.78	1.60	1.45	1.33	1.23	1.14	1.07	1.00	0.94	0.89	0.84	0.80	0.76	0.73	0.70	0.67	0.64	0.62
80	2.44	2.13	1.90	1.71	1.55	1.42	1.31	1.22	1.14	1.07	1.00	0.95	0.90	0.85	0.81	0.78	0.74	0.71	0.68	0.66
85	2.59	2.27	2.01	1.81	1.65	1.51	1.39	1.30	1.21	1.13	1.07	1.01	0.95	0.91	0.86	0.82	0.79	0.76	0.73	0.70
90	2.74	2.40	2.13	1.92	1.75	1.60	1.48	1.37	1.28	1.20	1.13	1.07	1.01	0.96	0.91	0.87	0.83	0.80	0.77	0.74
95	2.90	2.53	2.25	2.03	1.84	1.69	1.56	1.45	1.35	1.27	1.19	1.13	1.07	1.01	0.97	0.92	0.88	0.84	0.81	0.78
100	3.05	2.67	2.37	2.13	1.94	1.78	1.64	1.52	1.42	1.33	1.25	1.19	1.12	1.07	1.02	0.97	0.93	0.89	0.85	0.82

PENTOBARBITAL

(Nembutal)

(This table of doses is for the treatment of severe head injury)

IV loading dose:
2 - 15 mg/kg over 1 - 2 hrs

Mixture: 1000 mgPentobarbital / 250 mL NS

Concentration: 4 mg/mL

Infusion dose: 0.5 - 3 mg/kg/hr

mcg/kg/min = Infusion rate x concentration/60/pt wt

Table 6.36

Infusion rate (mL/hr)	Patient weight (kg)																			
	35	40	45	50	55	60	65	70	75	80	85	90	95	100	105	110	115	120	125	130
	Dose (mg/kg/hr)																			
5	0.6	0.5	0.4	0.4	0.4	0.3	0.3	0.3	0.3	0.3	0.2	0.2	0.2	0.2	0.2	0.2	0.2	0.2	0.2	0.2
10	1.1	1.0	0.9	0.8	0.7	0.7	0.6	0.6	0.5	0.5	0.5	0.4	0.4	0.4	0.4	0.4	0.3	0.3	0.3	0.3
15	1.7	1.5	1.3	1.2	1.1	1.0	0.9	0.9	0.8	0.8	0.7	0.7	0.6	0.6	0.6	0.5	0.5	0.5	0.5	0.5
20	2.3	2.0	1.8	1.6	1.5	1.3	1.2	1.1	1.1	1.0	0.9	0.9	0.8	0.8	0.8	0.7	0.7	0.7	0.6	0.6
25	2.9	2.5	2.2	2.0	1.8	1.7	1.5	1.4	1.3	1.3	1.2	1.1	1.1	1.0	1.0	0.9	0.9	0.8	0.8	0.8
30	3.4	3.0	2.7	2.4	2.2	2.0	1.8	1.7	1.6	1.5	1.4	1.3	1.3	1.2	1.1	1.1	1.0	1.0	1.0	0.9
35	4.0	3.5	3.1	2.8	2.5	2.3	2.2	2.0	1.9	1.8	1.6	1.6	1.5	1.4	1.3	1.3	1.2	1.2	1.1	1.1
40	4.6	4.0	3.6	3.2	2.9	2.7	2.5	2.3	2.1	2.0	1.9	1.8	1.7	1.6	1.5	1.5	1.4	1.3	1.3	1.2
45	5.1	4.5	4.0	3.6	3.3	3.0	2.8	2.6	2.4	2.3	2.1	2.0	1.9	1.8	1.7	1.6	1.6	1.5	1.4	1.4
50	5.7	5.0	4.4	4.0	3.6	3.3	3.1	2.9	2.7	2.5	2.4	2.2	2.1	2.0	1.9	1.8	1.7	1.7	1.6	1.5
55	6.3	5.5	4.9	4.4	4.0	3.7	3.4	3.1	2.9	2.8	2.6	2.4	2.3	2.2	2.1	2.0	1.9	1.8	1.8	1.7
60	6.9	6.0	5.3	4.8	4.4	4.0	3.7	3.4	3.2	3.0	2.8	2.7	2.5	2.4	2.3	2.2	2.1	2.0	1.9	1.8
65	7.4	6.5	5.8	5.2	4.7	4.3	4.0	3.7	3.5	3.3	3.1	2.9	2.7	2.6	2.5	2.4	2.3	2.2	2.1	2.0
70	8.0	7.0	6.2	5.6	5.1	4.7	4.3	4.0	3.7	3.5	3.3	3.1	2.9	2.8	2.7	2.5	2.4	2.3	2.2	2.2
75	8.6	7.5	6.7	6.0	5.5	5.0	4.6	4.3	4.0	3.8	3.5	3.3	3.2	3.0	2.9	2.7	2.6	2.5	2.4	2.3
80	9.1	8.0	7.1	6.4	5.8	5.3	4.9	4.6	4.3	4.0	3.8	3.6	3.4	3.2	3.0	2.9	2.8	2.7	2.6	2.5
85	9.7	8.5	7.6	6.8	6.2	5.7	5.2	4.9	4.5	4.3	4.0	3.8	3.6	3.4	3.2	3.1	3.0	2.8	2.7	2.6
90	10.3	9.0	8.0	7.2	6.5	6.0	5.5	5.1	4.8	4.5	4.2	4.0	3.8	3.6	3.4	3.3	3.1	3.0	2.9	2.8
95	10.9	9.5	8.4	7.6	6.9	6.3	5.8	5.4	5.1	4.8	4.5	4.2	4.0	3.8	3.6	3.5	3.3	3.2	3.0	2.9
100	11.4	10.0	8.9	8.0	7.3	6.7	6.2	5.7	5.3	5.0	4.7	4.4	4.2	4.0	3.8	3.6	3.5	3.3	3.2	3.1

PROPOFOL
(Diprivan)

Mixture: 500 mg Propofol / 50 mL emulsion

Concentration: 10 mg/mL (10,000 mcg/mL)

Infusion dose: Start infusion at 5 mcg/kg/min

Dose range is: 5 - 50 mcg/kg/min

IV loading dose: None

(mcg/kg/min = Infusion rate x concentration/60/pt wt)

Table 6.39

Infusion rate (mL/hr)	Patient weight (kg)																			
	35	40	45	50	55	60	65	70	75	80	85	90	95	100	105	110	115	120	125	130
	Dose (mcg/kg/min)																			
2	10	8	7	7	6	6	5	5	4	4	4	4	4	3	3	3	3	3	3	3
4	19	17	15	13	12	11	10	10	9	8	8	7	7	7	6	6	6	6	5	5
6	29	25	22	20	18	17	15	14	13	13	12	11	11	10	10	9	9	8	8	8
8	38	33	30	27	24	22	21	19	18	17	16	15	14	13	13	12	12	11	11	10
10	48	42	37	33	30	28	26	24	22	21	20	19	18	17	16	15	14	14	13	13
12	57	50	44	40	36	33	31	29	27	25	24	22	21	20	19	18	17	17	16	15
14	67	58	52	47	42	39	36	33	31	29	27	26	25	23	22	21	20	19	19	18
16	76	67	59	53	48	44	41	38	36	33	31	30	28	27	25	24	23	22	21	21
18	86	75	67	60	55	50	46	43	40	38	35	33	32	30	29	27	26	25	24	23
20	95	83	74	67	61	56	51	48	44	42	39	37	35	33	32	30	29	28	27	26
22	105	92	81	73	67	61	56	52	49	46	43	41	39	37	35	33	32	31	29	28
24	114	100	89	80	73	67	62	57	53	50	47	44	42	40	38	36	35	33	32	31
26	124	108	96	87	79	72	67	62	58	54	51	48	46	43	41	39	38	36	35	33
28	133	117	104	93	85	78	72	67	62	58	55	52	49	47	44	42	41	39	37	36
30	143	125	111	100	91	83	77	71	67	63	59	56	53	50	48	45	43	42	40	38
32	152	133	119	107	97	89	82	76	71	67	63	59	56	53	51	48	46	44	43	41
34	162	142	126	113	103	94	87	81	76	71	67	63	60	57	54	52	49	47	45	44
36	171	150	133	120	109	100	92	86	80	75	71	67	63	60	57	55	52	50	48	46
38	181	158	141	127	115	106	97	90	84	79	75	70	67	63	60	58	55	53	51	49
40	190	167	148	133	121	111	103	95	89	83	78	74	70	67	63	61	58	56	53	51

PROCAINAMIDE
(Pronestyl)

IV load: (see Stat Med chapter)

Mix: 1 g / 250 mL D5W

Concen: **4** mg/mL

Infuse: 1 - 4 mg/min

Infusion rate mL/hr	Dose mg/min
5	0.3
10	0.7
15	1
20	1.3
25	1.7
30	2
35	2.3
40	2.7
45	3
50	3.3
55	3.7
60	4
65	4.3
70	4.7
75	5

Table 6.38

VASOPRESSIN
(Pitressin)

For septic shock and for organ donor management

Mix: 20 units / 250 mL D5W,NS

Concen: **0.08** units/mL

Infuse: 0.02 - 0.1 unit/min

Infusion rate mL/hr	Dose units/min
8	0.01
15	0.02
22	0.03
30	0.04
38	0.05
45	0.06
52	0.07
59	0.08
67	0.09
76	0.1
82	0.11

Table 6.40

VASOPRESSIN
(Pitressin)

For variceal bleeding (Off Label)

Mix: 200 units / 250 mL D5W,NS

Concen: **0.8** units/mL

Infuse: 0.2 - 0.4 units/min

Infusion rate mL/hr	Dose units/min
11	0.15
15	0.2
19	0.25
22	0.3
26	0.35
30	0.4
34	0.45

Table 6.41

VERAPAMIL
(Calan, Isoptin)

IV Load: 2.5 - 5 mg over 2 minutes

Mix: 50 mg / 20 mL Verapamil + 180 mL D5W

Concen: **0.25** mg/mL

Infuse: 5 - 10 mg/hr

Infusion rate mL/hr	Dose mg/hr
10	2.5
12	3
14	3.5
16	4
18	4.5
20	5
22	5.5
24	6
26	6.5
28	7
30	7.5
32	8
34	8.5
36	9
38	9.5
40	10
42	10.5
44	11
46	11.5
48	12
50	12.5

Table 6.43

(Shaded) Doses outside the therapeutic range.

VECURONIUM
(Norcuron)

IV loading dose:
0.08 - 0.1 mg/kg

Mixture: 20 mg Vecuronium / 100 mL D5W or NS

Concentration: 200 mcg/mL

Infusion dose: 0.8 - 1.2 mcg/kg/min

(mcg/kg/min = Infusion rate x concentration/60/pt wt)

Table 6.42

Infusion rate (mL/hr)	Patient weight (kg) 35	40	45	50	55	60	65	70	75	80	85	90	95	100	105	110	115	120	125	130
	Dose (mcg/kg/min)																			
2	0.2	0.2	0.1	0.1	0.1	0.1	0.1	0.1	0.1	0.1	0.1	0.1	0.1	0.1	0.1	0.1	0.1	0.1	0.1	0.1
4	0.4	0.3	0.3	0.3	0.2	0.2	0.2	0.2	0.2	0.2	0.2	0.1	0.1	0.1	0.1	0.1	0.1	0.1	0.1	0.1
6	0.6	0.5	0.4	0.4	0.4	0.3	0.3	0.3	0.3	0.3	0.2	0.2	0.2	0.2	0.2	0.2	0.2	0.2	0.2	0.2
8	0.8	0.7	0.6	0.5	0.5	0.4	0.4	0.4	0.4	0.3	0.3	0.3	0.3	0.3	0.3	0.2	0.2	0.2	0.2	0.2
10	1.0	0.8	0.7	0.7	0.6	0.6	0.5	0.5	0.4	0.4	0.4	0.4	0.4	0.3	0.3	0.3	0.3	0.3	0.3	0.3
12	1.1	1.0	0.9	0.8	0.7	0.7	0.6	0.6	0.5	0.5	0.5	0.4	0.4	0.4	0.4	0.4	0.3	0.3	0.3	0.3
14	1.3	1.2	1.0	0.9	0.8	0.8	0.7	0.7	0.6	0.6	0.5	0.5	0.5	0.5	0.4	0.4	0.4	0.4	0.4	0.4
16	1.5	1.3	1.2	1.1	1.0	0.9	0.8	0.8	0.7	0.7	0.6	0.6	0.6	0.5	0.5	0.5	0.5	0.4	0.4	0.4
18	1.7	1.5	1.3	1.2	1.1	1.0	0.9	0.9	0.8	0.8	0.7	0.7	0.6	0.6	0.6	0.5	0.5	0.5	0.5	0.5
20	1.9	1.7	1.5	1.3	1.2	1.1	1.0	1.0	0.9	0.8	0.8	0.7	0.7	0.7	0.6	0.6	0.6	0.6	0.5	0.5
22	2.1	1.8	1.6	1.5	1.3	1.2	1.1	1.0	1.0	0.9	0.9	0.8	0.8	0.7	0.7	0.7	0.6	0.6	0.6	0.6
24	2.3	2.0	1.8	1.6	1.5	1.3	1.2	1.1	1.1	1.0	0.9	0.9	0.8	0.8	0.8	0.7	0.7	0.7	0.6	0.6
26	2.5	2.2	1.9	1.7	1.6	1.4	1.3	1.2	1.2	1.1	1.0	1.0	0.9	0.9	0.8	0.8	0.8	0.7	0.7	0.7
28	2.7	2.3	2.1	1.9	1.7	1.6	1.4	1.3	1.2	1.2	1.1	1.0	1.0	0.9	0.9	0.8	0.8	0.8	0.7	0.7
30	2.9	2.5	2.2	2.0	1.8	1.7	1.5	1.4	1.3	1.3	1.2	1.1	1.1	1.0	1.0	0.9	0.9	0.8	0.8	0.8
32	3.0	2.7	2.4	2.1	1.9	1.8	1.6	1.5	1.4	1.3	1.3	1.2	1.1	1.1	1.0	1.0	0.9	0.9	0.9	0.8
34	3.2	2.8	2.5	2.3	2.1	1.9	1.7	1.6	1.5	1.4	1.3	1.3	1.2	1.1	1.1	1.0	1.0	0.9	0.9	0.9
36	3.4	3.0	2.7	2.4	2.2	2.0	1.8	1.7	1.6	1.5	1.4	1.3	1.3	1.2	1.1	1.1	1.0	1.0	1.0	0.9
38	3.6	3.2	2.8	2.5	2.3	2.1	1.9	1.8	1.7	1.6	1.5	1.4	1.3	1.3	1.2	1.2	1.1	1.1	1.0	1.0
40	3.8	3.3	3.0	2.7	2.4	2.2	2.1	1.9	1.8	1.7	1.6	1.5	1.4	1.3	1.3	1.2	1.2	1.1	1.1	1.0

ECG

ECG

The Normal ECG

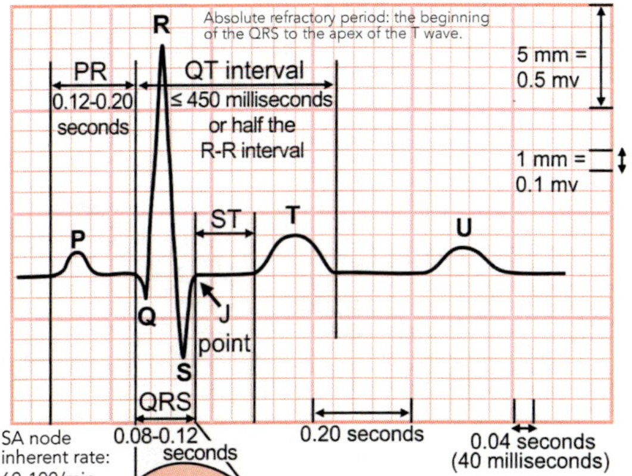

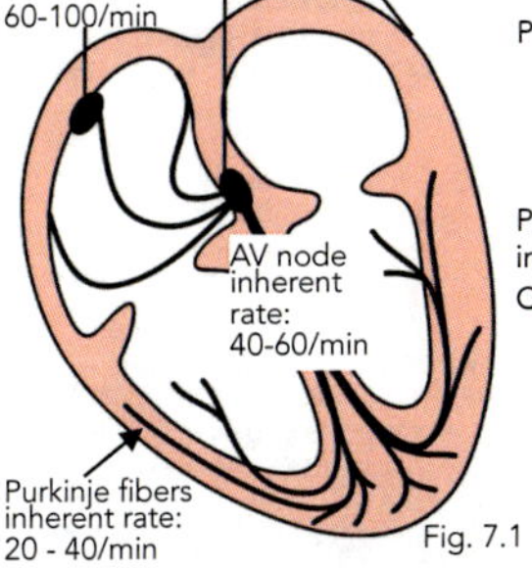

Fig. 7.1

P wave: Depolarization of the atria. Normal impulse from the SA node produces a normal shape. Impulse from another atrial focus produces an abnormal shape.

PR interval: Conduction delay at the atria, AV node, and bundle of HIS.

Q wave: The first negative deflection of the QRS represents depolarization of the interventricular septum. Normally, Q waves are < 0.03 seconds long, < 1 mm tall. Q waves that are > 1 mm signify pathology (ischemia, infarction).

R & S waves: Depolarization of the left and right ventricular walls. Normally, the R is positive in all leads except AVR, V1, V2. Normal impulse initiated by the AV node produces normal QRS configuration and duration. Ventricular conduction delay produces a wide QRS.

J Point: Where the S wave ends and the ST segment begins.

ST Segment: The beginning of ventricular repolarization. Normally isoelectric. Significant ST elevation or depression indicates myocardial injury.

T wave: Repolarization of the ventricles. T wave should be in the same direction as the QRS. Electrical stimulus during the T wave (R-on-T phenomenon) can cause ventricular arrhythmia.

QT interval: The distance from the onset of the Q to the end of the T wave. Represents the cycle of ventricular depolarization-repolarization. Prolonged if > 450 milliseconds in males, ≥ 460 ms in females, or more than one-half of the R-R interval. Short QT is ≤ 390 ms. Prolonged QT can increase the chance of R-on-T phenomenon, is caused by some electrolyte and metabolic imbalances.

U wave: Recovery of the Purkinje conduction fibers. Prominent U may be due to hypercalcemia, hypokalemia, digoxin toxicity.

Reentry: The presence of two conducting pathways, which allows impulses from one pathway to enter the second pathway, causing re-excitation. Reentry is a common cause of tachycardia.

http://www.medicine.mcgill.ca/physio/vlab/cardio/ecgbasics.htm, (accessed 2/5/2016)

Dubin D. Rapid Interpretation of ECG. Cover Publishing Co., 2000.

Basic ECG Analysis

4 Way to Count Rate:

1. Count the QRS's in a 6-second strip, then multiply by 10.
2. Determine the time between R to R, then divide into 60:
   Example: 60/(20 small boxes x .04 seconds each) = 75 bpm
3. Find a QRS that falls on a heavy line:

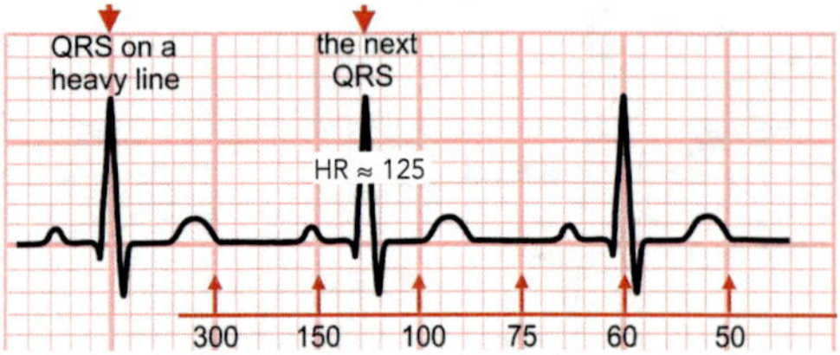

Fig. 7.2

If the next R is on or near the next heavy line, HR ≈ 300
If the next R is on or near the second heavy line, HR ≈ 150
If the next R is on or near the third heavy line, HR ≈ 100

4. With Marriott's exact ruler, find an R wave on a heavy line:

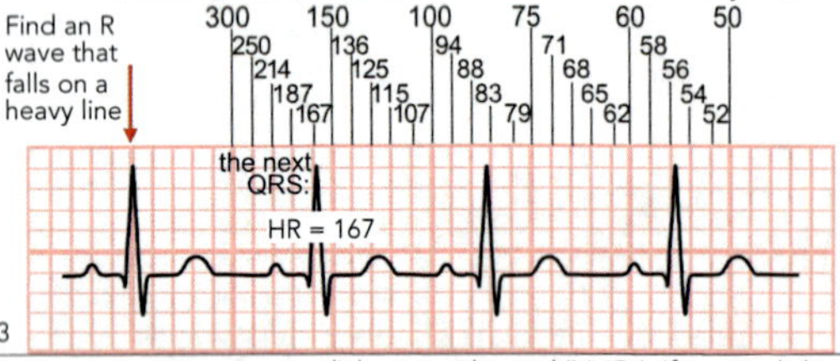

Fig. 7.3

Heart rate > 150:	Increases myocardial oxygen demand (MVO2). If myocardial O2 supply (MDO2) is limited, myocardial ischemia results. Decreases diastolic filling time, leading to decreased stroke volume, decreased CO, decreased BP. Decreases diastolic time -> ↓ coronary artery perfusion time.
Heart rate < 50:	Decreases cardiac output and blood pressure.
Loss of atrial contraction:	A fib/ A flutter, junctional rhythms, rhythms originating in the ventricles all lose the benefit of the atrial kick, which normally contributes 30% more volume to the filling of the ventricle at the end of diastole. Without the atrial kick, cardiac output may be inadequate
Retrograde depolarization of the atria:	Beats that originate in the AV node or in the ventricles may send a wave of depolarization that moves backward to the atria, causing the atria to depolarize. The P wave, however, will be negative (in Leads I, II, V4, V5, V6, AVF) and will occur either after the QRS, within the QRS, or so close to the QRS that the PR will be < 0.12 seconds.
Inherent rates:	Any cell in the heart may function as a pacemaker, but each of the following locations has an inherent rate: SA node: 60 - 100 AV node: 40 - 60 Ventricles: 20 - 40
Dysrhythmia analysis:	• Is the rate too slow or too fast? • Is the rhythm regular? • Are P waves present and do they have a normal shape? • Is the PR interval prolonged? • Do the QRS complexes have normal shape and duration? • What is the relationship between the P waves and QRS's?

Lead Placement: for a 3-Lead System

Manufacturers have standardized a color code for ECG monitoring leads to designate placement and polarity:

RA	=	Right arm	=	White
LA	=	Left arm	=	Black
G	=	Ground	=	Green or Red

Traditional placement for Leads I, II, III
Fig. 7.4

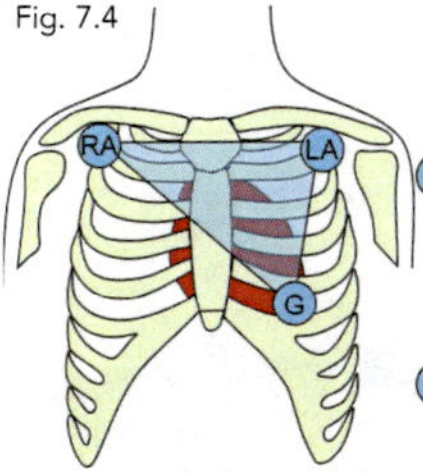

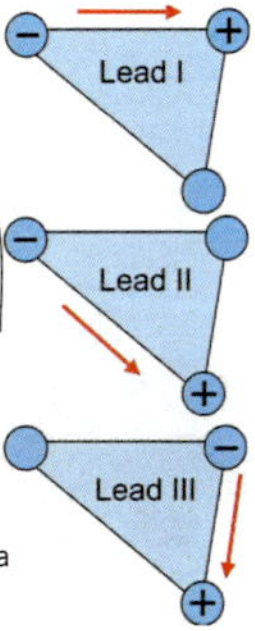

RA Right infraclavicular fossa
LA Left infraclavicular fossa
G 5 ICS, MCL

"When a wave of depolarization moves toward a positive electrode, it will write a positive R wave on the ECG"

Since Lead II places the positive electrode at the apex of the heart, and since the wave of depolarization moves toward the apex, Lead II is the lead where you will normally find the most upright R wave. This lead is the easiest one for the monitor to see and therefore accurately count HR.

When transporting patients with a portable ECG monitor, this lead is best.

Traditional placement for MCL1
Fig. 7.5

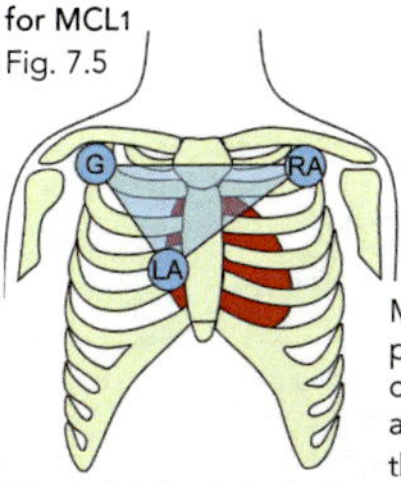

To get MCL1, select "Lead I" on the monitor:

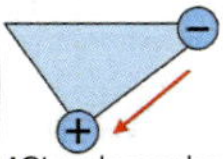

MCL1 places the positive electrode over the right atrium, to amplify the P wave.

RA Left infraclavicular fossa
LA 4 ICS, right of the sternum
G Right infraclavicular fossa

MCL1 is best for helping you detect the presence or absence of P waves, in order to distin-guish PVC's from atrial beats with aberrant conduction.

MCL1 approximates what you would see in V1 on a 12-lead ECG. Since the heart's wave of depolarization moves away from MCL1's positive electrode, it will write a negative R wave on the ECG. Therefore, this lead is harder for the monitor to see and count accurately.

Placement for MCL1/MCL6:
Fig. 7.6

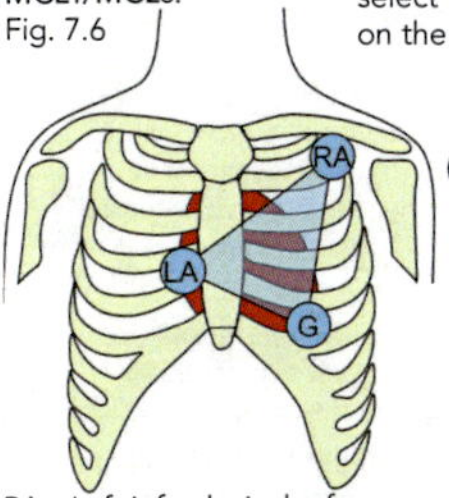

To get MCL1, select "Lead I" on the monitor:

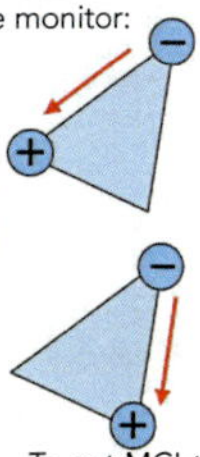

To get MCL6, select "Lead II" on the monitor.

RA Left infraclavicular fossa
LA 4 ICS, right of the sternum
G 5 ICS, mid axillary line

MCL6 views the heart at the same angle as Lead II and also approximates what you would see in V6 on a 12-lead ECG.

Select "Lead I" to get MCL1
Select "Lead II" to get MCL6
By configuring a 3-lead system this way, you can switch back and forth without having to move electrodes.
Some monitors allow you to monitor both "Lead I" and "Lead II" simultaneously.

Lead Placement: for a 5-Lead System

Manufacturers have standardized a color code for ECG monitoring leads to designate placement and polarity:

RA	=	Right arm	=	White
LA	=	Left arm	=	Black
RL	=	Right leg	=	Green
C	=	Chest	=	Brown

RA	Right arm	Right infraclavicular fossa
LA	Left arm	Left infraclavicular fossa
C	Chest	5th ICS, midclavicular line
RL	Right leg	Right lower chest or upper abdomen
LL	Left leg	Left lower chest or upper abdomen

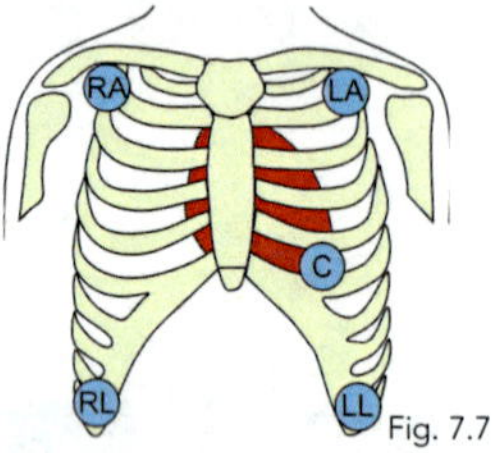

Fig. 7.7

When you select a limb lead (Lead I, II, or III), this illustration shows how the monitor will designate the polarity of each electrode.

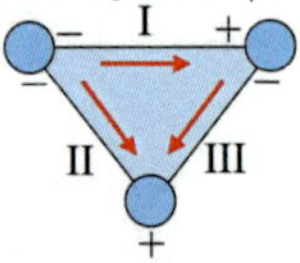

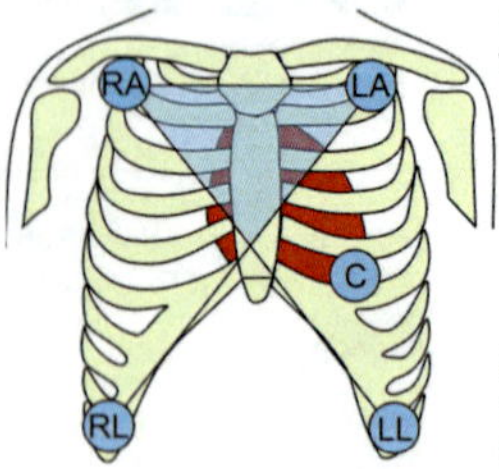

Fig. 7.8

Since Lead II places the positive electrode at the apex of the heart, and since the wave of depolarization moves toward the apex, Lead II is the lead where you will normally find the most upright R wave.

The C lead is equivalent to the V lead on 12-lead ECG and can be moved to any of the V lead sites:

V1	4th ICS, right sternal border
V2	4th ICS, left sternal border
V3	Midway between V2 and V4
V4	5th ICS, midclavicular line
V5	5th ICS, anterior axillary line
V6	5th ICS, midaxillary line

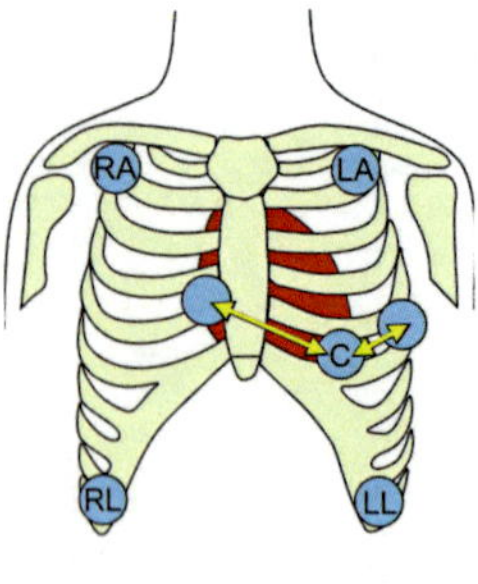

Fig. 7.9

To obtain Lead V1, move the chest lead to the 4th ICS, Rt sternal border.
Lead V1 is considered the best lead to:

- Assess right and left bundle-branch block
- Check the location of a right ventricular pacing lead (transvenous right ventricular pacing usually produces LBBB pattern).
- Distinguish ventricular tachycardia from SVT with aberrant ventricular conduction

Since the heart's wave of depolarization moves away from V1, the V1 lead will record a negative R wave on the ECG.

Move the C lead to other sites to identify the location of ischemia or infarction:

Lead V4:	Anterior wall ischemia
Lead I and V6:	Lateral wall ischemia
Lead II, III, AVF:	Inferior wall ischemia

Dysrhythmia	Characteristics	Significance
Sinus Bradycardia	Sinus rhythm in which the rate of impulses from the SA node is slowed P waves: normal shape, upright in Lead II Atrial rate: < 60 Atrial rhythm: may be slightly irregular QRS: normal	Normal in athletes and during sleep. May be caused by sinus node disease, increased parasympathetic tone, drug effect (e.g., digoxin, beta-blocker, calcium channel blocker). May occur with Inferior AMI (the right coronary artery supplies the SAnode). The slower heart rate can lower the cardiac output, may cause lower BP.
Sinus Tachycardia	Sinus rhythm in which the rate of discharge from SA node is increased. P waves: normal shape, but may be superimposed over the T wave Atrial rate: 100 - 150 Atrial rhythm: regular QRS: normal	Usually due to increased sympathetic discharge (due to pain/anxiety), but may also represent effort to maintain cardiac output when stroke volume is threatened (e.g., hypovolemia). May also be due to effects of stimulants (e.g., caffeine). Look for and treat the cause. Danger in CAD - tachycardia increases myocardial O_2 demand, and may also decrease diastolic filling time.
Sinus Arrhythmia	Sinus rhythm in which the sinus rate increases during inspiration and decreases during expiration. P waves: normal shape Atrial rate: 60 - 100, irregular Atrial rhythm: rate varies with respiration QRS: normal	A normal rhythm when associated with respiration. May cause patient anxiety. If not associated with respiration, beware the development of ectopic beats and bradycardia.

Fig. 7.10 Sinus Bradycardia

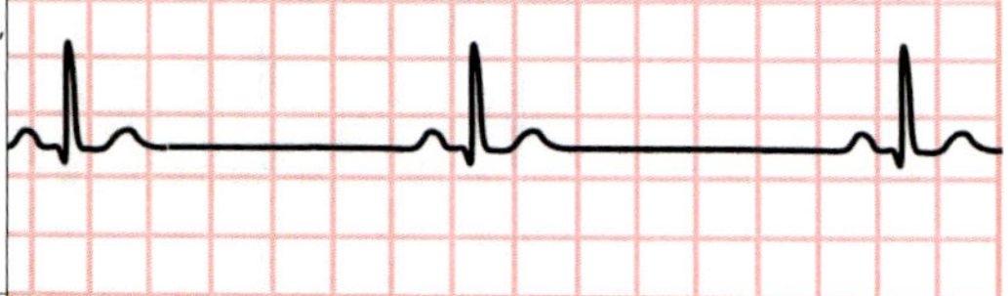

Fig. 7.11 Sinus Tachycardia

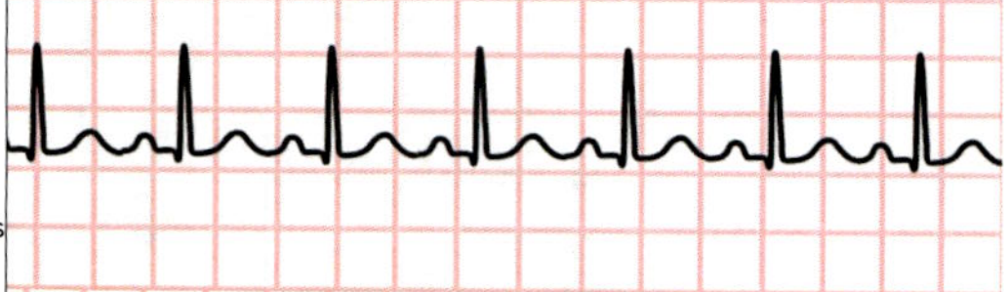

Fig. 7.12 Sinus Arrhythmia

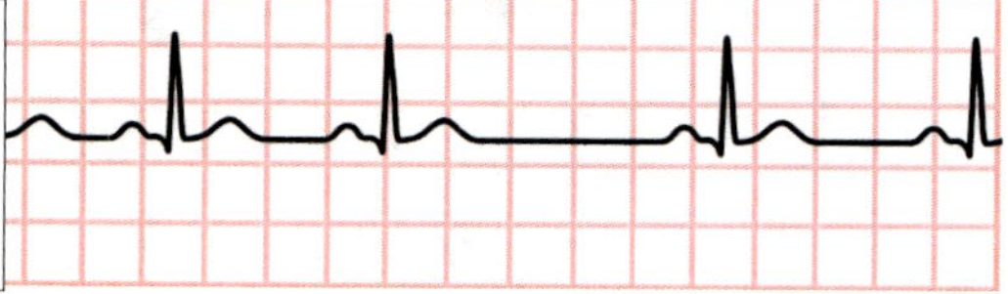

Dysrhythmia	Characteristics	Significance
Sinus Block	Impulse from the SA node is blocked, resulting in a missing P-QRS-T. The pause is a multiple of the R-R interval. P waves: none for the missed beat, shape is normal after the block QRS: none for the missed beat	Usually transient and causes no symptoms, but can decrease HR enough to affect CO. May be related to Sick Sinus Syndrome, hypokalemia, MI, digoxin or quinidine.
Sinus Arrest	SA node fails to generate an impulse, resulting in a missing P-QRS-T. The pause is not a multiple of the R-R interval, and if the escape rhythm is atrial, subsequent P waves will be different. P waves: shape is different or absent after the sinus arrest. Rhythm: irregular, due to the pause	Serious sinus node dysfunction or disease (e.g., Sick Sinus Syndrome, or sinus node ischemia associated with inferior AMI). Atrial, junctional, or ventricular escape beats may occur. Can result in syncope, falls, injury. Can be caused by digoxin, beta-blockers, procainamide. Treated as bradycardia.
Premature Atrial Contraction	Ectopic focus in the atria (rather than the sinus node) initiates the beat. P waves: configuration is different from the normal sinus beats, or may be lost in the previous T wave. PR: may vary, but is no less than 0.12 secs. If < 0.12 secs and the P has negative polarity, consider premature junctional with retrograde conduction to atria Rhythm: irregular, due to prematurity of abnormal beats	Can cause discomfort, anxiety, feeling of "heart skipping beats." Often caused by stress, anxiety, caffeine, alcohol, fever. Also due to valve disease, hypoxia, digoxin, electrolyte imbalance. In patients with heart disease, may precede AFlutter or AFib.

Fig. 7.13 Sinus Block

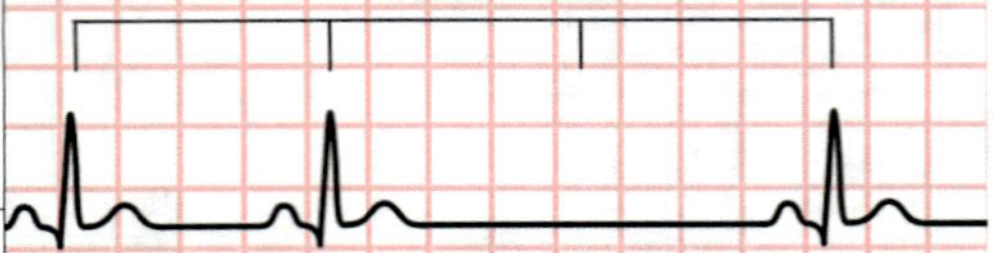

Fig. 7.14 Sinus Arrest

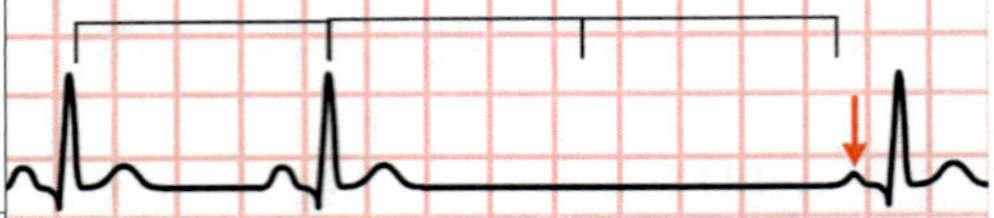

Fig. 7.15 Premature Atrial Contraction

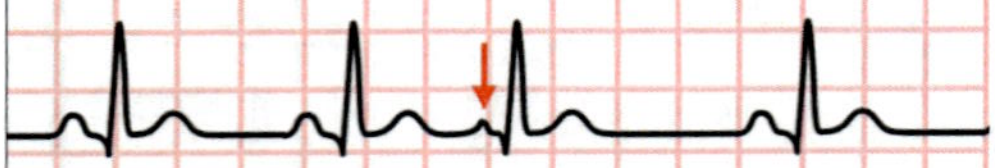

Dysrhythmia	Characteristics	Significance
Atrial Tachycardia	Rapid firing of an ectopic atrial pacemaker P waves: have a configuration different from the patient's normal P wave. May be buried in the previous T wave. Atrial rate: 150 - 250 Atrial rhythm: regular Vent. rate if no block occurs at AV node, the ventricular rate will equal the atrial rate.	Caused by caffeine, stimulants, electrolyte imbalance, hypoxia. If high heart rate results, can cause hemodynamic instability. If the onset is sudden, it is called paroxysmal atrial tach (PAT). Digoxin toxicity may cause PAT with block (some P's do not conduct). See ACLS for narrow complex tach.
Multifocal Atrial Tachycardia	Multiple atrial ectopic impulses pace the atria. P waves: All p waves vary in shape PR: may vary, but is no less than 0.12 seconds Atrial rhythm: irregular Rate: 100 - 250 QRS: normal, < 0.12 seconds	Due to atrial irritability, COPD, or heart disease. Associated with high mortality. High HR may cause hemodynamic compromise.
Atrial Flutter	An atrial ectopic focus fires in rapid succession. The result of a reentry circuit. P waves: "saw-tooth," all identical P:QRS more flutter waves than QRS's Atrial rate: 250 - 350 Atrial rhythm: usually regular Ventricular rate: Usually 125 - 175 Rate can be very high if most or all of the flutter waves conduct Ventric. rhythm: Regular if there is consistent block at the AV node	Almost always associated with heart disease or conditions that enlarge the atria (valve disease). High heart rate as well as loss of the atrial kick can decrease cardiac output and BP. See ACLS algorithms for synchronized cardioversion and medications.

Fig. 7.16 Atrial Tachycardia

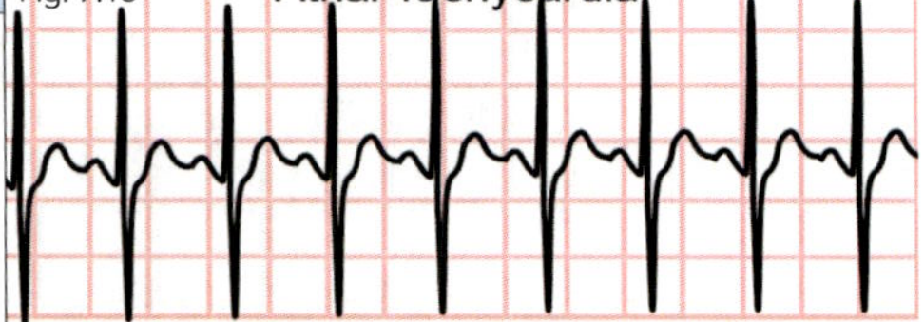

Fig. 7.17 Multifocal Atrial Tachycardia

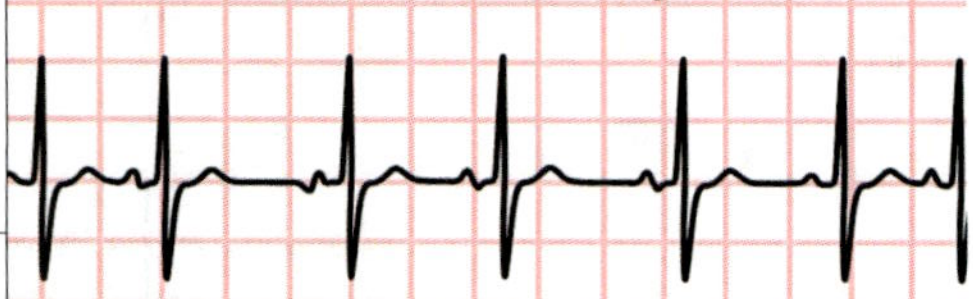

Fig. 7.18 Atrial Flutter

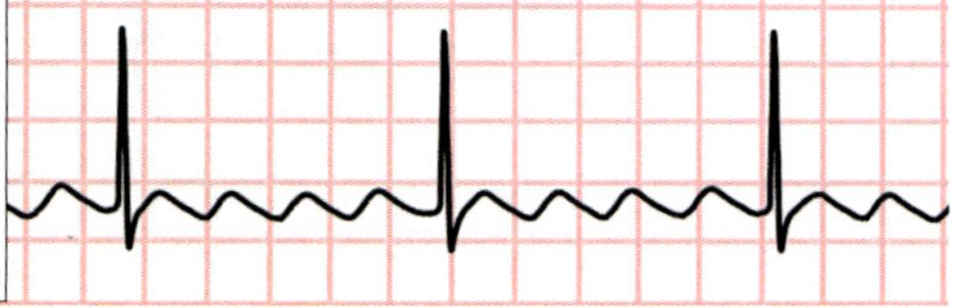

Dysrhythmia	Characteristics	Significance
Atrial Fibrillation	Continuous rapid-firing of multiple atrial foci or from multiple areas of reentry. P waves: coarse or fine fibrillating waves PR interval: none Atrial rate: 350 - 600 (no atrial contraction) Vent rate: 120 - 200 and irregular. Rate can be very high if most or all of the AFib waves conduct. Vent. rhythm: irregular as some of the fib waves conduct, others don't. QRS: Normal, < 0.12 seconds	Causes include CAD, pericarditis, hypoxia, increased atrial pressure, CHF, cardiac surgery. Loss of atrial kick, shortened diastole may cause hemodynamic crisis. Increased MVO_2 can trigger myocardial ischemia, infarction, heart failure. Synchronized cardio-version only if onset within last 3 days. See ACLS algorithms for narrow-complex tach.
Paroxysmal Supra-Ventricular Tachycardia	Normal QRS tachycardia with abrupt onset. Since P waves can't be identified, you won't be able to tell if the ectopic focus causing the PSVT is atrial or junctional. Episodes may end abruptly; vagal maneuvers may be used. P waves not identifiable. May be buried in the T wave or in the QRS. QRS: Normal Vent rate: 150 - 250 Vent rhythm: regular	Tolerated by the young. In the elderly and patients with heart disease, can precipitate myocardial ischemia, decreased BP, pulmonary edema. Adenosine is used to slow the rate, in order to distinguish this tach from AFib. See ACLS algorithm for narrow complex tachycardia.
Premature Junctional Contraction	Irritable ectopic focus in the AV node fires prematurely, inhibiting the SA node. P waves: inverted due to retrograde conduction or buried in the QRS Rhythm: premature beat irregularity QRS: normal	Occurs in normal individuals. Also caused by digoxin toxicity, caffeine, inferior MI, valve disease, AV node edema after cardiac surgery.

Fig. 7.19 Atrial Fibrillation

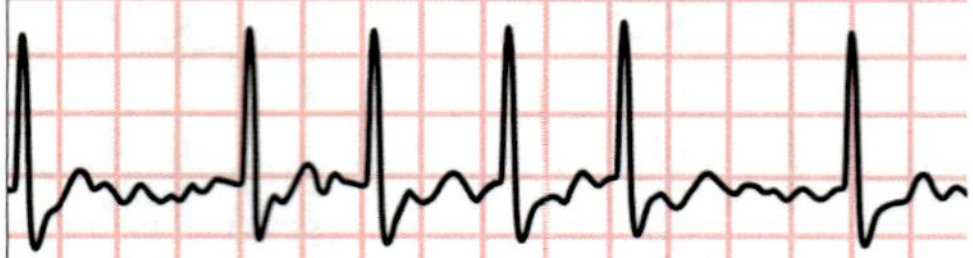

Fig. 7.20 Paroxysmal Atrial Tachycardia

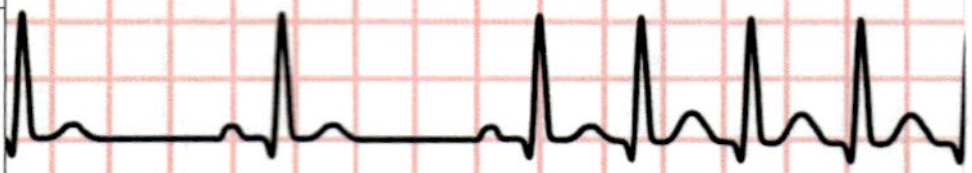

Fig. 7.21 Premature Junctional Contraction

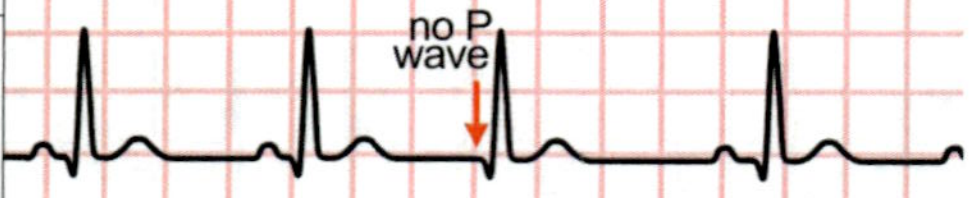

Dysrhythmia	Characteristics	Significance
Junctional Rhythm	Tissue near the AV node overrides the pacing rate of the SA node P waves: occur by retrograde conduction* Atrial rate: same as the junctional rate Junctional rate: 40 - 60 QRS: normal	May be caused by Sick Sinus Node, Digoxin toxicity, decreased K. Atrial kick is lost. Slow rate may cause hemodynamic compromise. See ACLS algorithm for bradycardia.
Accelerated Junctional Rhythm	Tissue near the AV node paces faster than the SA node. P waves: occur by retrograde conduction* Atrial rate: same as the junctional rate Junctional rate: 60 - 100 QRS: normal	Denotes increased automaticity of AV node, possibly due to digoxin toxicity, hypokalemia, acute myocardial infarction. Since HR may be near normal, cardiac output and blood pressure may remain acceptable
Junctional Tachycardia	Irritable AV node ectopic focus with enhanced automaticity overrides the SA node. P waves: occur by retrograde conduction* Atrial rate: same as junctional rate Junctional rate: 100 - 200, regular	Delayed atrial contraction may forfeit the atrial kick. Tachycardia may cause hemodynamic compromise, myocardial ischemia. See ACLS algorithm for narrow complex tachycardia.

* P waves, if visible, will be inverted in Leads II, III, AVF.
If retrograde P precedes the QRS, the PR may be too short to measure.
P waves may not be visible if buried in the QRS or T wave.
P waves after the QRS represent retrograde atrial contraction that may be too late to provide atrial kick. Dizziness, hypotension may result.

Fig. 7.22 Junctional Rhythm

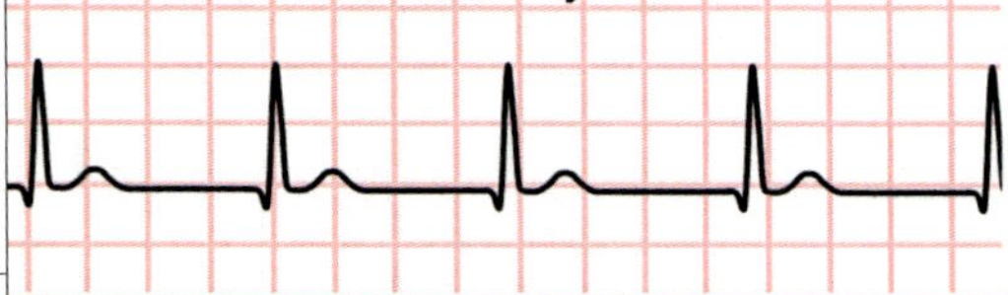

Fig. 7.23 Accelerated Junctional Rhythm

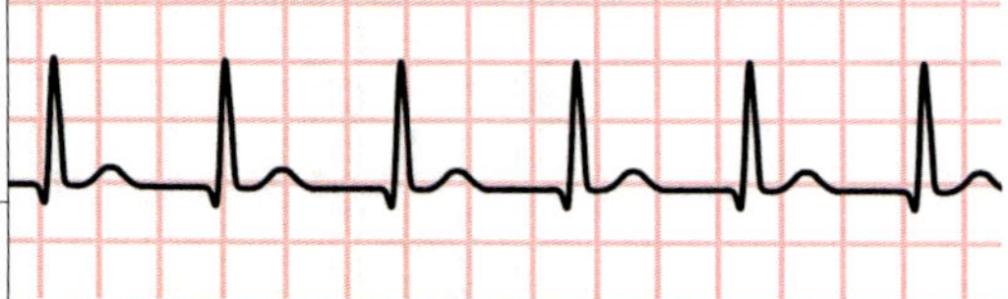

Fig. 7.24 Junctional Tachycardia

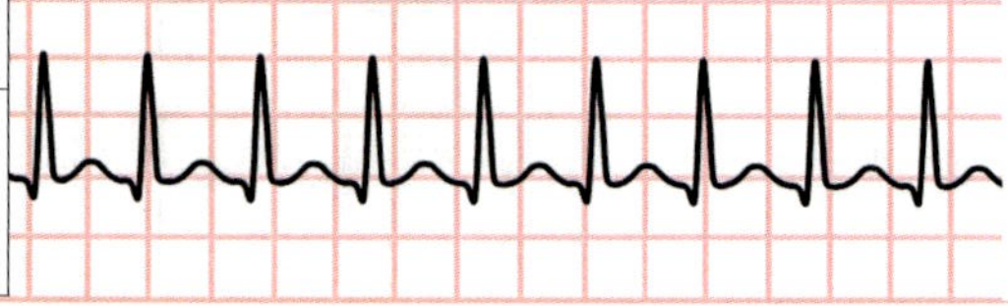

Dysrhythmia	Characteristics	Significance
1° AV block	Delay in conduction through the AV node. The delay is the same amount each cycle. P waves: normal, all conduct PR: Long, > 0.20 seconds QRS: normal, < 0.12 seconds Rhythm: regular	AVB's may be due to: lesions along the conduction pathway, medications that delay conduction (such as digoxin or verapamil), or electrolyte imbalance. 1° AVB is usually asymptomatic and is not treated, but monitor for progression to a more severe block.
2° AV block (Mobitz I) Wenckebach	The delay in conduction from atria to ventricles becomes progressively longer, until the AV node does not conduct at all. Then the cycle repeats. P waves: normal shape, but there are more P waves than QRS's. PR: progressively longer QRS: does not appear with the last P in the cycle Rhythm: irregular	Often due to vagal stimulation, or to digoxin, beta-blocker, CCB. Also associated with CAD & inferior MI. Usually a transient, benign arrhythmia (no treatment) unless it causes symptomatic bradycardia. May progress to a more serious block. Establish an IV and monitor patient's ECG.
2° AV block (Mobitz II)	A block occurs below the AV node, at the bundle of His or the bundle branches, resulting in P waves with no QRS's. Block may occur every other beat, every third, or every 4th. P waves: normal shape, more P's than QRS's, normal atrial rate PR: normal or prolonged, but length remains consistent QRS: wide if conduction through bundle branches is delayed.	Associated with degeneration of the conduction pathways, anterior wall MI, severe coronary artery disease. Has poor prognosis, since it can lead to 3° AVB. Often accompanied by PVC's. Bradycardia may reduce cardiac output enough to cause hypotension. See ACLS algorithm for bradycardia.

Fig. 7.25 1° AV Block

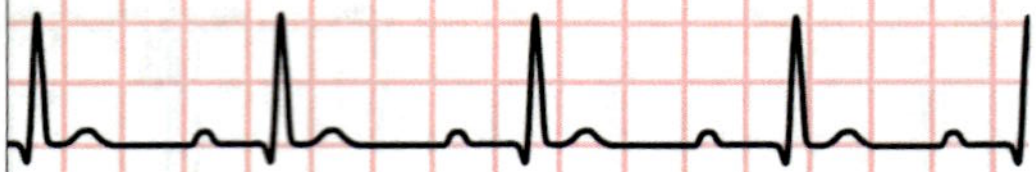

Fig. 7.26 2° AV Block Mobitz I

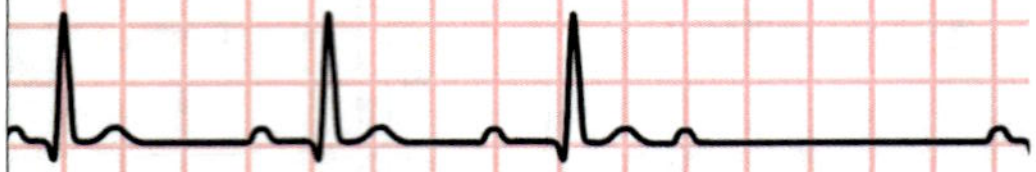

Fig. 7.27 2° AV Block Mobitz II

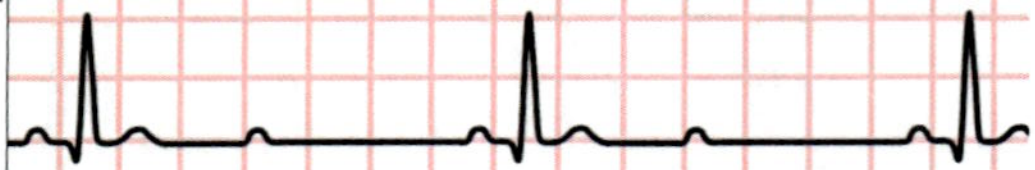

Dysrhythmia	Characteristics	Significance
3° AV block (Complete heart block, AV dissociation)	Impulses from the atria are completely blocked by the AV node. The atria and ventricles beat independently. P waves: normal, at rate of 60 - 100 PR: no consistent relationship to the QRS complexes. P:QRS ratio: usually more P's than QRS's QRS & Rate: Narrow QRS at rate 40 - 60 if escape rhythm is AV node Wide QRS at rate of 20 - 40 if escape rhythm is ventricular (Purkinje system)	If escape rhythm is junctional (with rate of 40 - 60) prognosis is good. If the escape rhythm is Purkinje system ("ventricular"), there is extensive conduction system disease/degeneration. Also a complication of anterior or inferior MI, use of CCB or beta-blockers, or digoxin toxicity. Slow rate can reduce CO, BP, LOC, and can cause chest pain. Episodes of asystole may be common. See ACLS algorithm for bradycardia.
Left Bundle Branch Block	Delay in the depolarization of the Left Bundle Branch. Lt ventricle depolarizes after the Rt ventricle, causing broad QRS, sometimes (R, R') in Leads V_5 and V_6 P waves: normal PR: normal QRS: Two R waves, or broad QRS > 0.12 seconds	Associated with CAD, conducting system degeneration, hypertensive disease, aortic stenosis. If BBB accompanies SVT, it may look like V tach. Also, AMI cannot be diagnosed in the presence of BBB, because the R, R' can obscure the Q wave and the ST segment.
Right Bundle Branch Block	Delay in the depolarization of the Right Bundle Branch. Rt ventricle depolarizes after the Lt ventricle, causing broad QRS, sometimes (R, R') in Leads V_1 and V_2 P waves: normal PR: normal QRS: Two R waves, or broad QRS > 0.12 seconds	Associated with Anterior MI, CAD, up to 67% of pts with pulmonary embolism. RBBB can be precipitated by PA catheter insertion. If your patient has LBBB and needs a PA catheter, have pacemaker at the bedside. See statement above in LBBB regarding SVT and dx of MI.

Fig. 7.28 3° AV Block

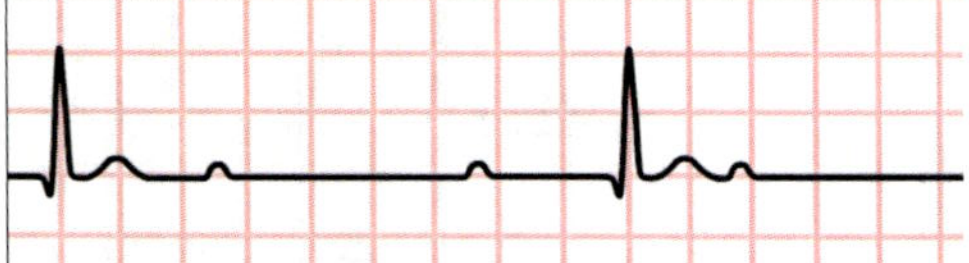

Fig. 7.29 Left Bundle Branch Block

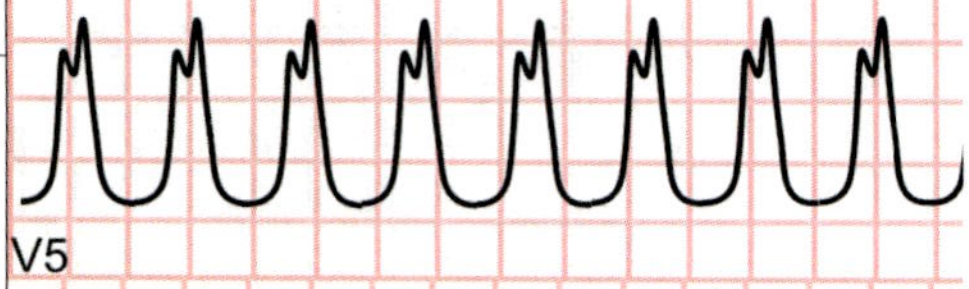

Fig. 7.30 Right Bundle Branch Block

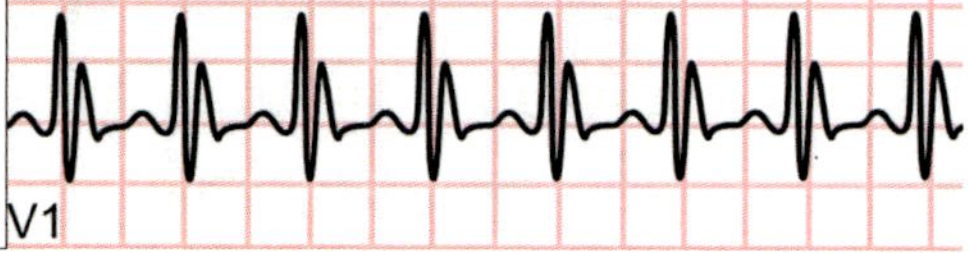

Dysrhythmia	Characteristics	Significance
Premature Ventricular Contraction	Initiated by ectopic focus in the ventricle P waves:: absent, retrograde, or buried QRS: > 0.12 seconds, appears wide and bizarre, often followed by a compensatory pause Rhythm: the premature beat interrupts the underlying rhythm T wave: Deflects opposite the direction of other QRS complexes	Can be benign. But serious arrhythmias may follow if the PVC's are multifocal, occur in pairs, fall on the preceding T, occur often, or reduce cardiac output. Caused by anxiety, stimulants, acidosis, hypoxia, electrolyte imbalance, drug toxicity, myocardial ischemia. Polymorphic PVC's and couplets may precede Torsades de Pointes.
Ventricular Tachycardia	Three or more successive beats of ventricular origin at a rate > 100. P waves: absent, retrograde, or buried; atrial rate can't be determined QRS: > 0.12 seconds, wide & bizarre Monomorphic: single ectopic focus, QRS shape remains the same Polymorphic: multiple ectopic foci, QRS shape constantly changes. T wave: Deflects opposite the QRS Rate: 100 - 200 Rhythm: Usually regular	May be well tolerated if duration is short, or may cause dire hemodynamic compromise. The atrial kick is absent and the high heart rate reduces diastolic filling tim Caused by heart disease (CAD, ischemia, infarction, valve disease, heart failure, myopathy), as well as by hypokalemia and drug toxicity (cocaine, digoxin, procainamide). See ACLS algorithm for wide complex tachycardia.
Fusion beat	Ventricle is depolarized in part by the normal pathways from the AV node, and in part by a ventricular focus. Occurs at the same R-R interval.	The presence of fusion beats helps confirm the diagnosis of V Tach.

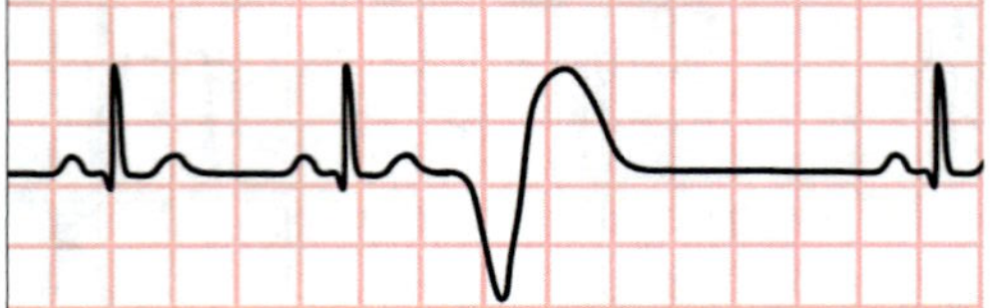

Fig. 7.31 Premature Ventricular Contraction

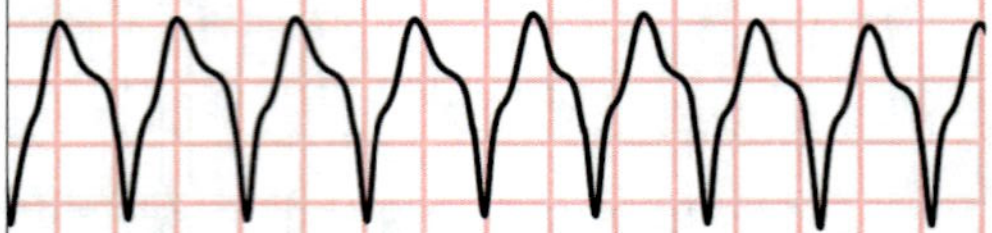

Fig. 7.32 Ventricular Tachycardia

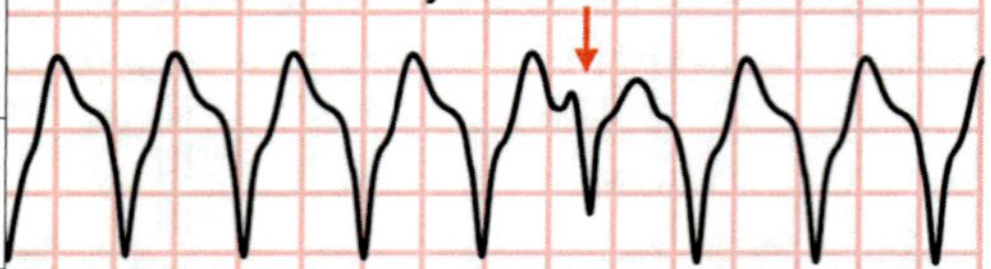

Ventricular Tachycardia with Fusion beat

Fig. 7.33

Dysrhythmia	Characteristics	Significance
Torsades de pointes	"Twisting about the points." A form of VTach in which the QRS complexes deflect down and up, rotating about the baseline, the morphology constantly changing. Rate: 150 - 250 Rhythm: Irregular May start and stop suddenly.	Most common cause is medication that prolongs the QT (anti-dysrhythmics, antibiotics, antipsychotics). Also due to myocardial ischemia, LV hypertrophy, severe bradycardia, electrolyte imbalance (hypokalemia, hypocalcemia, hypomagnesemia). Results in syncope and sudden death. Risk is high for patients with QT > 0.5 seconds or the duration is more than 1/2 the R to R.
Idioven-tricular	"The rhythm of last resort." If the SA node, atria, and AV node fail to pace, or conduction to the ventricles is blocked, cells of the His-Purkinje system may provide an escape rhythm. P: absent, retrograde, or buried QRS: > 0.12 seconds wide and bizarre T wave: deflects opposite the QRS QT: > 0.45 seconds Rate: 20 - 40	Associated with AMI, electrolyte imbalance, digoxin toxicity. The slow rate and loss of atrial kick reduces cardiac output, causing confusion, syncope, hypotension. A serious conduction defect, that may progress to Ventricular Fib. See ACLS algorithm for bradycardia and emergency transcutaneous pacing. Do not suppress this escape rhythm with antiarrhythmia medications.
Accelerated idioven-tricular	The ventricles compete with the atria as primary pacemaker. Unlike VTach, the mechanism is not due to reentry. P waves: present, absent, retrograde, or buried. T wave: deflects opposite the QRS QRS: > 0.12 sec., wide and bizarre Rate: 40 - 120	The most common reperfusion rhythm, strongly suggests success after thrombolytic therapy. Also caused by myocardial disease, hypertensive, rheumatic, and congenital heart disease, and by digoxin. May also occur in the absence of heart disease.

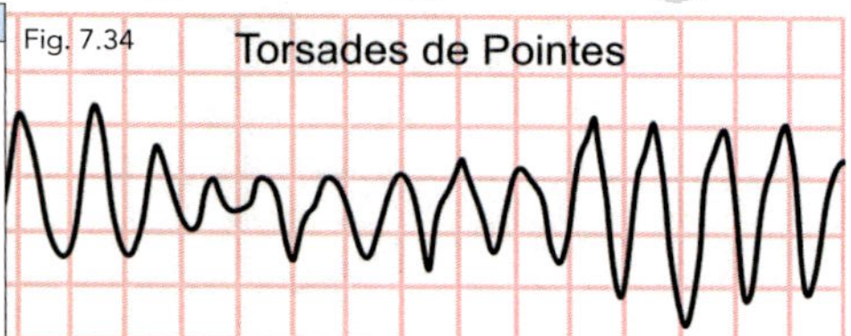

Fig. 7.34

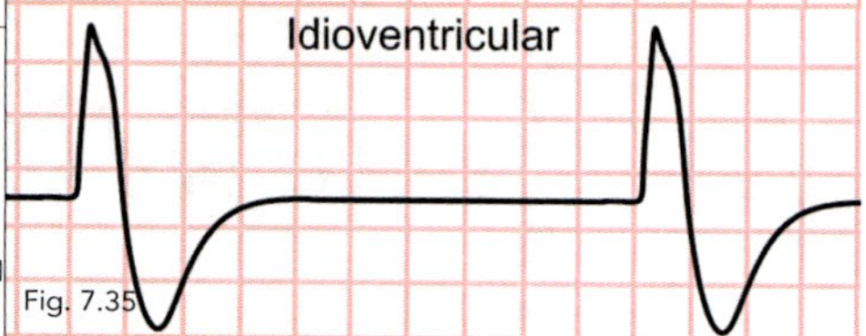

Fig. 7.35

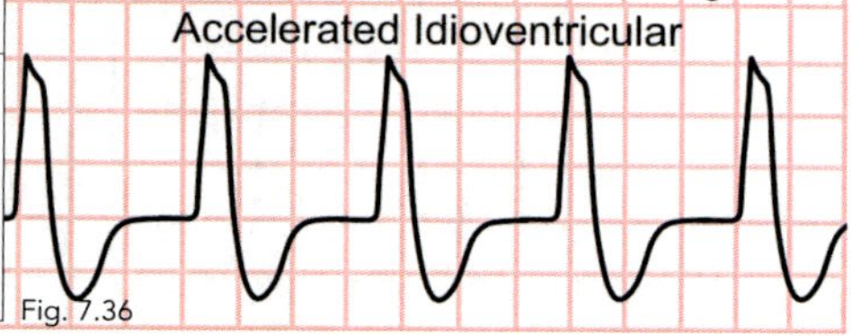

Fig. 7.36

Dysrhythmia	Characteristics	Significance
Ventricular Flutter	A form of Ventricular Tachycardia. A single ventricular ectopic focus and reentry phenomenon produce an extremely fast rate with smooth sinusoidal pattern. P waves: absent, retrograde, or buried QRS: wide, > 0.12 sec Rate: 250 - 350	The rapid rate prohibits cardiac filling or coronary artery perfusion. Considered a possible transition between VTach and VFib. Produces minimal cardiac output. Deteriorates into ventricular fib.
Ventricular Fibrillation	Continuous, rapid-rate discharges from numerous ectopic foci in the ventricles, producing no ventricular contraction. P, PR, QRS, T: none, indiscernible VF Rate: 350 - 450, no P's or QRS's Rhythm: none, no pattern, chaotic If Coarse VF: indicates a greater degree of electrical activity, is easier to convert.	Cardiac arrest. There is no ventricular contraction, no cardiac output, no blood pressure. Caused by myocardial ischemia, AMI, untreated VTach, CAD, hypo/hypercalcemia, electric shock, hyperkalemia. Perform emergency defibrillation to save life. See ACLS-VFib algorithm.
Asystole	Appears as a nearly flat line. Total absence of ventricular activity. There may be P waves (or pacer spikes if a pacer is active) Check 2 ECG leads to rule out fine V Fib (which is shockable).	Ventricular standstill. No electrical activity in the heart. No cardiac output, no blood pressure. The arrhythmia of death. Caused by MI, massive pulmonary embolus, prolonged hypoxemia, severe electrolyte or acid-base disturbance, electric shock, cocaine overdose. Beware misdiagnosing as fine V Fib, since shocking asystole may be harmful. See ACLS. Most cannot be revived.

Fig. 7.37 Ventricular Flutter

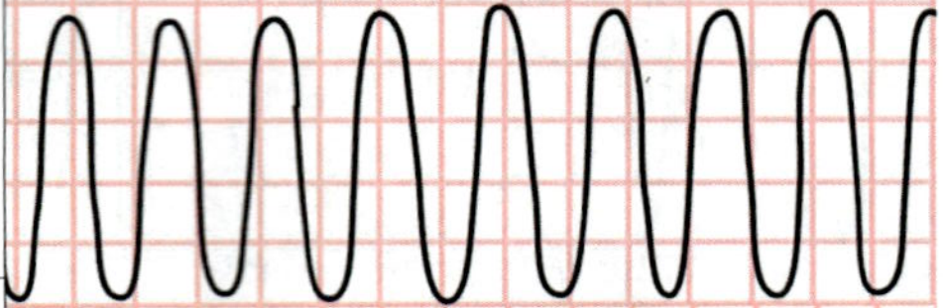

Fig. 7.38 Ventricular Fibrillation

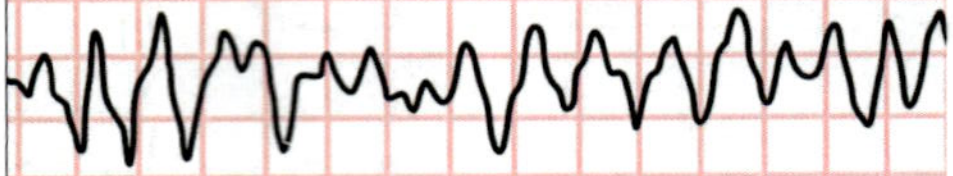

Fig. 7.39 Asystole

The Chest Leads

Fig. 7.40

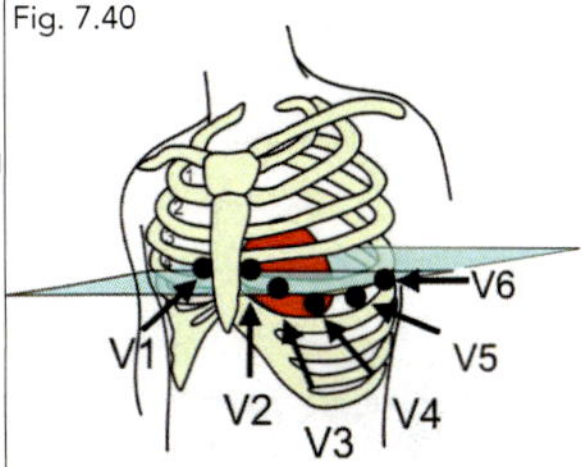

How to identify the location of cardiac ischemia:

Imagine each chest lead, according to its position on the chest, sees a particular part of the heart. V6, for example, when looking tpward the heart, sees the lateral wall of the left ventricle. V5 also sees the lateral wall.

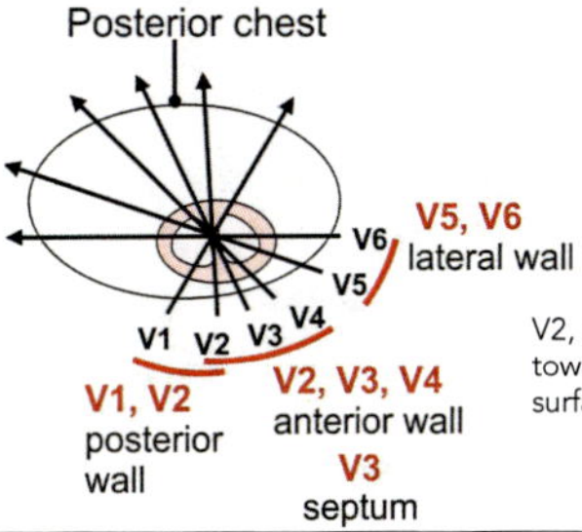

V2, V3, and V4, when looking toward the heart, see the anterior surface.

Fig. 7.41

The Limb Leads

Fig. 7.42

The limb leads also provide information on specific parts of the heart. Leads I and AVL see the lateral wall.

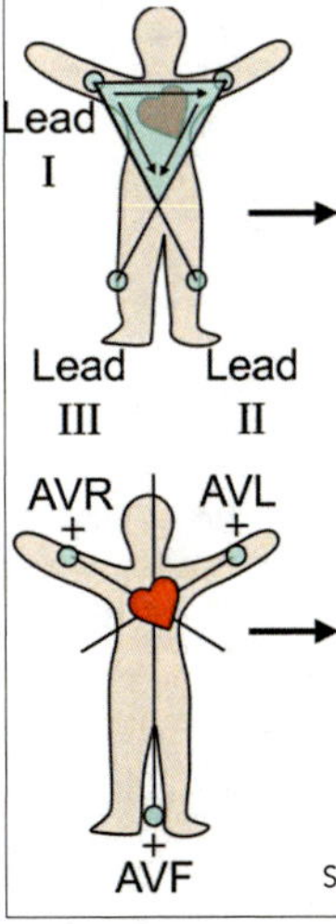

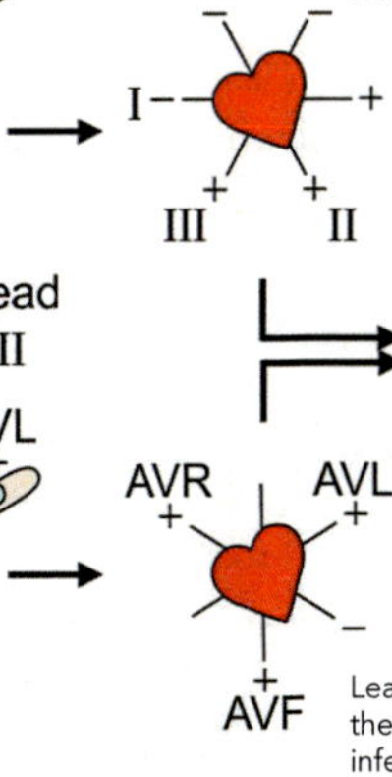

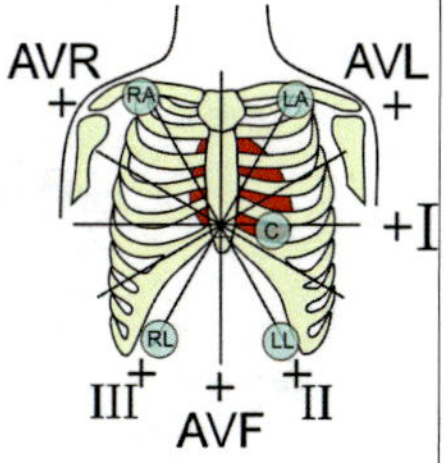

Leads II, III, and AVF "look up" from the feet (or lower chest) and see the inferior wall of the heart.

See the Summary of all 12-Leads on the next page →

12-Lead EKG to Localize Infarction

Diagnosis of STEMI is made when all 3 of the following are present:

1. Chest pain is characteristic of Acute Coronary Syndrome (ACS).
2. Cardiac biomarkers (Troponin or CK-MB) are elevated.
3. There is ST elevation ≥ 0.1 mV in 2 or more adjacent precordial or limb leads.

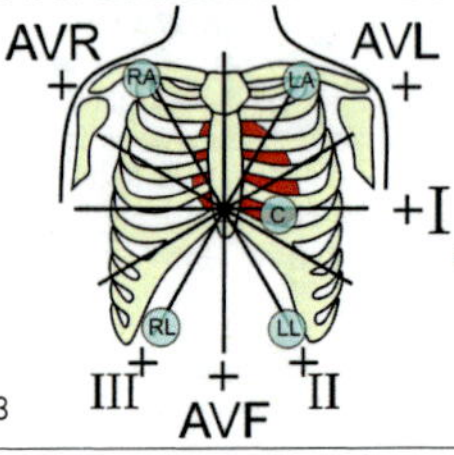

Fig. 7.43

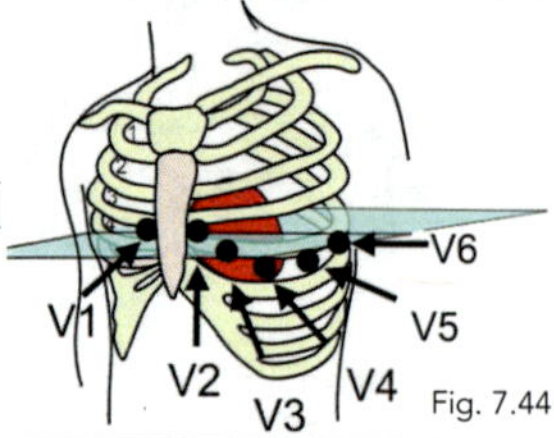

Fig. 7.44

The Limb Leads | **The Chest Leads**

Fig. 7.45

Lateral wall:

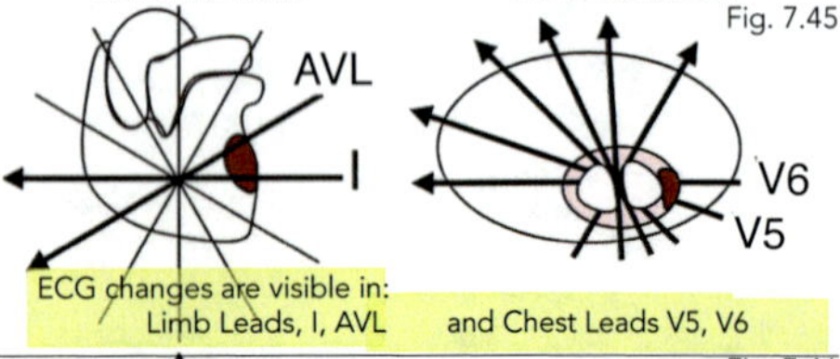

Fig. 7.46

Inferior wall:

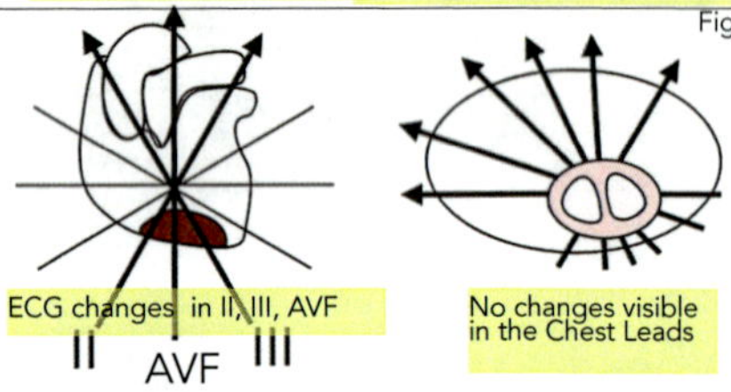

Fig. 7.47

Anterior wall:

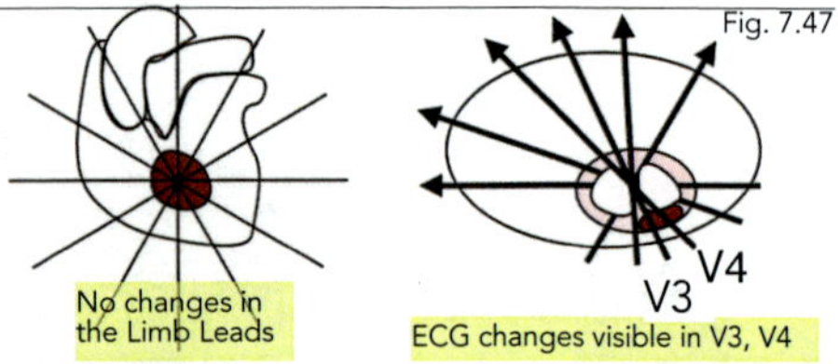

Fig. 7.48

Posterior wall:

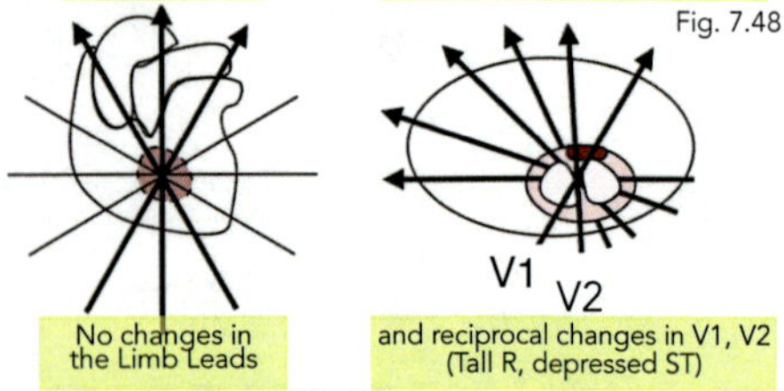

Axis

Principles: Axis is the general direction of the wave of depolarization. Remember that when a wave of depolarization moves toward a positive electrode, it writes a positive QRS on the ECG.

Normal Axis:

- Lead I is a positive electrode positioned on the left arm. Since the normal axis (wave of depolarization) is generally toward the patient's left, expect the QRS in Lead I to be positive.
- Lead AVF is a positive electrode positioned on the feet. Since the normal axis (wave of depolarization) is generally toward the pt's feet, expect the QRS in Lead AVF to be positive.
- Normal axis = positive QRS in Leads I & AVF

Fig. 7.49

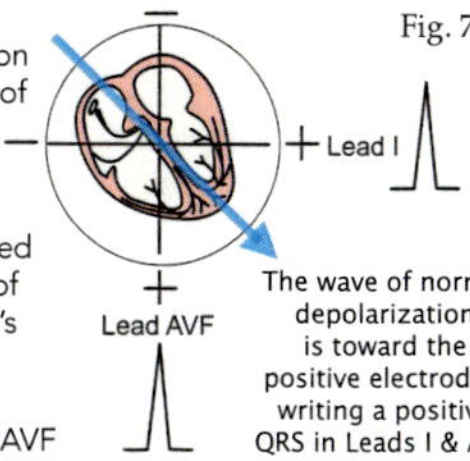

The wave of normal depolarization is toward the positive electrodes, writing a positive QRS in Leads I & AVF

Axis Shift: The wave of depolarization shifts *away* from areas of infarction. The wave of depolarization shifts *toward* areas of hypertrophy.

Right Axis Deviation:

- Right axis deviation is the shift of the axis to the patient's right.
- A patient with a lateral wall infarction shifts the general wave of depolarization away from Lead I and toward the right, causing the QRS in Lead I to be negative.
- Since the wave of depolarization remains generally toward the feet, the QRS in AVF would remain positive.
- Right Axis Deviation = negative QRS in Lead I and positive QRS in AVF.

Fig. 7.50

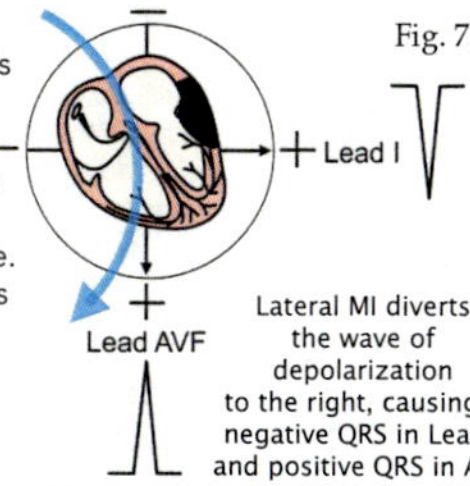

Lateral MI diverts the wave of depolarization to the right, causing a negative QRS in Lead I and positive QRS in AVF

Left Axis Deviation:

- Left axis deviation is the shift of the axis to the patient's far left. This could occur in a patient with inferior MI.
- The wave of depolarization still moves toward the left, so the QRS in Lead I would remain positive.
- Inferior MI shifts the axis away from the feet, so AVF would be negative.
- Left Axis Deviation = positive QRS in Lead I and negative QRS in AVF.

Fig. 7.51

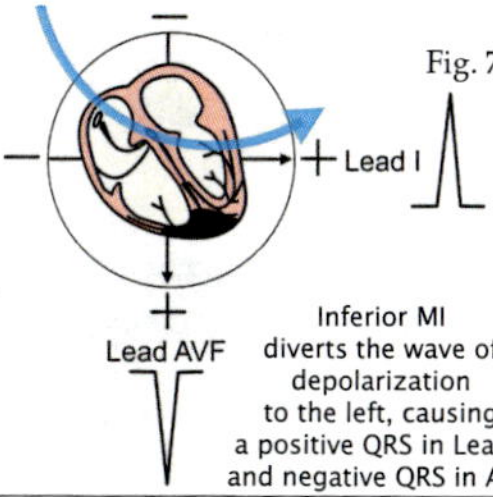

Inferior MI diverts the wave of depolarization to the left, causing a positive QRS in Lead I and negative QRS in AVF

Extreme Right Axis Deviation:

- Extreme right axis deviation is the shift of the axis to the pt's upper right.
- This can occur with Antero-lateral MI, as well as with RV hypertrophy.
- Since the wave of depolarization is in general away from the patient's left, the QRS in Lead I would be negative.
- Since the wave of depolarization is in general away from the pt's feet, the QRS in AVF would also be negative.
- Extreme right axis deviation = negative QRS in Leads I & AVF.

Fig. 7.52

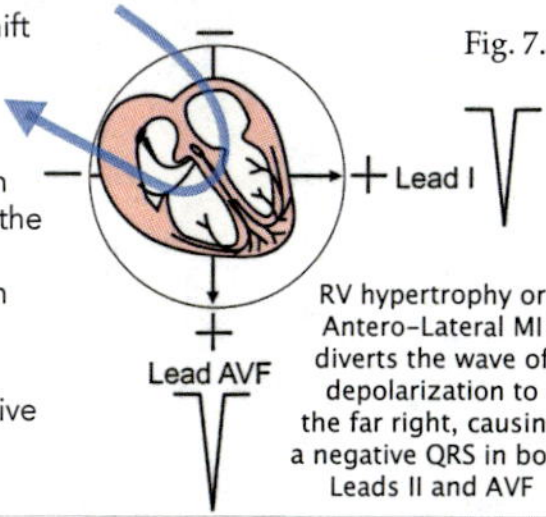

RV hypertrophy or Antero-Lateral MI diverts the wave of depolarization to the far right, causing a negative QRS in both Leads II and AVF

Summary of the 4 axis quadrants:

RAD = Right Axis Deviation
LAD = Left Axis Deviation

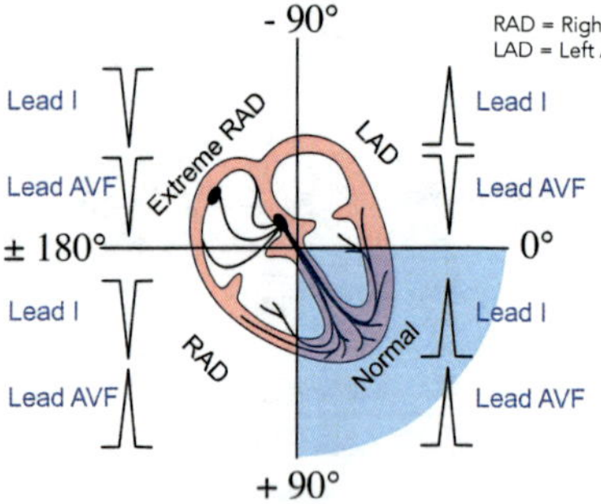

Fig. 7.53

Vector: The exact location of the axis (vector) can be located by using a 360° circle around the heart.

1. Locate the quadrant of the axis using the figure below.
2. Find the lead where the QRS is most isoelectric (the QRS is as much above the baseline as it is under the baseline). The wave of depolarization travels toward and then away from the isoelectric lead. The vector (axis) is therefore 90° to this lead.
   Example: If Lead III is the most isoelectric lead, the axis is 90° to Lead III, which is +30° (normal axis).
   Example: If Lead II is the most isoelectric lead, the axis is 90° to Lead II, which is -30° (left axis deviation).

Extreme Right Axis Deviation	
If the most iso-electric lead is	The Axis is
I	- 90°
AVL	- 120°
III	- 150°
AVF	- 180°

Left Axis Deviation	
If the most iso-electric lead is	The Axis is
I	- 90°
AVR	- 60°
II	- 30°
AVF	- 0°

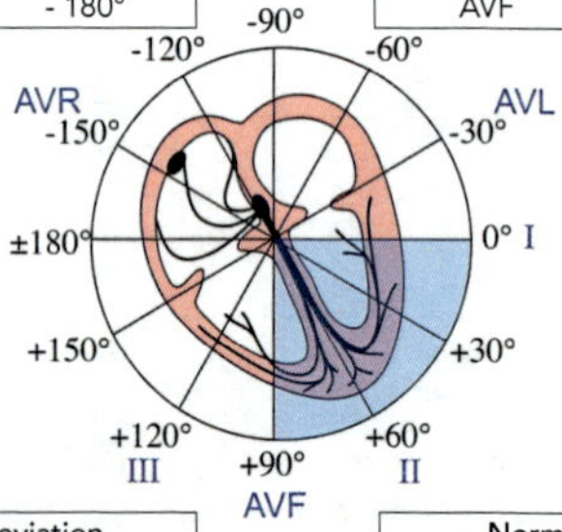

Fig. 7.54

Right Axis Deviation	
If the most iso-electric lead is	The Axis is
AVF	+180°
II	+150°
AVR	+120°
I	+ 90°

Normal Axis	
If the most iso-electric lead is	The Axis is
AVF	0°
III	+ 30°
AVL	+ 60°
I	+ 90°

ST Segment Monitoring

Description:

- The ST Segment represents ventricular repolarization (myocytes actively elongate in preparation for the next contraction).
- On the ECG, the ST is normally at or near the baseline.
- Baseline is identified as the end of the T to beginning of the P.

The J-point defined:

- The level of the point that is 0.6 seconds after the J point (the end of the QRS) is compared to the baseline) and any difference is measured. Normally the J point is at the baseline.
- Significant myocardial Ischemia is defined as ST elevation of at least 1 - 2 mm for at least 1 minute, or ST depression > 0.5 mm

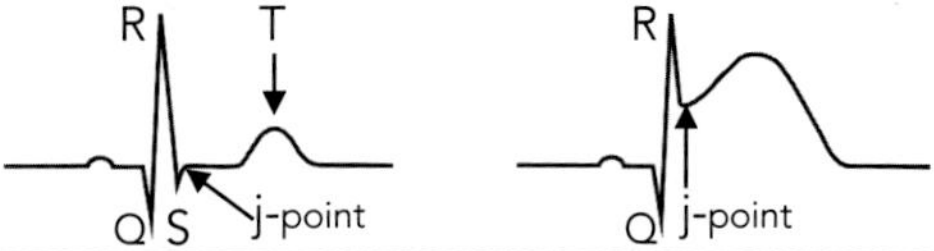

Significance of the ST:

- Patients have an individual ST fingerprint, a unique pattern of ST segment changes during ischemic episodes.
- Half of patients with potential ACS who have ST depression on the initial 12-lead ECG progress to MI within hours.
- Half of patients after PCI have transient ischemia, and are more likely to experience hypotension, AMI, death, abrupt closure of vessel, and longer hospital length of stay..
- A 50% decrease in peak ST elevation within the first hour of thrombolytics is used to predict vessel patency.
- ST changes occur in 20% of patients during vascular surgery and over 30% of these developed MI.
- ST changes are associated with 60% increased risk for failure to wean from mechanical ventilation.

The ST defined:

- The level of the point that is 0.6 seconds after the J point is compared to the baseline and any difference is measured.
- Baseline is identified as the end of the T to beginning of the P.
- Significant myocardial Ischemia is defined as if 1 - 2 mm elevation for at least 1 minute, or ST depression > 0.5 mm.

Indications for ST-Segment Monitoring:

- ACS (Acute Coronary Syndrome)
- Myocardial ischemia without chest pain
- Receiving thrombolytic therapy for STEMI
- Chest pain or angina-equivalent symptoms in the ED
- During/after percutaneous coronary intervention, particularly angioplasty without stent, PCI with suboptimal results
- Potential for vasospasm (e.g., Prinzmetal angina, cocaine)
- ↑ K^+, acute pericarditis, cardiac contusion or hypertrophy

Which Leads to Monitor:

- Patients with the following known areas of cardiac ischemia:

Anterior wall:	V2 or V3 preferred, then V4
Septum:	V1 and V2
Inferior wall:	III preferred, then aVF or II, V3R, and V4R
Lateral wall:	I, AVL, V5 preferred, or V6.
Low lateral:	V5, V6 or High lateral: AVL
Posterior wall:	V1-V3 for reciprocal changes (ST depression)

- Noncardiac patients undergoing surgery: V5

Procedural Info:

- Monitor patient in supine position.
- HOB elevation less than 45°.
- Mark ECG lead sites with indelible ink pen.
- Good skin prep with soap/water (no alcohol) to remove oil.
- Abrade skin lightly with dry cloth.
- Set the alarm for ST deviation of 1 - 2 mm
- If the patient is high risk, set the ST deviation alarm at 1 mm.

When ST monitoring is not beneficial

Pericarditis or myocardial contusion	LBBB, RBBB
ST segment depression due to digoxin	Paced rhythm
ST obscured by AFib or AFlutter	Agitated state

Notes

Pacing

Pacing

Pacing Modes

Available for Temporary Pacing

The AHA system for classifying different types of pacing asks three questions: Which chambers are paced, Which chambers are sensed, The pacer's response.

* A = Atrium	D = Dual (both A & V)	I = Inhibited
V = Ventricle	O = none	

	chamber paced	chamber sensed	pacer response	
Atrial fixed rate	A	O	O	The atria are paced but not sensed. Atrial pacing fixed rate occurs at the set (fixed) rate, regardless of the inherent atrial rhythm the patient may have.
Atrial demand	A	A	I	Patient must have functioning AV node for this demand mode. The atria are sensed. Atrial pacing will occur if no P wave is sensed during the time interval needed to match the HR set on the pacemaker. Sensed P wave inhibits atrial pacing. The mode of choice when atrioventricular conduction is intact but the natural pacemaker (the SA node) is unreliable.
Ventricular fixed rate	V	O	O	The ventricles are paced but not sensed. Ventricular pacing occurs at the set (fixed) rate, regardless of any inherent ventricular rhythm.
Ventricular demand	V	V	I	The ventricles are sensed. Ventricular pacing will occur only if no QRS is sensed during the time interval needed to match the rate set on the pacer. Sensed QRS will inhibit pacing. This mode is suitable when no synchronization with the atrial beat is required (e.g., atrial fibrillation).
AV Sequential fixed rate	D	O	O	The atria and ventricles are paced but neither the atria nor ventricles are sensed. AV pacing occurs at the set (fixed) rate, regardless of any atrial or ventricular rhythm the patient may have.
AV Sequential ventricular demand	D	V	I	The ventricles are sensed, the atria are not. Atrial pacing occurs at the set (fixed) rate, regardless of whatever inherent atrial rhythm the patient may have. Ventricular pacing will occur only if no QRS is sensed at the time interval needed to match the rate set on the pacemaker. AV Sequential combines Atrial Fixed Rate with Ventricular demand.
AV Sequential dual demand	D	D	I	Pacing in both the atria and ventricles. Sensing in both the atria and ventricles. Inhibited in both chambers.
Dual Demand	D	D	D	Senses and paces both atria and ventricles. Maintains AV synchrony and atrial kick. Will follow the intrinsic atrial rate only as far as the preset upper limit.

Ventricular Pacer: Controls*

Refer to you pacer operating manual for instructions specific to your device.

Cable/Electrode Connection (at top of pacer)
This pacer allows you to connect the electrodes to a connecting cable, or if the cable is unavailable, to insert the wires/pins directly into the separate "heart wire" sockets.

Fig. 8.1

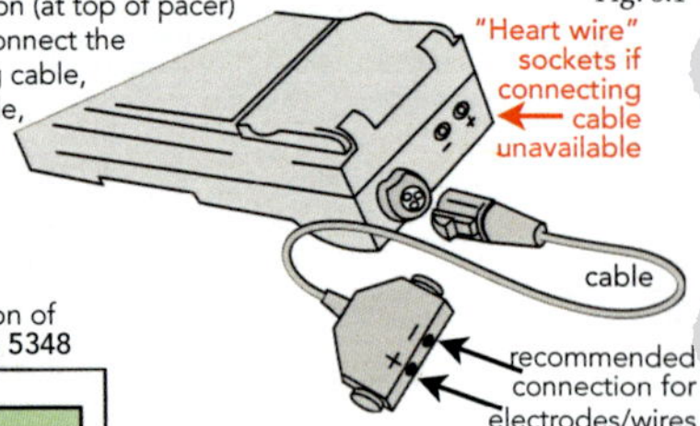

Fig. 8.2 representation of the **Medtronic Model 5348**

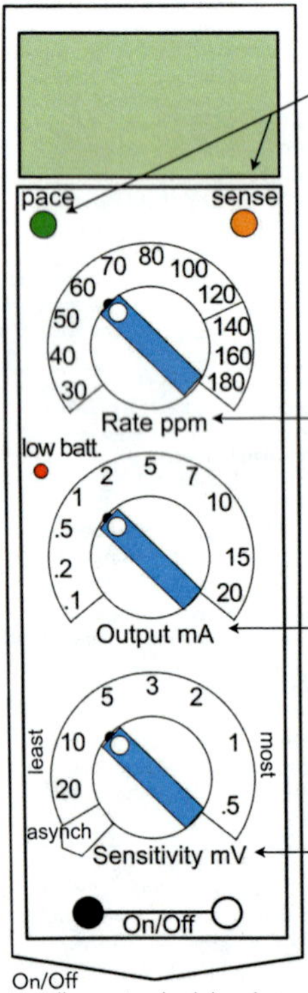

Pacing/Sensing Indicator
Flashes each time the pacemaker delivers an impulse each time it senses the patient's R wave. Does not indicate if the pacing stimulus resulted in capture (depolarization). You must check the ECG for pacer spike followed by wide QRS.

Rate
30 - 180 ppm (pulses per minute)
Usually set on 70-100 for fixed rate (asynchronous). For demand pacing, set at 10 beats/minute under patient's rate or set at 60 ppm.

Output
0.1 - 20 mA (milliamps)
The amount of current delivered to the ventricle. Usually 1.5 mA is enough to capture (depolarize) the chamber.
Minimum pacing threshold (MPT) is the minimum output needed to cause capture (depolarization) in each patient.
Output is usually set at 2 times MPT.
MPT is increased by anesthetics, acidosis, hypoxia, fibrosis on the tip of the catheter.
MPT is decreased by exercise, low blood sugar, steroids, catecholamine.

Sensitivity
0.5 - 20 mV (millivolts)
Ability to sense cardiac activity.
The millivolt setting represents the size of the sensed R wave. If set on 0.5 mV, the pacer will sense R waves as small as 0.5 mV. Thus the pacer is very sensitive and will be inhibited by the sensed beats (i.e., demand pacing).
If set on 20 mV, the pacer will not sense the R unless the R wave voltage is ≥ 20 mV (the pacer is not very sensitive to the presence of inherent cardiac activity).
If set on "asynch," the pacer is completely insensitive to the presence of any QRS, and paces at a fixed rate based on the rate set on the RATE control.

On/Off
Usually requires both hands to turn pacer off.

Clear plastic cover protects pacer from accidental changes in settings.

Refer to your pacer operating manual for detailed, specific instructions.

Transvenous Pacing

Indications:	
Acute MI:	Asystole Bradycardia with hypotension Bilateral Bundle Branch Block New Bifasicular block with 1° AVB Mobitz type II 2° AVB
Bradycardia without MI:	Asystole Bradycardia with hypotension 2° or 3° AV Block Bradycardia induced ventricular tachyarrhythmias
Cardiac Surgery:	Aortic surgery Tricuspid surgery Closure of VSD

Insertion of Transvenous Electrode:

1. Establish IV access.
2. Monitor ECG with 4 limb leads. Connect C (Chest) lead to pacing electrode, (this will allow monitoring of electrode position.
3. Have access to defibrillator and emergency meds.
4. Assemble customary items for venous cannulation.
5. Check pacemaker, replace batteries.
6. Pacing electrodes, connecting cables, and alligator clips.

Atrial ECG: is used to track the position of the pacing electrode without using fluoroscopy.

Fig. 8.3

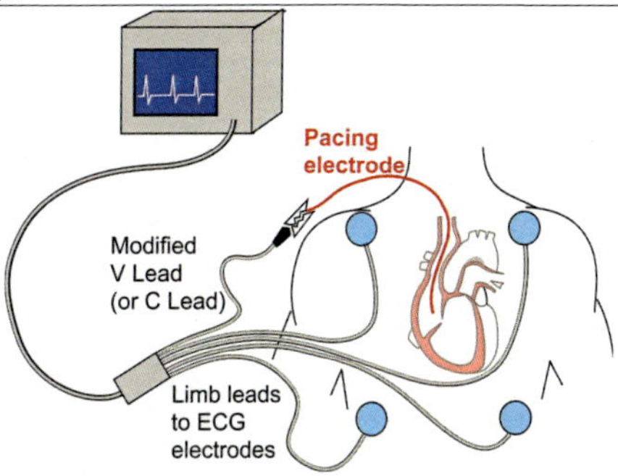

Run strip recorder and observe ECG monitor during placement:

- When the electrode is in the atrium, the P waves will be large.
- When the electrode is in the ventricle, the QRS will be large.
- When the ST segment elevates, contact has been made with the endocardium.

Fig. 8.4

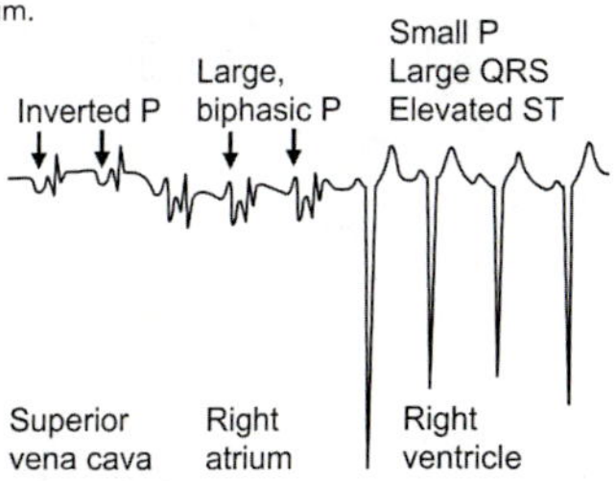

Ventricular Pacing: Connections

Transvenous Ventricular Pacing:

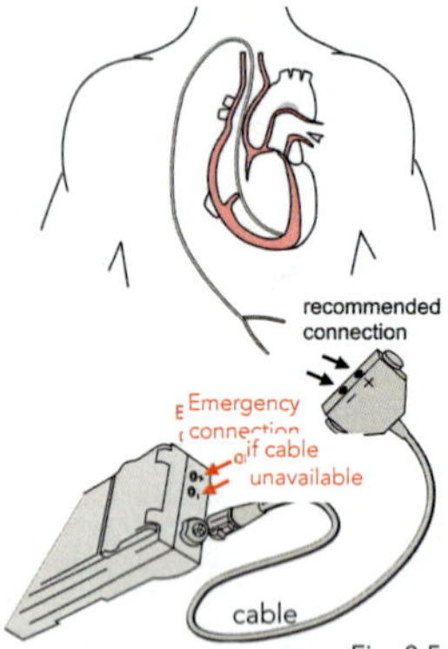

Fig. 8.5

1. Connect patient cable to top of pacer, then insert pacing leads into the cable. Tighten thumbwheels to hold the leads securely in place.
2. In an emergency, if the connecting cable is unavailable, the pacing leads may be placed directly into separate "heart wire" sockets at the top of the pacer. Although the wires will be snug in the sockets, the wires cannot be locked in place.
3. Cover any exposed electrode wire or contacts with nonconducting material.

The pacing stimulus is discharged from the pacer's negative pole. The stimulus is then conducted by this (negative) lead wire to the end of the electrode. The current then flows to the positive electrode, and then back to the pacer's positive terminal.

Epicardial Ventricular Pacing:
Surgeon's rule on positioning pacing wires:
Wire/s which exit to the left (patient's left) of the sternum are ventricular.
Wire/s which exit to the right (patient's right) of the sternum are atrial.
A wire with one end imbedded in the skin (either stitched or attached to a curved needle), serves as the positive electrode for a unipolar epicardial lead.

Bipolar epicardial lead

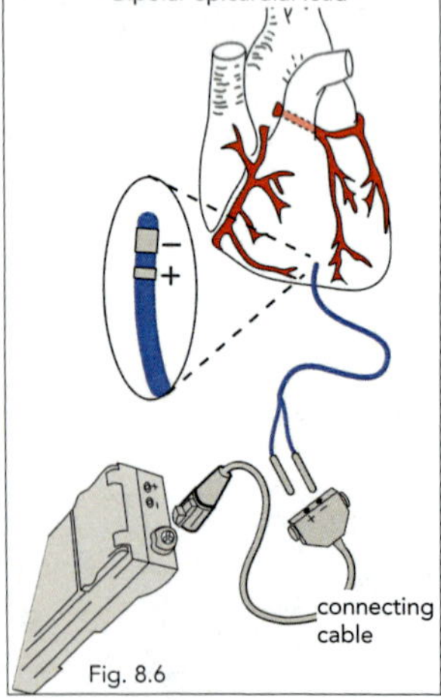

Fig. 8.6

Unipolar epicardial lead

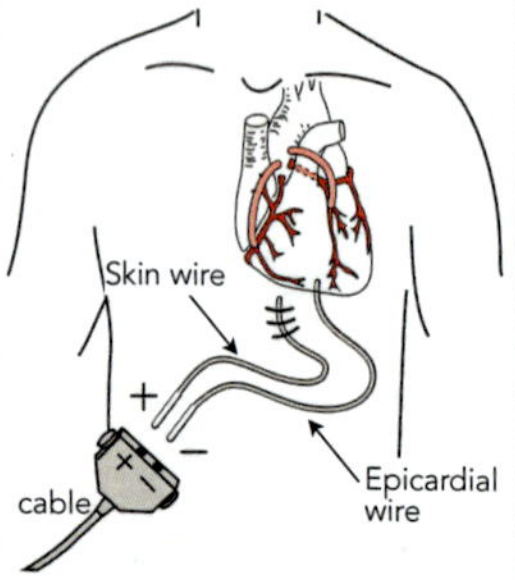

The electrode of the epicardial lead is sutured to or is embedded in the epicardium, and must be connected to the negative pole of the pacer. The skin wire (or ground wire) must be connected to the positive pole of the pacer.

Fig. 8.7

First connect the cable to the pacer, then connect the leads to the cable. Match negative pin to the negative receptacle, and the positive pin to the positive receptacle.

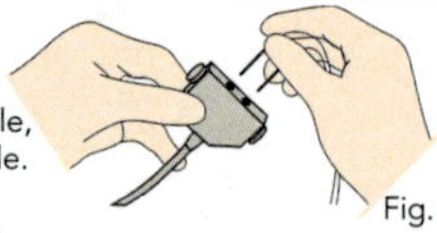

Fig. 8.8

Settings for EMERGENCY PACING

The patient is asystolic or has symptomatic bradycardia.

1. Set rate at 80 - 100.
2. Set output at 20 mA.
3. Set sensitivity on "asynch" (> 20 mV).
4. Turn pacer on.
5. Note pacing indicator is flashing "pace."
6. Identify pacing spikes on EKG.
   Look for capture (depolarization).
7. When patient more stable,
   slowly reduce mA to identify
   minimum pacing threshold (MPT).
   Increase mA to at least 2 times the MPT.

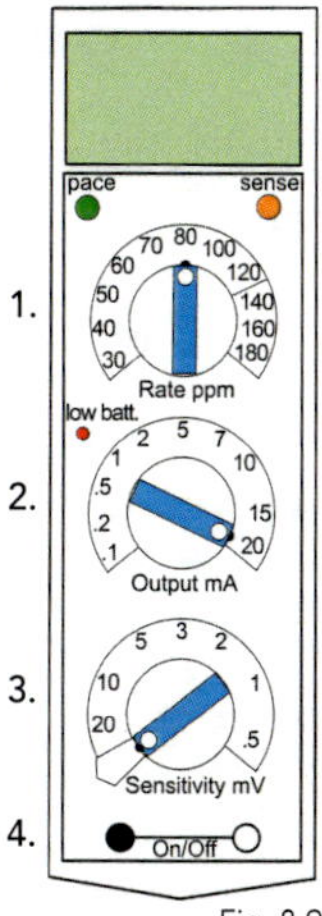

Fig. 8.9

Settings for Demand Pacing (see next page) ⟶

Pacemaker Safety Precautions

- Have defibrillator on hand during insertion of pacing leads.
- Wear gloves whenever handling pacemaker or wires. You could conduct a microshock (which is imperceptible to you) to the patient's heart, causing dysrhythmia, and even cardiac arrest.
- Check to be sure that all equipment in the room is properly grounded.
- Cover all exposed wires with nonconductive material. Secure, cover, protect wires at the insertion site.
- To prevent accidental changes in the pacer settings and to discourage pacer tampering, cover the pacer controls.
- Secure all connections. To prevent accidental disconnect/pacing failure, secure pacer to patient's arm or consider suspending pacer from an IV pole.
- Set a policy that specifies pacers position, so that the pacer may be quickly accessed by other clinicians if emergency occurs.
- Check batteries each shift. If "sense" or "pace" indicators no longer flash, change batteries. Change 9 volt batteries once per week.
- Be sure that the EKG monitoring lead that you use correctly counts the R waves, not the pacing spikes.
- Remember the margins of safety for synchronous (demand) pacing:
- Sensitivity (mV) is set at one-half the sensitivity threshold.
- Output (mA) is set at 2 times pacing threshold.
- If the patient deteriorates during pacing:
  1. Verify Sense and Capture
  2. Increase the rate (ppm)
  3. If AV pacer, adjust the AV interval

Factors which affect Minimum Pacing Threshold (MPT)

MPT is increased by	MPT is decreased by
Acidosis	Exercise
Hypoxia	Low blood sugar
Electrolyte imbalance	Steroids
Anesthetics	Catecholamines
	Fibrosis on tip of pacing lead

Set Pacer for Demand (Synchronized) Pacing

VVI, AAI

First, Set the Sensing Threshold: Leave these settings as they are.

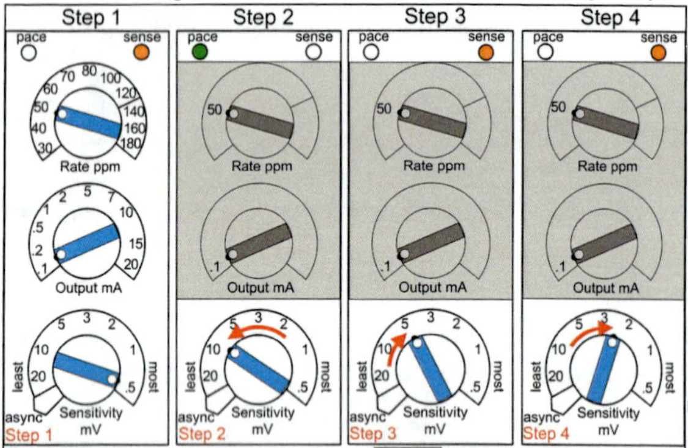

Fig. 8.10 Leave these settings as they are

Step 1	Step 2	Step 3	Step 4
Start with these settings: Rate is less than pt's HR. Output 0.1 mA. Sensitivity 0.5 mV. Pacer will flash "sense."	Turn sensitivity to the left to stop the sensing of intrinsic heart rate. "Pace" will flash, spikes will appear on ECG but no capture (the mA is too low)	Slowly turn sensitivity to the right until sensitivity restored (no pacer spikes on ECG). This is the Sensing Threshold. In this example, 5.	Slowly continue to turn sensitivity to the right (clockwise) to a value that is half the Sensing Threshold, In this example, 2.5 mV

Second, Set the Pacing Threshold: Leave these settings as they are.

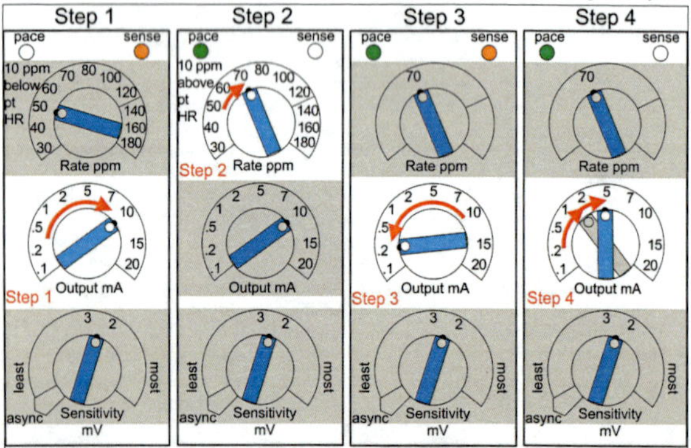

Fig. 8.11 Leave these settings as they are

Step 1	Step 2	Step 3	Step 4
After Sensitivity is set, increase the output to 10 mA. No pacing will occur yet, the set rate is too low.	Turn rate to 10 above the pt's rate. Observe pacing and capture occur. Pace light flashes. Note spike and capture on ECG.	Slowly turn mA down until there is loss of capture. Pace and Sense lights flash intermittently.	Slowly turn mA up until capture occurs. This is the Pacing Threshold. For margin of safety, turn mA up, to 2 times this value.

Ventricular Pacing: Troubleshooting

Fail to Capture: No depolarization after delivery of pacing spike

Fig. 8.12

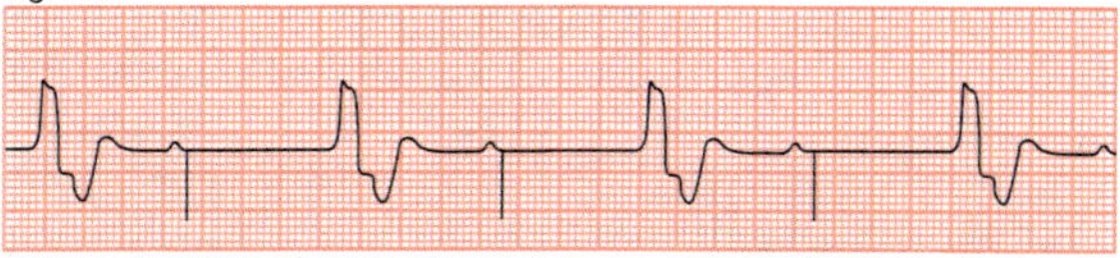

- Output (mA) is too low. Patient conditions can increase the pacing threshold: electrolyte imbalance, tissue changes, medication effect, fibrosis around the electrode. Correct any electrolyte imbalances, reassess the pacing threshold.
- Catheter tip may not be in contact with endocardium. Reposition patient. Physician may need to reposition the pacing wire.
- Battery or pacer failure. Change either or both.

Fail to Sense: Pacer does not detect intrinsic rhythm and delivers pacing stimulus (spike) at the wrong time. Also, the sense indicator does not flash although ECG shows intrinsic rhythm. VTach or V Fib could result if pacer fires during the QT interval.

Fig. 8.13

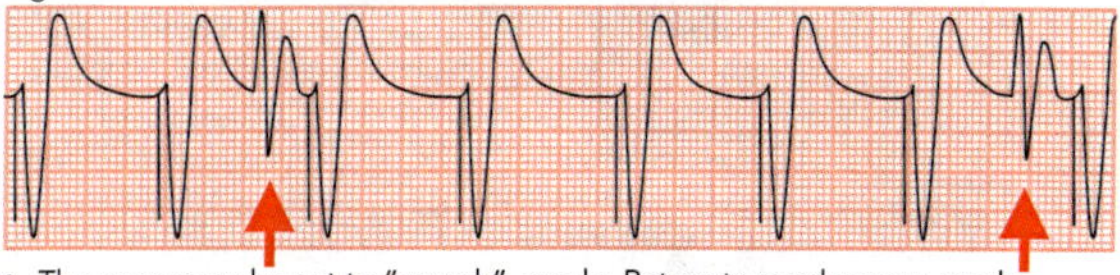

- The pacer may be set to "asynch" mode. Return to synchronous mode.
- Pacer's set sensitivity is not enough. Reassess Sensing Threshold.
- If the patient's QRS voltage is too low to be detectable, increase the mV.
- Electrode/s not in contact with endocardium. Reposition patient and/or wire.
- Check equipment in the room for proper grounding.
- Check for break in connections, electrode fracture, or battery failure.
- If pacer continues to fire on the QT, inform physician. May need to stop the pacer. Have atropine on hand. Consider transcutaneous pacing.

Fail to Pace: Pacer does not release a stimulus (spike) when it should

Fig. 8.14

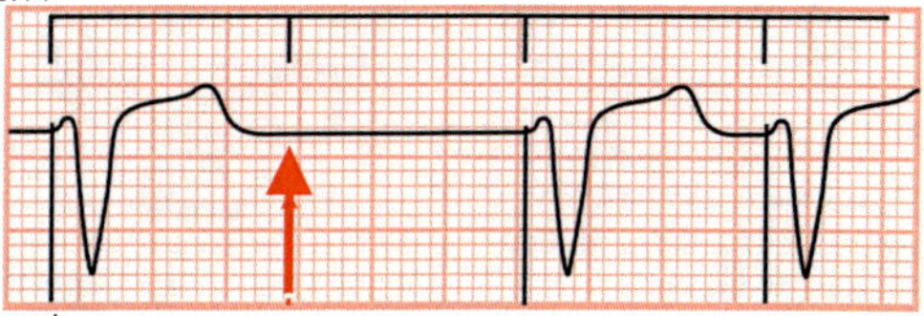

Oversensing:

- Pacer may be too sensitive and thus inhibited by other electrical signals (P or T wave) or by muscle activity. Decrease the sensitivity (turn mV to the left, to a higher number). Retest sensing threshold, and set sensitivity at 1/2 threshold.
- If AV pacing, decrease the atrial mA setting.
- Verify lead position with X-ray (may be sensing P waves).
- Check for possible insulation break in the cable/s; replace cable if necessary.
- Pacer Malfunction:
    1. if pace or sense flashing: check connections, electrode placement, integrity of the pacer and pacing wires or cables
    2. if pace or sense not flashing: change the battery.

The AV Sequential Pacer

Pace/Sense Indicators
The "A" indicators flash when a P wave is sensed and/or atria are paced. The "V" indicators flash when an R wave is sensed and/or ventricles are paced.

Fig. 8.15

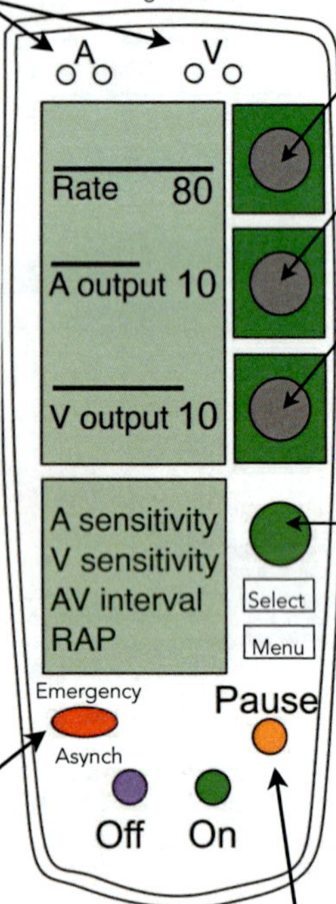

Representation of the Medtronic 5388

Emergency ASYNC
For emergency high-output, dual chamber, asynchronous pacing.

Pause
Press and hold to suspend pacer activity for up to 10 seconds, to allow assessment of the patient's inherent rhythm. After 10 seconds, pacemaker resumes function.

On/Off
Some pacers require both hands to turn pacer off. On this model, press OFF twice.

* Refer to your pacer operating manual for detailed, specific instructions.

Connections at top of pacer

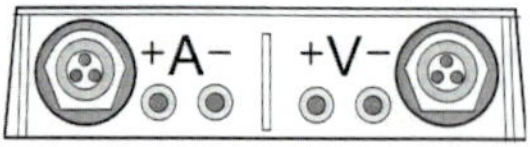

Fig. 8.16

Rate
30 - 200 pulses per minute

Atrial Output
0.1 - 20 milliamps (mA)
The amount of current delivered to the atria. Set at 10 ma or 2 - 3 times the patient's minimum pacing threshold.

Ventricular Output
0.1 - 25 milliamps (mA)
The amount of current delivered to the ventricles. Set at 10 mA or 2 times minimum pacing threshold, which is the minimal output needed to cause capture (depolarization). MPT is ↑ by anesthetics, acidosis, hypoxia, fibrosis on the electrode tip and is ↓ by exercise, low blood sugar, steroids, catecholamine.

Dial for lower screen menu
To set the following parameters:

1. Atrial Sensitivity
   0.4 - 10 millivolts (mV)
   Ability to sense atrial activity. If set on a low setting (0.4), the P does not have to be very tall to be sensed, therefore the pacer is very sensitive to the intrinsic cardiac activity. If set on a high setting, the P has to be tall to be sensed.
2. Ventricular Sensitivity
   0.8 - 20 mV millivolts (mV)
   Ability to sense ventricular activity. If set on a low setting (0.8), the R does not have to be very tall to be sensed, therefore the pacer is very sensitive (demand pacing). If set on a high setting, the R has to be tall to be sensed. If set higher than 20 mV, the pacer functions as fixed rate (asynchronous) and will fire at the rate set on the rate dial.
3. AV Interval
   50 - 250 milliseconds (msec)
   The time interval between atrial and ventricular pacing (equivalent to a PR interval). Usually set at 170 msec. Proper timing results in good atrial/ventricular synchrony and an optimal cardiac output.
4. Rapid Atrial Pacing* (by physician only). Pressing and holding SELECT initiates rapid pacing of the atria.

AV Sequential Pacing: Connections

Multipurpose PA Catheter

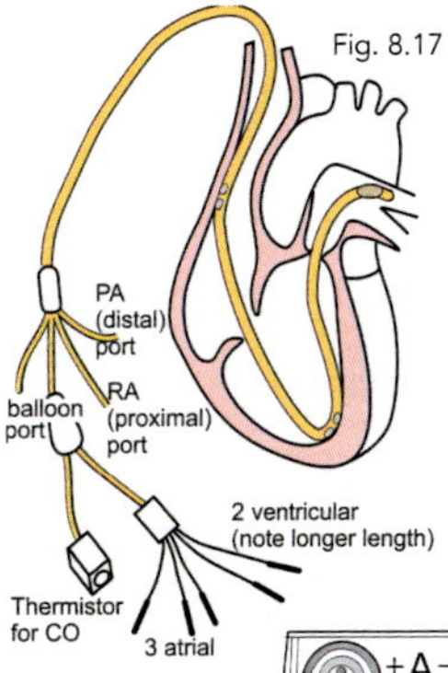

Fig. 8.17

Transvenous AV Pacing Catheter

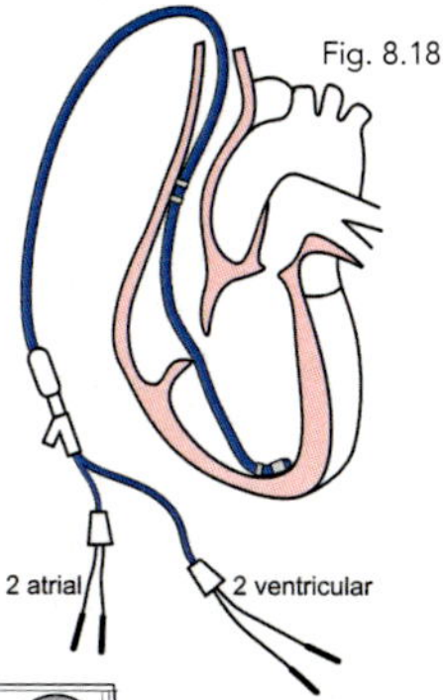

Fig. 8.18

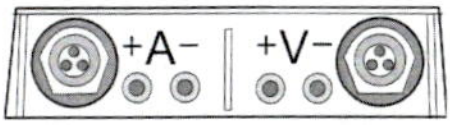

Fig. 8.19

Be absolutely certain that: A leads are connected to A terminal/s
V leads are connected to V terminal/s

Current flows out of the negative pole and returns via the positive pole.

AV Epicardial Bipolar Pacing Leads (for cardiac surgery patients)

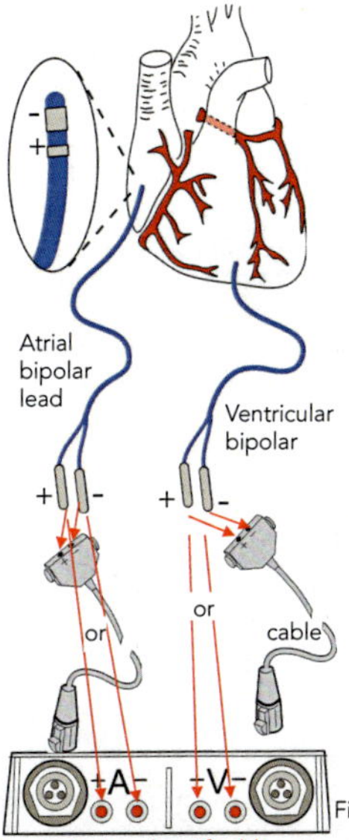

Fig. 8.20

"heart wire" sockets if cable not available

1. The wire located to the right of the sternum is the atrial bipolar lead. The wire located to the left of the sternum is the ventricular bipolar lead. (Unipolar leads are contraindicated in AV pacing, because of limitations in sensing)
2. First connect the cables to the pacer. Then insert leads into the connecting cable, matching the atrial leads to the cable attached to "A," and the ventricular leads to the cable attached to "V,"and matching + to +, and - to -.
3. In an emergency, if a connecting cable is unavailable, the leads may be inserted directly into the separate "heart wire" sockets at the top of the pacer.
4. Do not insert pins into the cable sockets, they are intended for the cable only.
5. Lead placement by the surgeon must:distance the atrial lead from the AV node, as well as the right ventricle;avoid crossing over vascular grafts;avoid tension on the leads to allow pt.movement without dislodging the leads; avoid the thin anterior ventricular wall; position the wires to permit ease of removal.

AV Sequential Pacing - Start Up

Description: Pacing of both the atria and ventricles in sequence can increase the cardiac output 20 - 50 % over ventricular pacing alone.
If the pacer is set for DVI pacing (demand pacing):

1. As long as the pacer senses a heart rate that is greater than the rate set on the pacer, atrial and ventricular pacing are inhibited
2. If the patient's heart rate slows below the rate set on the pacer, an atrial impulse is delivered and the AV interval begins.
3. At the end of the set AV internal, if the pacer does not sense an R wave, the pacer emits a ventricular impulse.

If the pacer is set for DOO pacing (fixed rate pacing): The pacer will pace both chambers, regardless of intrinsic rhythm, and according to the set ventricular rate and AV interval.

Indications:
Symptomatic sinus bradycardia
Bradycardia with heart failure
Complete heart block
Atrial or ventricular arrhythmias
Sick Sinus Syndrome
Hemodynamic support of the cardiac surgery patient

Contraindications:

- AV pacing is ineffective and contraindicated in AFib or AFlutter.
- Single chamber atrial pacing is contraindicated in patients with AV block.
- Asynchronous pacing is contraindicated in patients with an intrinsic rhythm.
- Unipolar leads are contraindicated in AV pacing because the current path of one can interfere with the current path of the other.

Connections:

1. Wear gloves to electrically isolate yourself from patient. Don't touch exposed metal leads, wires, or terminal or allow them to contact conductive or wet surfaces
2. Insert new battery, turn pacer on, test pacer, turn OFF
3. Connect pacing cable to the pacer, then connect leads to cable.(In an emergency and when connecting cable is unavailable, pacing leads may be inserted directly into the top of pacer.
4. See illustrations on how to make the connections to: Transvenous, Epicardial, or Multipurpose PA catheter.

Pacer Presets: Some pacers have automatic settings which can be selected. These settings are activated when the pacer is turned on:

If Emergency Pacing is selected:
DOO Dual Chamber, Asynchronous, Fixed Rate Pacing:

Base rate	80 pps
A output	20
V output	25
A sensitivity	asynch
V sensitivity	asynch
AV interval	not applicable

If Demand Pacing is selected:
DDD Dual Chamber Sensing and Pacing (Demand):

Base rate	80 pps
A output	10
V output	10
A sensitivity	0.5 mV
V sensitivity	2 mV
A tracking	ON
A-V interval	170 msec

No Pacing: Some clinicians deactivate the presets, and start with no pacing:
Turn A and V rate down to less than patient's intrinsic rate.
Turn A and V sensitivity to its most sensitive setting (0.5 mV).
Adjust A and V output to the lowest setting (0.1 mA).

Set Sensing and Pacing Thresholds for AV Pacing

Start with pacer on and A & V output down to lowest setting before connecting to patient. Set sensing threshold first, then set pacing threshold.

Set Atrial and Ventricular Sensing Threshold:

The sensing threshold is the minimum sensitivity needed to consistently sense intrinsic atrial and ventricular activity.

1. Set **Rate** at least 10 ppm below patient's intrinsic rate. This ensures no pacing. Sense indicator flashes (If the ventricular sense indicator is not flashing, it may be necessary to increase the AV interval.
2. Set A and V **Output** to 0.1 mA, to prevent risk of competitive pacing.
3. Decrease the **Sensitivity** by slowly turning sensitivity dial counterclockwise (increasing the mV value) until pace indicator flashes consistently.
4. Increase the **Sensitivity** by slowly turning the sensitivity dial clockwise (decreasing the mV value) until sense indicator flashes consistently. This value is the sensing threshold.
5. Set **Sensitivity** to half the threshold value. If threshold value is 5 mV, set sensitivity to 2.5 mV. This provides at least a 2:1 safety margin. Failure to follow this procedure can lead to asynchronous pulses. However, be aware that setting the sensitivity value too low (too sensitive) could result in inappropriate sensing of far-field signals (e.g., sensing of R- or T-waves on the atrial channel or P-waves on the ventricular channel), leading to inappropriate inhibition of pacing pulses. The simultaneous use of high output and maximum sensitivity (the lowest mV value) should be avoided.

Set Atrial and Ventricular Pacing Threshold:

The stimulation threshold is the minimum output pulse needed to consistently capture (depolarize) the heart.

1. Set **Rate** at least 10 ppm above patient's intrinsic rate. This ensures pacing. Pace indicator flashes. (If ventricular pacing does not occur, it may be necessary to decrease the AV interval).
2. Slowly decrease **Output** by turning the output dial counterclockwise until ECG shows loss of capture. Pace and sense indicators flash intermittently.
3. Slowing increase the **Output** by turning the output dial clockwise until ECG shows consistent capture. Pace indicator flashes; sense indicator stops flashing. This value is the pacing (stimulation) threshold.
4. Set **Output** to two times greater than the pacing threshold value.

Problems with AV Pacing:

- Fail to Sense
- Fail to Capture
- Fail to Pace
- Oversensing
- Crosstalk: inappropriate sensing of 1 chamber of a pacing discharge that was intended for the other chamber. Occurs when pacer is set on maximum sensitivity (lowest mV) and high ouput (mA).
- Pacemaker induced tachyarrhythmias (can be atrial or ventricular). (Occurs only in DDD mode). A too-long AV interval, as well as sensing of retrograde P-waves, PVC's, or artifacts, can trigger pacing of the ventricle during the vulnerable QT. This should be managed by increasing the PVARP (Post Ventricular Atrial Refractory Period). The PVARP is the period of time when the pacer does not respond to any incoming signals.

Complications of Pacing

Adverse effects:

- Asystole, which may or may not be temporary, following abrupt cessation of pacing. When discontinuing pacing, set pacer to demand mode, then gradually reduce the pacing rate below the patients intrinsic rate.
- Pacer inhibition in the presence of strong electromagnetic interference
- Pacemaker induced tachyarrhythmias
- Pacemaker self-inhibition
- High atrial pacing thresholds

Complications related to lead system:

- Complications of central venous catheterization: hemothorax, pneumothorax,infection, subclavian artery injury, hematoma
- Inappropriate lead connections or inadvertent disconnection of the lead system, resulting in no pacing
- Lead fracture or displacement causing intermittent or complete loss of capture and/or sensing
- Cardiac perforation, cardiac tamponade, septal perforation
- Myocardial irritability resulting in fibrillation
- Infarction
- Pericarditis
- Body rejection phenomena (local tissue reaction)
- Stimulation of skeletal muscle, diaphragm
- Bleeding/pericardial tamponade following epicardial lead removal
- Inability to remove epicardial lead, resulting in lead retention

What interferes with operation:

- Electrosurgical equipment, if within 15 cm (6 inches) of pacer and leads
- Diathermy equipment
- Some telemetry devices (if within 3 feet)
- Communications devices and transmitters, such as cell phones, walkie talkies, ambulance communication systems
- MRI (Magnetic Resonance Imaging)

About the battery:

- Alkaline battery (9 volt) last about 9 days of continuous operation.
- Common hospital policy is to change this type battery once per week.
- Lithium battery lasts about 16 days.
- In some pacers, removing the battery and reinstalling causes all settings to revert to preset values.

If cardioversion or defibrillation required:

- Although the pacer will not be affected by cardioversion, it is nevertheless recommended that the pacer be turned off and be disconnected from the patient. Protect any exposed metal electrodes, wires, pins.
- Paddles/pads should be positioned at least 15 cm (6 inches) away from pacer and leads.

Possible pacer failures (most common cause is low battery):

- No output or erratic output
- No sensing or erratic sensing
- False indicator light signals
- Inappropriate variance in rate, output pulse width, or output amplitude
- Reversion to asynchronous mode
- Loss of control of rate, output, sensitivity, or power

Resp

Resp

Respiratory Assessment

Inspect	Mental status:	Level of consciousness, mentation.
	Color:	Skin, mucous membranes, conjunctivae, nail beds.
	Character of respirations:	Rate, depth, rhythm, ease, symmetry of chest wall movement, nasal flaring.
	Inspiration:Expiration time:	The ratio is normally 1:3
	Use of accessory muscles:	Intercostals, abdominal, sternocleido-mastoids, trapezius, abdomen.
	Retractions:	Suprasternal, sternal, supraclavicular.
	Clubbing of fingers:	Nail bed angle (normal is 160°) may be increased to 180° by chronic hypoxemia.
Palpate	Position of the trachea:	Is there deviation left or right.
	PMI:	Is there deviation left or right.
	Location of:	Deformities, tenderness, pain, crepitus.
	Vocal fremitus:	Vibrations felt on the chest wall when the pt vocalizes "99." Strong vibrations imply that underlying lung is fluid filled
Percuss	Normal:	Resonant and low pitched.
	Hyperresonant:	Higher pitch, more air than solid tissue. may indicate air trapping, emphysema, or pneumothorax.
	Tympany:	Fluid-filled sound = more fluid than air.
	Dullness:	Less resonant, dense tissue, little air = consolidation of underlying lung.
	Flatness:	No resonance = consolidation or pleural effusion.
Auscultate	Tracheal:	Loud, tubular, high pitched, harsh, heard over the trachea, during both inspiration and expiration.
	Bronchial:	Loud, tubular, hollow, high pitched, heard over the manubrium, at 2nd ICS next to the sternum, longer in expiration than inspiration, with no sound between inspiration and expiration
	Vesicular:	Low pitch, light and breezy, heard over alveoli, mostly during inspiration.
	Broncho-vesicular:	A combination of bronchial & vesicular, heard where there is a combination of alveoli and larger airways. Normally heard over, and to either side of, the sternum, between scapulae, with vesicular sound heard on inspiration and bronchial sound heard on expiration.

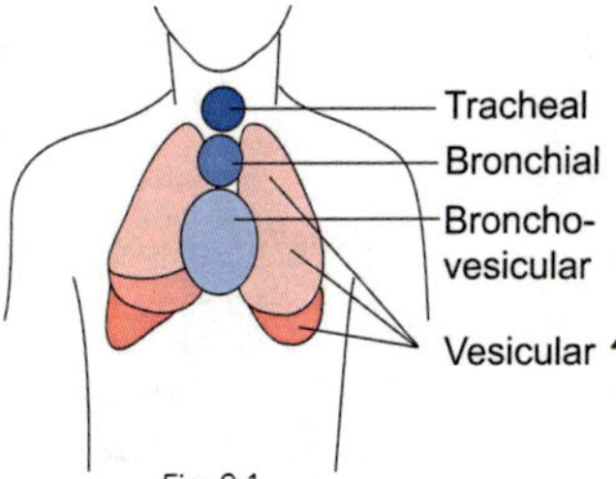

Fig. 9.1

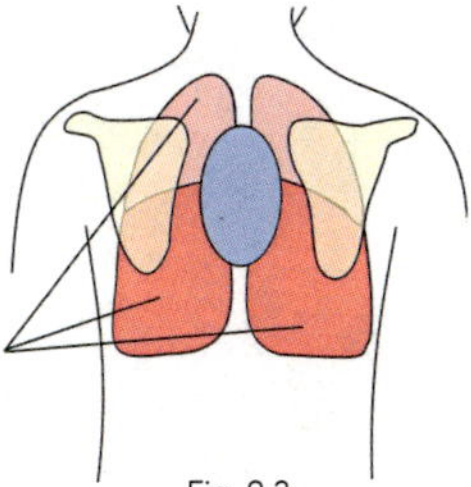
Fig. 9.2

Abnormal Breath Sounds

Decreased breath sounds	Fluid, air, or increased tissue interferes with the transfer of sound to the chest wall.
Absent breath sounds	Major or minor airway obstruction obstructs air flow.
Crackles	Occur when fluid-filled alveoli reinflate or small airways reopen, and occur only during inspiration.
Fine crackles	Crackling sound, at end-inspiration, due to inflammation or congestion of alveoli. Coughing does not clear the sound.
Medium crackles	Moist, rattling sound due to air passing through secretions in bronchioles or due to the separation of adherent bronchiolar walls.
Coarse crackles	Loud, bubbling, gurgling, due to vibration of secretions in the larger airways, occur during early inspiration, usually clear with coughing.
Rhonchi	Continuous, low-pitched, snoring sounds due to air passing through fluid-filled, narrowed airways. Occur during both inspiration and expiration.
Sibilant rhonchi	High-pitched, musical, almost squeaky.
Wheezing	Whistling sound due to air passing through airways that are narrowed or partially filled with fluid/mucus.
Friction rub	A rubbing, squeaking sound (like new leather being bent or twisted) due to inflammation of the pleural membranes.

Stethoscope placement and progression when listening to breath sounds:

Fig. 9.3

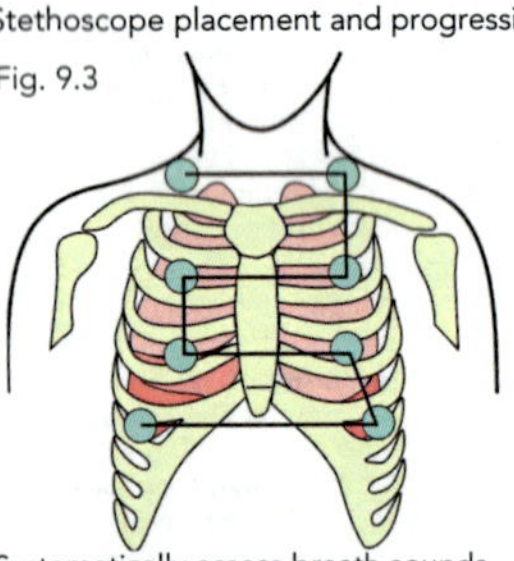

Systematically assess breath sounds, moving the stethoscope from the apex to the base of the lungs, comparing left to right. There should be vesicular breath sounds when the stethoscope is placed in the locations noted above.

Fig. 9.4

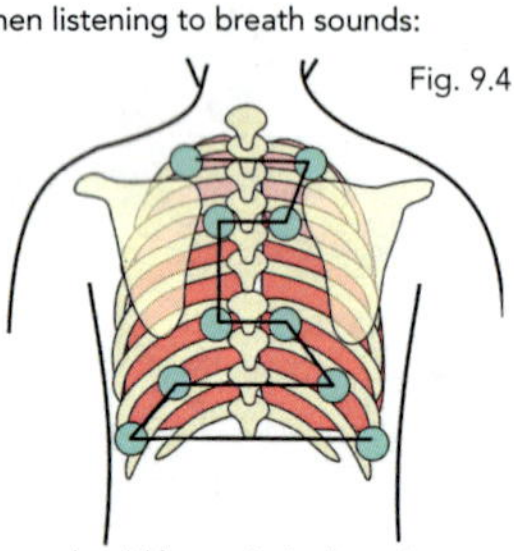

There should be vesicular breath sounds except between the scapulae, which is a location over bronchioles and alveoli, and which therefore produces the combination of bronchial and vesicular sounds .

Fig. 9.5

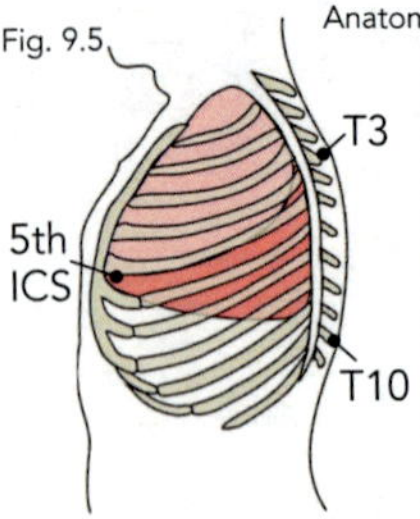

Anatomic landmarks for auscultating the lobes of the lungs

LLL:	T3 & T10 to the Left 5th ICS
RML:	Right Rib 4 to Right Rib 6 anteriorly
RLL:	T3 & T10 to the Rt anterior axillary line

Fig. 9.6

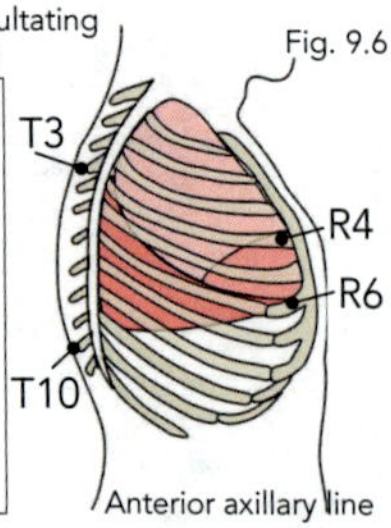

Arterial Blood Gases: Oxygenation

	Arterial		Venous	
Normal ABG's: (at sea level)	PaO_2	= 90 - 95 mm Hg	PvO_2	= 40 mm Hg
	SaO_2	= > 95 %	SvO_2	= 60 - 80 %
	pH	= 7.35 - 7.45	pH	= 7.36
	$PaCO_2$	= 35 - 45 mm Hg	$PvCO_2$	= 40 - 50 mm Hg
	HCO_3	= 22 - 26 mEq/L	HCO_3	= 22 - 26 mEq/L

PaO_2
- PAO_2 is the O_2 in Alveoli. PaO_2 is the O_2 dissolved in arterial blood.
- Normal PAO_2 (the pressure of O_2 in the Alveoli) depends on 4 factors:
  1. FiO_2
  2. Barometric Pressure
  3. $PaCO_2$
  4. Water vapor
- Considering these 4 factors, you can use the Alveolar Air Equation to determine "normal" PAO_2 where you live.

$$PAO_2 = (\text{Barometric pressure} - \text{Water Vapor pressure}) \times FiO_2 - \frac{PaCO_2}{\text{Resp quotient}}$$

PAO_2 at Sea Level
[(760 - 47) x .21] - 40/0.8
[713 x .21] - 50
100

PAO_2 in Denver CO
[(630 - 40 mm Hg) x .21] - 40/0.8
[590 x .21] - 50
74

- Sea Level: 80 - 100 mm Hg. Denver: 65 - 80 mm Hg
- Knowing the pressure of O_2 is in the Alveoli, you can now estimate the normal PaO_2 (i.e., how much O_2 made it into arterial blood):
- On room air, expect the PaO_2 to be 5 - 10 mm Hg less than the PAO_2.
- On 100 % FiO_2, expect the PaO_2 to be 50 mm Hg less than the PAO_2
- A quick way to determine what the PaO_2 should be at sea level is to use the "rule of 5." Multiply your patient's FiO_2 by 5 (this is not exact, but it will give you a general idea). For example:
  - FiO_2 x 5 = What the minimum PaO_2 should be
  - 21 % x 5 = 100 mm Hg
  - 50 % x 5 = 250 mm Hg

SaO_2
- SO_2 is the percentage of hemoglobin that is saturated with O_2.
- The degree of saturation of arterial hemoglobin (SaO_2) depends on:
  1. The PO_2 in the pulmonary capillary.
     - Low PO_2 in the lungs results in incomplete saturation of Hgb
     - Higher PO_2 in the lungs promotes complete saturation of Hgb.
  2. The affinity of hemoglobin for oxygen:
     - The affinity is ↑ by: hypothermia, alkalosis, ↓ 2,3-DPG*
     - The affinity is ↓ by: hyperthermia, acidosis, ↑ $PaCO_2$
- The oxyhemoglobin curve describes the relationship between PO_2 and SO_2. A higher PO_2 produces a higher SO_2; a lower PO_2, produces a lower SO_2. A pulse oximeter that displays SaO_2 = 90% implies the PaO_2 is at best 60 mm Hg. A venous oximeter that displays SvO_2 = 35%, implies the PvO_2 is at best 20 mm Hg (see pg. 6 of this chapter).

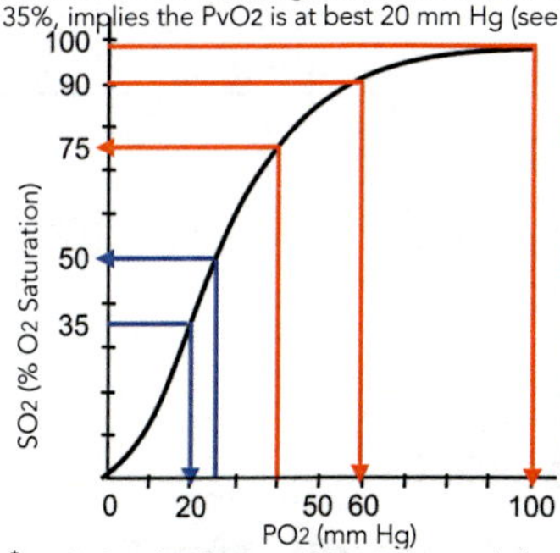

If SO_2 is	PO_2 is
99 %	100
97 %	90
95 %	80
93 %	70
90 %	60
85 %	50
75 %	40
60 %	30
50 %	26
40 %	22
35 %	20
10 %	10

*2,3-diphosphoglycerate (2,3-DPG) is made by the red blood cells; It facilitates release of oxygen by the hemoglobin.

Causes of Hypoxemia

1. **Decreased FiO_2:** High altitude, inhalation of gas absent in oxygen.
2. **Hypoventilation:** Pulmonary alveoli are inadequately ventilated. $PaCO_2$ is also increased, and is the hallmark of hypoventilation.
   Causes: Respiratory center depression
   Respiratory muscle weakness, fatigue, paralysis
   Treatment: Increase the respiratory rate and/or the volume
   Increase the FiO_2 (but this does not correct the ↑ $PaCO_2$).
3. **Diffusion Defect:** Disease or injury of the alveolar-capillary membrane which delays the diffusion of O_2 from alveolus to capillary.
   Causes: Interstitial fibrosis, Asbestosis, Sarcoidosis, Hyaline membrane, Severe emphysema, Lupus Erythematosus, Scleroderma, Carcinoma
   Treatment: Increase the FiO_2
4. **Decreased Perfusion** (↑ "Dead Space"): Anatomic dead space represents the conducting airways that do not participate in gas exchange. Normal "Dead Space Volume" is 110 - 150 mL, but can increase if the perfusion of functional alveoli is reduced or absent.

   Causes: Pulmonary embolism, Pulmonary vasoconstriction, ALI/ARDS
   Treatment: Increased FiO_2 may temporarily improve PaO_2 and SaO_2, but the low perfusion must be corrected.
5. **Shunt:** Blood flow past nonfunctional alveoli. The arterial blood will be a mixture of poorly oxygenated blood (from the areas of shunt) and normally oxygenated blood (from areas without shunt).
   Causes: The shunt may be anatomic (e.g., due to VSD), or physiologic (pneumonia, pulmonary edema, pneumothorax, ALI/ARDS)
   Treatment: Since shunted blood contacts no air, increasing the FiO_2 will have no effect on the nonventilated alveoli, but can improve the oxygenation of blood via the functioning alveoli.
6. **Ventilation-Perfusion Inequality:** The most common cause of hypoxemia is a combination of both shunting and increased dead space ventilation. A portion of the lungs is relatively underventilated, while another portion is relatively overventilated. This characterizes the normal lungs from apex to base, and in the extreme form, almost all critically ill patients who require mechanical ventilation.

Fig. 9.10

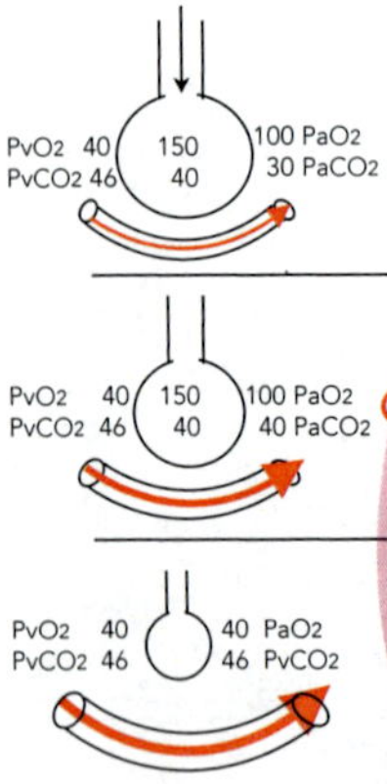

pulmonary capillary blood flow

High V/Q ratio: $\frac{\text{Ventilation}}{\text{Perfusion}} \quad \frac{0.25}{0.07} = 3.6$

Normal V/Q ratio: $\frac{\text{Ventilation}}{\text{Perfusion}} \quad \frac{0.5}{0.63} = 0.8$

Low V/Q ratio (< 0.8): $\frac{\text{Ventilation}}{\text{Perfusion}} \quad \frac{0.8}{1.3} = 0.62$

Also, shunt reduces the P/F ratio to < 300

Shunt (example) $\frac{PaO_2}{FiO_2} = \frac{60}{.50} = 120$

O_2 Delivery Devices

Nasal Cannula (NC)	Allows patient to eat, drink, talk. Works even if patient is mouth breathing. No need to add humidification if O_2 flow is < 5 LPM
Nasal Cannula Reservoir (NCR)	Stores 100% O_2 in a 20 mL reservoir, allowing higher FiO_2 at lower flow rates. The reservoir also captures exhaled water vapor, which is returned on inhalation. No need to add humidification.
Face Mask (FM)	Although the face mask allows the mixture of O_2 and room air, the mask itself serves as an O_2 reservoir, allowing an FiO_2 35 - 50% at flow rates of 5-10 LPM. O_2 flow rate must be maintained at ≥ 5 LPM to flush exhaled CO_2 from the mask. High flow rate may cause facial irritation, dry mucous membranes.
Partial Rebreather (PR)	A simple face mask with a reservoir, allowing higher FiO_2 at lower O_2 flow rates. The O_2 reservoir is used when the patient's inspiratory flow rate exceeds that of the O_2 source. The flow must be fast enough to keep the reservoir 1/3 to 1/2 full.
Non Rebreather (NR)	The patient breathes in a high concentration of O_2 from the full reservoir. A valve between the mask and reservoir bag prevents exhaled air from returning to the bag, while side vents in the mask allow exhaled CO_2 to escape.

Liters per minute (LPM) flow determines the FiO_2 delivered by each device:

O_2 Delivery Device \ LPM	1	2	3	4	5	6	8	10
NC	24%	28%	32%	35%	37%	41%	-	-
NCR	31%	35%	38%	41%	45%	48%	-	-
FM	-	-	-	-	35%	40%	45%	50%
PR	-	-	-	-	-	40%	55%	70%
NR	-	-	-	-	-	60%	80%	90%

% O_2 delivered by each device

Ventimask Any one of 6 air entrainment devices is selected to administer a precise oxygen concentration (24%, 28%, 31%, 35%, 40%, 60%) which is unaffected by O_2 flow rate, variations in breathing pattern, or mask fit. Exhalation valves prevent rebreathing of CO_2. A safety device prevents clothing or bedding from obstructing the entrainment of room air. Humidification is unnecessary.
For patients with chronic hypercarbia with moderate hypoxemia.

High-Flow/High-Humidity Nasal Cannula O_2 Therapy

Description:

- Nasal cannula system that delivers 21% - 100% oxygen, at a rate up to 60 LPM (which can match the patient's peak inspiratory flow), heated to 37° C, and with humidification that is equal to that of the airways.
- Oxygen and humidity fill the anatomic dead space, creating anatomic reservoirs of oxygen and humidity.
- Every 10 LPM delivered results in about 1 cm/H_2O of positive pressure. Much greater patient acceptance and comfort compared to oxygen masks.

Indications:

- Hypoxemia (to avoid intubation or tolerate recent extubation)
- Noninvasive treatment of mild to moderate respiratory distress
- Facilitate weaning from mechanical or non-invasive ventilation
- Maintain oxygenation immediately post extubation
- Prevention of hypoxia following surgery

Caution in those with:

Inability to follow commands
Respiratory acidosis
Medical instability
Nasal obstruction
Agitation
Swallowing impairment
Recent upper GI surgery
Recent airway surgery
Neuro surgery
Facial burns

Contra-indications

Hypercapnea
Inadequate respiratory drive
Inability to protect airway
Severe facial or head trauma
Basilar fracture of anterior cranial fossa

Oxygen Delivery

Fig. 9.8 **Normal oxygen transport to tissue:**

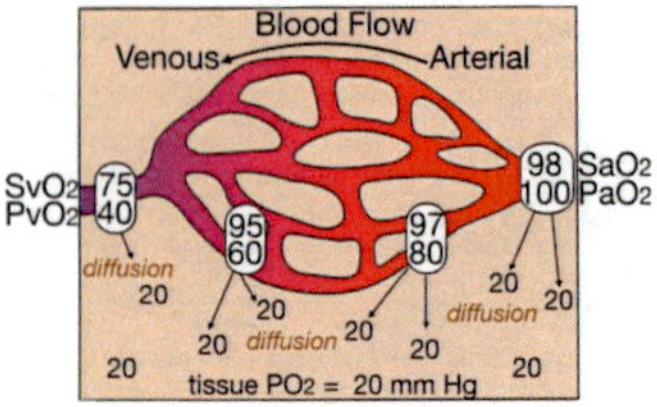

1. The PaO_2 of the arteriole is 100 mm Hg. The PO_2 of tissue is < 20 mm Hg. Diffusion gradient moves O_2 out of the capillary and into tissue.
2. As blood flows through the capillary and O_2 continues to move into tissue, capillary PO_2 falls, which prompts hemoglobin to unload (desaturate). The rate of unloading is described by the O_2/Hgb dissociation curve).

Fig. 9.9 **Inadequate oxygen transport:**

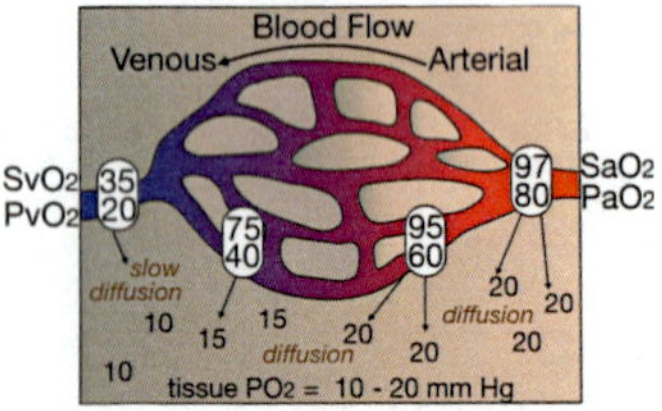

1. Starting with a lower PaO_2 narrows the diffusion gradient between blood vessel and tissue, and thus slows the diffusion of O_2.
2. When delivered O_2 is less, venous O_2 will be less.
3. When PvO_2 is < 20 mm Hg (with SvO_2 < 35%), poor diffusion gradients cannot support adequate oxygen-ation of tissue. Anaerobic metabolism begins.

In order to support the oxygenation of tissue, diffusion gradients must be maintained. This requires not only adequate amounts of dissolved oxygen, and adequate amounts of hemoglobin to carry the oxygen, but also adequate blood flow to deliver the oxygen at a sufficient rate every minute to meet the demand of the tissues. (Consider that oxygen demand can increase 4-fold over the resting state. That situation is shown on page 7, item 4.

O_2 Delivery is O_2 Content + Cardiac Output:

CaO_2	1. The oxygen content of arterial blood (CaO_2) is the amount (mL) of O_2 in each deciliter of blood. 2. Since O_2 is carried in blood in two ways: dissolved in plasma (measured as PaO_2), and attached to hemoglobin (measured as SaO_2), then 3. CaO_2 can be calculated by adding the mL of O_2 carried as SaO_2 to the mL of O_2 carried as PaO_2: CaO_2 = O_2 attached to Hgb + O_2 dissolved in plasma = (1.34 x Hgb x SaO_2) + (0.0031 x PaO_2) = (1.34 x 15 x .98) + (0.0031 x 90 mm Hg) = (19.7) + (0.3) = 20 mL O_2/dL blood 4. Of the two ways O_2 is carried in blood, the CaO_2 equation shows that most of the oxygen is carried attached to hemoglobin.
DO_2I	1. DO_2I is the amount of oxygen delivered to each square meter of tissue each minute, and is calculated as blood flow x CaO_2: DO_2I = CI x O_2 Content x 10 = CI x CaO_2 x 10 = 3 x 20 x 10 = 600 mL $O_2/min/m^2$ (this is normal DO_2I at rest) Remember that CI = CO/BSA 2. Beware that if conditions cut the patient's CI to half normal or the Hgb to half normal, DO_2I will be cut to half normal. 3. Meanwhile, many conditions increase tissue O_2 demand (see p. 8). 4. Maintaining at least a <u>minimum</u> DO_2I is critical, and what that amount must be, depends on the oxygen demands of the patient.

Oxygen Supply/Demand Balance

Fig. 9.11

"The tissues control the cardiac output according to the need for oxygen."
A. Guyton

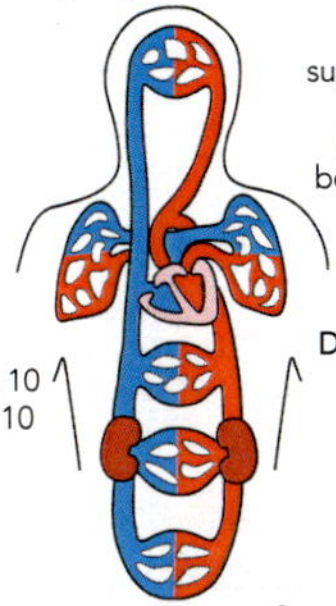

ScvO2 is sampled in the superior or inferior vena cava. SvO2 is sampled in the pulmonary artery and is the better measure of venous O2 saturation, but requires a PA catheter.

RO2I = Venous O2 Return
= CI (Venous O2 content) 10
= CI (1.34 x Hgb x SvO2) 10
= 3 (1.34 x 15 x .75) 10
= 3 (15) 10
= 450 mL O2/min/m^2

DO2I = Arterial O2 Delivery
= CI(Arterial O2 content)10
= CI (1.34 x Hgb x SaO2)10
= 3 (1.34 x 15 x .99) 10
= 3 (20) 10
= 600 mL O2/min/m^2

150 mL/min/m^2
Tissue O2 Consumption (VO2I)
(Tissue O2 Demand)

1. At rest, the cardiorespiratory system normally delivers 600 mL O2/min/m^2, the tissues consume 150 mL/min/m^2 (resting metabolic rate), and blood flow returns oxygen to the heart at the rate of 450 mL/min/m^2.
2. Because oxygen delivery is normally 4 times O2 consumption (600:150), supply/demand balance is said to be 4:1 and oxygen extraction is 25%.
3. SvO2 (mixed venous oxygen saturation) is the venous return of oxygen to the heart. The normal value of 75% (the normal range is 60 - 80%) reflects the balance of 4:1 and mirrors the tissue O2 extraction of 25%.
4. When tissue oxygen demands increase, the central nervous system normally increases oxygen delivery, maintaining the 4:1 balance and an SvO2 of 75%:

   RO2I= CI (1.34 x Hgb x SvO2) 10
   = 4 (1.34 x 15 x .75) 10
   = 600 mL/min/m^2

   DO2I= CI (1.34 x Hgb x SaO2) 10
   = 4 (1.34 x 15 x .99) 10
   = **800** mL/min/m^2

   VO2I = **200**

5. Many patients have conditions which decrease O2 delivery, such as left ventricular failure, anemia, and respiratory failure.

   RO2I = CI (1.34 x Hgb x SvO2) 10
   = 2 (1.34 x 10 x **.39**) 10
   = **105** mL/min/m^2

   DO2I= CI (1.34 x Hgb x SaO2) 10
   = 2 (1.34 x 10 x .95) 10
   = **255** mL/min/m^2

   VO2I = **150**

   In this example, assume the patient has a resting metabolic rate while DO2I falls to 255 ml/min/m^2. The SvO2 would fall to 39%.

6. If O2 delivery falls *and* tissue O2 demands increase, the fall in SvO2 can be extreme, and can be rapid if the increase in O2 demand occurs suddenly.

   RO2I = CI (1.34 x Hgb x SvO2) 10
   = 2 (1.34 x 10 x **.28**) 10
   = **75** mL/min/m^2

   DO2I= CI (1.34 x Hgb x SaO2) 10
   = 2 (1.34 x 10 x .95) 10
   = **255** mL/min/m^2

   VO2I = **180**

7. Resting metabolic rate (and thus tissue O2 demand) varies according to age:

Age	Resting VO2 (mL/min/m^2)
13 - 30	175
30 - 50	150
50 - 60	135
> 65	125

Because the elderly have a lower metabolic rate, normal oxygen delivery is proportionately lower. The normal values for age > 65 years are:

RO2I = CI (1.34 x Hgb x SvO2) 10
= 2.5 (1.34 x 15 x .75) 10
= 375 mL/min/m^2

DO2I= CI (1.34 x Hgb x SaO2)10
= 2.5 (1.34 x 15 .99) 10
= **500** mL/min/m^2

VO2I = **125**

Oxygen Supply/Demand Balance (cont'd)

Conditions which ↑ VO_2	% Increase
Fever (each 1° C)	10
Agitation	18
Fractures (each)	10
↑ work of breathing	40
Infection	50
Chest trauma	60%
Systemic Sepsis	50 - 100
Shivering	50 - 100
Seizing	100
Burns	100
Head injury, sedated	89
Head injury, unsedated	138

Conditions which ↓ VO_2	% Decrease
Hypothermia (each 1° C)	10
Morphine 0.5 mg/kg	9 - 21
Morphine 0.2-0.5 mg/kg/hr	21
Anesthesia	30
Anesthesia in burn pts	50
Assist/control	30
Propranolol in head injury	32

Neuromuscular blockade abolishes any ↑ in VO_2 caused by muscular activity.

Procedures which ↑ VO_2	% Increase
Dressing change	10 - 25
Nursing assessment	12
ECG	16
Extremity movement	18
Physican exam	20
Visitors	22
Bath	23
Chest-xray	25
ET Suctioning	27
Turn in bed	31
Chest PT	20 - 35
Weight on sling scale	35
Nasal intubation	25 - 40
Out of bed to chair	40 - 50

Medications which ↑ VO_2	Dose mcg/kg/min	% Increase
Norepinephrine	0.10 - 0.31	10 - 21
Dopamine	5	6
Dopamine	10	15
Dobutamine	10	19
Epinephrine	0.1	23 - 29

Interpretation of SvO_2

	Due to	Physiologic Cause	Example Pathologies
↓ SvO_2	↓ O_2 Delivery	↓ CI	LV dysfunction/failure Myocardial depression Positive end-expiratory pressure
		↓ SaO_2	Respiratory failure Airway obstruction, ET Suctioning Disconnect from O_2 source
		↓ Hgb	Uncompensated Anemia Acute blood loss, Hemodilution
	↑ O_2 Demand	↑ VO_2	Shivering, Hyperthermia, Pain/Agitation/Posturing Catecholamine administration ↑ Work of breathing
↑ SvO_2	↑ O_2 Delivery	↑ CI	Hyperdynamic septic shock Inotropic support/IABP Fluid volume replacement Afterload reducing agents
		↑ SaO_2	PEEP, ↑ FiO_2
		↑ Hgb	Transfusion, Hemoconcentration
	↓ O_2 Demand	↓ VO_2	Hypothermia Paralysis, Pain relief Sleep/Sedation/Anesthesia
	Other	Ventricular septal defect	Left to right cardiac shunting arterialization of venous blood
		↓ O_2 utilization by tissues	Sepsis or other causes of poorly distributed capillary blood flow. Cyanide toxicity

Prolonged supply/demand imbalance and low SvO_2 predict poor outcome.

SvO_2 value:	Significance
> 80 %	O_2 demand is low, or there is shunting of blood flow
60 - 80 %	Supply/demand balance is 4:1
50 %	Supply/demand balance is 2:1 (minimum acceptable level)
35 % or less	Anaerobic metabolism, organ dysfunction, death.

Acid-Base Imbalance

Respiratory Acidosis $\uparrow$ $PaCO_2$ $\rightarrow$ $\downarrow$ pH	Respiratory Alkalosis $\downarrow$ $PaCO_2$ $\rightarrow$ $\uparrow$ pH
CO_2 is a waste product of aerobic cellular metabolism. The CO_2 level in blood is monitored by aortic chemoreceptors, which signal the brain to increase or decrease ventilatory rate and depth (minute ventilation) according to blood pH. Hypoventilation retains CO_2 in blood, where it combines with water to form carbonic acid: $CO_2 + H_2O \rightarrow H_2CO_3$	Hyperventilation expels CO_2, causing CO_2 in blood to fall. Less carbonic acid results in a rising pH. Beware that low $PaCO_2$ causes cerebral vasoconstriction, which can threaten those patients who have cerebral pathology.
Every 10 mm Hg $\uparrow$ in $PaCO_2$ causes the pH to $\downarrow$ by 0.08 $PaCO_2$ pH 40 $\rightarrow$ 7.40 50 $\rightarrow$ 7.32 60 $\rightarrow$ 7.24 70 $\rightarrow$ 7.16	Every 10 mm Hg $\downarrow$ in $PaCO_2$ causes the pH to $\uparrow$ by 0.08 $PaCO_2$ pH 40 $\rightarrow$ 7.40 35 $\rightarrow$ 7.44 30 $\rightarrow$ 7.28 25 $\rightarrow$ 7.52
Causes include: Hypoventilation due to any cause (coma, narcotic effect. Airway obstruction due to asthma. Alveolar dysfunction such as atelectasis, pulmonary edema, fibrosis., Compensatory effort to decrease the pH in the setting of metabolic alkalosis.	Causes include: Hyperventilation due to any cause. Mechanical ventilation, during which the respiratory rate, tidal volume, and PEEP increase minute volume. Compensatory effort to increase the pH when the pH is decreased by metabolic acidosis (e.g., Kussmaul respiration seen in ketoacidosis.

Metabolic Acidosis $\downarrow$ HCO_3 $\rightarrow$ $\downarrow$ pH	Metabolic Alkalosis $\uparrow$ HCO_3 $\rightarrow$ $\uparrow$ pH
HCO_3 is a base that is regulated by the kidneys and used to buffer metabolic acids (eg. HCl or lactic acid). When HCO_3 combines with H+ ions in the buffering process, HCO_3 level falls. Beware that metabolic acidosis triggers hyperventilation in the effort to correct the pH.	Excess of HCO_3 alkalinizes the blood Beware that metabolic alkalosis triggers hypoventilation, in order to raise the PCO_2 and thus bring down the pH.
Every 10 mm Hg $\downarrow$ in HCO_3 causes the pH to $\downarrow$ by 0.15 HCO_3 pH 24 $\rightarrow$ 7.40 19 $\rightarrow$ 7.325 14 $\rightarrow$ 7.25	Every 10 mm Hg $\uparrow$ in HCO_3 causes the pH to $\uparrow$ by 0.15 HCO_3 pH 24 $\rightarrow$ 7.40 34 $\rightarrow$ 7.55 44 $\rightarrow$ 7.70
Causes include: Consumption of HCO_3 by excess acid. Excess loss of HCO_3 from the GI tract. Hypokalemia. Hyperchloremia. Renal failure, which impairs the ability of the kidneys to regulate HCO_3. Compensatory effort to decrease the pH when pH is increased by a low PCO_2.	Causes include: Loss of normal body acid (eg., loss of HCl via vomiting or NG suctioning). Excess administration of $NaHCO_3$. Hypokalemia, Hypochloremia. Compensatory effort to increase the pH when the pH is decreased by a rising PCO_2.

On the next page, see how the body compensates for any 1 of the 4 acid-base imbalances shown on this page.

Acid-Base Imbalance with Compensation

Respiratory Acidosis (↑ $PaCO_2$ → ↓ pH) is compensated by Metabolic Alkalosis (↑ HCO_3 → ↑ pH)	Respiratory (↓ $PaCO_2$ → ↑ pH) is compensated by Metabolic Acidosis ↓ HCO_3 → ↓ pH)
Hypoventilation results in ↑ $PaCO_2$ (more carbonic acid in blood), which leads to ↓ pH): pH = 7.24 $PaCO_2$ = 60 HCO_3 = 24 The pH can be improved if the kidneys **conserve** HCO_3: Metabolic alkalosis compensates for Respiratory acidosis: pH = 7.39 $PaCO_2$ = 60 HCO_3 = 34 The $PaCO_2$ is the same, but the rise in HCO_3 brought the pH of 7.24 up to a more tolerable level of 7.39	Hyperventilation results in ↓ $PaCO_2$ (less carbonic acid in blood), which leads to ↑ pH) pH = 7.56 $PaCO_2$ = 20 HCO_3 = 24 The pH can be improved if the kidneys **remove** some HCO_3: Metabolic acidosis compensates for Respiratory alkalosis: pH = 7.41 $PaCO_2$ = 20 HCO_3 = 14 The $PaCO_2$ is the same, but the fall in HCO_3 brought the pH of 7.56 down to a more tolerable level of 7.41

Metabolic Acidosis (↓ HCO_3 → ↓ pH) is compensated by Respiratory Alkalosis (↓ $PaCO_2$ → ↑ pH)	Metabolic (↑ HCO_3 → ↑ pH) is compensated by Respiratory Acidosis (↑ $PaCO_2$ → ↓ pH)
Metabolically produced acids consume HCO_3, leading to ↓ pH) pH = 7.25 $PaCO_2$ = 40 HCO_3 = 14 The pH can be improved if the lungs **decrease** CO_2 (by hyperventilation) thus decreasing the level of carbonic acid: Metabolic acidosis compensated by Respiratory alkalosis: pH = 7.37 $PaCO_2$ = 25 HCO_3 = 14 The HCO_3 is the same, but the fall in $PaCO_2$ (by means of hyperventilation) decreased the $PaCO_2$, which brought the pH of 7.25 up to a more tolerable level of 7.37	Metabolically retained HCO_3 or excessive administration of HCO_3, leads to ↑ pH. pH = 7.55 $PaCO_2$ = 40 HCO_3 = 34 The pH can be improved if the lungs **retain** some CO_2 (by hypoventilation), thus increasing the amount of carbonic acid: Metabolic alkalosis compensated by Respiratory acidosis: pH = 7.43 $PaCO_2$ = 55 HCO_3 = 34 The HCO_3 is the same, but the rise in $PaCO_2$ (by means of hypoventilation) increased the $PaCO_2$, which brought the pH down to a more tolerable level of 7.43

The Endotracheal Tube

Cuff Pressure: Ischemia vs Aspiration

- Inflation of high volume/low pressure (HVLP) cuff does not protect the airway from aspiration.
- Inspiratory effort increases laryngeal diameter.
- Folds in the ETT cuff , as well as underinflation permit aspiration.
- Changes in body and head position alter cuff pressure.
- Changes in lung compliance and intrathoracic pressure alter cuff pressure.
- 5 cm PEEP may delay the leakage, but the lower airway is eventually contaminated with oral secretions within 24 hours of intubation.
- Ideal ETT cuff pressure is 20 - 30 cm H_2O
- During mechanical ventilation, periodic measurement of cuff pressure during the inspiratory phase is recommended.

  Cuff pressure that is:
  1. < 20 cm H_2O (15 mm Hg) is associated with an increased risk of aspiration and a 2.5-fold increase in VAP.
  2. > 30 cm H_2O (22 mm Hg) or > 34 cm H_2O in hypertensive patients, impedes capillary blood flow, causing damage of the tracheal wall mucosa.
  3. > 50 cm H_2O results in total obstruction of capillary blood flow at the cuff.

Fig. 9.13

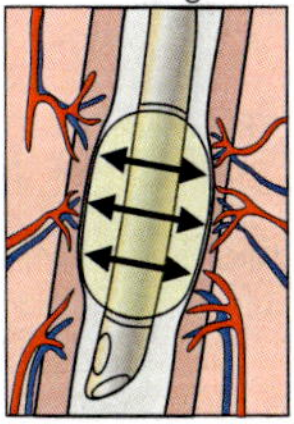

- Oral care and frequent suctioning of the oropharynx is recommended to reduce the incidence of VAP.
- Continuous aspiration of subglottic secretions (CASS) may reduce the incidence of VAP.

Instillation of Normal Saline into the ETT prior to suctioning:

- Normal saline does not thin or mobilize secretions. ET suctioning after NS instillation recovers only 18.7% of the amount instilled.
- Up to 5 times as many colonies are dislodged from the ETT when normal saline is instilled, contributing significantly to lower airway contamination.
- But NS instillation is associated with decreased oxygenation, doubled recovery time, and patient anxiety, fear, and dread.
- Causes coughing which may increase intracranial pressure, increase bleeding, or increase tissue oxygen demands.
- Causes tachycardia, which may increase myocardial oxygen demand or adversely affect cardiac output.
- Normal saline instillation may be useful when it is necessary to elicit a cough, or for clearing the catheter after suctioning.

Unplanned extubation:

- Incidence is 3 - 14%
- Most have low level of sedation (Ramsay score 2.42) prior to self extubation.
- Most (> 75%) are restrained. Physical restraints increase the risk 3-fold.
- 89% occur when the nurse is away from bedside
- Proper pain management is important to preventing self extubation.

Strong predictors of extubation failure: ineffective cough, prior history of mechanical ventilation lasting > 7 days, severe LV dysfunction. (Thille AW, Boissier F, Ghezala HB, et al. Risk factors for and prediction by caregivers of extubation failure in ICU patients. CCM, 2015;43(3):613-620.)

Criteria for Reintubation:

1. Respiratory or cardiac arrest
2. Neurologic deterioration
3. Hemodynamic instability
4. Upper airway obstruction with stridor
5. Unmanageable tracheobronchial secretions
6. Respiratory distress, (SpO_2 < 90%, respiratory rate > 35/min., use of accessory respiratory muscles, or presence of thoracoabdominal paradox).

> 100% high-flow O_2 by nasal cannula offers an O_2-enriched environment that moderates hypoxemia during intubation.

Complications of Reintubation:

Upper airway trauma, hypotension, hypertension, new arrhythmia, bradycardia, cardiac arrest, death.

Mechanical Ventilation: Start-Up

Indications for Intubation and Mechanical Ventilation: when spontaneous ventilation is inadequate to sustain the patient.

Signs/Symptoms	Causes
Hypercapnea (↑ $PaCO_2$) $PaCO_2$ > 50 mm Hg and pH < 7.5	Reduced respiratory rate and/or depth Respiratory muscle fatigue Respiratory depression Chest wall injury or abnormality Closure of small airways
Hypoxemia (↓ PaO_2) PaO_2 < 55 mm Hg despite supplemental O_2 A-a DO_2 is on 100% O_2 is > 450	Alveolar/capillary injury Intrapulmonary shunt Ventilation-perfusion mismatch Decreased Functional Residual Capacity
Work of Breathing has become intolerable/ineffective. The patient is exhausted.	Tachypnea (respiratory rate > 30 bpm) Vital Capacity is < 15 mL/kg Minute ventilation is > 10 L/min PaO_2 < 85 mm Hg despite supplemental O_2

Initial Ventilator Settings:

1 Rate:	10 - 12/min		
FiO_2	100 %		
Tidal Volume*	Normal:	10 - 12 mL/kg	
	COPD:	10 mL/kg	
	ALI:	6 - 8 mL/kg	
PEEP:	Shunt > 25%	5 cm H_2O	

* Remember that normal TV in spontaneous breathing is 5 - 8 mL/kg.

2 Evaluate the P/F ratio:

If P/F ratio is > 200:	If the patient's oxygenation is good enough to permit a reduction in the FiO_2, the P/F ratio (PaO_2/FiO_2) can be used to identify what FiO_2 would be best. For example, If the patient's PaO_2 is 225 mm Hg while on 100% O_2, (P/F ratio is 225/1), what FiO_2 would it take to achieve a PaO_2 of 100 mm Hg? Answer: 44% $\frac{PaO_2}{FiO_2}$ $\frac{225}{1} = \frac{100}{x}$ $225x = 100$ $x = 0.44$ Reduce FiO_2 by 10 percentage points every 5-10 min. Goal: PaO_2 60 - 100 mm Hg with FiO_2 50%.
If P/F ratio is < 200:	Peep ≥ 5 cm and advanced modes of ventilation are required.

3. Support O_2 Supply/Demand Balance:
   Support/optimize cardiac output.
   Correct anemia, particularly in those with marginal or low cardiac output.
   Reduce tissue oxygen demands (sedate, paralyze, pain control).

Care "Bundle" is started soon after mechanical ventilation is started.	Hazards of Intubation and Mechanical Ventilation include:
• HOB elevation to 30 - 40° • Mouth/ETT care with chlorhexidine • Lung protective ventilator strategies • A plan to discontinue mechanical ventilation ASAP • Appropriate analgesia and sedation • Daily interruption of sedation • Early mobilization • DVT prophylaxis • GI stress prophylaxis • Balanced IV fluid administration	• Ventilator associated lung injury • Ventilator associated pneumonia • Accidental extubation or disconnect • Patient anxiety/panic • O_2 supply/demand imbalance • Inadequate ventilation, culminating in respiratory acidosis • Excessive ventilation, culminating in respiratory alkalosis • Ventilator dependence

Raoof S. Baumann MH. Ventilator associated events: the new definition. AJCC, 2014;23(1):7-9.

Modes of Ventilation

	ACV Assist Control Ventilation	APRV Airway Pressure Release Ventilation
Description	Simple and most effective way to provide mechanical ventilation. If inspiratory effort exceeds the set sensitivity, the ventilator delivers a fixed tidal volume. If inspiratory effort is weak, the ventilator delivers a minimum number of breaths.	An expiratory valve allows the patient to breathe spontaneously during the prolonged periods of elevated airway pressure.
Indications	Patients with normal respiratory drive but weak respiratory muscles. Patients who need ventilatory support, not control. Patients emerging from anesthesia. Most commonly used initial mode.	For patients with severely decreased compliance (ARDS), or unresponsive to PEEP that is > 15 cm H_2O. To reduce pulmonary shunt without barotrauma.
Advantages	Augments breathing without completely controlling it. Less fighting with the ventilator. Does not result in respiratory muscle atrophy like CMV does. Lets patient change respiratory rate when CO_2 levels change.	Reduces work of breathing and oxygen cost of breathing while offering the lung-protective effects of IRV (Inverse Ratio Ventilation). Less cardiac compromise. Need for vasopressors is less.
Disadvantages	Can cause anxiety and increased work of breathing if sensitivity to the pt's inspiratory effort is too low. Can lead to hyper-ventilation. Can decrease the cardiac output, since every breath is a positive pressure breath.	Can't use in patients with increased airway resistance (asthma, COPD). Gas trapping can result from the very short periods of exhalation. No studies have shown improved outcome with APRV or IRV.

	BiPAP BiLevel Positive Airway Pressure	CPAP Continuous Positive Airway Pressure
Description	Is CPAP with 2 preset pressures: 1. positive pressure on inspiration 2. positive pressure on expiration. Must be able to breathe spontaneously and maintain airway. Requires face or nasal mask.	Constant positive pressure is applied throughout respiratory cycle to support oxygenation and reduce work of breathing. The patient initiates all breaths.
Indications	Obstructive sleep apnea, cardiogenic pulmonary edema (must be hemodynamically stable), weaning from mechanical ventilation, terminally ill respiratory failure, spinal cord injury, hypercapnic hypoxemic failure.	To wean without removing the ventilator and having to connect to additional equipment. Treatment for Auto-PEEP. Also used for spinal cord injury patients and for sleep apnea.
Advantages	Noninvasive (employs face or nasal mask). Increases FRC by recruiting collapsed alveoli. May be able to avoid ET intubation and mechanical ventilation in some patients, reducing length of stay.	Offers patient the psychological security of the ventilator being there. Can be delivered by tight face mask or artificial airway. Takes advantage of the ventilator alarm systems.
Disadvantages	Mask must fit well. Slight leaks result in blast of gas into eyes and loss of therapeutic effect. Mask may cause anxiety or agitation. Cannot use if patient very agitated or cannot protect his airway.	Not all ventilators are equipped with CPAP. Patient may sense resistance when breathing through ventilator tubing.

(more modes of ventilation) →

Modes of Ventilation

	CMV Continuous Mandatory, or Control Mode Ventilation	IMV Intermittent Mandatory Ventilation
Description	Delivers a set tidal volume at a set rate regardless of patient's attempt to breathe on his/her own. Patient must be sedated, paralyzed, and receiving anxiolytics.	Delivers a set tidal volume at a set rate, while also allowing the patient to initiate an independent breath from a reservoir of humidified oxygen. Ventilator rate is set at lowest level that will maintain ABG's. The set tidal volume is delivered regardless of the pt's efforts and position in the respiratory cycle.
Indications	Apnea due to CNS or neuromuscular dysfunction (e.g., head injury, Guillain-Barre Syndrome, drug OD, or anesthesia. To reduce paradoxical chest wall motion of Flail Chest.	Patients who temporarily need positive pressure ventilatory support but are expected to return to spontaneous unassisted ventilation soon. Commonly used during weaning.
Advantages	If the patient is apneic, the ventilator does all of the work of breathing.	Allows patient to do some of the work of breathing. Having some control helps reduce anxiety. Fewer ventilator breaths mean lower intrathoracic pressure and less risk for barotrauma and ↓ CO. Lessens the need for sedation paralysis. Produces lower mean airway pressures.
Disadvantages	Since the patient cannot initiate a breath, anxiety and fighting against the ventilator may result. If $PaCO_2$ increases, the patient cannot increase ventilatory rate. If airflow obstruction and ventilator does not allow sufficient expiratory time, hyperinflation → ↑ CO_2. Carries risk of causing barotrauma. Respiratory muscles may atrophy. Accidental disconnect is life threatening.	Must set peak inspiratory pressure limit to < 10 cm above the patient's peak inspiratory pressure, to prevent "stacked breaths" (ventilator breath delivered on top of a patient breath), which increases risk for barotrauma. Danger if rate is set low and patient's own respiratory rate slows or stops. (more modes of ventilation) →

What is Auto-PEEP?	
Description	Auto-PEEP is gas trapped in the alveoli at end expiration.
Causes	Inadequate expiratory time Mucus plugging Bronchoconstriction
Consequences	Increased work of breathing Use of inspiratory reserve muscles, which significantly increases work of breathing
Remedy	CPAP, at a level higher than the auto-PEEP, given via mask or endotracheal tube, "splints" the airways open. The amount of CPAP must exceed the amount of auto-PEEP. Patient may sense resistance to breathing.

Modes of Ventilation

	IRV Inverse Ratio Ventilation	PEEP Positive End-Expiratory Pressure
Description	Controlled positive pressure ventilation that reverses the normal Inspiratory/Expiratory (I:E) ratio of 1:2, by ↑ inspiratory time and ↓ expiratory time, to as much as 4:1.	Maintains a preset positive airway pressure during the expiratory phase. Best PEEP: 1. ↑ PaO_2 so that FiO_2 may be ↓ 2. Does not reduce cardiac output 3. Minimizes pulmonary shunt 4. Decreases airway resistance
Indications	Severely decreased compliance (ARDS), or fails to respond to Peep that is > 15 cm H_2O. To reduce pulmonary shunt without barotrauma.	To treat PaO_2 < 60 mm Hg when FiO_2 is > 50 mm Hg, by recruiting dysfunctional alveol. Also used to increase intrapulmonary pressure to decrease intrathoracic bleeding after cardiac surgery.
Advantages	Recruits collapsed alveoli, allows more time for gas exchange so that gas may move from fast-filling to slow-filing alveoli. Short expiratory time induces intrinsic (auto) PEEP	Improves PaO_2 and SaO_2, while allowing FiO_2 to be decreased. Keeps airways and alveoli from closing at end-expiration, especially in patients with surfactant deficiency. Decreases work of breathing, helps preserve functional residual capacity.
Disadvantages	At ratio 4:1, can decrease cardiac output, especially if patient is hypovolemic. Gas trapping may cause pneumothorax (risk increases with the length of time on IRV). Uncomfortable mode for the patient. Sedatives and NMBA's required.	Increases FRC, increasing the risk for barotrauma. Contraindicated in patients with hypovolemia, drug induced decrease in cardiac output, unilateral lung disease, COPD. May increase ICP; must insure CO_2 is maintained at 30 - 35 mm Hg. Can cause increased dead space.

	SIMV Synchronized Intermittent Mandatory Ventilation	TGI Tracheal Gas Insufflation
Description	Incorporates a demand valve that must be patient activated. A set tidal volume delivered at a set rate is synchronized to occur when triggered by the patient's inspiration. If the ventilator does not sense spontaneous breathing, it will give a breath according to the preset rate. If spontaneous breaths occur faster	An adjunct to mechanical ventilation. Through a small catheter or through channels in the wall of an endo-tracheal tube, stream of fresh gas (4-8 L/min) is directed into the lower trachea, flushing the CO_2-laden gas out of the lower airways prior to the next inspiration.
Indicate	Same as IMV	Patients with increased dead-space, hypercapnea, or acidosis.
Advant:	Same as IMV	Can control $PaCO_2$ while still taking advantage of lower tidal volume
Disadvantages	If there is lag between the patient's inspiratory effort and when the ventilator gives the breath, SIMV can increase anxiety, work of breathing. If the rate is set too slow, may lead to dyspnea, increased work of breathing. Danger if rate is set low and pt's own respiratory rate slows or stops.	Desiccation of secretions. Airway mucosa injury. Accumulation of secretions. Development of auto-PEEP.

Modes of Ventilation

	NPPV Noninvasive Positive Pressure Ventilation	PAV Proportional Assist Ventilation
Description	As an alternative to endotracheal intubation, NPPV is the delivery of positive pressure breathing utilizing a tight-fitting mask. Works well with Proportional Assist Ventilation.	Promotes pt/ventilator synchrony, by providing inspiratory flow and pressure in proportion to pt's effort. Allows the patient to attain his/her ventilation and breathing pattern. Available on selected ventilators.
Indications	Provide ventilatory assistance minus the problems of an artificial airway, particularly in those with COPD, acute cardiogenic pulmonary edema, or immunocompromise. May be used during bronchoscopy or to oxygenate critically ill patients prior to intubation. But NPPV in the treatment of ARDS/ALI or pneumonia report failure rates up to 50%.	To facilitate weaning from mechanical ventilation. To increase comfort and tolerance in patients with chronic respiratory failure due to COPD.
Advantages	Avoids the complications of the artificial airway and invasive mechanical ventilation. Decreases the incidence of ventilator associated pneumonia. Less ventilatory assistance required compared to pts who are intubated.	Some studies showed that, PAV compared to pressure support, reduces the work of breathing. The constant computer interaction with the patient's changing breathing pattern automates pt. assessment and ventilator adjustment.
Disadvantages	Contraindicated in uncooperative, agitated, delirious, or obtunded pts, and in those unable to protect the airway or have copious secretions. Danger of vomiting -> aspiration. Leaks from the face mask prevent adequate ventilatory assist. Failure rate is high in those who have respiratory failure with hemodynamic compromise. Increased commitment and time by nurses and RT's.	Some studies showed that PAV, compared to pressure support, reduces the work of breathing. The constant computer interaction with the patient's changing breathing pattern automates patient assessment and ventilator adjustment.

	PSV Pressure Support Ventilation
Description	For pts with spontaneous breathing. When patient initiates a breath, ventilator does not deliver a set volume, but rather a preset positive pressure for the duration of inspiration. The patient determines inspiratory flow rate, time, and respiratory rate. Helps overcome the airway resistance of the ET tube.
Indications	Patients on long-term mechanical ventilation. Often used with IMV/SIMV. May reduce work of spontaneous breathing. Useful method to wean.
Advantages	Increases spontaneous tidal volume and reduces work of breathing while maintaining respiratory muscle tone. The patient determines inspiratory time, respiratory rate, and minute volume, improving patient-ventilator synchrony. PSV limits the distending pressure of the lung. This mode can theoretically benefit patients with acute lung injury.
Disadvant.	Tidal volume varies depending on the resistance and elasticity of the respiratory system. Danger if patient's respiratory rate slows or stops. PSV is therefore often used with IMV or SIMV. Can be used with PEEP or CPAP but increases risk for ↓ CO and for barotrauma.

Acute Respiratory Distress Syndrome

"The Berlin Definition" of ARDS:
Compared to the definition from the AECC (American European Consensus Conference definition, 1994), the Berlin Definition (2012) offers a more current definition of ARDS and better predicts mortality rate:

1. Hypoxemia:
   - mild ARDS: PaO_2/FIO_2 = 200 to ≤ 300 mm Hg
   - moderate ARDS: PaO_2/FIO_2 = 101 to ≤ 200 mm Hg
   - severe ARDS: PaO_2/FIO_2 ≤ 100 mm Hg.
2. Progressive x-ray severity (pulmonary infiltrates often peak within 3 days)
3. Decreased respiratory system compliance (≤ 40 mL/cm H_2O).
4. High levels of positive end-expiratory pressure are required (≥ 10 cm H_2O).
5. Corrected expired volume per minute (≥ 10 L/min).

Ferguson ND, et al. ARDS The Berlin Definition. JAMA,2012;307(23):2526-2533.

Description:

- Development of acute dyspnea and hypoxemia, usually within 12 - 48 hrs of an inciting event, affecting the integrity of both alveolus and pulmonary capillary endothelium. The alveoli are unable to remain dry, the interstitium becomes too wet, and the lungs become stiff.
- The result is life-threatening interruption in adequate gas exchange, and lungs that become difficult to oxygenate and ventilate.
- 40% of patients with ARDS die, mostly due to multiple organ failure.
- Those who live develop fibrosing alveolitis and must also overcome extensive muscle wasting. Fortunately, changes in treatment have improved outcome.

Causes:

- Direct lung injury: pneumonia, aspiration, inhalation injury, pulmonary contusion, near drowning, fat embolism, reperfusion injury.
- Indirect lung injury: sepsis, shock, acute pancreatitis, multiple transfusion, burns, cardiopulmonary bypass.

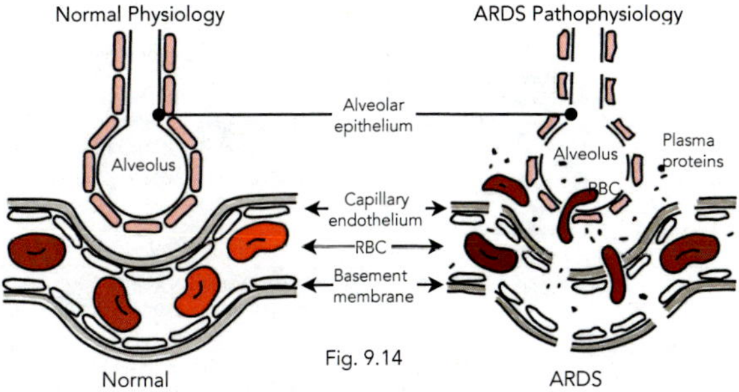

Fig. 9.14

Alveolus Injury	Influx of protein-rich fluid into the alveolar space. Injury to type II cells, causing less surfactant production, decreased alveolar compliance, alveolar collapse, and pulmonary shunting. Noncompliant lungs increase the work of breathing, causing the muscles of respiration to demand as much as 50% more oxygen. Fibrin deposits in the interstitium further restrict alveolar ventilation. Unaffected alveoli are overdistended by positive pressure breathing, raising the risk for pneumothorax.
Pulmonary Capillary Injury	Pulmonary capillary leak allows plasma into the interstitium, increasing the diffusion distance between capillary and alveolus, further impairing gas exchange. Lymphatic outflow is overwhelmed. Aggregated platelets, agglutinated WBC's, vasoconstrictive chemical mediators, and hypoxemia lead to impaired pulmonary blood flow, increased pulmonary vascular resistance, pulmonary hypertension.

Acute Respiratory Distress Syndrome (cont'd)

Stage	Time frame	Physiologic Phases	The Physiologic Result
1	1 - 7 days	Exudative Phase	Interstitial and alveolar edema, atelectasis, intrapulmonary shunting, hypoxemia, stiff lungs, hypoxemia
2	1 - 2 weeks	Reparative or Proliferative Phase	Lungs are dense and fibrous. The patient will repair/recover or succumb to proliferative disease.
3	2 - 3 weeks	Fibrotic or Chronic Phase	Alveolar walls are thickened by connective tissue.

The inciting event is most often Sepsis.

Tidal Volume:	Mortality rate
6 mL/kg IBW:	34%
12 mL/kg IBW:	42%

Treatment of ARDS:

ARDSnet Protocol

- Volume assist-control mode
- Initial TV of **6 - 8** mL/kg IBW (reduce to 4 mL/kg if possible).
- Inspiratory plateau pressure should be limited to ≤ 30 cm H_2O (higher levels significantly elevate the risk for alveolar over-distension and "alveolar volutrauma").
- Ventilator rate may be set up to **35** bpm, to keep pH 7.3 - 7.45
- PEEP set to at least 5 cm H_2O and FiO_2 set to keep PaO_2 55 - 85 mm Hg or SaO_2 88 - 95%. Titrate FiO_2 to < 70% if feasible.
- Over < 4 hrs, reduce tidal volumes to 7 mL/kg, then 6 mL/kg.
- If inspiratory plateau pressures remain high, may reduce TV in 1 mL/kg increments, to as low as 4 mL/kg.
- Consider other causes of noncompliant lungs (pleural effusion, pneumothorax), or noncompliant chest wall (burns, obesity).

PCV?

If high inspiratory pressures produce low tidal volume, then pressure-controlled ventilation (PCV) should be considered.

Fluids and Blood:

- A conservative approach works best.
- Some recommend monitoring urinary output and giving diuretics to maintain negative fluid balance.
- Central venous O_2 monitoring is helpful in titrating fluids, but using CVP or PA catheters do not influence patient outcome.
- Hgb ≤ 8 g/dL may require erythropoetin or blood transfusion.

NMBA and/or Sedative:

Early administration of cisatracurium with sedative may offer survival benefit to patients with severe ARDS.
During the stage when lung compliance is low and ventilator pressures are hight, heavy sedation may be needed.

Edema:

- Albumin may be used to mobilize interstitial edema.
- Studies are underway to determine if β_2-agonists (Dopamine, Dobutamine) can enhance alveolar fluid clearance.

Prevent other insults:

- Incidence of VAP in ARDS patients may be as high as 55%.
- Follow CDC guidelines (see the last topic in this chapter).
- Reduce risk of VAP by using an in-line suction catheter system.
- H_2 antagonist may be given to reduce gastric acid production.

Steroid?

Methylprednisolone given 7 days after ARDS onset did not improve mortality; given after 14 days, mortality increased.

Prone:

In patients with P/F ratio < 150 - 200 mm Hg, prone positioning for ≥ 10 hrs significantly reduces mortality. Does require a coordinated team effort. Lee JM et al. CCM, 2014;42:1252-1262.

Nutrition:

- Nutritional support, preferably given enterally, should be started after 48 - 72 hours of mechanical ventilation.
- Carbohydrate is restricted in order to control the production of CO_2 while a high-fat/high-protein formula supports the structure and function of respiratory muscles.
- Including anti-inflammatory and vasodilating elements such as omega-3 and omega-6 fatty acids along with antioxidants improved outcome in some studies of ARDS patients.

Preventing Ventilator Associated Events

Definition:	VAE (Ventilator Associated Event) is anything that results in a significant and sustained deterioration in oxygenation, defined as 1. > 20% daily increase in the FiO_2 to maintain oxygenation, or 2. An increase of at least 3 cm H_2O in the daily minimum PEEP needed to maintain oxygenation
3 New expressions:	1. VAC: Ventilator-associated condition: the patient develops hypoxemia for a sustained period of more than 2 days. 2. IVAC: Infection-related Ventilator-Associated Complication, described as hypoxemia that develops in the setting of generalized infection or inflammation, and antibiotics are instituted for a minimum of 4 days 3. VAP: Ventilator-Associated Pneumonia - in patients with IVAC, white blood cells are present in respiratory secretion, or respiratory pathogens are present on culture,.
Disturbing Facts just on VAP:	Studies have shown that without aggressive, preventative measures, Ventilator Association Pneumonia (VAP): • may be present (on average) in 25% of patients by day 4 of mechanical ventilation • may Increase length of hospital stay by 5 - 7 days. • may be associated with a mortality rate of 25- 45%. • treatment cost may average $50,000 per episode: VAP prevention program can cut the incidence of VAP in half.
Risk factors for VAP:	Endotracheal tube in place for 48 hours Reduced level of consciousness ARDS, COPD, Immunosuppression Reintubation (increases the likelihood of VAP 6-fold) Gastric tube (increases risk for gastric reflux and aspiration)

Regarding the Artificial Airway:

- Avoid endotracheal intubation whenever possible by trying noninvasive ventilation with face or nose mask.
- Perform oral care (chlorhexidine oral wash) at the time of intubation (see procedure "Oral Hygiene" on next page).
- Orotracheal rather than nasotracheal approach to intubation is preferred.
- Nasotracheal intubation carries higher risk for colonization of the lungs than does orotracheal intubation.
- Some use ET tubes that provide subglottic aspiration port, which was found to reduce incidence of VAP by 45 - 50%. Secretions that pool above the cuff create biofilm. Within 12 hours, biofilm harbors large amounts of bacteria. 100 - 150 mL can accumulate in the posterior oropharynx in 24 hrs.
- Maintain minimum cuff pressure of 20 cm H_2O (but don't count on the cuff to protect the patient from aspiration).
- Authorities recommend against saline lavage of the ETT, it does not thin or help mobilize secretions, and has been shown to disseminate bacteria.
- Some are employing silver nitrate coated endotracheal tubes.
- Prevent accidental extubation. Repeat intubation carries high risk.
- Suction oropharynx prior to extubation.
- When replacing tracheostomy tube, replace with one that has been sterilized or treated with high-level disinfection.
- Sterilize resuscitation bags between patients.

And the Ventilator:

- Maintain closed circuitry, including in-line suction catheter and nebulizer.
- No routine tubing change (no more often than q 48 hrs).
- Use sterile fluid for nebulized medications, handle aseptically.
- Periodically drain and discard condensate in the tubing.
- When lowering HOB, drain condensate to prevent movement of condensate toward the patient.
- Wean and extubate ASAP. VAP rate increases with duration of intubation.
- Weaning procedures can also increase aspiration risk.

Preventing Ventilator Associated Events

Body Position:

- Supine position during the first 24 hours of mechanical ventilation is a major risk factor for the development of VAP.
- ICU mortality is greater for patients kept flat supine (30%) than for those kept semi-recumbent (30% vs. 9% mortality).
- Elevate head of bed 30°- 45°. HOB elevation of 30° can decrease incidence of VAP by 34%.
- High risk patients should be turned every 2 hr.
- Prone positioning (10 - 18 hours!) for pts with acute hypoxemic respiratory failure resulted in a significant reduction in mortality

Oral Hygiene:

- This may be the single most important measure for the prevention of VAP.
- Pathogenic bacteria in dental plaque provide the nidus of infection. Micro-aspiration occurs in 20 - 40% of intubated pts.
- In 76% of patients, the bacteria colonizing the mouth and the lungs are the same.
- At the University of Michigan Hospital and Medical Center, efforts to reduce incidence of VAP failed until the following protocol was implemented:
  Every 2 hours provide mouth hydration and suction mouth and oropharynx. Then twice/day:
  1. Use toothpaste and soft toothbrush to cleanse teeth, gums, tongue. Rinse and suction.
  2. Rigorously apply Chlorhexidine 15 mL to the buccal, pharyngeal, gingival, tongue and tooth surfaces for 30 seconds. Suction excess.
  3. Apply mouth moisturizer.

Gastric Tube and feeding:

Insert gastric tubes orally, rather than nasally.
Start enteral feeding the first day of mechanical ventilation.
Start at 20 mL/hr, progress to 60 mL/hr.
Check residual volume regularly.

GI prophylaxis:

famotidine, pantoprazole, lansoprazole, ranitidine, omeprazole, or sucralfate

Progressive Activity:

If P/F ratio is < 200, consider lateral rotation therapy.
Carefully titrate the amount of sedatives and narcotics.
Have patient sit in chair as much as possible.
Promote weight bearing when transferring from/to bed.

Problems with the Bath:

- ICU patients who receive daily baths with chlorhexidine are less likely to become infected with methicillin-resistant Staphylococcus aureus (MRSA) and vancomycin-resistant Enterococcus (VRE).
- One study found that "some form of bacteria grew in 98 % of the (bath basins) samples: enterococci (54 %), gram-negative organisms (32 %), Staphylococcus aureus (23 %), vancomycin-resistant enterococci (13 %), methicillin-resistant Staph Aureus (8 %), Pseudomonas aeruginosa (5 %), Candida albicans (3 %), and Escherichia coli (2 %)."(Johnson D, Lineweaver L, Maze LM. Patients' bath basins as potential sources of infection.AJCC,2009;18(1): 31-40.
- Disinfecting the wash basin after bathing was found to reduce the incidence of nosocomial infection.

Raoof S, Baumann MH. Critical Care Collaborative (AACN, ACCP, ATS, SCCM). Ventilator-Associated Events: The new definition. AJCC, Jan 2014;23(1):7-9.
Muscedere J, Sinuff T, Heyland DK, et al. The clinical impact and preventability of ventilator associated conditions in the critically ill mechanically ventilated patients. Chest. 2013;144(5): 1453-1460.

Wean from Mechanical Ventilation

Facts:

- 40 - 50 % of the time spent on a ventilator is spent weaning.
- Failure to wean may occur in up to 25% of patients.
- Studies have demonstrated that the use of a weaning protocol by nonphysician health-care professionals can improve weaning success and reduce the duration of MV.
- Weaning Failure is caused by imbalance between respiratory capacity and respiratory workload.

↓ Respiratory Capacity

1. Respiratory muscle strength/endurance undermined by:
   - Electrolyte imbalance (decreases in Phos, Ca, Mg, or K)
   - Respiratory muscle wasting
   - Nutritional deficits
2. Pulmonary gas exchange altered by V/Q mismatch
3. Respiratory drive altered by neurologic deficit or injury, medications, sleep deprivation.
4. Peripheral gas exchange undermined by inadequate cardiac reserve to meet the extra demand of working to breathe.

↑ Respiratory Workload

Sudden removal of positive pressure breathing.
Additional burden of now working with airway resistance.

1. Wake Up: the Spontaneous Awakening Trial (SAT)

Screen for SAT Safety:
- No agitation
- No paralytics
- No myocardial ischemia
- No neurologic depression
- No decrease in Ca, Mg, K, Phos,

Monitor for SAT Failure:
- Development of anxiety, agitation, pain
- SaO_2 falls to < 88 %
- Respiratory rate increases to > 35 bpm
- Respiratory distress develops
- Cardiac arrhythmia develops

2. Assess Readiness for the Spontaneous Breathing Trial (SBT)

While the patient is still being ventilated, test for SBT Safety:
- No agitation
- $PaO_2 > 60$
- $SaO_2 > 90$
- $FiO_2 \leq 50\%$
- PEEP ≤ 8 cm H_2O
- Hgb ≥ 8 g/dL
- Minimal, thin secretions
- No myocardial ischemia
- Hemodynamically stable
- No vasopressors
- No electrolyte imbalance
- Inspiratory effort is good
- No respiratory depressants
- Free of conditions that increase metabolic rate
- No abdominal distention
- Oxygen deliver to tissue is good (CO, Hgb, SaO_2)

Choose SBT method: T-Piece, or SIMV, or CPAP 5 - 8 cm H_2O

Stay connected? Some advise maintaining connection to the ventilator, for monitoring purposes and to maintain positive airway pressure. Others advise against staying connected, since it is believed to ↑ work of breathing.

continued on next page →

Esteban A, Frutos F, Tobin MJ, et al. A comparison of four methods of weaning patients from mechanical ventilation. NEJM, 1995;332:345-350.
Robertson TE, Sona C, Schallom L, et al. Improved extubation rates with implementation of a daily spontaneous-breathing trial protocol. J Am Coll Surg 2008;206(3):489–495.

Wean from Mechanical Ventilation

3. Use the Rapid Shallow Breathing Index (RSBI), which is calculated during spontaneous breathing (no mechanical ventilation)

RSBI = Respiratory rate/tidal volume in liters.

- Elevate head of bed 30 - 45°. Allow spontaneous breathing for 2 - 3 mins (through a T-tube circuit). Calculate the Rapid Shallow Breathing Index.
- If RSBI > 105, stop the weaning attempt, return patient to a comfortable form of ventilatory support, reassess for and correct reversible factors.
- If RSBI < 105, proceed with 2 hour trial of spontaneous breathing T-tube.

4. The 2-Hour Spontaneous Breathing Trial:

Monitor closely for SBT failure, evidenced by any 1 of the following:

RR > 35 or < 8
SaO_2 < 90%
Heart rate > 140
Systolic BP < 90 or > 180 mm Hg
Development of diaphoretic, pale state
Respiratory distress (tachypnea RR > 35 bpm, dyspnea, use of accessory muscles, or presence of asynchronous breathing pattern)
Shallow breathing, TV < 5 mL/kg
Deterioration in mental status
Development of anxiety, agitation, panic, exhaustion
Development of cardiac arrhythmia

If the patient fails the SBT, return to mechanical ventilation and:

1. Attend to potentially remediable factors:
2. Reduce CO_2 production, reduce metabolic rate.
3. Attend to bronchoconstriction/secretions.
4. Improve pulmonary compliance.
5. Improve level of consciousness.
6. Assess for reversible causes of respiratory muscle weakness.
7. Use a comfortable, safe, well-monitored mode of MV, such as PSV.
8. If there are repeated failures, measure pulmonary mechanics.
9. Change to pressure support slow weaning protocol (SIMV with PS).

If the patient passes the SBT, consider the following problems:

1. Prior to extubation, absence of air leak around ET tube (with cuff deflated) suggests laryngeal edema.
2. 70% of patients who develop dyspnea after extubation will require re-intubation.
3. 15% of patients will require reintubation (re-intubation rate is higher in neurologically impaired patients).
4. For extubation failure, some recommend NPPV (noninvasive positive pressure ventilation) as a means of avoiding re-intubation.
5. If re-intubation is necessary:
6. Carries an 8-fold higher odds ratio for nosocomial pneumonia
7. Carries a 6-fold to 12-fold increased mortality risk.
8. But 50% who self-extubate do not require re-intubation.

Placing patients at higher risk for re-intubation on NIPPV immediately after extubation may reduce the likelihood that re-intubation may be required.

Prolonged MV: patient spends ≥ 21 straight days on a ventilator for ≥ 6 hrs/day.
Permanent ventilator dependency: > 3 months of failed weaning attempts.

McConville JF, Kress JP. Weaning patients from the ventilator. NEJM 2012; 367:2233-2239.

Pulmonary Embolism

Description:
- Obstruction of some part of the pulmonary circulation, most often as a complication of venous thromboembolism.
- PE should be suspected in any patient with unexplained chest pain, dyspnea, tachypnea, or any patient with risk factors for PE.
- Half of patients who have PE have atypical presentation.
- Patients with PE often decompensate suddenly.
- 70% of those who suffer cardiac arrest (most often as pulseless electrical activity) do not survive.
- Left untreated, 30% who survive PE will die from a 2nd episode.
- Postmortem studies have shown that 70% of unexpected deaths in a hospital setting died from massive PE.
- Pulmonary embolism is present in 60-80% of patients with DVT, even though more than half of these patients are asymptomatic.

Risk Factors:

Venous Stasis	Endothelial Injury	Hypercoagulable State
Immobility Paralysis Obesity Atrial fibrillation Heart failure Long-distance travel Venous insufficiency	Major trauma, surgery or severe burns, Recent central venous instrumentation, Hypertension Atherosclerosis	Carcinoma History of heavy smoking Pregnancy or Postpartum Estrogen therapy Sepsis, Polycythemia, Deficiency of protein C, protein S, antithrombin II

Source of the clots:
- Most emboli originate from deep veins of the lower extremities.
- Other sources include the pelvic veins, or upper extremity veins.
- Some are due to clots from the right heart as the result of A Fib.

Patho-physiology:
- Obstructed pulmonary blood flow results in increased alveolar dead space (ventilated but not perfused), pneumoconstriction, hypoxemia, and hyperventilation. After 24 hours, decreased surfactant production causes atelectasis. Infiltrates also appear.
- Major PE (> 50% reduction in pulmonary blood flow) results in ↑ pulmonary vascular resistance, ↑↑ PAP's, right heart strain, coronary artery constriction, ↓ CO, ↓ BP.
- Cardiac arrest (usually PEA) occurs when the left ventricle is unable to maintain adequate cardiac output.

Signs and Symptoms: The degree and duration of pulmonary artery occlusion determines the acuity, as well as the signs and symptoms:

Respiratory	Cardiovascular
Acute onset tachypnea (96% of pts) Acute onset of dyspnea (73% of pts) Pleuritic chest pain (66% of pts) Rales (58% of pts) Cough, possible hemoptysis Decrease in oxygen saturation Possible pleural friction rub Fever > 37.8° C (43% of pts)	Tachycardia (44%), Fainting S3 gallop, accentuated P2 (53%) Hypotension, syncope, diaphoresis, pallor New murmur of tricuspid regurgitation Increase in CVP, or jugular vein distention Systolic murmur of tricuspid regurgitation Homan sign (pain on dorsiflexion) is present in only 30% of the cases.

ECG:
- Most have tachycardia and nonspecific ST-T wave changes.
- Only 20% have classic ECG changes of right ventricular strain:
- S wave in Lead I, Q wave in Lead III, T wave inversion in Lead III (known as "S1, Q3, T3" pattern), Right axis deviation, new RBBB, or tall peaked P waves in Lead II (P pulmonale)
- T-wave inversion in Leads V1 - V4 occurs in 2/3 of massive PE cases. T-wave corrects with resolution of the RV strain.

Lab:
- D-dimer (a product of clot degradation by plasmin) is positive in most patients with PE, but is negative (< 500 ng/mL) in 15% of cases.
- Cardiac troponin can be up as much a 50% in moderate to severe PE, probably the result of acute right ventricular strain.
- WBC may be elevated (to as high as 20,000).
- Ischemia-modified albumin predicts outcome better than D-dimer.

Other: Right ventricular dysfunction is seen on cardiac ultrasound

Smithburger PL, Campbell S, Kane-Gill SL. Acute pulmonary embolism in the intensive care unit. Critical Care Nurse. 2013;33(2):17-27.

Pulmonary Embolism (cont'd)

Chest x-ray:
- Often abnormal; may reveal other causes of chest pain.
- Within 24 - 72 hrs of embolization, may have atelectasis, infiltrates, pleural effusion, elevation of a hemidiaphragm.

Angiogram:
- There is segmental perfusion defect with normal ventilation.
- Presence of intraluminal filling defect or abrupt termination of a vessel greater than 2 - 5 mm.
- Appearance of RV enlargement is a risk factor for death.

Echocardiography:
- 95% of unstable patients have evidence of right ventricular hypocontractility. If cardiac troponins are also elevated, the risk for complications and death is increased.

V/Q scan: Following the inhalation of a radioactive gas and IV injection of labeled albumin, concurrent images of blood flow (perfusion scan) and alveolar ventilation (ventilation scan) are obtained. The cardinal sign of pulmonary embolism is an underperfused part of the lungs, while the ventilation scan remains normal,

Treatment of PE

Oxygenate:
- O_2 by cannula, mask, or artificial airway to support SpO_2.
- ↑ HOB to 30°. Position Lt or Rt to maintain best SaO_2.

Fluids?
- In hypotensive patients, fluids may help or hurt. Test for fluid responsiveness with a small bolus while carefully monitoring systolic and diastolic blood pressure, and if possible, CVP.

Thrombolytic Therapy in Select Patients:
- Only patients with acute massive PE, who are at high risk for death and have no contraindications, are eligible for fibrinolytic therapy.
- High risk patients are those who have:
  1. marked dyspnea, anxiety, and low oxygen saturation
  2. elevated troponin, indicating right ventricular microinfarction
  3. right ventricular dysfunction on echocardiography, and
  4. right ventricular enlargement on chest CT.

For those receiving Thrombolytic	For those not receiving Thrombolytic
• Unfractionated heparin (UFH) should not be given at the same time as fibrinolytic therapy in acute massive pulmonary embolism. • But if there will be diagnostic delays, then UFH should be given and then stopped prior to fibrinolytic therapy after aPTT is < 80 seconds. • The FDA-approved alteplase regimen: 100 mg over 2 hours (50 mL/hr). • Subq Heparin may be used instead of UFH when the pts perfusion is stable.	• If acute pulmonary embolism is highly suspected, a parenteral anticoagulant should be given and not be delayed by diagnostic tests. • Intravenous unfractionated heparin is used if there is ↓ BP (which decreases SQ absorption). • Normotensive patients are given subq low molecular weight heparin (fondaparinux or enoxaparin). • Some choose Tinzaparin (Innohep) since it is dosed once/day.

- Warfarin 5 - 10 mg po should be started the same day as parenteral heparin, dosed to achieve INR 2 - 3. Delaying the start of Warfarin is not advised. Subcutaneous anticoagulants are usually continued for a minimum of 5 days, (and up to 10 days). The INR must by 2.0 for at least 24 h before subcutaneous anticoagulants are stopped.
- Warfarin is continued for 3 months, But if PE recurs, lifetime Warfarin
- Newer Direct Thrombin Inhibitors may replace Heparin + Warfarin regimen.

Additional Treatment of PE

- IVC filter is indicated only in pts who have contraindications to anticoagulant therapy. No IVC filter may be placed in patients treated with anticoagulants.
- Surgical embolectomy is usually reserved for patients in unstable condition who have contraindications to thrombolytic therapy.

Complications:

Sudden cardiac death	Cor pulmonale
Obstructive shock	Severe hypoxemia
Pulseless electrical activity	Intracardiac shunt
Pulmonary hypertension	

Bates SM et al. Diagnosis of DVT. Antithrombotic Therapy and Prevention of Thrombosis, 9th ed: ACCP Evidence-Based Clinical Practice Guidelines. Chest, 2012;141(2supp):351-418.

Pleural Effusion

Description:
- Fluid, blood, chyle, or products of infection in the pleural space.
- Most common causes, in order of frequency: congestive heart failure, pneumonia, malignancy, pulmonary embolism, cirrhosis with ascites, pancreatitis, tuberculosis.
- Simple pneumonic effusions have a greater potential to become complicated (empyema; fibroblasts grow into the effusion, producing an inelastic membrane that entraps the lung).

Pathophysiology: *Transudative* pleural effusion - the result of noninflammatory conditions, producing an accumulation of protein-poor and cell-poor fluid (may be called a hydrothorax) and is due to:
- Increased pulmonary capillary hydrostatic pressure (Heart failure is the most common cause of effusion)
- Decreased colloid osmotic pressure due to low serum albumin (e.g. cirrhosis, nephrosis)

Exudative pleural effusion - the result of inflammatory process, producing an accumulation of protein-rich fluid, due to:
- Increased pulmonary capillary permeability (e.g. pulmonary embolism, pneumonia, pancreatitis, sepsis). Develops in 30 - 40% of patients with bacterial pneumonia.
- Failure of pulmonary lymphatics to clear pleural fluid (e.g. malignant neoplasm)

Signs and Symptoms:
- Signs and symptoms related to the underlying disease process.
- Dyspnea is the most common symptom, indicates the effusion is at least 500 mL. Dyspnea is due more to distortion of the diaphragm and chest wall than to hypoxia.
- Chest pain, which may be mild or severe, is described as sharp or stabbing, aggravated by deep breath, pleuritic. Often the pain becomes less severe as the effusion increases in size.
- These physical findings do not manifest until volume > 300 mL:
  Decreased breath sounds; Dullness to percussion
  Decreased tactile fremitus; Pleural friction rub
  Asymmetric expansion of the chest
- Mediastinal shift if effusion volume is more than 1000 mL.
- Sometimes distended neck veins, S3 gallop.

Diagnostics: Chest xray is the primary diagnostic tool (available, accurate)

Treatment:
- Head of bed elevation 30 - 40°, supplemental oxygen.
- Thoracentesis
  1. Pneumothorax is the most common complication (3 - 12%). Incidence is reduced with ultrasound guidance or with aspiration through a catheter rather than needle.
  2. A chest tube 8 - 14 Fr. is better tolerated and easier to position successfully than larger 20 - 36 Fr.
  3. Aspiration that generates negative pressure < -20 cm can cause reexpansion pulmonary edema.
  4. Removal of 400 - 500 mL of fluid is usually sufficient. Removal of > 1200 mL may cause mediastinal shift.
  5. Hypoxemia is common after thoracentesis. O_2 should be given during and for several hours after thoracentesis.
  6. Risks increase with repeated thoracentesis.
- Treatment of the cause.

Normal Pleural fluid	Exudative Effusion
pH 7.60 - 7.64 Protein count < 2% (1-2 g/dL) LDH < 50% of plasma WBCs < 1000/mm^3 Glucose similar to that of plasma Na, K, Ca similar to interstitial fluid	pH < 7.2 needs urgent drainage Protein > 2.9 g/dL LDH is > 2/3 of the upper limit of normal serum LDH

Pneumothorax

Review of the Mechanics of Breathing:

1. The visceral pleura attached to the lungs and the parietal pleura attached to the inside of the chest wall glide over each other during ventilation.
2. The elastic recoil of the lungs and the outward pull of the ribs are opposing forces that create negative pressure between the pleural membranes.
3. During inspiration, the contraction of the diaphragm and the outward expansion of the chest wall further increase the negative pressure.
4. Negative intrathoracic pressure is transmitted throughout the chest cavity and facilitates venous return to the chest, especially during inspiration.
5. The loss of negative intrathoracic pressure results in reduced inspiratory volume, reduced venous return to the heart, ↓ CO, and subsequently ↓ BP.

Simple Pneumothorax:

1. A defect in the visceral pleural membrane allows alveolar air to leak into the pleural space. Loss of negative intrapleural pressure allows the lung to recoil/collapse and, if severe, results in decreased venous return to the heart.
2. The defect in the pleura usually does not continue to leak.
3. Pneumo that involves < 20% of the affected hemithorax will not require a chest tube unless the patient is to receive positive pressure breathing. (Positive pressure will likely increase in the size of the pneumo)

Fig. 9.15

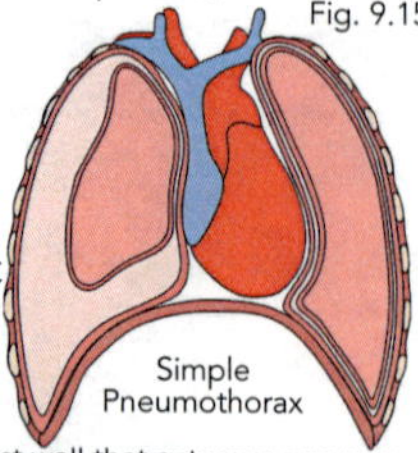

Assessment:

- Chest pain, shortness of breath
- Decreased breath sounds
- Hyperresonant percussion

Management:

- If pneumo > 20%, chest tube placed 2 ICS, MCL
- If pneumo < 20%, monitor for increase in size
- Lung should reexpand in 24 - 48 hours.

Tension Pneumothorax:

1. A defect in the trachea, bronchus, lung, or chest wall that acts as a one-way valve, allowing air to enter the pleural space during inspiration, but prohibiting its escape during expiration.
2. A tension pneumothorax enlarges with each breath.
3. Positive pressure builds in the pleural space, causing reduced venous return, mediastinal shift away from the affected lung, and compression of the unaffected lung. Blood pressure and PaO_2 fall, $PaCO_2$ rises.
4. Tension pneumo can develop slowly, can occur spontaneously, or expand rapidly, especially if the patient is receiving positive pressure breathing.

Fig. 9.16

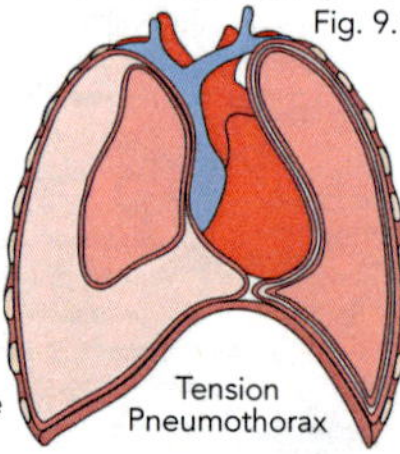

Assessment:

- Chest pain, Agitation, Decreased LOC
- Progressive dyspnea
- ↓ SaO_2/PaO_2, cyanosis, ↓ breath sounds
- Hyperresonance on the affected side
- Distended neck veins, ↑ CVP, ↓ BP, PEA.
- Tracheal deviation, PMI shift away from growing volume of trapped air
- Abdominal distention, due to downward displacement of the diaphragm
- If mechanically ventilated, progressive increase in pressure to ventilate.

Management:

- Stat needle thoracostomy/pleural chest tube at 2 ICS MCL or 5th ICS AAL.
- Added suction, manually or with equipment set at 20 - 30 cm suction.
- If defect is large, pleural chest tube may demonstrate continued pleural leak, which may require surgery.
- Conservative attempts to stop the leak may include application of PEEP onto the chest tube. Jet ventilation sometimes used for persistent leak.
- Avoid clamping the chest tube (e.g., for transport). Pneumo could recur.

Chest Tubes

Description Placement of large bore tubing into the pleural space, to evacuate air, fluid, or blood, or to administer medication.

Indications:

Hemothorax	Pleural effusion	Empyema
Pneumothorax	Chylothorax	Chemotherapy

Relative Contra-indications
Prolonged bleeding time.
Previous thoracotomy with adhesions, diaphragmatic elevation.
Massive hemothorax (if accumulated blood tamponades the source of bleeding, draining the blood may precipitate uncontrollable bleeding. The pleural tubes should be inserted in the OR).

Tube sizes Adult 28 - 36 Fr., Teen 28 - 32 Fr., Child 18 - 24 Fr., Infant 10 - 12 Fr.

Insertion Procedure:

1. If the patient is hemodynamically stable, give analgesic.
2. Some order 3 doses of cephalosporin: prior to insertion, and at 8 hours and 16 hours post insertion.
3. Insure IV access and availability of O_2, ambu bag, intubation supplies, and ventilator.
4. Position patient affected side up, arm flexed over the head.
5. May need HOB elevated 20° - 30° if short of breath.
6. For hemothorax, prep the area around the 5-6th ICS, anterior or mid-axillary line.
7. For pneumothorax, prep the area around the 2nd ICS MCL, or 5th ICS AAL.
8. Lidocaine 1% - 2%, as much as 30 - 40 mL, 22 g needle: the skin, around the rib, subcutaneous tissue and pleura is infiltrated.
9. The skin is incised with a scalpel.
10. The subcutaneous tissues and intercostal muscle are dissected, carefully avoiding vessels along the lower border of the rib.
11. A tunnel is made with the index finger through the chest wall.
12. The parietal pleura is palpated, then punctured.
13. A Kelly clamp is used to guide the tube into the pleural space.
14. You should see condensation on the walls of the tube, or drainage of blood or fluid, or hear a sucking sound.
15. Connect tube to a drainage system and secure connections.
16. Added suction to the drainage system may be required.
17. The tube is sutured to the skin and occlusive dressing applied.
18. Obtain a post-insertion chest x-ray.

Complications

- Incidence of complications is 1%.
- Insufficient treatment of hemo or pneumo may occur if the tube is small, kinked, obstructed or improperly positioned.
- Subcutaneous emphysema may occur if tube not inserted far enough (one drainage hole is outside the pleural space).
- Bleeding from skin or intercostal vessel.
- Pulmonary laceration. Intercostal nerve injury.
- Injury of the pulmonary artery, vein, or thoracic aorta.
- Injury to the diaphragm or abdominal organs.
- Pain/splinting may - hypoventilation, atelectasis, pneumonia.
- Pain may trigger a vasovagal response (↓ HR, ↓ BP, ↓ LOC).
- If large, long-standing pleural effusion is rapidly drained, re-expansion pulmonary edema may result.
- Insertion site infection.
- Bronchopleural fistula (large, persistent air leak).

Removal:

1. PCT removal is OK if no air leak and < 200 mL drainage/24 hr.
2. Premedicate with Morphine 4 mg IV 20 minutes ahead.
3. DC suction, clamp the chest tube. Remove dressing and suture.
4. Provide towel onto which to place the pulled tube.
5. The patient should be asked to take a deep breath and valsalva.
6. If the patient is being ventilated, tube is pulled at end-inspiration.
7. Apply vaseline gauze dressing. Some order chest x-ray.
8. Check breath sounds, vital signs, color, SaO_2.

Chest Tube Drainage Unit

Description:
Chest tubes remove both fluid and air trapped in the pleural space (hemothorax, hydrothorax, pleural effusion, pneumothorax). To manage chest tubes, you must understand:

1. the mechanic of breathing
2. the danger of exposing the patient's pleural space to atmospheric pressure
3. the dangers of a chest drainage unit

How It Works:
Chest drainage units for critical care usually have 3 chambers:

1. The "Collection Chamber," where fluid drainage is collected. In some units, this chamber can be removed when full, and replaced with a new chamber. The collection chamber also connects to the chamber 2.
2. The waterseal chamber, allows the patient's respirations to move air that has been trapped in the pleural space, through the water seal, which releases it to the atmosphere, while also prohibiting outside air from entering the patient's pleural space. The amount of water that is placed in the chamber (2 cm) is critical to the the function of chamber 2. Bubbles can be seen in this chamber whenever air is moved out of the pleural space.
3. The suction control chamber, for controlling the amount of suction applied to a patient's chest tube, when needed to promote drainage. By adding or removing water in the suction control chamber, the chest drain effectively controls the amount of suction imposed on the patient.
   The lower the water content, the lower the imposed suction.
   The higher the water level, the greater the imposed suction.
   Suction set at -20 mm Hg is the usual amount.
   Suction greater than - 40 mm Hg is not recommended.

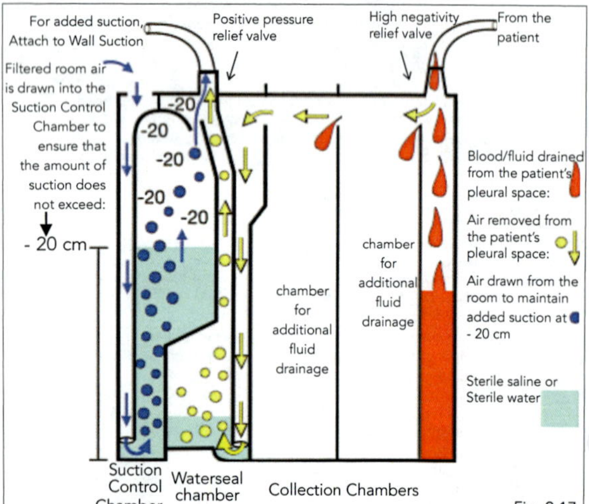

Fig. 9.17

Pressure Release Valves:
Chest drainage units for critical care also have 2 pressure relief valves:

1. Positive pressure release - to vent excessively high intrathoracic pressure
2. Negative pressure release - limits negativity to about -50 cm H_2O to prevent lung injury when "stripping" or "milking" the chest tubes.

Warning: when operating on gravity drainage (no added suction) do not depress the POSITIVE PRESSURE relief valve, as pneumothorax may occur.

Chest Tube Drainage (cont'd)

Water fluctuation in the water seal chamber:

- During spontaneous respiration:
  Inhalation: the water level rises due to negative intrapleural pressure
  Exhalation: the water level returns to where it started, or falls further with forced exhalation or a cough. Air bubbles appear if a leak remains in the pleura. Then the water level return to where it started.
- During positive pressure breathing:
  Inhalation: the water level falls, due to increased intrathoracic pressure, and will be accompanied by air bubbles if a leak remains in the pleura.
  Exhalation: the water level returns to where it started.
- If suction has been added to the suction control chamber: fluctuations in the waterseal chamber will probably not be visible.

When someone asks "Is there an air leak?"

- This can mean one of 2 things:
  1. Does the patient's pleura still leak air (i.e., the pleura has not healed yet) as evidenced by air bubbles emitted (by the patient) into the waterseal chamber,
     or
  2. Is there a leak in the drainage system that might explain why the chest x-ray revealed unevacuated air in the thorax.
- To find out, first apply suction to the suction control chamber, then momentarily clamp the chest tube. If air bubbles still appear in the water seal chamber, these bubbles are not from the patient. Check for a leak in the system, somewhere below where you placed the clamp.
- Promptly unclamp the chest tube after completing this test.

Care and Maintenance:

1. If suction is ordered, connect the suction port to a suction source. -20 mm Hg suction is usual. More than -40 mm Hg suction is not recommended.
2. Eliminate dependent loops in the connecting tubing.
3. Keep tubing straight or coiled. Ensure there are no kinks in any of the tubing.
4. Check the water seal chamber. The presence of air bubbles indicates the system is still removing air from the patient's pleural space.
5. When suction has been added to the suction control chamber, adjust the wall suction to a level of suction that produces gentle bubbling. High level suction will cause turbulent bubbling and a lot of noise, and will accelerate evaporation of the water from the suction control chamber.
6. Check the waterseal chamber and the suction control chamber for evaporative water loss and replenish the supply.

Replace the Drainage Unit:

- Follow the manufacturer's instructions to set up a new Drainage Unit.
- Clamping the chest tubes will be required, and clamp time must be brief. Clamping a pleural chest tube in a patient with a persistent pleural leak, particularly if the patient is receiving positive pressure breathing, can result in the development of a pneumothorax.
- When the Drainage unit is ready:
  1. Clamp the patient's chest tube.
  2. Disconnect the chest tube from the connecting tubing.
  3. Quickly connect the patient's chest tube to the connecting tubing of the new drainage unit.
  4. Quickly unclamp the chest tube.
- The One-way water seal is now reestablished.
- Assess the patient, then assess the operation of the new drainage unit.
- Attach added suction if it is ordered.

Autotransfusion:	of blood collected in a chest drainage unit is no longer recommended.

Notes

Renal/Endo

Renal/Endo

Acute Kidney Injury (AKI)

Definition: An abrupt decrease in glomerular filtration rate (GFR), with failure of the kidney to remove nitrogen wastes, maintain fluid and electrolyte balance, and acid-base homeostasis.

Facts:

- Acute Renal Failure occurs in 15-25% of all critically ill patients
- The mortality rate is 40 - 80%. The most common causes of death are sepsis, cardiac failure, or pulmonary failure.
- Among the survivors, 30% will require long-term dialysis

Causes: The 3 causes if i GFR occur "Before, Within, or After" the Kidney:

1. Prerenal: inadequate renal blood flow
2. Intrarenal: injury to the glomerulus and/or tubules
3. Postrenal: obstruction located beyond the nephrons

Significant Risk Factors: Advanced age, history of renal dysfunction, surgery/trauma, volume depletion, exposure to nephrotoxic agent/s,

1. Prerenal AKI

Definition: Inadequate renal blood flow.

Patho-physiology:

- Glomerular filtration rate (GFR) is directly related to glomerular hydrostatic pressure, which is threatened if MAP is < 60 mm Hg. ↓ BP poses an even greater risk to pts with chronic hypertension.
- Inadequate blood flow stimulates sympathetic-adrenal response, with renal artery vasoconstriction, decreased GFR, conservation of Na and water, and reduced clearance of urea and creatinine.
- Nephron function initially is intact. If treatment is prompt, there will be no permanent damage; renal function returns to normal.
- When RBF is low, the kidneys are especially vulnerable to further insults (considered "the 2nd hit").

Causes: Any of the causes of hypovolemia, pump failure, or vasodilation. Renal vascular obstruction (renal artery thrombosis). ↓ autoregulation of renal blood flow (e.g., due to NSAIDS).

Treatment: Depends on the cause of the reduction in renal blood flow:

- Hypovolemia: Fluids to restore CVP to 5 - 8 mm Hg, Blood is usually given if Hgb ≤ 8 g/dL. Albumin is given if serum albumin is low.
- Cardiac performance is optimized.
- Vasodilated (septic shock) pts need careful fluid management, inotropes, vasoconstrictors (see "Hemo" chapter for details).

2. Postrenal AKI

Definition:	Reduced GFR due to diseases or conditions that affect the ureters, bladder, or urethra, and resulting in obstructed outflow of urine.
Patho-physiology:	Increased tubular pressure decreases the filtration driving force. Bilateral obstruction results in hydronephrosis with progressive decline and ultimate cessation in glomerular filtration, along with azotemia, acidosis, fluid overload, and hyperkalemia.
Causes:	Ureteral or tubular obstruction by calculi, clots, crystals, strictures. Collecting system compression by tumor, infection, mass, or prostatic hypertrophy. Bladder stone or clot Foley catheter obstruction Neurogenic bladder
Assessment:	Sudden cessation of urinary output or anuria Symptoms of urgency, frequency, hesitancy Flank pain and hematuria
Treatment:	1. If complete obstruction is relieved within 48 hours of onset, recovery of GFR can occur within a week. 2. In the presence of normal kidney function, expect a diuretic phase, with dilute urine and hypokalemia, lasting 2 - 4 days. 3. Fluids are given as D_5 0.45NS to replace 2/3 of the previous hour's urine output + 30 mL to replace insensible loss. 4. Prolonged obstruction can lead to irreversible renal fibrosis.

Initial Assessment of AKI

The 3 types of renal failure distinguished by the lab results.

	Normal values	1 Prerenal	2 Postrenal	3 Intrarenal
Incidence:	% of all cases →	50%	< 10 %	40%
General cause:	----	↓ kidney perfusion	Urinary tract obstruction	Parenchyma damage
Urine volume:	500 - 2500 mL/d (> 0.5 mL/kg/hr)	oliguria 100-400 mL/d	usually anuria < 100 mL/d	oliguria, normal, or high
Urinary Na:	10 - 30 mEq/L	< 10	10 - 40	> 40
Sediment:	None	None	Organisms may be present	Casts: of tubule, white and red cells
Proteinuria:	No	No	No	Yes
Sp. gravity:	1.010 - 1.030	> 1.020	normal - 1.010	< 1.010
Urine osmolalty	500 - 800 mOsm	> 500	< 350	< 300
BUN:	5 - 20	> 25	> 25	> 25
Creatinine:	0.5 - 1.5	Normal	Normal or ↑	> 1.5
$\frac{BUN}{Cr}$ ratio	5	> 20 (as high as 40)	Normal or > 10	< 20
FeNa:	----	< 1 %	> 1 %	> 2 %

Changes in serum Creatinine reflect changes in Glomerular Filtration Rate:

Cr (mg/dL)		% ↓ in GFR		GFR (mL/min)
Cr is < 1	=	Normal GFR	=	125
Cr is 1.5	=	25% ↓ in GFR	=	94
Cr is 2	=	50% ↓ in GFR	=	63
Cr is 4	=	75% ↓ in GFR	=	25
Cr is 8	=	95% ↓ in GFR	=	6

Fractional excretion of sodium (FeNa) is used to differentiate between Prerenal versus Intrarenal ARF. FeNa ↑ before oliguria occurs.

$$FeNa = \frac{\text{Urine Na/Serum Na}}{\text{Urine Cr/Serum Cr}} \times 100$$

< 1% = prerenal ARF

> 2% = ATN/intrarenal ARF

If all Glomerular filtration stops:

K	↑	0.3-0.5 mEq/L/d
HCO3	↓	1-2 mEq/L/d
BUN	↑	10-20 mg/dL/d
Cr	↑	1-2 mg/dL/d

Fig. 11.1

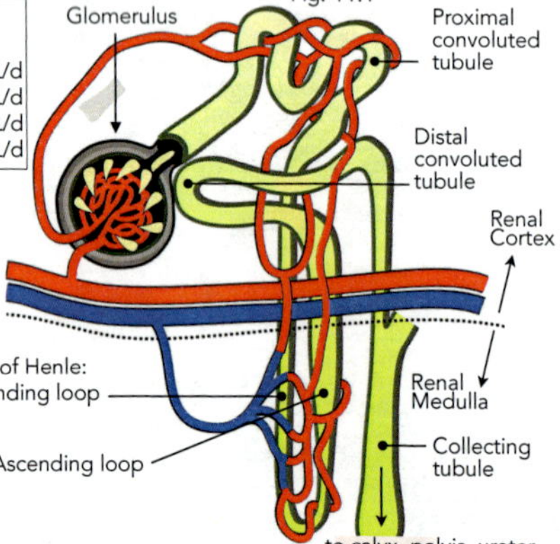

Assessment of Risk and Severity:

The RIFLE Assessment	Serum Cr is ↑	or GFR is ↓	Urinary Output (UO)
Risk is present if there is:	x 1.5	> 25%	< 0.5 mL/kg/h x 6 h
Injury is present::	x 2	> 50%	< 0.5 mL/kg/h x 12 h
Failure is present:	x 3, or ≥ 4 mg/dL	> 75%	< 0.3 mL/kg/h x 24 h
Kidney failure:	has been present >4 weeks		
End-stage disease:	kidney failure has been present > 3 months		

3. Intrarenal AKI

Definition: Injury to the glomerulus or tubules, from any or all of 3 sources:

1. Prolonged period of renal hypoperfusion (prerenal AKI) culminating in acute tubular necrosis (ATN)
2. Nephrotoxin exposure accounts for 30 - 40% of ARF cases:
   - Aminoglycosides, amphotericin, carbenicillin, cephalosporin,
   - NSAIDS, cyclosporine, ACEI's, acyclovir, tetracycline, contrast media, chemotherapy, anesthetics.
   - Endogenous substances (e.g., myoglobin)
   - Immunosuppressive therapy
   - Organic solvents, heavy metals

   (Recovery from uncomplicated nephrotoxic injury is more likely and is more rapid than from ischemic ATN)
3. Inflammatory disease: Infection, Auto immune disease.

Pathophysiology:

- Acute Tubular Necrosis (ATN) is the most common form of intrarenal ARF, accounting for 75% of all cases.
- Tubule cells swell, necrose, slough into the tubular lumen, forming cylindrical casts (made up of white blood cells, red blood cells, or kidney cells) and obstructing tubular flow.
- Cell swelling obstructs capillary flow, which perpetuates the ischemic process.
- 50% are oliguric (UO < 400 mL/day), 50% are nonoliguric.
- Glomerulonephritis accounts for 25% of cases.
- Inflammation of or injury to the glomerulus produces increased permeability, allowing RBC's and albumin into the urine.
- Nonoliguric intrarenal ARF (UO > 400 mL/day, but BUN and Cr are elevated) represents less severe injury, and carries a
- lower morbidity/mortality than does oliguric renal failure.

Risk Factors: Hypertension, CHF, diabetes, pre-existing renal disease, recent trauma, hypovolemia, IAP > 20 mm Hg, chronic infection.

Diagnostic Tests: Currently, the presence of urine sediment and FeNa > 2 are the earliest and most sensitive indicators of ATN.
The rise of serum Cr may not occur until 50% of the GFR is lost.
The kidneys are salt wasting, urine Na is > 40 mEq/L.
Heavy loss of protein in the urine (> 3 grams/day).
Ultrasound, CT, MRI are extremely useful.

Assessment: Uremia becomes symptomatic when BUN reaches 100 mg/dL.

General:	Easily fatigued, muscle weakness
Neuro:	Confusion, apathy, lethargy, obtundation, coma, headache, vertigo, twitching, asterixis, hyperreflexia, seizure.
GI:	Anorexia, nausea, vomiting, hiccups gastric ulcers, GI bleeding, ileus, constipation.
Resp:	If metabolic acidosis, Kussmaul respiration. If volume excess, pulmonary edema. Pneumonia, Acute Respiratory Distress.
CV:	Dysrhythmias due to electrolyte imbalances. Hypertension due to fluid excess. AMI, Pericarditis, Heart failure, Cardiac arrest.
Skin:	Edema due to Na and albumin losses.
Hematologic:	Anemia. 35 - 40 % have thrombocytopenia. Platelet dysfunction, purpura, coagulopathy.
Immune:	T-Cell suppression, decreased WBC activity. Infection (lungs, wounds, urinary tract)
Metabolic:	Catabolic state
Electrolytes:	↑ K, ↑ Phos, ↑ Mg, ↓ Na, ↓ Ca, ↓ HCO_3, ↓ pH K and Phos must be measured frequently.

Treatment of Intrarenal AKI

General Approach: Prerenal and Postrenal causes of ARF must be ruled out or treated. All nephrotoxic medications must be discontinued. The treatment goals are prevention, avoidance of further kidney injury, treatment of underlying condition, aggressive treatment of complications.

Diuretics vs Normal Saline:

- Normal Saline is used to convert oliguria to nonoliguria by h GFR and by preventing casts from obstructing the tubules. (Oliguria has a higher mortality than nonoliguria.)
- Diuretics are not given until hypovolemia has been treated andcardiovascular function optimized. Beware that overly aggressive fluid resuscitation lead to edema, ARDS.
- Furosemide 100 - 200 mg (as much as 600 mg/day) given by IV infusion (not by IV push) promotes sustained diuresis, with less danger of ototoxicity. A positive response offers optimism. If the pt. is unresponsive to diuretic, it should be discontinued.
- Outcome is worse in patients with contrast-induced AKI if furosemide is given. But infusion of NaCl is very beneficial.

Agents that cause harm: Dopamine, nesiritide, fenoldopam, mannitol, radiocontrast agents, nephrotoxic antibiotic, cancer agents, NSAIDs.

Early dialysis: Starting dialysis when BUN = 40 mg/dL offers better outcome than waiting until BUN = 95 mg/dL.

Electrolytes:

Na is ↓:	Normal saline infusion, to maintain Na and volume.
K is 5.5 - 6.5:	Restrict dietary K to < 50 mEq/day. Kaexylate 25 g + 70 % Sorbitol 15 mL q 3 - 6 h. Kaexylate oral is preferable (longer contact with GI tract for K exchange to occur). Beware, for each 1 mEq K removed, 1 mEq of sodium is retained. Sorbitol is given to prevent constipation.
K is (> 6.5):	Calcium (for cardioprotection) given as 10 mL of 10 % Calcium Gluconate for 1 - 3 doses. Glucose and Insulin given as: 1 - 2 amps D50W and 5 - 10 U regular insulin IV Effect occurs within 30 minutes. Beware, these measures move K into cells. As effects dissipate, expect plasma K to rise again.
Ca is ↓:	IV Calcium may be needed.
Phos is ↑:	Restrict phosphate intake, give phosphate-binders

Acid-Base: pH is ↓: Dialysis (rarely bicarbonate) if HCO_3 < 15 mEq/L.

Pulmonary: Hypoxia is common during dialysis, probably due to alveolar hypoventilation and to WBC sequestration in the lungs. Monitor SaO_2; O_2 by nasal cannula; Strict pulmonary care.

CV: Dysrhythmias and hypertension are common.
There is risk for heart failure, pericarditis, cardiac arrest.
Hemodynamic instability occurs in 25% of patients during dialysis.
Anemia undermines O_2 delivery; some prescribe Epogen.

Infection: Strict care of airway, pulmonary, wounds, invasive devices.
Remove foley catheter. Minimize intravascular catheters.
Beware that fever and WBC response will be less pronounced.

Bleeding Risk: GI bleed occurs in 1/3 of patients (usually mild) but accounts for 3 - 8% of deaths. Monitor H/H, platelets, PT, PTT.
Guaiac test of stool, NG aspirate, vomitus.

Nutrition: Early, aggressive nutritional support improves survival.
Most have marked increase in protein catabolism.
Carbohydrate: 300 g/day to prevent protein catabolism.
Calories: 35 Kcal/kg/day (or 1800 - 2500 Kcal/day)
Protein: 0.6 - 0.7 g/kg/day (1 - 2 g/kg/day if pt on CRRT)
Restrict: High-K foods (see next page).

↓ K, ↓ Phos: In the polyuric phase of AKI, potassium and phosphorus may be depleted. IV and/or dietary supplement may be needed.

Treatment of Intrarenal AKI

The Phases of Oliguria:

Phase	Duration	Description	Cr Clearance
Onset:	0 - 2 days	Fall in urinary output.	-----
Oliguria:	10 - 16 days	Urine volume < 400 mL/day Weight loss 0.2 - 0.5 kg/day	< 5 mL/min
Early Diuretic:	5 - 10 days	Sharp increase in UO, to > 400 mL/day (but may be as high as several L/day). BUN/Cr stop rising.	5 mL/min
Late Diuretic:	1 - 3 weeks	Slow decrease in BUN and Cr, independent of dialysis.	25 mL/min
Recovery:	3 - 12 months	Normal UO and electrolytes GFR usually returns to 70 - 80% of normal within 1 - 2 years. Stable BUN and Cr indicate the pt. has reached his best renal function.	50 mL/min

Indications for Dialysis:	Non-ARF indications for Continuous Renal Replacement Therapy (CRRT):
Oliguria (urine output < 200 mL/12 h) BUN > 40 - 80 mg/dL, Cr > 10 mg/dL Hyperkalemia (K > 6.5 mEq/L) Marked metabolic acidosis (pH < 7.1) Na > 160 or < 115 Uremic complications (encephalopathy, pericarditis, neuropathy, myopathy) Diuretic resistant volume overload, pulmonary edema or cardiac failure	Severe hyper/hyponatremia (Na > 160 or < 115 mEq/L) Overdose with dialyzable toxin Hyperthermia (> 39.5° C) CRRT is contraindicated if: Hct > 45%
Restrict High-Potassium Foods: Apricots, dried — Figs, dried Avocados — Lima beans Bananas — Molasses Celery — Nuts of all kinds Chocolate — Potato chips, fries Coffee, instant — Prunes Cucumbers — Raisins Dates — Veal Dried fruit Yams	**Hold Meds Prior to Intermittent Hemodialysis:** Avoid giving hypotensive agents: Vasodilators Beta-blockers Calcium channel blockers ACE inhibitors Narcotics Avoid meds which obscure neuro status Avoid giving dialyzable drugs.

Calculations used in CRRT:

Fractional excretion of sodium (FeNa)	$\frac{\text{Urine Na/ Plasma Na}}{\text{Urine Cr/ Plasma Cr}} \times 1000$	< 1 % = prerenal > 1 % = renal
Renal Failure Index (RFI)	(Urine Na x Plasma Cr)/Urine Cr	< 1 % = prerenal > 2 % = renal
Anion Gap	(Na + K) - (Cl + HCO_3)	N = 16 $\pm$ 4
Replacement fluids in CRRT	Hourly Total Out (exclude dialysate) - Hourly Total In (exclude RF's) - Desired Hourly Fluid Balance	
Filtration Fraction in CRRT	$\frac{\text{UF mL/min}}{\text{(Blood flow mL/min - prefilter Hct)}}$	maintain < 30 %
Blood flow in CRRT	pumped = SV x rpm not pumped = (UF mL/min x Hct out)/(Hct In - Hct out)	
Calculated Serum osmolality	[2 x (Na + K)] + BUN/2.8 + Glucose/18	N = 285-295 mOsm/kg

Creatinine Clearance	male	$\frac{(140 - \text{age}) \times \text{wt (kg)}}{72 \times \text{serum creatinine}}$
	female	$\frac{(140 - \text{age}) \times \text{wt (kg)}}{72 \times \text{serum creatinine}} \times 0.85$

Normal	>	100 (mL/min)
Mild ARF	=	40 - 60
Moderate	=	10 - 40
Severe	=	< 10

Continuous Renal Replacement Therapies (CRRT)

Description:

- Designed for critically ill patients, CRRT is dialysis that utilizes a slow and continuous process over a duration of 2 - 3 days, so that hemodynamic stability can be maintained.
- By comparison, Intermittent Hemodialysis removes 2 - 3 liters of fluid during a 4 hr treatment. CRRT removes the same amount over 24 hours.
- CRRT employs a hemofilter and a blood pump, sometimes in combination with fluids and/or dialysate, to:
  1. remove excess blood volume
  2. remove unwanted solutes such as K, Na, urea, Cr, uric acid (particle size < 50,000 Daltons)
  3. in some cases, remove toxins
- The patient's blood is pumped into the filter, where it flows against a semipermeable membrane, the surface area of which averages about 1 m^2
- Return blood flow is pumped packed to the patient.
- Sometimes "Replacement fluids" and/or "Dialysate" are used to intensify the removal of solutes and/or fluids, according to specific patient needs.
- Anticoagulation with either Heparin or Citrate maintains filter patency. But if the patient has prolonged bleeding times, then only NS flush q 1 h is used.
- Compared to intermittent hemodialysis, CRRT allows enhanced nutritional support with more protein and less restriction on fluids and electrolytes.

The Mechanisms of CRRT include:

- Ultrafiltration: Hydrostatic pressure (i.e., blood flow, blood pressure, and resistance within the filter) against the semipermeable membrane removes fluid (called "Ultrafiltrate"). 100 - 400 mL/hr to as high as 2,000 mL/hr can be removed from the patient. The degree of membrane permeability of the filter is called the "ultrafiltration coefficient".
- Osmosis: Moving fluid from an area of low solute concentration (e.g., patients with volume excess) across the membrane to an area of high concentration.
- Diffusion: Moving solutes from an area of high concentration (the patient's blood) to an area of low concentration, namely the other side of the membrane, which is bathed in dialysate tailored made for the patient.
- Convection: Using water (called "replacement fluids") to help move (or "drag") a greater amount of solutes across a semipermeable membrane.
- Adsorption: Some substances, such as inflammatory cytokines and some medium-weight molecules, adhere to the membrane surface, particularly after placement of a new AN69 filter.

About Replacement Fluids (RF's):

- RF's do sometimes replace the fluids removed from some patients, but the real job of RF's is to provide the "convection effect" that removes solutes.
- RF's expand the volume and pressure presented to the filter, which
  1. promotes the filtering of large amounts of water, which also
  2. carries unwanted solutes into the filtrate ("solute drag").
- RF's sometimes are also used to maintain the patient's electrolytes.
- If RF's are given "prefilter," they provide a continuous flush for the hemofilter
- Increasing the rate of replacement fluid increases the volume of ultrafiltrate and the clearance of both water and unwanted solutes.
- Unfortunately, pre-filter replacement fluids invalidate post-filter lab samples.

What is Filtered?

- The semipermeable membrane of a hemofilter permits molecules of < 50,000 Daltons in size to pass through.
- Adding Replacement Fluids and/or Dialysate speeds the process.
- Using a high-permeability hemofilter allows the removal of cytokines

Small Molecules	Medium Molecules		Large Molecules	
(all < 200 Daltons)		Daltons	(cannot pass through the filter's membrane)	
Electrolytes	Vitamin B12	1,350		
Glucose	Insulin	6,000		Daltons
Creatinine	Myoglobin	17,000	Albumin	70,000
Uric acid	LMWH	1,000 - 10,000	Dextran 70	70,000
Urea	Heparin	3,000 - 30,000	IgG	150,000

Continuous Renal Replacement Therapies (CRRT)

Fig. 11.2 SCUF

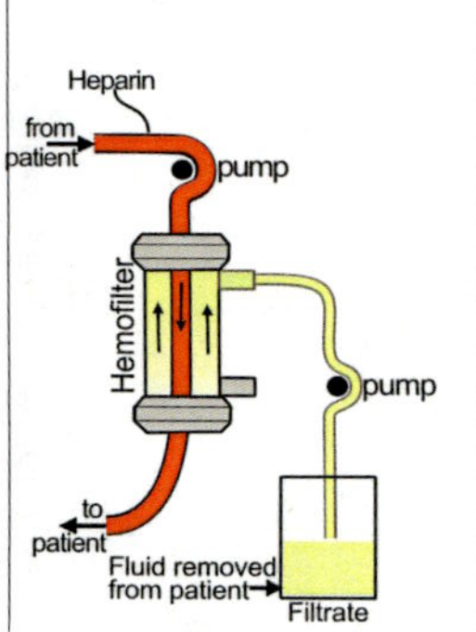

No replacement fluids or dialysate. Solute removal is minimal. For pts with fluid overload, but without uremia or electrolyte imbalance

Blood flow rate:	50 - 200	mL/min
Replace fluids:	0	L/day
Dialysate flow:	0	mL/min
Filtrate flow:	100	mL/hr
Urea clearance:	1.7	mL/min

Fig. 11.3 CVVH

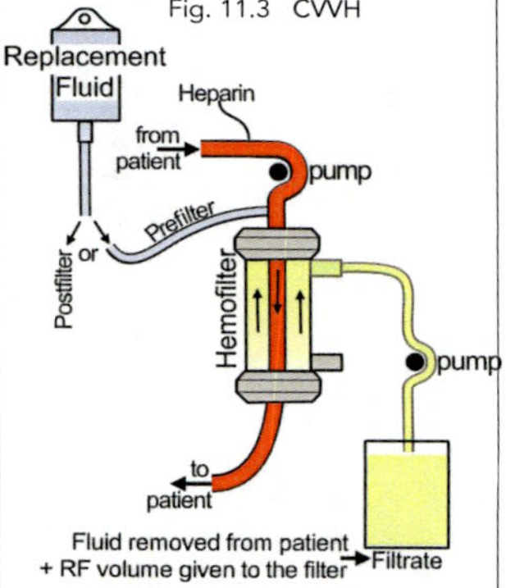

RF convection removes large quantity of solutes while maintaining an even fluid balance in the patient. For uremic patients, with severe pH or electrolyte imbalance.

Blood flow rate:	50 - 200	mL/min
Replace fluids:	21.6	L/day
Dialysate flow:	0	mL/min
Filtrate flow:	1000	mL/hr
Urea clearance:	12 - 36	mL/min

Fig. 11.4 CVVHD

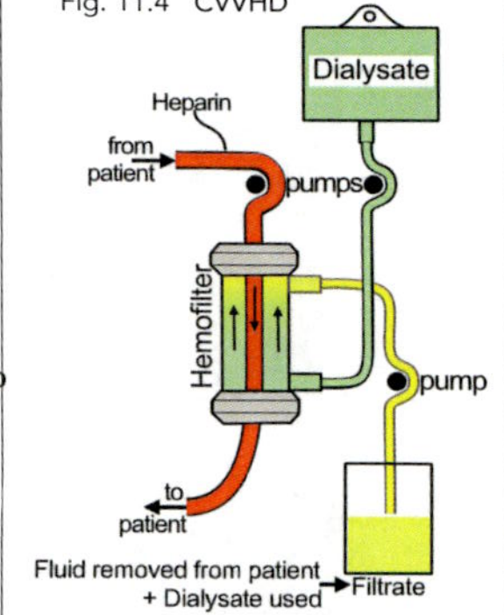

Dialysate uses diffusion to remove small solutes. No RF's -> less volume removal. Used to remove solute; the dialysate is tailored to maintain electrolyte balance.

Blood flow rate:	50 - 200	mL/min
Replace fluids:	0	L/day
Dialysate flow:	10 - 20	mL/min
Filtrate flow:	300	mL/hr
Urea clearance:	14 - 36	mL/min

Fig. 11.5 CVVHDF

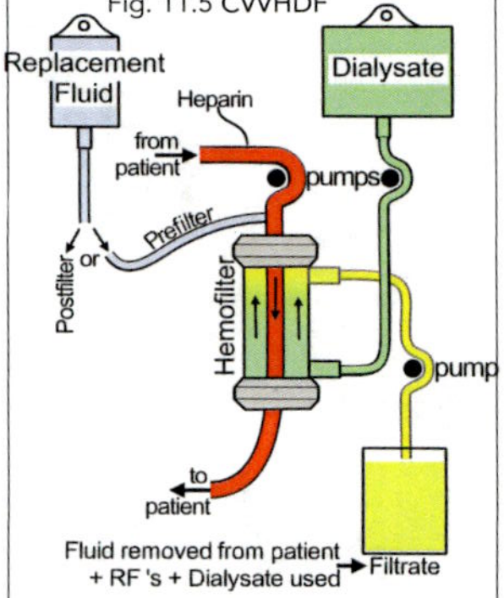

Uses both replacement fluids *and* dialysate to remove small and medium solutes as well as volume, all at a faster rate.

Blood flow rate:	50 - 200	mL/min
Replace fluids:	16.8	L/day
Dialysate flow:	10 - 20	mL/min
Filtrate flow:	800	mL/hr
Urea clearance:	30	mL/min

Continuous Renal Replacement Therapies (CRRT)

Vascular Access:

- Venovenous techniques require 8 Fr. double-lumen, non-tapered venous catheter via subclavian, femoral, or internal jugular (IJ) vein.
- Catheter lifespan in the subclavian or IJ is 7 - 10 days; 5 days for femoral.
- If CRRT suspended, instill Heparin (flush dose) into each lumen, in an amount that just fills the lumen. Every 2 days, remove and replace the Heparin.
- A CRRT control unit to which is connected a hemofilter/tubing cassette system has automated a very labor intensive procedure. However, preparation of the hemofilter, anticoagulant, replacement fluids, dialysate, whether the therapy will be machine-controlled or nurse/patient controlled, is similar.
  1. Connect, prime, and debubble the access line, blood pump line, and the hemofilter with flush solution of 1000 mL NS + Heparin 5000 units.
  2. Connect anticoagulant infusion and replacement fluids.
  3. Connect and prime dialysate line and ultrafiltrate line.
  4. Use strict aseptic technique to connect to vascular access.

CRRT control unit:

- Displays instructions for priming, initiating dialysis, and trouble shooting.
- Loads and primes the set automatically.
- Pumps blood through the blood flow path.
- Delivers anticoagulant into the blood flow path.
- Controls fluid removal from the patient.
- Pumps sterile replacement solution.
- Pumps sterile dialysate and effluent.
- Displays the amount of delivered replacement solution, dialysate used, effluent volume, actual patient fluid removed.
- Monitors the system and alarms in response to procedural problems.

CRRT Control unit alarms:

- Access Pressure Alarm: Access catheter occlusion, kink, malposition
- Return Pressure Alarm: Disconnection, position change, tubing kink or occlusion, clotted access.
- Filter Pressure: Sudden increase indicates filter will be clogged or clotted soon (with 2 hours). Low pressure indicates that blood pump speed is slow.
- Blood Leak Detectors: Blood in the effluent/filtrate indicates leak in the filter. Cease treatment, change filter.
- Air In Line: stops the blood pump if air is detected in the line that returns blood to the patient
- Fluid and Effluent Pump Alarms: sound when fluids are empty or effluent is full, if clamp is left close, bag is improperly spiked.

Anticoagulation vs Hemofilter Life:

- Anticoagulation is not recommended for patients at risk for bleeding:
- Platelets < 50,000, INR > 2, aPTT > 60, Active bleeding or episode of active bleeding in last 24 h, Severe hepatic dysfunction, recent liver transplantation, or cardiopulmonary bypass or ECMO within previous 24 h. In these patients, filter clotting can be prevented by routine flushing with 50 - 100 mL NS q 1 hr.
- In all other patients, Heparin 2500 units IV prior to start, then prefilter infusion of 8 - 10 units/kg/hr, a low dose that sustains life of the filter. 75% of the heparin is removed by the filter, having little effect on the pt's coagulation.
- Systemic UFH is reserved for patients who have other indication for anticoagulation (i.e., DVT, mechanical cardiac valve).
- Citrate given pre-filter is another option. It anticoagulates by binding to Calcium. Requires giving continuous calcium infusion into a central line. Eliminates HITT risk and does not cause systemic anticoagulation. Must monitor Ca levels and titrate CaCl infusion accordingly. Dialysate and replacement fluids must be calcium free. More expensive.
- Regional Heparinization entails pre-filter UFH 1000 units/hr + post-filter Protamine (ratio of Protamine to Heparin is 10:1). Probably effective but side effects of protamine may be prohibitive.
- Filter life of 24 hours can easily be achieved. Most recommend changing filter by 48 hours. At 72 hours, most dialysis units warn against continued use.

Continuous Renal Replacement Therapies (CRRT)

Technical Problems

Clotting of hemofilter:

1. Although blood flow rate > 200 mL/min risks hemolysis, blood flow rate < 100 mL/min risks clotting.
   The ideal blood flow rate is 150 -180 mL/min.
2. If no blood pump is used, blood flow rate through the hemofilter is determined by:
   - Patient's mean arterial pressure (MAP)
   - Catheter length, diameter, patency
   - Blood viscosity
   - Patency of the hollow fibers of the filter
3. Maintain Filtration Fraction (FF) as follows:
   - If replacing fluids pre filter, keep FF < 15 %
   - If replacing fluids post filter, keep FF < 30 %
   - Filtration fraction is the % of plasma water being removed by
   - ultrafiltration. FF should be high enough to provide adequate solute/fluid removal, but not so high as to allow clotting or
   - increased oncotic pressure to impair filter performance.
4. Anticoagulate filter with Heparin or Citrate, given pre-filter, or flush with 100 mL NS q 1 - 2 h at rate of 10 mL/min.

↓ Removal of Plasma Volume:

1. Causes:
   - Ultrafiltration coefficient of the hemofilter
   - ↓ Blood flow rate
   - ↑ Hct, ↑ Intravascular oncotic pressure
   - Clots and protein deposits on the membrane
2. If using gravity to drain UF (no UF pump), UF collection bag must be positioned an adequate distance below the filter. Negative "siphon" effect by the UF collection device is 0.75 mm Hg per cm of distance that the collection device is positioned below the filter. Place collection device 40 cm below the filter.

↓ Removal of Solute:

- Over time, proteins deposits on the membrane -> ↓ permeability.
- Ratio of Filtrate urea nitrogen/Blood urea nitrogen goal is > 0.8
  FUN/BUN = 92/100 = 0.92 -> Continue with current filter
  FUN/BUN = 42/66 = 0.64 -> Replace current filter
- Increase Solute Removal in two ways:
  1. Replacement fluid administered at high flow rate to remove more solute with convective force.
  2. Use of dialysate to create diffusion gradients that prompt solutes to cross the dialyzing membrane and into the effluent. Not uncommon to cause ↓ Na, ↓ Ca, ↓ Mg, ↓ Phos.

Replace filter if:

- The filter is over 72 hours old.
- The trans-membrane pressure is consistently above 250 mm Hg.
- Ultrafiltrate volume is less than 500 mL/hr.
- Urea, creatinine, K levels start to rise. FUN/BUN ration is < 0.65
- Hemofilter is clotted.
- Membrane is leaking (blood is in the filtrate).
- If filter is discontinued without flushing with NS to return RBC's, or if hemofilter is clotted, patient loses about 130 mL of blood.

The Meds: Meds and nutritional support should be infused at a site that is distant from the access port of the dialysis catheter.

Transport:

1. Place CRRT control unit on standby.
2. Clamp both lumens of the patient's access.
3. Disconnect the patient from CRRT/hemofilter system.
4. Cover the access ports with sterile dead-ender caps.
5. In the ICU maintain system with continuous flush until the patient returns.

Stop CRRT when:

- Creatinine clearance is at the least > 20 mL/min.
- BUN and Cr are not rising.
- Patient's urinary output can maintain fluid balance.

Continuous Renal Replacement Therapies (CRRT)

Elements measured in blood	Normal levels in blood	Premixed Dialysates: Gambro Prismasate with Calcium	Premixed Dialysates: Gambro Prismasate Calcium-Free	Premixed Dialysates: NxStage Pureflow (lactate as buffer)	Element weight
Potassium K	3.5 - 5	0	2	2	mEq/L
Calcium Ca	2.3 - 2.6	3.5	0	3	mEq/L
Magnesium Mg	1.4 - 2	1	1	1	mEq/L
Sodium Na	135 - 145	140	140	140	mEq/L
Chloride Cl	100 - 108	109.5	108	110	mEq/L
Bicarbonate HCO_3^-	22 - 26	32	32	0	mEq/L
Lactate	0.5 - 2.2	3	3	45	mEq/L
Dextrose	70 - 110	0	110	100	mg/dL
Osmolarity	280 - 296	287	292	297	mOsm/L

http://www.gambro.com/PageFiles/7980/306100332_1_PrismaSATEBroch-hi.pdf
http://www.nxstage.com/criticalcare/products/fluids

Problems	Causes	Intervention
Hypotension	Removal of too much fluid Hypovolemia Rapid change in electrolytes LV dysfunction Bleeding Sepsis	Frequent assessment of: peripheral pulses, capillary refill, mucous membranes, level of consciousness, HR/rhythm, JVD, CVP, CO, Temp Look for evidence of bleeding. Infuse Normal Saline ASAP, inotrope may be needed.
Bleeding, Blood Loss	From access site, Into the thorax or abdomen, Anticoagulant effect (skin, GI tract, cranium), Accidental disconnect from CRRT blood circuit, Clotted filter (130 mL loss)	Monitor hemodynamics, Hgb/Hct, Frequent physical assessment is imperative, particularly of the access site, all connections, and patient's condition.
Electrolyte Imbalance	Overcorrection of K, NaCL replacement fluids can h Na and Cl, Excess Cl leads to i HCO_3	Closely monitor lab work, Accurate Intake/Output, Discuss plan with the physician.
Hypothermia	Exposure of blood flow to room temperature	Beware CRRT cooling effect may mask fever. Warm the CRRT fluids.
Hyperglycemia	Glucose in the dialysate, Physiologic stress	Blood glucose monitoring.
Acid-Base Imbalance	Poor perfusion, Respiratory acidosis, Electrolyte imbalance	Treatment with bicarb is not recommended until pH < 7.1, Treatment of poor perfusion, Treatment of h pCO_2
Infection	Contamination of invasive lines, catheters, tubes, wounds. Immunosuppression due to renal disease.	Meticulous care of access site. Meticulous skin, mouth, oral, and wound care. Prevention of VAP. Monitor WBC, temperature, heart rate, respiratory rate.
Medication blood levels may ↑ ↓	Particularly antibiotics and anticonvulsants	Consult with clinical pharmacist, especially on meds that do or don't pass through the hemofilter.
Pulmonary edema	Capillary leak syndrome, heart failure, i serum protein Excess fluid replacement	Monitor respiratory status, particularly rate, breath sounds, work of breathing, SpO_2.

Potassium

Normal serum level: 3.5 - 5 mEq/L
Normal daily requirement: 70 - 100 mEq (4.7 g)
Functions of Potassium: The major positive ion inside the cells, responsible for the generation of electrical impulses that power cell function and enable neuromuscular transmission.

	Causes	Signs/Symptoms	Treatment
↓ K	Malnutrition, Diuretics, GI loss: vomiting, diarrhea, suction, Alkalosis, Severe hypoglycemia, Treatment of DKA, Corticosteroids, Prolonged stress, Cushing's disease, Sweating. Symptoms do not occur until K level is ≤ 2.5 mEq/L.	Flat or inverted T, ↓ ST, peaked P, prolonged PR, prominent U, asystole, ventricular arrhythmia, ↓ myocardial contractility, muscles weak -> flaccid -> paralysis -> apnea, weak or absent reflexes, paresthesia, leg cramps, N/V, paralytic ileus, abdominal distention, anorexia, digoxin sensitivity or toxicity.	Cardiac monitoring is required. Alkalosis should be corrected. Underlying cause should identified and managed. Peripheral and Central line administration guides and infusion tables are on the next 2 pages →
↑ K	Excess intake, Cell injury or lysis (rhabdomyolysis, burns, ischemia), Chronic Renal failure, Blood transfusion, GI hemorrhage, Untreated DKA (Insulin deficient), Metabolic acidosis, Addison disease (↓ aldosterone). Symptoms do not occur until K level is ≥ 7 mEq/L.	Tall, peaked T waves, wide QRS, ↓ ST, long PR, flattened P, escape beats, VTach/Fib, ↓ height of R wave, heart block, bradycardia, idioventricular rhythm, asystole when K > 8.5 diastolic cardiac arrest, N/V, diarrhea, ileus, intestinal colic, hyperactive reflexes, weakness, ascending paralysis, respiratory failure.	AHA recommendations: 1. $NaHCO_3$ 50 mEq over 5 minutes 2. Regular Insulin 10 units 3. $D_{50}W$ 1 amp (50 mL) 4. Calcium Chloride 500 - 1000 mg (5 - 10 mL of 10% solution) over 2-5 mins. unless Digoxin toxicity is a possibility, then Magnesium sulfate 2 g over 5 minutes. PO, NG, or per rectum: Kaexylate 15 - 50 g + 20% Sorbitol 100 mL Furosemide 40 - 80 mg IV. Dialysis Off Label: Albuterol 10-20 mg nebulized over 15 minutes

Magnesium

Normal serum level: 1.3 - 2.2 mEq/L
Normal daily requirement: 320 - 420 mg
Functions: Structural element of bone, Catalyzes some enzymatic reactions. Influences Na/K pump.

	Causes	Signs/Symptoms	Treatment
↓ Mg	Malnutrition, GI fluid loss, Pancreatitis, Alcoholism, Burns, Diuretics, DKA.	T wave changes, prolonged QT, PVC's, Torsades de pointes, VFib, anorexia, nausea, tremor, hyperactive reflexes, muscle cramps, tetany, ataxia, seizures, death.	For symptomatic Torsades: $MgSO_4$ 1 - 2 g in 50 - 100 mL D_5W over 30 - 60 mins. For cardiac arrest due to Torsades: $MgSO_4$ 1 - 2 g in 10 mL D_5W over 5 - 20 minutes.
↑ Mg	Renal failure with excess intake of Mg based antacids, Hyperparathy-roidism Acute acidosis.	According to Mg level: 2 - 4: N/V, weakness/fatigue 4 - 5: ↓ deep tendon reflexes 5 - 6: ↓ BP, vasodilation 8 - 10: paralysis, AFib, 1° AVB, ventricular conduction delay, heart block, asystole, stupor, coma, resp. arrest.	Withhold Magnesium. Normal Saline and Furosemide 1 mg/kg, CaCl 10% 500 - 1000 mg slow IV, Glucose + Insulin, Hemodialysis for Mg > 8 mEq/L

Intravenous Potassium

Facts:

- Undiluted Potassium given IV push can be lethal. JCAHCO statement: "No concentrated K^+ vials are ever to leave the pharmacy."
- Premixed Potassium solutions are strongly recommended.
- Potassium infusion requires an infusion pump in order to control infusion rate. Every effort must be made to prevent accidental uncontrolled infusion.
- In general care units, the concentration of K is limited to 30 mEq/1000 mL and the administration rate is limited to 10 mEq/hr.
- In acute care areas, a central line and careful cardiac monitoring allow higher concentrations and faster administration rates.
- Doses must be reduced in patients with renal insufficiency or after cardiac surgery.
- The usual maximum total dose of K in a 24 hour period is 240 mEq.
- However, as much as 400 mEq may be administered in a 24-hour period while monitoring blood electrolyte concentrations.
- Expect serum K^+ to h by about 0.25 mEq/L for each 20 mEq KCl infused.
- Infusion rate > 20 mEq/hr may cause injury to the cardiac conduction system and its use is restricted to patients with serum $K^+ < 2$ <u>and</u> with signs of imminent death.
- The Route of Administration dictates the maximum concentration and the maximum infusion rate allowed, as follows:

Route	Maximum Concentration	Maximum infusion rate	Warnings
Peripheral line	0.1 mEq/mL	10 mEq/hour	Check IV site q 2 - 4 hours.
Central line, in patient with serum K^+ = 2 - 3.5 mEq/L	0.2 mEq/mL	20 mEq/hour	Cardiac monitoring required. See next page.
Central line, in patient with serum **K^+ < 2 mEq/L, death is imminent**	0.4 mEq/mL	40 mEq/hour	Some advise against this concentration and infusion rate. See dosing in "Life-threatening Hypokalemia" on next page. →

Potassium via Peripheral Line

The following 3 mixtures have a concentration of 0.08 mEq/mL:

$\frac{20 \text{ mEq } K^+}{250 \text{ mL D5W or NS}} = 0.08$ mEq/mL

$\frac{40 \text{ mEq } K^+}{500 \text{ mL D5W or NS}} = 0.08$ mEq/mL

$\frac{80 \text{ mEq } K^+}{1000 \text{ mL D5W or NS}} = 0.08$ mEq/mL

Dosing table for 0.08 mEq/mL:

Dose mEq/hr	Infusion rate mL/hr
2	25
4	50
6	75
8	100
10	125

The following 2 mixtures have a concentration of 0.1 mEq/mL:

$\frac{10 \text{ mEq } K^+}{100 \text{ mL D5W or NS}} = 0.1$ mEq/mL

$\frac{20 \text{ mEq } K^+}{200 \text{ mL D5W or NS}} = 0.1$ mEq/mL

Dosing table for 0.1 mEq/mL:

Dose mEq/hr	Infusion rate mL/hr
2	20
4	40
6	60
8	80
10	100

Maximum <u>concentration</u> for a peripheral line: **0.1 mEq/mL**
Maximum administration <u>rate</u> into a peripheral line: **10 mEq/hr**

Potassium Via Central Line

Maximum concentration for a central line in a nonemergency: 0.2 mEq/mL
Maximum administration rate into a central line in a nonemergency: 20 mEq/hr
Careful ECG Monitoring is required.

Each of the following 3 mixtures have a concentration of 0.2 mEq/mL:

$\frac{10 \text{ mEq } K^+}{50 \text{ mL D5W or NS}}$ = 0.2 mEq/mL
(premixed)

$\frac{20 \text{ mEq } K^+}{200 \text{ mL D5W or NS}}$ = 0.2 mEq/mL
(premixed)

$\frac{40 \text{ mEq } K^+}{200 \text{ mL D5W or NS}}$ = 0.2 mEq/mL

Dose, mEq/hr	Infusion rate, mL/hr
4	20
6	30
8	40
10	50
12	60
20	100
22	110
24	120

(Shaded:) Dangerous dose and infusion rate

This infusion table can be used to select the infusion rate according to the desired dose, or to identify the dose according to the current infusion rate.

Potassium via Central Line
for Life Threatening Hypokalemia

1. the patient's K is < 2 mEq/L, and
2. there are ECG changes, and/or
3. there is muscle paralysis, and/or
4. cardiac arrest is believed to be imminent.

Maximum concentration for a central line in an emergency: 0.4 mEq/mL
Maximum administration rate into a central line in an emergency: 40 mEq/hr
Infusion of > 20 mEq/hr may cause injury to the cardiac conduction system.
Some advise against this concentration and this administration rate.
ECG Monitoring is required. Physician must be in attendance.

Each of the following 3 mixtures have a concentration of 0.4 mEq/mL:

$\frac{10 \text{ mEq } K^+}{25 \text{ mL D5W or NS}}$ = 0.4 mEq/mL

$\frac{20 \text{ mEq } K^+}{50 \text{ mL D5W or NS}}$ = 0.4 mEq/mL
(premixed)

$\frac{40 \text{ mEq } K^+}{100 \text{ mL D5W or NS}}$ = 0.4 mEq/mL

Dose, mEq/hr	Infusion rate, mL/hr
10	25
12	30
14	35
16	40
18	45
20	50
22	55

(Shaded:) Dangerous dose and infusion rate

This infusion table can be used to select the infusion rate according to the desired dose, or to identify the dose according to the current infusion rate.

Sodium

Normal serum level: 135 - 145 mEq/L
Normal daily intake: 2 - 3 g (2.4 g = 1 teaspoon salt)
Functions of Sodium: As the major extracellular cation, sodium maintains extracellular volume.
Serum sodium determines the osmolality of blood.
Generation of electrical impulses.
Regulation of acid-base balance.

	Causes	Signs/Symptoms	Treatment
↓ Na	Mild: 130-135 mEq/L Mod: 120-129 mEq/L Severe: < 120 mEq/L Na loss due to Vomiting, Diarrhea, GI suction, SIADH. Draining fistulas, Nephritis, Thiazide diuretics, Na dilution due to Hypotonic fluids, water excess in CHF, cirrhosis, nephrotic syndrome	Signs of either ECF deficit (dry membranes, ↑ HR) or excess (peripheral edema). urine specific gravity < 1.0 HA, confusion, lethargy, nausea, muscle cramps, hyperactive reflexes, disorientation, malaise, seizures, coma, signs of cerebral edema and ↑ ICP leading to brainstem herniation, respiratory arrest, and death.	NaCl 0.9% unless *severe symptoms*, then use 3% NaCl to ↑ serum Na by 4 - 6 mEq/L in 1 - 2 hr. Then raise serum Na no faster than 0.5 mEq/hr or 12 mEq/day (given too fast, can cause cerebral pontine myelinolysis, or severe damage to the myelin sheath). Vasopressin is given for dilutional hyponatremia.
↑ Na	Hypernatremia is usually caused by 1. dehydration due to impaired access to water, or 2. water loss (severe watery diarrhea, sweating, diabetes insipidus), or 3. excess Na intake (such as ingestion of sea water)	Hypernatremia produces cellular dehydration (particularly in the brain). Extreme thirst, fever, flushed skin, restlessness, irritability, delirium, lethargy, stupor, coma, spasticity, seizures, dry/sticky mucous membranes, weakness	Treatment must be careful. Rapid change in serum osmolality may cause cerebral edema, seizures, coma, death. Mortality rate is > 50%. D5 1/2NS (which contains 77 mEq/L of sodium) may be given. Correct the serum Na no faster than 1 mEq/hr.

Chloride

Normal serum level: 98 - 108 mEq/L
Normal daily requirement: 80 - 120 mEq/day
Functions: Chloride is the body's most abundant negative ion.
Chloride moves in and out of cells opposite the movement of positive electrolytes (Na and K).
Hydrogen and Chloride form hydrochloric acid (gastric acid).
Cl maintains acid/base balance by exchanging with HCO_3.
Chloride enables RBC's to transport CO_2 away from tissues.

	Causes	Signs/Symptoms	Treatment
↓ Cl	Prolonged vomiting or GI suction (which causes loss of HCL), or pt has history of water excess (which causes dilution of the chloride in blood), or loss of salt due to excessive sweating.	Metabolic alkalosis, compensatory respiratory acidosis (shallow, slowed breathing), muscle excitability, hyperirritability, tetany, hypotension due to fluid loss.	Treatment of the cause. Fluids that contain sodium chloride and potassium chloride. Ammonium chloride may be used EXCEPT for patients with liver disease or liver failure.
↑ Cl	Dehydration, Renal failure, Salicylate intoxication, Diabetes insipidus, Diuretics, Overactive parathyroid gland, Excessive infusion of hypertonic saline.	Metabolic acidosis leading to respiratory alkalosis (deep, rapid Kussmaul breathing) Weakness, lethargy diminished cognitive ability, progressing to coma.	For metabolic acidosis, infusion of bicarbonate, acetate, citrate, or phosphate instead of NaCl. (Normal Saline contains Chloride 154 mEq/L and Sodium 154 mEq/L).

Calcium

Normal total calcium: 9 - 10.5 mg/dL (2.2 - 2.6 mmol/L)
Normal ionized calcium: 4.5 - 5.6 mg/dL (1.1 - 1.4 mmol/L)
The narrow range of calcium in the blood is maintained by parathyroid hormone (calcitonin).
Normal daily requirement: 1000 - 1200 mg
Functions: Bone formation, Blood coagulation, Cell membrane integrity, Muscle and nerve function, Major role in the regulation of heart contractility and rhythm, and SA node automaticity.
Antagonizes K and Mg.

	Causes	Signs/Symptoms	Treatment
↓ Ca	Ionized calcium level < 4.4 mg/dL (or < 1.1 mmol/L), should prompt a search for the possible cause: Blood transfusion, Pancreatitis, Renal failure, Hypoparathyroidism, Damage or removal of parathyroid glands during thyroid surgery Soft tissue infection, Sepsis/Septic shock, Intestinal or pancreatic fistula, Respiratory Alkalosis. ↑ phosphorus, ↑ magnesium, Malabsorption	Symptoms occur when ionized Calcium is < 2.5 mg/dL (<0.8 mmol/L). **Neuro:** tingling in the fingers/toes, carpopedal spasms, hyperactive reflexes, paresthesias, muscle cramps, tetany, twitching, seizures. **Cardiovascular:** long QT and ST segments on ECG, heart block, heart failure, ↓ HR, ↓ BP. Hematologic: prolonged clotting time, bleeding. **Resp:** prolonged contraction of the respiratory and laryngeal muscles (bronchospasm) causes stridor, cyanosis.	Seizure precautions, Airway precautions, 1 - 3 g Calcium Gluconate in 100 mL D5W, given no faster than 50 mg/min., or 1 g Calcium Chloride in 100 mL D5W, given no faster 50 mg/min. (too fast → N/V, ↓ HR, Heart block, ↑ BP, chest pain).
↑ Ca	Acidosis, Malignancy, Vitamin A and D intoxication, ↓ renal excretion, Immobility, Thyrotoxicosis, Hyperparathyroidism, Adrenal insufficiency Renal transplantation, Thiazide diuretics.	Hypoactive reflexes, confusion, memory loss, stupor, coma. Shortened QT, Prolonged PR and QRS, bradycardia, ↑ BP, weakness, fatigue, anorexia, nausea, vomiting, constipation, hypoactive reflexes, ↓ K, ↓ Mg, ↓ Na,	Correct underlying cause. NaCl 3 - 5 L in 24 hr, to achieve urinary output 200 - 300 mL/hr. K and Mg supplements. Oral phosphates if serum Phos < 1.2 mmol/L.

Phosphorus

Normal serum level: 2.4 - 4.1 mg/dL (0.8 - 1.4 mmol/L)
Normal daily requirement: 800 - 1200 mg
Functions: Formation of ATP, Acid-base buffer, Component of neuronal myelin sheath, Required for protein synthesis, fluid balance.
Major component of bone, teeth, and cell structure.

	Causes	Signs/Symptoms	Treatment
↓ Phos	Malnutrition, alcohol abuse (i absorption), Hyperparathyroidism, Renal dysfunction, Respiratory alkalosis. Diabetic ketoacidosis.	Confusion, lethargy, muscle weakness. difficulty weaning from ventilator, anemia, paresthesias, heart failure.	Potassium Phosphate given via central line: 12 mmol over 1 hr, or 24 mmol over 6 hr, or 36 mmol over 8 hr. Beware of causing hypocalcemia.
↑ Phos	Kidney disease, High intake of Phos without adequate intake of Calcium.	Diarrhea, calcification of organs and soft tissue, hypocalcemia with tetany or seizures.	Balance the intake of phosphorus and calcium. (excess Phos without Ca leads to osteoporosis)

Adrenal Insufficiency and Adrenal Crisis

Normal control of the adrenal cortex:

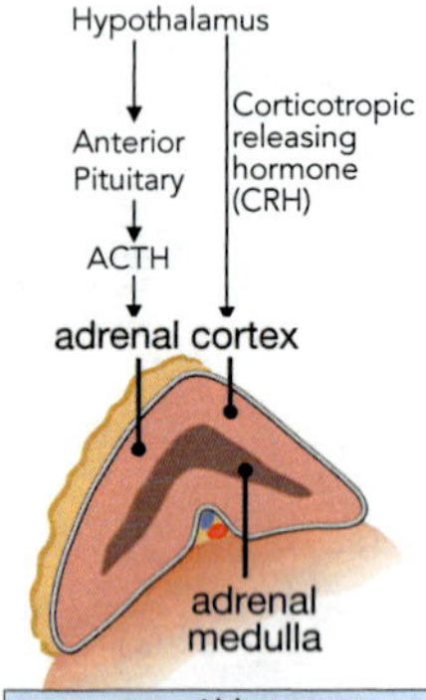

Description:

- Deficiency of glucocorticoid and aldosterone, that culminates in hypovolemia with shock, hyponatremia, hypoglycemia, coma.
- Reported incidence in critically ill patients is 0 - 28%, but may be as high as 50 - 75% in patients with septic shock. Can easily be missed or misdiagnosed.
- Primary Adrenal Insufficiency: (aka Addison disease) is caused by injury to the adrenal cortex due to sepsis, autoimmune disease, cancer, adrenal hemorrhage, medications.
- Secondary Adrenal Insufficiency is caused by
  1. Disease of the hypothalamus or pituitary
     or
  2. Steroid suppression of the HPA axis, (hypothalamus, pituitary, adrenal gland) and then abrupt discontinuation of that therapy
     or
  3. Stress in the patient on high-dose steroid

Aldosterone	Glucocorticoid
Normally, the adrenal cortex releases aldosterone in response to sympathetic discharge, decreased renal perfusion, or decreased serum Na. The function of Aldosterone is to reabsorb Na and H_2O. For each Na ion reabsorbed, either Cl or HCO_3 is also absorbed.	Cortisol promotes tissue breakdown (catabolism) to form amino acids, and increases liver gluconeogenesis and glycogenolysis to maintain blood sugar. Mobilizes fat from adipose tissue, and increases extracellular fluid volume. Sensitizes blood vessels to vasopressors. Suppresses the immune response.
Without sufficient aldosterone, the excretion of Na and H_2O is increased, causing hypovolemia & hyponatremia. Reduced excretion of K^+ results in hyperkalemia. The rise in K^+ promotes reabsorption of H^+, causing acidosis.	Decreased cortisol impairs the regulation of glucose (causing hypoglycemia), impairs the ability to maintain circulatory blood volume, and impairs the control of the inflammatory response.

Signs:

- Neuro: Weakness, malaise, fatigue, confusion, psychosis.
- CV: ↑ HR, ↓ CO, orthostatic hypotension, hypovolemia, ↓ BP refractory to catecholamine or volume.
- GI: Nausea, vomiting, diarrhea or constipation, anorexia, abdominal pain, weight loss.
- Other:Arthralgias, hyperpigmentation of tongue, palms, and scars.
- Lab: ↓ Na, ↑ K, ↑ Ca, ↓ BG, ↓ HCO_3, ↓ pH, ↓ H/H, ↑ BUN.

Cortisol level: Normal diurnal pattern (lowest concentrations 10 pm - 2 am, highest levels at about 8 am) is lost in stressed, critically ill pts.

Treatment:

- D5NS, to protect blood glucose and to volume replace.
- If hemodynamically unstable, spot cortisol is drawn. If < 15 mcg/dL, Dexamethasone 1 - 4 mg IV may be given. (It does not interfere with subsequent ACTH stimulation test and can be life saving while awaiting lab results).
- If cortisol = 15 - 34 μg/dL, cosyntropin (synthetic ACTH) 250 mcg (some recommend a lower dose) is given IV and cortisol rechecked in 30 minutes and in 1 hour.
- If serum cortisol does not increase by at least 9 μg/dL, Hydrocortisone 50 - 100 mg IV q 6 - 8 hour is started (patients who have been on steroid therapy chronically may need reduced dose). Should see better BP within 6 hours, but may need vasopressor support until then.
- Fludrocortisone 0.05 - 0.2 mg (a mineralocorticoid) may be added (Hydrocortisone has some mineralocorticoid effect).

Diabetic Ketoacidosis

Description:
- Most often precipitated by infection, stress, or noncompliance with the insulin and dietary regimen.
- DKA is a syndrome of hyperglycemia, dehydration, acidosis, ketogenesis, and severe electrolyte abnormalities.
- Mortality rate 4 - 10% with treatment; 100% if left untreated.

Pathophysiology:
- Insulin deficiency prevents the uptake of glucose by the muscle, fat, and liver. This shifts metabolism away from carbohydrate and to the metabolism of fat (lipolysis).
- The ketone products of lipolysis cause metabolic acidosis.
- Hepatic ketogenesis contributes further to the acidosis.
- Accumulating H ions move into the cells, causing K to move out of the cells, resulting in a temporary increase in serum K. But total body K deficit may exceed 3 - 5 mEq/kg.
- The hyperglycemia causes osmotic diuresis, whereby the kidneys remove sodium, potassium, phosphates, water.
- Hyperglycemia also shifts fluid from the intracellular to the intravascular space, causing dilutional hyponatremia.
- DKA patients often have a fluid deficit of 5 - 10 L.
- Hepatic gluconeogenesis and glycogenolysis infuse the blood with more glucose. Blood glucose rises to > 250 mg/dL.
- Serum sodium falls about 1.6 - 2.4 mEq/L for every 100 mg/dL of glucose elevation above the normal levels.
- The fluid and electrolyte deficits may be life-threatening.
- During treatment, serum K can drop precipitously with insulin treatment and with the dilutional effects of fluid management.
- Treatment that reduces BG will cause serum sodium to rise.
- Too rapid fluid administration can cause intracellular fluid shift that can result in cerebral edema (high mortality in kids).
- Protein breakdown (catabolism) -> increased urea production.

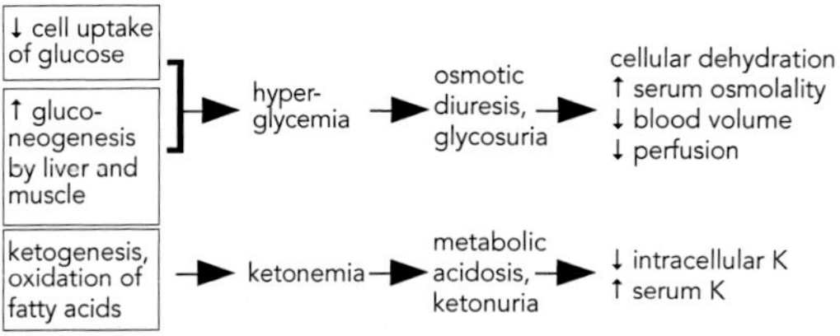

Signs and Symptoms:
Thirst, polydipsia
Polyuria, nocturia, dysuria
Anorexia, nausea, vomiting
Weakness, malaise, lethargy, fatigue
Confusion, decreased reflexes, unresponsiveness
Hypotension, tachycardia
Poor skin turgor, dry skin, dry mucous membranes
Shortness of breath, tachypnea, ketone breath
Kussmaul respiration, unless severe acidosis depresses the CNS
Chest pain, abdominal pain (sometimes severe)
Signs of infection, fever, chills

Lab:
Blood glucose > 250 mg/dL
pH < 7.3, HCO_3 < 18 mEq/L
ketonemia, ketonuria, glycosuria
↓ Na to start, ↑ Na with treatment
↑ K to start, ↓ K with treatment

Ketone tests:
Ketone dipsticks are great screening tools for DKA, but do not measure the more common ketone, beta-hydroxybutyrate.
Lab test for beta-hydroxybutyrate is available.

Diabetic Ketoacidosis Treatment

Fluids First:
- 0.9% NaCL 15-20 mL/kg (1-2 L) should be given in the first hr.
- 4 - 8 L fluid may be necessary during the first 24 hours.

Fluid benefits:
- Hemodilutes the hyperglycemic state.
- Improves excretion of glucose and ketones.
- Reduces the stress response.

Insulin:
Loading dose (considered optional by some) of Regular insulin 0.15 units/kg IV push (10 U), then Continuous infusion:

$$\frac{\text{100 units regular insulin}}{\text{100 mL of 0.9\% NaCL}} = \text{1 unit/mL}$$

Dose: 0.1 unit/kg/hr or about 5 - 7 units/hr

Insulin: Transports glucose into cells
Converts glucose to glycogen in liver and muscle
Converts fatty acids to triglycerides

Expect BG to fall 50 - 75 mg each hr that insulin is given

Potassium:
- Serum K will fall significantly due to fluids, glucose, insulin.
- When K falls to < 5 mEq/L, K should be added to the fluids:
  If K = 4 - 5 mEq: 20 mEq should be added to each Liter
  If K = 3 - 4 mEq: 40 mEq should be added to each Liter
  If K < 3, hold all insulin, continue fluids, and give 10 - 20 mEq K per hour. When K > 3.5 mEq/L , it is safe to resume insulin.

Sodium:
- As K moves back into the cells, Na moves out of the cells.
- Expect significant increase in Serum Na. If Na > 150 mEq, should switch from NS 0.9% to NS 0.45%

Magnesium: Low Mg decreases cellular uptake of K. Restore Mg if low.

BG:
- Monitor blood glucose (BG) q 1 hour.
- Goal is to reduce BG by 50 - 75 mg/dL each hr insulin is given.
- When BG falls to 200 mg/dL, dextrose should be added to the IV fluids. The BG goal is 150 - 200 mg

When Na, K, HCO3, pH normalize:
- Subcutaneous insulin may be started, and 1 - 2 hours later insulin infusion can be weaned.
- Remain vigilant monitoring the anion gap.

If serum Na > 150 mEq/L, switch to NaCl 0.45%
If serum Na is low, continue with NaCL 0.9%

NS vs 1/2 NS:

Normal Saline 0.9%	Half Normal Saline 0.45%
pH = 5 Na = 154 mEq/L Cl = 154 mEq/L 300 mOsm/L (equivalent to 1.6 teaspoon of salt in 1 L	pH = 4.5 Na = 77 mEq/L Cl = 77 mEq/L 154 mOsm/L (equivalent to 0.8 teaspoon of salt in 1 L)

Treatment Hazards:
- Pass into hypoglycemia without regaining consciousness.
- Slide rapidly from hyperkalemia to hypokalemia
- Fluids move into hypertonic brain cells -> cerebral edema
- Interrupt Kussmaul breathing with mechanical ventilation. Without respiratory alkalosis, metabolic acidosis -> ↓↓ pH.
- Vomiting in presence of ↓ LOC can result in aspiration pneumonia and/or ARDS.

Insulin Type	Insulin Preparation	Onset (hours)	Peak (hours)	Duration (hours)
Rapid acting:	Humalog (Lispro)	0.25 - 0.5	0.5 - 1.5	3 - 5
Short acting	Regular (Humulin R)	0.5	2 - 5	5 - 8
Intermediate	NPH (Humulin N) Lente (Humulin L)	1 - 2 1 - 2.5	4 - 12 3 - 10	18 - 24 18 - 24
Long acting:	Ultralente	0.5 - 3	10 - 20	20 - 36

Kerr J, Moore M, Frank D, Gujral Rashmeet. Management of diabetic ketoacidosis and other hyperglycemic emergencies. SCCM Crit Connections, Dec/Jan 2013,11(6)16-17

Hyperthyroidism and Thyrotoxicosis (Storm)

Definition: Excess secretion of thyroid hormone, producing a hypermetabolic state, that carries an overall mortality rate of 10%. Thryrotoxicosis (Thyroid storm) is an exaggerated form that can kill in < 2 hrs.

Patho-physiology:

- The hypothalamus releases TRH (thyrotropin releasing hormone).
- In response, the anterior pituitary releases TSH (thyroid stimulating hormone) which stimulates thyroid secretion.
- The thyroid secretes thyroxin (T4), triiodothyronine (T3), and thyroid hormone (90% T4 + 10 % T3) (all contain iodine), and Calcitonin. Elevation in Thyroid hormones causes ↓ TSH (Normal TSH = 0.4 - 4.8 μIU/mL).
- T3 & T4 increase metabolic rate and oxygen consumption, resulting in increased production of CO_2 and heat.
- Protein synthesis and protein catabolism are increased.
- Carbohydrate, lipid metabolism, growth rate are accelerated.
- Sensitivity to catecholamine is heightened.

	Causes	Signs and Symptoms
Hyper-thyroidism:	Graves disease Toxic goiter Thyroid carcinoma Thyroid adenoma Thyroiditis Amiodarone (up to 10 % of patients)	Tremors, restlessness, insomnia, emotional lability, nervous, anxious, sweating, flushing (to dissipate heat). Thyroid bruit. Heat intolerance. ↓ SVR, ↑ HR, ↑ SV, ↑CO, tachypnea weight loss, ↑ appetite, exophthalmia. total body loss of Ca and Phos.
	Precipitating Factors	**Signs and Symptoms**
Thyroid Storm:	Infection Stress Thyroid ablation Surgery/trauma Metabolic crisis (e.g., DKA)	Nausea, vomiting, diarrhea, progressive agitation, irritability, delirium, stupor, coma, seizures, pronounced HR ↑, PAT, SVT, A Fib, systolic murmur, palpitations, hypertension, pulmonary edema, ventricular hypertrophy, heart failure, Fever (39° - 41° C), dyspnea, diaphoresis (as much as 4 L/day), hypoglycemia (ominous sign). TSH < 0.1 μIU/mL.

Treatment of Thyrotoxicosis (Storm)

Problem	Rx Strategy	Treatment
Dysrhythmias and ↑ BP	β-blockers to ↓ adrenergic activity	Caution giving β-blocker if there is heart failure. Propranolol 0.5 - 1 mg IVP (may repeat) or Esmolol (short-acting and easy to titrate) 500 mcg/kg over 1 min, then 50-100 mcg/kg/min
Fever	Antipyretics	Tylenol po or suppository. (No ASA - it may ↑ T3 levels) Cooling blankets, Core temp monitoring.
Hypovolemia	IV fluids	D5NS to replace fluids lost by sweating, vomiting, diarrhea. The dextrose prevents and treats hypoglycemia.
Excess Thyroid hormone	Inhibit T4 synthesis	Methimazole 80 mg, then 40 - 80 mg po q 12 h. Propylthiouracil (PTU) only for patients who cannot take Methimazole.
	Inhibit thyroid production	Hydrocortisone 100 mg q 8 h or Dexamethasone 2 mg q 6 h.
	Block release of thyroid hormone	Telapague (iopanoic acid) 1 g orally q d, or SSKI 1 - 5 drops orally q 8 h, or Lithium 800 - 1200 mg orally q d.
	Remove thyroid hormone	Dialysis, Plasmapheresis Radioactive iodine to ↓ thyroid size/activity

Hypothyroidism

Description: Deficiency of thyroid hormone, resulting in hypometabolism. If left untreated, myxedema coma may lead to fatal hypotension. Primary hypothyroidism: failure or loss of the thyroid gland. Autoimmune disease is the most common cause. Other causes include inadequate dietary iodine, surgical removal, radio-iodine ablation, drug induced (Amiodarone, Lithium, α-interferon). Secondary hypothyroidism: caused by pituitary insufficiency. Even with early diagnosis and treatment, myxedema coma mortality rate is as high as 60%, due to AMI, arrhythmia.

Assessment:	Hypothyroidism	Myxedema Coma
Face	Facial bloating	Periorbital edema
Neuro	Fatigue, Weakness Slowed mentation Muscle cramps Personality change	Psychosis ("myxedema madness") ↓ cerebral blood flow, stupor Seizures (occur in 25 - 50% of patients) Obtundation, Coma.
CV	Bradycardia Hypertension	Pericardial effusion (in 1/3 of patients) ↓ HR, ↓ SV, ↓ CO, ↑ SVR, ↓↑ BP, Rarely, dilated cardiomyopathy
ECG	Bradycardia, 1° AVB Low voltage QRS	Flat or inverted T, low voltage, AV Block, Prolonged QT or PR
Resp	Deep, husky voice	Hypoventilation due to: ↓ respiratory muscle function, ↓ RR, ↓ response to PO_2 and PCO_2.
GI	Constipation	Ileus, Megacolon, GI Bleeding
Renal	Nonpitting edema Normal BUN/Cr	Dilutional hyponatremia (occurs in 50% of patients). Hypoglycemia.
Metabolic	Cold intolerance Cool, dry skin	Temp < 32° C in 75% of pts. Fall in temp is progressive, to as low as 24° C.
Precipitating Factors:	Pulmonary or urinary infection, cold stress, stroke, trauma, surgery, CHF, sedatives, antidepressants, tranquilizers, narcotics, hypovolemia due to bleeding or excess diuretic.	
Lab:	↑ TSH (> 20 μIU/mL), ↓ T4, ↓ T3, anemia, Iron and B12 deficiency	

Treatment of Myxedema Coma:	
Hypothermia:	*Passive* rewarming with blankets. (Active rewarming with hyperthermia units can cause vasodilation, shock, CV collapse). Warm no faster than 0.5° C per hour. If temp < 28° C, VFib is the major threat.
Hypoventilation:	Early intubation and mechanical ventilation.
Adrenal insufficiency:	5 - 10% have coexisting adrenal insufficiency. Hydrocortisone 100 mg IV q 8 h.
Give Thyroid:	Levothyroxine (LT4) 200 - 300 mcg IV bolus. May repeat to total of 500 mcg in first 24 h. then 50 - 100 mcg q 24 hours until stable. or Liothyronine 12.5 mcg IV q 6 h. Monitor for cardiac ischemia and arrhythmia.
Hypoglycemia:	Check BG q 4 hrs. IV fluids containing dextrose may be needed.
Decreased Na:	The hyponatremia is dilutional. Fluids and free water must be restricted. Hypertonic saline is given for severe hyponatremia.
Decreased BP:	$D_{10}NS_{0.45}$ (or $D_{10}NS$ if Na low). Within 6 - 36 hrs of receiving thyroid hormone, BP and temp rise, mentation improves.
Medications:	Hypometabolism slows the elimination of medications. It may be necessary to moderate the dosages.

Lab/IVs/Bld

Lab/IVs/Bld

Chemistry

LAB	Conventional Units		SI Units*	
Albumin	3.5 - 5	g/dL	33 - 50	g/L
Alkaline phosphatase	40 - 120	U/L	40 - 120	U/L
ALT, SGPT	1 - 45	U/L	1 - 45	U/L
AST, SGOT	1 - 36	U/L	1 - 36	U/L
Ammonia	10 - 50	μmol/L	10 - 50	μmol/L
Amylase	25 - 125	U/L	25 - 125	U/L
Anion gap	8 - 16	mEq/L	8 - 16	mmol/L
Bilirubin, conjugated	< 0.4	mg/dL	≤ 7	μmol/L
Bilirubin, total	0.1 - 1.3	mg/dL	2 - 18	μmol/L
BUN	10 - 25	mg/dL	3 - 9	mmol/L
Calcium	8.5 - 10.5	mg/dL	2.1 - 2.65	mmol/L
Calcium, ionized	4.25 - 5.25	mg/dL	1.1 - 1.3	mmol/L
Carbon dioxide (CO_2)	22 - 32	mEq/L	22 - 32	mmol/L
Chloride	98 - 108	mEq/L	98 - 108	mmol/L
Cholesterol	< 200	mg/dL	-	-
HDL cholesterol	< 50	mg/dL	-	-
LDL cholesterol	< 100	mg/dL	-	-
Cortisol 8 AM:	4 - 22	μg/dL	110 - 607	nmol/L
4 PM:	3 - 16	μg/dL	80 - 469	nmol/L
10 PM:	< 50%	of AM val	< 50 % of AM value	
C-reactive protein	negative		negative	mmol/L
Creatine (M)	0.2 - 0.5	mg/dL	15 - 40	μmol/L
(F)	0.3 - 0.9	mg/dL	25 - 70	μmol/L
Creatine kinase (M)	55 - 170	U/L	55 - 170	U/L
(CK, CPK) (F)	30 - 135	U/L	30 - 135	U/L
Creatinine, serum	0.7 - 1.4	mg/dL	50 - 110	μmol/L
Folate	2 - 9	ng/mL	4.5 - 20.4	nmol/L
Glucose	70 - 115	mg/dL	3.9 - 6.1	nmol/L
GGT	5 - 40	U/L	5 - 40	U/L
Iron, serum	25 - 170	μg/dL	4 - 30	μmol/L
Iron binding capacity	240 - 410	μg/dL	45 - 73	μmol/L
Lactic acid	9 - 16	mg/dL	1 - 1.8	mmol/L
LDH	110 - 220	U/L	110 - 220	U/L
Lipase	7 - 60	U/L	0.12- 1	U/L
Magnesium	1.5 - 2.5	mg/dL	0.75 - 1.2	mmol/L
Osmolality, serum	275 - 305	mOsm/kg	275 - 305	mOsm/kg
Phosphorus (Adult)	2.5 - 4.5	mg/dL	0.8 - 1.45	mmol/L
Potassium	3.5 - 5	mEq/L	3.5 - 5	mmol/L
Protein, total	6 - 8.5	g/dL	60 - 85	g/L
Pyruvate	0.3 - 0.9	mg/dL	0.03 - 0.09	mmol/L
Sodium	135 - 145	mEq/L	135 - 145	mmol/L
T3 (Triiodothyronine)	70 - 190	ng/dL	1 - 2.9	nmol/L
T4 (Tyroxine)	5 - 12	μg/dL	58 - 154	nmol/L
Thyroglobulin	3 - 42	μ/mL	3 - 42	μg/L
TSH	0.4 - 4.8	μIU/mL	0.4 - 4.8	mIU/L
Transferrin	188 - 341	mg/dL	1.88 - 3.41	g/L
Triglycerides	40 - 150	mg/dL	2.26	mmol/L
Uric acid (M)	4 - 8.5	mg/dL	238 - 506	μmol/L
(F)	2.5 - 7.5	mg/dL	149 - 446	μmol/L

*Systeme Internationale Units

Cardiac Biomarkers	Description	Time from CP onset	Test result on admit is	Repeat test is	Implication
hs-cTnI	Better test for pts who present < 3 h from CP onset	< 3 h	< 5 ng/L 0.5-26 ng/L > 26 ng/L	< 3 ng/L elevated elevated	May rule out AMI Suspicious Risk for MI/death
hs-cTnT	Better test for pts who present > 3 h	> 3 h	≤14 ng/L ≥ 52 ng/L	< 3 ng/L ↑ ≥ 5 ng/L	May rule out AMI Probable AMI
CK-MB	A marker of myocardial cell death.	> 4 - 5 h	> 5 mcg/L	elevated	Peak: in 12 - 24 h Possible AMI
Myoglobin	Early onset. But may be zero if pt delays care > 1 d.	1 - 2 h	>100 mcg/L	NA	Peak: in 8 - 12 h Consider AMI Normal in: 24 h

Lab

Hematology

Hematology		Conventional Units		SI Units*	
RBC	(M)	4.6 - 6.2	million/mm^3	4.6 - 6.2	x 10^{12}/L
	(F)	4.2 - 5.4	million/mm^3	4.2 - 5.4	x 10^{12}/L
MCH		26 - 34	pg/cell	26 - 34	pg/cell
MCHC		32 - 36	g/dL	320 - 360	g/L
MCV		80 - 96	µm^3	80 - 96	fL
Hgb	(M)	13 - 18	g/dL	8.1 - 11.2	mmol/L
	(F)	12 - 16	g/dL	7.4 - 9.9	mmol/L
Hct	(M)	39 - 50	mL/dL	0.40 - 0.54	
	(F)	36 - 44	mL/dL	0.37 - 0.47	
Methemoglobin		30 - 130	mg/dL	19 - 80	µmol/L
Sedimentation rate		0 - 15	mm/hr	--	
WBC		4.5 - 11	thousand/mm^3	4.5 - 11	x 10^9/L
Neutrophils		52 - 62	%	3000 - 5800	x 10^6/L
Bands		3 - 5	%	150 - 400	x 10^6/L
Eosinophils		1 - 3	%	50 - 250	x 10^6/L
Basophils		0 - 1	%	15 - 50	x 10^6/L
Lymphocytes		25 - 33	%	1500 - 3000	x 10^6/L
Monocytes		3 - 7	%	300 - 500	x 10^6/L
Platelets		150 - 350	thousand/mm^3	150 - 350	x 10^6/L
PT		12 - 14	seconds	12 - 14	seconds
aPTT		20 - 35	seconds	20 - 35	seconds
FSP (FDP)		< 10	µg/mL	< 10	mg/L
d-dimer		< 250	µg/L	< 250	µg/L
INR		< 2		--	
Fibrinogen		200 - 400	mg/dL	2 - 4	g/L
Bleeding time		2 - 8	minutes	2 - 8	minutes
ACT		90 -150	seconds	--	

*Systeme Internationale Units

Drug Levels

Medication	Therapeutic Level		Toxic Level	
Acetaminophen	10 - 20	µg/mL	> 250	µg/mL
Amiodarone	1 - 2	µg/mL	> 2	µg/mL
Digitoxin	15 - 25	ng/mL	> 35	ng/mL
Digoxin	1 - 2	ng/mL	> 2.4	ng/mL
Diltiazem	0.05 - 0.2	µg/mL	--	µg/mL
Disopyramide	2 - 5	µg/mL	> 7	µg/mL
Disopyramide	40 - 190	ng/mL	--	ng/mL
Lidocaine	1.5 - 5	µg/mL	> 7	µg/mL
Lithium	0.6 - 1.2	mmol/L	> 2	mmol/L
Milrinone	150 - 250	ng/mL	--	ng/mL
Nicardipine	0.028 - 0.050	µg/mL	--	µg/mL
Nitroprusside	< 10	mg/dL	> 10	mg/dL
Phenobarbital	15 - 40	µg/mL	> 45	µg/mL
Phenytoin	10 - 20	µg/mL	> 20	µg/mL
Procainamide	4 - 10	µg/mL	> 15	µg/mL
Propranolol	50 - 100	ng/mL	--	ng/mL
Quinidine	2.5 - 5	µg/mL	> 5	µg/mL
Salicylate	100 - 250	µg/dL	> 300	µg/dL
Tegretol	8 - 12	µg/mL	> 15	µg/mL
Theophylline	10 - 20	µg/mL	> 20	µg/mL

Antibiotics

Antibiotics	Therapeutic	Toxic Peak	Toxic Trough	
Amikacin	25 - 30	> 35	> 10	µg/mL
Gentamycin	5 - 10	> 10	> 2	µg/mL
Tobramycin	5 - 10	> 10	> 2	µg/mL
Vancomycin	5 - 10	> 40	> 10	µg/mL

Ethanol

Intoxication Level	as mg/dL	as %	as mmol/L
Intoxicated	> 100	> 0.1 %	> 22
Very Intoxicated	300 - 400	0.3 - 0.4	65 - 87
Stupor	400 - 500	0.4 - 0.5	87 -109
Coma	> 500	> 0.5	> 109

Lab

Blood Gases

Arterial		Venous	
PaO_2	80 - 100 mm Hg	PvO_2	35 - 45 mm Hg
O_2 Sat	98 - 99 %	O_2 Sat	60 - 80 %
$PaCO_2$	34 - 45 mm Hg	$PvCO_2$	40 - 50 mm Hg
pH	7.35 - 7.45	pH	7.31 - 7.41
HCO_3	22 - 26 mEq/L	HCO_3	22 - 26 mEq/ L

Urinalysis

Specific Gravity 1.001 - 1.035
pH 4.6 - 8
Negative for: bilirubin, blood, acetone, glucose, protein, bacteria
Occasional: epithelial cells, hyaline casts

24 hr Urine

	Conventional Units		Systeme International Units	
Aldosterone	3 - 20	µg/24 hr	8.3 - 55	nmol/d
Amylase	< 17	U/hr	< 17	U/hr
Calcium	100 - 240	mg/24 hr	< 6.3	nmol/d
Chloride	110 - 250	mEq/24 hr	110 - 250	mmol/d
Creatinine (M)	110 - 150	mL/min	110 - 150	mL/min/1.73 m^2
Clearance(F)	105 - 132	mL/min	105 - 132	mL/min/1.73 m^2
Creatinine	15 - 25	mg/kg/24 hr	0.13 - 0.22	mmol/kg/d
Glucose	< 250	mg/24 hr	< 250	mg/d
Magnesium	6 - 10	mEq/24 hr	3 - 5	mmol/d
Osmolality	38 - 1400	mOsm/kg	38 - 1400	mOsm/kg
Phosphate	0.4 - 1.3	g/24 hr	13 - 42	mmol/d
Potassium	25 - 125	mEq/24 hr	25 - 125	mmol/d
Protein	10 - 150	mg/24 hr	10 - 150	mg/d
Sodium	60 - 260	mEq/24 hr	60 - 260	mmol/d
Urea Nitrogen	12 - 21	g/24 hr		
Urate	250- 750	mg/24 hr	1.5 - 4.4	mmol/d

Cerebrospinal Fluid

	Conventional Units		Systeme International Units	
Pressure	70 - 180	mm H_2O	78 - 180	mm H_2O
Albumin	20 - 48	mg/dL		
Ammonia	25 - 80	mg/dL		
Bicarbonate	20 -24	mEq/L		
Calcium	2.1 - 3	mEq/L		
Cell count	0 - 5	cells/mm^3	< 5	x 10^6/L
Chloride	116 - 122	mEq/L		
Glucose	50 - 80	mg/dL	2.8 - 4.2	mmol/L
Magnesium	2 - 2.5	mEq/L		
Osmolality	292 - 297	mOsm/L		
Phosphorus	1.2 - 2.0	mEq/L		
Potassium	2.7 - 3.9	mEq/L		
Protein	15 - 45	mg/dL	150 - 450	mg/L
Sodium	137 - 145	mEq/L		
Urea	4.4 - 4.8	mmol/L		
Uric acid	0.23 - 0.27	mg/dL		

Immunology

	Conventional Units		Systeme International Units	
Complement, C3	85 - 175	mg/dL	0.85 - 1.75	g/L
Complement, C4	15 - 45	mg/dL	150 - 450	mg/L
Complement, total	150 - 250	U/mL	150 - 250	U/mL
IgG	I620 - 1400	mg/dL	6.4 - 14.3	g/L
IgA	80 - 350	mg/dL	0.7 - 3.1	g/L
IgM	45 - 250	mg/dL	0.2 - 1.4	g/L
IgD	0.3 - 3	mg/dL	< 80	mg/L
IgE	0.002 - 0.2	mg/dL	0.1 - 0.4	mg/L

	Percentage	Absolute
Total T cells	56 - 77 %	860 - 1880
Total B cells	7 - 17 %	140 - 370
Helper induced cells	32 - 54 %	550 - 1190
Suppressor-cytoxic	24 - 37 %	430 - 1060
Activated T cells	5 - 14 %	70 - 310
E rosette T cells	73 - 87 %	1040 - 2160
Natural Killer Cells	8 - 22 %	130 - 500

IV Fluids - Crystalloids

Abbrv.	Solution	Description	Uses	Advantages	Disadvantages
D5W	5% Dextrose in Water	50 grams of Dextrose/L 200 calories/L Osmolality 380 mOsm/L	To provide fluid with small amount of substrate. Used as a keep-open or flush	Rehydrate when serum Na and Cl are concentrated.	Excess D5W can dilute electrolytes and plasma proteins -> electrolyte imbalance, interstitial and cellular edema. Do not use in patients with head injury.
0.45 NS	0.45% Hypotonic Saline	Sodium 77 mEq/L Chloride 77 mEq/L Osmolality 154 mOsm/L	To volume replace.	Rehydrate without increasing serum Na or Cl.	Interstitial and intracellular edema.
0.9 NS	0.9% Normal Saline	Na = 154 mEq/L Cl = 154 mEq/L Osmolality 308 mOsm/L pH = 5.0	To replace loss of body fluid (e.g., for bowel obstruction, peritonitis, GI suction) when red cell mass is adequate.	↑ plasma volume without changing Na concentration or serum osmolality.	Dilutes RBC's and plasma proteins, Lowers osmotic pressure which can result in pulmonary edema. Can cause hypernatremia and hyperchloremic metabolic acidosis
RL	Ringer's Lactate	Na = 130 mEq/L Cl = 109 mEq/L K = 4 mEq/L Ca = 1.4 mEq/L Lactate = 27 mEq/L Osmolality 274 mOsm/L pH = 6.5	For early stages of hemorrhagic shock. As an imitation of interstitial fluid, which shifts into cells and into vasculature during hemorrhage.	Isotonic, cheap, electrolytes are balanced to interstitial fluid, K and Ca promote myocardial contractility, Ca aids clotting, lactate is converted to glucose and carbonic acid. Doesn't increase serum Na or Cl.	Dilutes RBC's and plasma proteins, Lowers osmotic pressure which can result in pulmonary edema. Can't give with blood, the Ca can neutralize the citrate anticoagulant in bank blood.
3% HS	3% Hypertonic Saline	Sodium 512 mEq/L Chloride 513 mEq/L Osmolality 1026 mOsm/L	To increase plasma volume. To increase serum sodium. Fluid resuscitate patients with severe head injury.	Hypertonic, takes less to resuscitate. Solid evidence that HS improves cardiac output, as well as regional and microcirculatory blood flow.	Given too fast can lead to ↑ Na, ↓ K, dysrhythmias, seizures
5% HS	5% Hypertonic Saline	Sodium 855 mEq/L Chloride 855 mEq/L Osmolality 1710 mOsm/L	May moderate the inflammatory response in shock/trauma patients.	Given as either a bolus or continuous infusion can be more effective than mannitol in reducing episodes of elevated ICP.	Same as 3% HS

IV Fluids - Colloids

Solution	Description	Uses	Advantages	Disadvantages
Albumin 5%	Albumin 50 g/L in NS Osmolality 300 mOsm/L	Rapidly volume expand. Mobilize interstitial (pulmonary) edema.	Increases osmotic pressure, Stays intravascular longer, Takes less too resuscitate.	Expensive. Can increase edema in the presence of capillary leak syndrome. Curtails albumin synthesis.
Albumin 25 %	Albumin 240 g/L Osmolality 1500 mOsm/L 5 times the albumin content of plasma.	Increase plasma colloid osmotic pressure, for patients with hypoproteinemia.	Rarely associated with allergic reaction or transmission of hepatitis.	Risk of volume overload. Limit rate to < 4 mL/min.
Dextran 40 (Rheomadrodex)	Synthetic colloid, with glucose polysaccharides in NS or D5W Molecular wt = 40,000	Rapidly volume expand. Prevent formation of microthrombi.	Volume expands 100 %. Can prevent microemboli by decreasing platelet adhesiveness. Associated with less allergic reaction than Dextran-70.	Anticoagulant properties. May cause allergic reaction in low flow states. 70% is excreted unchanged in urine. Can cause osmotic nephrosis and ATN. Expensive. Alters urine sp. gr. and osmolarity
Dextran 70 (Rheomadrodex)	Molecular weight of 70,000	Rapidly volume expand. Mobilize interstitial edema.	Has identical weight to albumin, but much larger molecules. Increased plasma volume is maintained up to 24 hrs.	Higher incidence of allergic reactions.
Hespan (HES)	Synthetic colloid made from corn	Rapidly volume expand. Mobilize interstitial edema.	Volume expand (up to 50%) Effects last 24 - 36 hours.	May increase serum amylase, serum glucose. Decreases clotting factor VIII. Prolongs PT, aPTT, may decrease platelets. Dilutes RBC's.
11/25/2013 FDA issued box warning for Hespan:	• Do not use HES in critically ill or septic adult patients, • Avoid use in patients with pre-existing renal dysfunction. • Discontinue use of HES at the first sign of renal injury. • Monitor renal function for ≥ 90 days in all who receive HES		• Monitor coagulation of pts undergoing open heart surgery with cardio-pulmonary bypass. Discontinue use of HES at the first sign of coagulopathy. • Do not use HES products in patients with severe liver disease. • Monitor liver function in patients receiving HES products.	
Plasmanate (Plasma protein fraction)	5% solution of human plasma proteins in NS. Albumin 44 g/L Osmolality 290 mOsm/L	Increase serum colloid osmotic pressure	Like 5% albumin, has low risk of transmitting hepatitis.	Risk of allergic reaction. May cause hypotension if given > 10 mL/min. Expensive.

Blood and Blood Products

Component	Volume	Filter	Infusion rate	Description	Uses	Additional Information
Cryoprecipitate	10 mL	Component filter	10 mL/min	Clotting factors V, VII, XIII, von Willebrand's factor, and fibrinogen.	Hemophilia A, von Willebrands disease, fibrinogen deficiency. Blood bank needs 1 hr. to prepare.	Usually given as pool of 10 - 20 units.
Fresh Frozen Plasma (FFP)	150 - 200 mL	Blood filter or component filter	10 - 15 mL/kg at 10 mL/min	Plasma, all clotting factors (II, V, VII, IX, X, XI, XII, XIII) Contains no RBC's, WBC's, or platelets. Must administer within 4 hrs of being defrosted.	When need for blood is > 6 - 8 units, to replace clotting factors. For bleeding disease of unknown cause. For Coumadin intoxication.	Risk of allergic reaction, volume excess, lung injury 1 - 2 units given for every 5 units PRBC's given.
Frozen and thawed RBC's	200 mL	Blood filter	within 2 hrs	Frozen for up to 3 years in a glycerol solution. Has RBC's, minimal WBC's and platelets, no plasma.	To store extremely rare blood types. Less antigenic for organ transplant pts For pts who want to store blood for their own use for a future surgery.	Blood bank needs 1 hr.
Granulocytes	250 - 300 mL	Blood filter	over 2 - 3 hrs	Granulocytes and hydroxyethyl starch	Granulocyte count < 500/mm^2	Volume overload, pulmonary congestion.
Leukocyte - poor RBC's	200 - 250 mL	Blood filter	within 2 hrs	Most WBC's and platelets are removed to reduce the antigens	Previous febrile transfusion reactions. Patient requires multiple transfusions (leukemia). Potential organ transplant pt.	Blood bank needs 1 hr.
Packed Red Blood Cells (PRBC's)	250 - 300 mL	Blood filter	within 2 hrs	80% of the plasma has been removed. Lacks clotting factors and platelets.	For acute and chronic anemia. Given with NS and FFP as replacement in hemorrhagic shock.	Should ↑ Hgb by 1 gram, and ↑ Hct by 3%.
Platelets	50 mL/unit	Special component filter	1 unit q 30 minutes	1 pack or unit represents the platelets removed from 1 unit of whole blood.	Plt count: < 20,000 in nonbleeding patient Plt count: < 50,000 in preop or bleeding pt	1 unit should ↑ platelet count by 6,000. Usually given in pools of 6-10 units
Washed RBC's	300 mL	Blood filter	within 2 hrs	Like Leukocyte-poor except almost *all* WBC's removed.	Same as Leukocyte-poor RBC's.	Much more expensive.
Whole blood	500 mL	Blood filter	2 - 4 hrs/unit (or 1200 mL/ min in massive bleeding)	Contains all elements: RBC's, WBC's, Plasma. If blood is > 24 hrs old, platelets and clotting factors are no longer functional.	Not for routine use, due to excess volume. Used for acute, massive bleeding.	See complications of transfusion on next page.

Complications of Blood Transfusion

Complication	Pathophysiology	Manifestations	General Treatment
Hemolytic reaction	Rapid destruction of RBC's due to incompatibility of the ABO blood group.	Chills, fever, chest and back pain, oozing from wounds, hemoglobinuria, ATN.	Stat IV fluids, NS 1500 - 2000 mL, Diuretics (Mannitol), $NaHCO_3$.
Allergic reaction	Patient's antibodies react to the antigens of white cells and platelets.	Urticaria, chills, fever, abdominal pain, diarrhea, anaphylaxis.	Give antihistamine, corticosteroids, Washed RBC's for future transfusions.
Hyperkalemia	In the unit of stored cells, K^+ ↑ 1 mEq/day. pH in a unit of blood is < 6.0, due to citrate and anaerobic metabolism of the RBC's.	Signs and symptoms of hyperkalemia. pH change evident on arterial blood gas.	Withhold K^+ $NaHCO_3$ according to lab results.
Hypothermia	Bank blood is stored at 4° C.	Reduces cardiac contractility, Prolongs clotting times, ↑ Hgb affinity for O_2	Use blood warmers, give blood with warm NS, warm the environment.
Disease transmission	Contaminated blood, although rare, is possible.	Fever, severe abdominal cramps, diarrhea vomiting, increased respiratory rate, ↓ BP	Treatment of specific organism.
Microemboli	By the time the unit expires, 1/2 of the RBC's have ruptured. A standard blood filter does not remove all of the RBC debris.	Pulmonary sequestration that could result in acute lung injury.	Microfilters have not been shown to make a difference.
Coagulopathy	Blood that is > 24 hrs old has no functional platelets or clotting factors. Citrate is used in bank blood to bind ionized calcium to prevent clotting during storage. Hypothermia suppresses coagulation.	Oozing from surgical wounds and venipuncture sites, hematuria, blood tinged sputum.	FFP 1 - 2 units for every 5 units PRBC's, or if PT/PTT > 1.5 times control. Blood warmers or warm NS. Cryoprecipitate. Platelets if platelet count < 100,000. Routine CaCl is not recommended.
Hypocalcemia	Due to citrate binding of ionized Calcium.	Signs and symptoms of hypocalcemia.	CaCl according to lab results.
Decreased 2,3 DPG	Dysfunctional RBC's fail to make this enzyme. The affinity of hemoglobin for oxygen increases, which can result in reduced tissue oxygenation.	Venous blood may appear "too red" due to increased saturation of hemoglobin. Causes increased $ScvO_2$ and SvO_2.	Fresh (< 24 hrs old) blood.
Hypotension (mild to profound)	Due to: Hypothermic myocardial depression, Allergic reaction (histamine), Infection from contaminated blood, septic shock.	(manifestations will depend on the cause of the hypotension).	Depends on the cause.

Fahrenheit = Celsius

F	C	F	C
65.0	18.3	99.0	37.2
70.0	21.1	99.2	37.3
75.0	23.9	99.4	37.4
80.0	26.6	99.6	37.5
85.0	29.4	99.8	37.6
90.0	32.2	100.0	37.7
92.0	33.3	100.2	37.9
92.2	33.4	100.4	38.0
92.4	33.5	100.6	38.1
92.6	33.6	100.8	38.2
92.8	33.7	101.0	38.3
93.0	33.9	101.2	38.4
93.2	34.0	101.4	38.5
93.4	34.1	101.6	38.6
93.6	34.2	101.8	38.7
93.8	34.3	102.0	38.9
94.0	34.4	102.2	39.0
94.2	34.5	102.4	39.1
94.4	34.6	102.6	39.2
94.6	34.7	102.8	39.3
94.8	34.9	103.0	39.4
95.0	35.0	103.2	39.5
95.2	35.1	103.4	39.6
95.4	35.2	103.6	39.7
95.6	35.3	103.8	39.8
95.8	35.4	104.0	40.0
96.0	35.5	104.2	40.1
96.2	35.6	104.4	40.2
96.4	35.7	104.6	40.3
96.6	35.9	104.8	40.4
96.8	36.0	105.0	40.5
97.0	36.1	105.2	40.6
97.2	36.2	105.4	40.7
97.4	36.3	105.6	40.8
97.6	36.4	105.8	41.0
97.8	36.5	106.0	41.1
98.0	36.6	107.0	41.6
98.2	36.7	108.0	42.2
98.4	36.9	109.0	42.7
98.6	37.0	110.0	43.3
98.8	37.1	111.0	43.8

F = (C x 1.8) + 32
C = (F - 32) x 0.555

Feet/inches=Inches=Centimeters

Ft	inches	Inches	Cm	Ft	inches	Inches	Cm
2	0	24	61	5	0	60	152
2	1	25	64	5	1	61	155
2	2	26	66	5	2	62	157
2	3	27	69	5	3	63	160
2	4	28	71	5	4	64	163
2	5	29	74	5	5	65	165
2	6	30	76	5	6	66	168
2	7	31	79	5	7	67	170
2	8	32	81	5	8	68	173
2	9	33	84	5	9	69	175
2	10	34	86	5	10	70	178
2	11	35	89	5	11	71	180
3	0	36	91	6	0	72	183
3	1	37	94	6	1	73	185
3	2	38	97	6	2	74	188
3	3	39	99	6	3	75	191
3	4	40	102	6	4	76	193
3	5	41	104	6	5	77	196
3	6	42	107	6	6	78	198
3	7	43	109	6	7	79	201
3	8	44	112	6	8	80	203
3	9	45	114	6	9	81	206
3	10	46	117	6	10	82	208
3	11	47	119	6	11	83	211
4	0	48	122	7	0	84	213
4	1	49	124	7	2	85	216
4	2	50	127	7	3	86	218
4	3	51	130	7	4	87	221
4	4	52	132	7	5	88	224
4	5	53	135	7	6	89	226
4	6	54	137	7	7	90	229
4	7	55	140	7	8	91	231
4	8	56	142	7	9	92	234
4	9	57	145	7	9	93	236
4	10	58	147	7	10	94	239
4	11	59	150	7	11	95	241

1 inch = 2.54 cm
1 cm = 0.4 inches

Lbs = Kgs

Lb	Kg
20	9.08
22	9.99
24	10.90
26	11.80
28	12.71
30	13.62
32	14.53
34	15.44
36	16.34
38	17.25
40	18.16
42	19.07
44	19.98
46	20.88
48	21.79
50	22.70
52	23.61
54	24.52
56	25.42
58	26.33
60	27.24
62	28.15
64	29.06
66	29.96
68	30.87
70	31.78
72	32.69
74	33.60
76	34.50
78	35.41
80	36.32
82	37.23
84	38.14
86	39.04
88	39.95
90	40.86
92	41.77
94	42.68
96	43.58
98	44.49

Lb	Kg
100	45.40
102	46.31
104	47.22
106	48.12
108	49.03
110	49.94
112	50.85
114	51.76
116	52.66
118	53.57
120	54.48
122	55.39
124	56.30
126	57.20
128	58.11
130	59.02
132	59.93
134	60.84
136	61.74
138	62.65
140	63.56
142	64.47
144	65.38
146	66.28
148	67.19
150	68.10
152	69.01
154	69.92
156	70.82
158	71.73
160	72.64
162	73.55
164	74.46
166	75.36
168	76.27
170	77.18
172	78.09
174	79.00
176	79.90
178	80.81

Lb	Kg
180	81.72
182	82.63
184	83.54
186	84.44
188	85.35
190	86.26
192	87.17
194	88.08
196	88.98
198	89.89
200	90.80
202	91.71
204	92.62
206	93.52
208	94.43
210	95.34
212	96.25
214	97.16
216	98.06
218	98.97
220	99.88
222	100.79
224	101.70
226	102.60
228	103.51
230	104.42
232	105.33
234	106.24
236	107.14
238	108.05
240	108.96
242	109.87
244	110.78
246	111.68
248	112.59
250	113.50
252	114.41
254	115.32
256	116.22
258	117.13

Lb	Kg
260	118.04
265	120.31
270	122.58
275	124.85
280	127.12
285	129.39
290	131.66
295	133.93
300	136.20
305	138.47
310	140.74
315	143.01
320	145.28
325	147.55
330	149.82
335	152.09
340	154.36
345	156.63
350	158.90
360	163.44
370	167.98
380	172.52
390	177.06
400	181.60
410	186.14
420	190.68
430	195.22
440	199.76
450	204.30
460	208.84
470	213.38
480	217.92
490	222.46
500	227.00
525	238.35
550	249.70
575	261.05
600	272.40
625	283.75
650	295.10

1 lb = 0.454 kg
1 kg = 2.2 lbs

Ideal body weight in pounds:
men: 106 + 6(height in inches - 60)
women: 105 + 5(height in inches - 60)

Body Surface Area

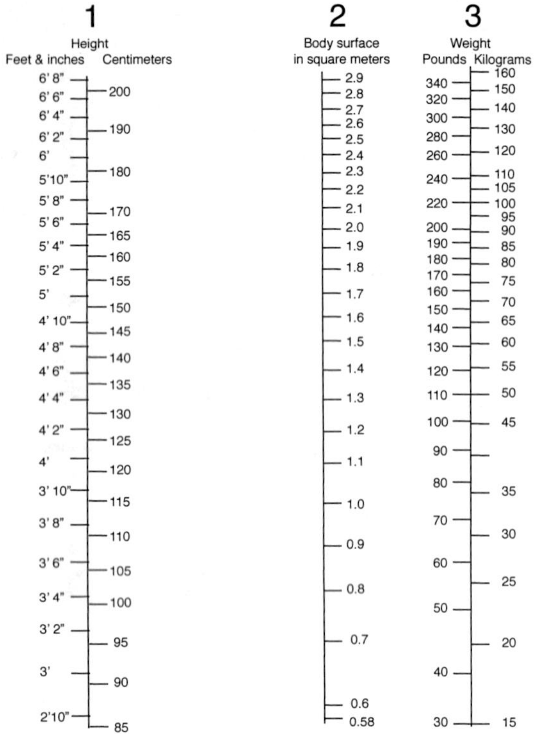

Fig. 12.1

A body surface chart. To find the body surface area of a person,

1. Locate the height in feet and inches or in centimeters on scale 1.
2. Locate the person's weight in pounds or kilograms on scale 3.
3. Place a ruler or straight edge connecting these two points.
4. The ruler crosses scale 2 at the person's body surface area.

(used with permission from Meschan I, and Ott DJ: Introduction to diagnostic imaging. Philadelphia: WB Saunders, 1984.)

The Mosteller formula:

$BSA\ (m^2) = ([Height\ (cm) \times Weight\ (kg)]/3600)^{1/2}$

$BSA\ (m^2) = ([Height\ (in) \times Weight\ (lbs)]/3131)^{1/2}$

The DuBois formula:

$BSA\ (m^2) = 0.007184 \times Height\ (cm)^{0.725} \times Weight\ (kg)^{0.425}$

About the Book and the Author

Thirty years of experience in critical care nursing, teaching, writing, and research have convinced Kathy that being a critical care nurse is a tremendous challenge. First you must build an in-depth knowledge base on how to care for every type of critically ill patient. Then you must continue to keep up with all of the changes.

There are excellent textbooks and journals to help you, as well as references on line. But there isn't time to hunt down the information you need. There are excellent educators and clinical mentors among your colleagues. But when you are at the bedside, all alone, any hour of the day or night, help may be too far away. You need something you can carry with you. A bedside reference.

Not just any reference. It must be packed with information, yet concise and relevant. There should be frequent updates whenever there are changes in the standards of practice. The illustrations must enhance and speed understanding. Critical information on specialty practice must be available. And it must all be backed by medical evidence and by real-world experience.

When creating Fast Facts, Kathy drew upon her experience:
As a critical care nurse, in these positions:
Staff nurse, Med-Surg ICU, Baylor Medical Center, Dallas Tx
Staff nurse, Emergency Room, Parkland Hospital, Dallas Tx
Instructor, Nursing Internship, Parkland Hospital, Dallas, Tx
Nurse Coordinator, Critical Care, Methodist Medical Center, Dallas Tx
Clinical Nurse Specialist, Critical Care, Methodist Medical Center, Dallas Tx
Staff Nurse, Critical Care, University of South Alabama, Mobile AL

Upon her experience as a nationally recognized speaker:
1984 - 2006 at the National Teaching Institute of the AACN
1984 - 2001 courses on "SvO2 & O2 Transport" across the USA & Canada
1980 - 2001 courses on "Trauma Care" across the USA and Canada

Upon her experience as an author, with contributions to:

These journals:
- Nursing
- American Journal of Nursing
- Journal of Emergency Nursing
- Heart and Lung
- Cardiovascular Nursing
- Critical Care Clinic of North America
- AACN Clinical Issues

These Text books:
- Critical Care Nursing
- Hemodynamic Monitoring
- Essentials of Critical Care Nursing

"As an ICU nurse, I often questioned myself on what could go wrong with my patient. What signs had I missed, misinterpreted, or underestimated. What did I not see, that could stall the patient's recovery. And worst of all, was the patient going down and I didn't know enough to recognize it.

Time to treatment is everything in the critically ill patient. If we are armed with the knowledge of great nursing care and we recognize, or better yet, anticipate, the subtle clues of a threat to the patient, our swift action can avert catastrope.

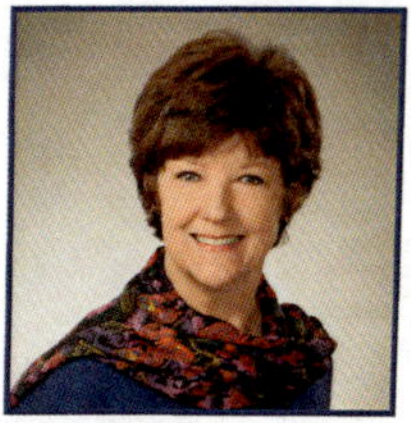

For the ICU patient, each of us is capable of making a huge difference, not only in the course of the patient's care, but also in the patient's eventual outcome."

Kathleen M. White, RN, MS

Notes

Pedi

Pedi

Normal Pediatric Vital Signs

Age	lbs	kg	Resp Rate	Heart Rate	Sys BP	Dias BP	MAP
Premature	3	1.5	40 - 70	120 - 170	55 - 75	35 - 45	50
0 - 3 months	7.5	3.5	35 - 55	100 - 150	65 - 85	45 - 55	58
3 - 6 months	12 - 16	5 - 7	30 - 45	90 - 120	70 - 90	50 - 65	64
6 - 12 months	17 - 22	8 - 10	25 - 40	80 - 120	80 - 100	55 - 65	70
1 - 3 years	22 - 32	10 - 15	20 - 30	70 - 110	90 - 105	55 - 70	74
3 - 6 years	32 - 45	15 - 20	20 - 25	65 - 110	95 - 110	60 - 75	79
6 - 12 years	45 - 90	20 - 41	14 - 22	60 - 95	100 - 120	60 - 75	81
over age 12	> 90	> 41	12 - 18	60 - 85	110 - 135	65 - 85	90

adapted from: Kliegman RM, et al. Nelson's Textbook of Pediatrics, 18th edition. Philadelphia: Saunders Elsevier, 2007: 389.

Immediate Attention Required

Abnormal Vital Signs

Age	Resp Rate	Heart Rate	Sys BP
Infant	< 20 or > 60	< 90 or > 160	< 60 mm Hg
1 month - 12 months	< 24 or > 50	< 80 or > 150	< 70 mm Hg
1 - 10 years old	< 10 or > 40	< 70 or > 150	< 2 times age + 70
≥ 10 years old	< 10 or > 30	< 70 or > 150	< 90 mm Hg

www.kathywhite.com

Abnormal Assessment Findings

Assessment	Findings	
Level of Consciousness	Responds only to physical stimuli, or only to pain, or is unresponsive.	
Oxygenation and Work of Breathing	Nasal flaring Prolonged expiration Sternal retraction Cyanosis or ↓ SpO_2	Intercostal muscle retraction Supraclavicular fossa retraction Contraction of neck muscles Grunting, gasping, stridor
Response to O_2	Poor, absent, or worsening response to oxygen. High flow O_2 required to maintain $SpO_2 \geq 94\%$.	
Fever	Especially with petechiae, tachycardia, bounding pulses.	
Trauma	Loss of consciousness (or history of), weak pulses, capillary refill > 2 seconds, pallor, mottled, GCS ≤ 8, absent or abnormal motor, distended abdomen.	
Burns	Involving more than 10% of body surface area.	

Initial Emergency Approach

	ABCD
A	If the airway cannot be maintained, or if prolonged assisted ventilation is anticipated, consider endotracheal intubation.
B	If child is breathing adequately, administer high-flow O_2 with non-rebreather mask or blow-by. If child is not breathing or breathing is inadequate, assist ventilations using a BVM, high-flow (100%) oxygen and nasal or oral airway.
C	If symptomatic tachycardia or bradycardia, or pulseless, proceed to PALS. If signs of shock: Establish vascular access (Intravenous or Intraosseous). Administer fluid bolus of NS 20 mL/kg over 5 - 20 minutes. Reassess after initial bolus. If signs of shock persist, repeat fluid bolus to maximum total of 60 mL/kg.
D	If low blood glucose, glucose is given slowly (10 mL/min): Neonate with BG < 40: $D_{10}W$, 3 mL/kg IV/IO. < 2 yrs old with BG < 60: $D_{25}W$, 2 mL/kg IV/IO. > 2 yrs old with BG < 80: $D_{50}W$, 1 mL/kg IV/IO.

Rapid Sequence Intubation

Rapid Sequence Intubation (RSI) is the sequential administration of a sedative, paralyzing agent, vagolytic, and cerebroprotective agent, given 2 minutes (or less) prior to emergency endotracheal intubation, to prevent major complications or even death due to hypoxia, hypercapnea, or acidosis.

Indications:	Respiratory arrest, apnea, agonal or gasping respirations. Cannot maintain airway; potential airway obstruction exists. Hypoxemia in spite of supplemental oxygen. Hypercapnea. Chest or head injury. Immediate need for ventilatory support.
Contra-indications:	Limited cervical mobility, receding mandible, major facial or laryngeal trauma, limited jaw opening, upper airway obstruction, distorted facial or airway anatomy. Alert anesthesiology.
ET tube size:	Uncuffed tube internal diameter = 4 + (age/4). After 2 years of age, uncuffed ET tube is no longer used. Cuffed tube internal diameter = 3.5 + (age/4).
Tube depth:	= ET tube size (i.e., mm internal diameter) x 3

	ET Tube Sizes (mm)		*Laryngoscope size & type blade*	*ET Depth (cm lip to tip)*	*Suction cath (Fr.)*
	uncuffed	*cuffed*			
Premature	2.5	x	# 0 or # 1 straight	6 + Wt. Kg	6
Newborn	3.0	x	# 1 straight blade	6 + Wt. Kg	6
6 months	3.5	x	# 1 straight blade	11	8
1 yr	4.0	x	# 1 straight blade	12	8
3 yr	x	4.5	# 2 curved or straight	14	8
5 yr	x	5.0	# 2 curved or straight	15	10
7 yr	x	5.5	# 2 curved or straight	16	10
9 yr	x	6.0	# 2 curved or straight	18	10
11 yr	x	6.5	# 2 curved or straight	19	10
12 yr	x	7.0	# 3 curved or straight	21	12
14 yr	x	7.5	# 3 curved or straight	22	12

Supplies:	3 ET tubes (one of the expected size, one larger, one smaller) Tonsil tip suction, Suction catheters — Laryngoscope and light Atropine, a sedative, and Lidocaine — ECG monitor Neuromuscular blocking agent — SpO_2 oximeter Pedi Resusbag + mask + O_2 reservoir — End tidal CO_2 monitor
Preoxygenate:	100% oxygen by mask. If pt is hypoventilating or apneic, use bag/mask ventilation. Gentle cricoid pressure may be used to prevent aspiration (beware excess pressure can cause tracheal obstruction)
Medicate in sequence:	1. Atropine 0.02 mg/kg to prevent bradycardia. 2. Lidocaine 1 mg/kg IV push if there is known or suspected elevation in ICP, or to patients with reactive airways (asthma). 3. Rocuronium 0.6 - 1 mg/kg, or Succinylcholine 1 - 2 mg/kg 4. Etomidate or ketamine or thiopental as the sedative
Intubate:	C-spine immobilization is maintained. Intubation is attempted when there is full relaxation of the airway muscles, usually 45 seconds after rocuronium or succinylcholine has been given. Limit time for intubation attempt to < 30 seconds. Place tube to proper depth. Ventilate with bag while ET tube is secured.
Confirm tube placement:	Breath sounds are present over lateral chest, high in the axillae, but absent over epigastric area. Visible expansion of chest with ventilation, vapor in the tube, improved SpO_2 when FiO_2 returned to previous setting (beware the SpO_2 elevation on 100% O_2 may persist for 3 minutes), positive indicator by $PetCO_2$. Obtain ABG's. Obtain chest x-ray. ET tube tip should be no lower than 1 - 2 cm above the carina and no higher than the first rib.
Cuff Pressure:	If cuffed tube used, keep cuff pressure < 20 cm H_2O.
Position Head:	Neck flexion may push tube down, extension may pull the tube out of the trachea. Keep the patient's head in a neutral position.

Intraosseous Access

Description:	Insertion of a needle/cannula through the bone cortex and into the marrow, to establish access for the administration of fluids medications, and blood products. The cannula can be inserted in 30-60 seconds, is safe and effective, and allows treatment when vascular access can't be achieved. Because the absorption rate is the same as IV access, the IO is preferred over the ET tube as a means of drug delivery. The cannula may also be used to aspirate samples for T & C, chemistry, blood gases. Intended for short-term use (< 24 hr).
What meds and Fluids?	Drugs infused via the IO route include cardiac medications, sedatives, and paralytics. Hypertonic solutions and strongly alkaline agents should be avoided.
Insertion sites:	In children, the favored insertion site is the anterior-medial aspect of the proximal tibia, 2 - 3 cm below the kneecap. The distal tibia and the head of the humerus are alternative sites. Contraindicated sites include extremities with history of recent injury, bone disorders, or in areas of cellulitis or infection.

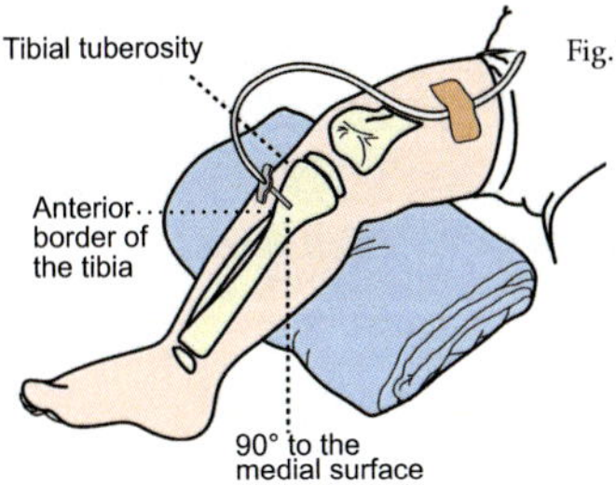

Fig. 16.1

IO Site for Infants. Illustration used with permission. The American Heart Association & The American Academy of Pediatrics. ***Pediatric Advanced Life Support*** 1997-1999, Fig 4, p. 5-6.

Supplies:	Intraosseous infusion needle/cannula, which may be inserted via hand-power, battery power, or spring-loaded device. Gauze, kling, and tape, to support the needle after insertion. Sterile saline flush solution with administration set. Pressure infusion bag or pump may be needed.
Procedure for proximal tibia insertion:	Place a firm towel or pad of linen under the knee, then secure the leg with towel/pad to an armboard. Cleanse the site with antiseptic. 1% lidocaine may be injected. Grasp the posterior thigh, knee, & lower limb to stabilize the site. The needle/cannula must be directed 90° to the tibia. Angulation toward the tibia head risks injury to epiphyseal plate. Hand powered insertion requires a firm twisting/drilling motion. The needle is in the bone marrow cavity when there is a sudden decrease in resistance, the cannula can remain upright without support, aspiration returns bloody bone marrow, and a 10 mL saline flush encounters no resistance. Evacuate air from IV administration set and connect to cannula. Begin continuous infusion, and assess for signs of infiltration: Increased firmness of surrounding tissue Increased circumference of the soft tissue of the extremity Increased resistance to injection. Stabilize the cannula by supporting with a bulky dressing. If the cannula becomes obstructed, it can be replaced with a second cannula, as long as there is no evidence of infiltration. If infiltrated, remove cannula, select an alternative insertion site.
Complications:	Occur in < 1 % of patients, but include: Infiltration, Cellulitis, Fracture, Osteomyelitis, Skin necrosis, Compartment syndrome.

Pediatric Advanced Life Support (PALS)

American Heart Association, 2010

Kleinman ME, Chameides L, Schexnayder SM, et al. Part 14: Pediatric advanced life support: 2010 American Heart Association Guidelines for Cardiopulmonary Resuscitation and Emergency Cardiovascular Care. Circulation. 2010;122:S876 –S908.

	About IV, IO, ET medication administration in children:
IV:	Drugs given by peripheral IV should be given at the port closest to the catheter and should be followed by a bolus of at least 5 mL NS.
IO:	Rapid, safe, effective route. Can give meds, fluids, blood. Onset of drug action is the same as if given intravenously. Can also obtain samples for T & C, chemistry, and blood gases.
ET:	Only lipid-soluble drugs can be given ET and include Lidocaine, Epinephrine, Atropine, Naloxone ("LEAN"). ET administration requires doses that are 2 - 3 times higher than IV doses. Instill via catheter that is passed beyond the tip of the ET tube, follow with 2 - 5 mL NS, then give 5 positive pressure breaths.

After Advanced Airway Placement: Stop CPR cycles, 2 rescuers switch to 100 compressions/min and 8 - 10 breaths/minute, without pause for breaths.

With each algorithm, **search for and treat possible causes:**

Hypovolemia	Hypo/hyperkalemia	Toxins/poisons/drugs
Hypoxia	Hypoglycemia	Tamponade, cardiac
Hydrogen ion (acidosis)	Hypothermia	Tension pneumothorax
	Trauma	Thrombosis (coronary or pulmonary)

Tachycardia with Poor Perfusion

American Heart Association, 2010

Assess and maintain **airway, breathing, circulation.**
Administer 100 % **oxygen**
Attach monitor/pacer. Prepare for possible cardioversion.
Establish IV/IO access. Consider expert consultation.
Evaluate duration of the QRS:

Sinus Tachycardia QRS ≤ 0.09 sec.	**Supraventricular Tach** QRS ≤ 0.09 sec.	**Wide Complex SVT or Ventricular Tachycardia** QRS > 0.09 sec.
History suggests cause. P waves are present and upright in leads I, aVF. Physical activity affects the heart rate. Variable R-R interval. Constant P-R interval. Infant: HR usually < 220 Child: HR usually < 180	History is nonspecific, or there is history of abrupt changes in heart rate. Absent or negative P waves in leads II, III, and aVF. HR is unrelated to the patient's physical activity Infant: HR usually ≥ 220 Child: HR usually ≥ 180	**If the SVT is causing adverse effects** (acutely altered LOC, hypotension, signs of shock) proceed to synchronized cardioversion 0.5 - 1 joule/kg. If ineffective, increase to 2 joules/kg. Sedate if possible, but don't delay treatment.
Identify and manage possible causes. (Verapamil 0.1 - 0.3 mg/kg may be effective in treating SVT in older children, but in infants, is not used without first seeking expert opinion).	Consider vagal maneuvers, e.g., blow through a straw. Adenosine 0.1 mg/kg IV, (max of 6 mg) rapidly. If no response, Adenosine 0.2 mg/kg (max of 12 mg) rapidly. *or* **If hemodynamically unstable, proceed to** Synchronized cardioversion 0.5 - 1 joule/kg. If ineffective, increase to 2 joules/kg. Sedate if possible, but don't delay treatment.	**If the SVT is causing no adverse effects, the rhythm is regular, and the QRS is monomorphic:** Adenosine 0.2 mg/kg (max of 12 mg) rapidly. *or* Amiodarone 5 mg/kg IV over 20 - 60 minutes *or* Procainamide 15 mg/kg over 30 - 60 minutes. Expert consultation is strongly recommended.

Fast Facts for

Pediatric Acute Care

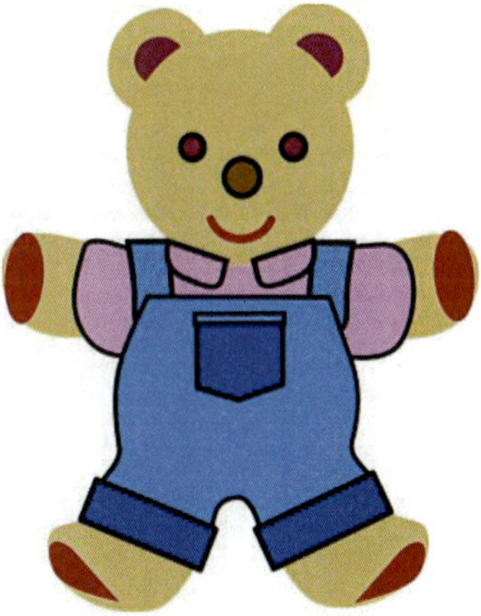

A Specialty Chapter on the Management of the Acutely Ill Pediatric Patient

FAST FACTS for Critical Care®

The references for ***Fast Facts for Pediatric Acute Care*** are available at www.kathywhite.com. Some of the major sources of information include:

Rogers Handbook of Pediatric Intensive Care
Pediatric Critical Care Medicine
Pediatrics (The Journal)
The Journal of Trauma
Critical Care Medicine
Journal of Neurotrauma
AACN Advanced Critical Care
Critical Care Nurse

Fast Facts for Pediatric Acute Care

Printed in the United States of America

Kathy White Learning Systems
PO Box 41113
Mobile, Alabama 36640
Toll free: 1-800-940-0895
Local phone: 251-438-2175
Fax number: 251-438-1959
Internet address: http://www.kathywhite.com

Kathy White Learning Systems
638 Saddlebrook Dr.
Killen, AL 35645

The author, reviewers, and publisher have made a conscientious effort to ensure that the information, medications, and treatment schedules in this chapter are correct and accurate, and compatible with standards generally accepted at the time of publication. Nevertheless, many medications, treatment protocols, and diagnostic regimens are the subject of ongoing research, may be controversial, and are subject to frequent change. As new information becomes available, changes in diagnostic and treatment protocols and in the use of drug therapy become necessary. In view of the possibility of human error or changes in the medical sciences, neither the authors nor the publisher nor any other party who has been involved in the preparation of the publication of this work warrants that the information contained herein is in every respect accurate or complete and they disclaim all responsibility to any errors or omissions or for the results obtained from the use of the information contained in the work. The reader is strongly advised to consult the instructions, information, and warnings included in the package insert (prescribing information) of each medication or therapeutic agent before administration, and to consult accepted and published textbooks, journals, and standards of clinical practice for more detailed explanations, recommendations, and instructions on diagnostic and treatment regimens. The author, reviewers, and publisher disclaim all responsibility for any liability, loss, injury, or damage incurred as a consequence, directly or indirectly, of the use and application of any of the contents of this volume.

ISBN # (Printed version): 978-0-9835750-6-1
ISBN # (eBook version): 978-0-9835750-7-8

Normal Pediatric Vital Signs

Age	lbs	kg	Resp Rate	Heart Rate	Sys BP	Dias BP	MAP
Premature	3	1.5	40 - 70	120 - 170	55 - 75	35 - 45	50
0 - 3 months	7.5	3.5	35 - 55	100 - 150	65 - 85	45 - 55	58
3 - 6 months	12 - 16	5 - 7	30 - 45	90 - 120	70 - 90	50 - 65	64
6 - 12 months	17 - 22	8 - 10	25 - 40	80 - 120	80 - 100	55 - 65	70
1 - 3 years	22 - 32	10 - 15	20 - 30	70 - 110	90 - 105	55 - 70	74
3 - 6 years	32 - 45	15 - 20	20 - 25	65 - 110	95 - 110	60 - 75	79
6 - 12 years	45 - 90	20 - 41	14 - 22	60 - 95	100 - 120	60 - 75	81
over age 12	> 90	> 41	12 - 18	60 - 85	110 - 135	65 - 85	90

adapted from: Kliegman RM, et al. Nelson's Textbook of Pediatrics, 18th edition. Philadelphia: Saunders Elsevier, 2007: 389.

Immediate Attention Required

Abnormal Vital Signs

Age	Resp Rate	Heart Rate	Sys BP
Infant	< 20 or > 60	< 90 or > 160	< 60 mm Hg
1 month - 12 months	< 24 or > 50	< 80 or > 150	< 70 mm Hg
1 - 10 years old	< 10 or > 40	< 70 or > 150	< 2 times age + 70
≥ 10 years old	< 10 or > 30	< 70 or > 150	< 90 mm Hg

Abnormal Assessment Findings

Assessment	Findings	
Level of Consciousness	Responds only to physical stimuli, or only to pain, or is unresponsive.	
Oxygenation and Work of Breathing	Nasal flaring Prolonged expiration Sternal retraction Cyanosis or ↓ SpO_2	Intercostal muscle retraction Supraclavicular fossa retraction Contraction of neck muscles Grunting, gasping, stridor
Response to O_2	Poor, absent, or worsening response to oxygen. High flow O_2 required to maintain $SpO_2 \geq 94\%$.	
Fever	Especially with petechiae, tachycardia, bounding pulses.	
Trauma	Loss of consciousness (or history of), weak pulses, capillary refill > 2 seconds, pallor, mottled, GCS ≤ 8, absent or abnormal motor, distended abdomen.	
Burns	Involving more than 10% of body surface area.	

Initial Emergency Approach

	ABCD
A	If the airway cannot be maintained, or if prolonged assisted ventilation is anticipated, consider endotracheal intubation.
B	If child is breathing adequately, administer high-flow O_2 with non-rebreather mask or blow-by. If child is not breathing or breathing is inadequate, assist ventilations using a BVM, high-flow (100%) oxygen and nasal or oral airway.
C	If symptomatic tachycardia or bradycardia, or pulseless, proceed to PALS. If signs of shock: Establish vascular access (Intravenous or Intraosseous). Administer fluid bolus of NS 20 mL/kg over 5 - 20 minutes. Reassess after initial bolus. If signs of shock persist, repeat fluid bolus to maximum total of 60 mL/kg.
D	If low blood glucose, glucose is given slowly (10 mL/min): Neonate with BG < 40: $D_{10}W$, 3 mL/kg IV/IO. < 2 yrs old with BG < 60: $D_{25}W$, 2 mL/kg IV/IO. > 2 yrs old with BG < 80: $D_{50}W$, 1 mL/kg IV/IO.

Rapid Sequence Intubation

Rapid Sequence Intubation (RSI) is the sequential administration of a sedative, paralyzing agent, vagolytic, and cerebroprotective agent, given 2 minutes (or less) prior to emergency endotracheal intubation, to prevent major complications or even death due to hypoxia, hypercapnea, or acidosis.

Indications:	Respiratory arrest, apnea, agonal or gasping respirations. Cannot maintain airway; potential airway obstruction exists. Hypoxemia in spite of supplemental oxygen. Hypercapnea. Chest or head injury. Immediate need for ventilatory support.
Contra-indications:	Limited cervical mobility, receding mandible, major facial or laryngeal trauma, limited jaw opening, upper airway obstruction, distorted facial or airway anatomy. Alert anesthesiology.
ET tube size:	Uncuffed tube internal diameter = 4 + (age/4). After 2 years of age, uncuffed ET tube is no longer used. Cuffed tube internal diameter = 3.5 + (age/4).
Tube depth:	= ET tube size (i.e., mm internal diameter) x 3

	ET Tube Sizes (mm) *uncuffed*	*cuffed*	*Laryngoscope size & type blade*	*ET Depth (cm lip to tip)*	*Suction cath (Fr.)*
Premature	2.5	x	# 0 or # 1 straight	6 + Wt. Kg	6
Newborn	3.0	x	# 1 straight blade	6 + Wt. Kg	6
6 months	3.5	x	# 1 straight blade	11	8
1 yr	4.0	x	# 1 straight blade	12	8
3 yr	x	4.5	# 2 curved or straight	14	8
5 yr	x	5.0	# 2 curved or straight	15	10
7 yr	x	5.5	# 2 curved or straight	16	10
9 yr	x	6.0	# 2 curved or straight	18	10
11 yr	x	6.5	# 2 curved or straight	19	10
12 yr	x	7.0	# 3 curved or straight	21	12
14 yr	x	7.5	# 3 curved or straight	22	12

Supplies:	3 ET tubes (one of the expected size, one larger, one smaller) Tonsil tip suction, Suction catheters — Laryngoscope and light Atropine, a sedative, and Lidocaine — ECG monitor Neuromuscular blocking agent — SpO2 oximeter Pedi Resusbag + mask + O2 reservoir — End tidal CO2 monitor
Preoxygenate:	100% oxygen by mask. If pt is hypoventilating or apneic, use bag/mask ventilation. Gentle cricoid pressure may be used to prevent aspiration (beware excess pressure can cause tracheal obstruction)
Medicate in sequence:	1. Atropine 0.02 mg/kg to prevent bradycardia. 2. Lidocaine 1 mg/kg IV push if there is known or suspected elevation in ICP, or to patients with reactive airways (asthma). 3. Rocuronium 0.6 - 1 mg/kg, or Succinylcholine 1 - 2 mg/kg 4. Etomidate or ketamine or thiopental as the sedative
Intubate:	C-spine immobilization is maintained. Intubation is attempted when there is full relaxation of the airway muscles, usually 45 seconds after rocuronium or succinylcholine has been given. Limit time for intubation attempt to < 30 seconds. Place tube to proper depth. Ventilate with bag while ET tube is secured.
Confirm tube placement:	Breath sounds are present over lateral chest, high in the axillae, but absent over epigastric area. Visible expansion of chest with ventilation, vapor in the tube, improved SpO2 when FiO2 returned to previous setting (beware the SpO2 elevation on 100% O2 may persist for 3 minutes), positive indicator by PetCO2. Obtain ABG's. Obtain chest x-ray. ET tube tip should be no lower than 1 - 2 cm above the carina and no higher than the first rib.
Cuff Pressure:	If cuffed tube used, keep cuff pressure < 20 cm H2O.
Position Head:	Neck flexion may push tube down, extension may pull the tube out of the trachea. Keep the patient's head in a neutral position.

Intraosseous Access

Description:	Insertion of a needle/cannula through the bone cortex and into the marrow, to establish access for the administration of fluids medications, and blood products. The cannula can be inserted in 30-60 seconds, is safe and effective, and allows treatment when vascular access can't be achieved. Because the absorption rate is the same as IV access, the IO is preferred over the ET tube as a means of drug delivery. The cannula may also be used to aspirate samples for T & C, chemistry, blood gases. Intended for short-term use (< 24 hr).
What meds and Fluids?	Drugs infused via the IO route include cardiac medications, sedatives, and paralytics. Hypertonic solutions and strongly alkaline agents should be avoided.
Insertion sites:	In children, the favored insertion site is the anterior-medial aspect of the proximal tibia, 2 - 3 cm below the kneecap. The distal tibia and the head of the humerus are alternative sites. Contraindicated sites include extremities with history of recent injury, bone disorders, or in areas of cellulitis or infection.

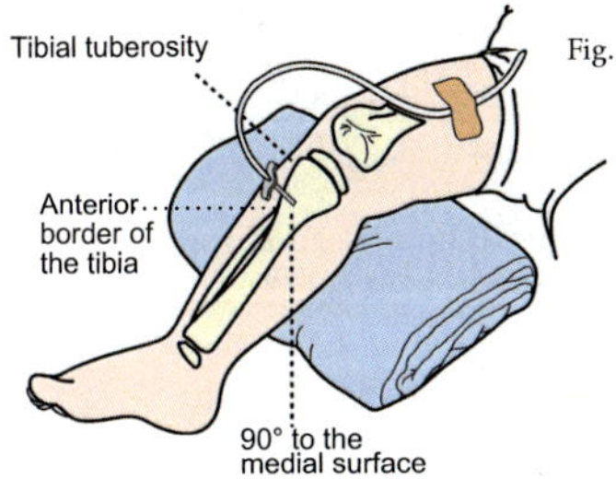

Fig. 16.1

IO Site for Infants. Illustration used with permission. The American Heart Association & The American Academy of Pediatrics. ***Pediatric Advanced Life Support*** 1997-1999, Fig 4, p. 5-6.

Supplies:	Intraosseous infusion needle/cannula, which may be inserted via hand-power, battery power, or spring-loaded device. Gauze, kling, and tape, to support the needle after insertion. Sterile saline flush solution with administration set. Pressure infusion bag or pump may be needed.
Procedure for proximal tibia insertion:	Place a firm towel or pad of linen under the knee, then secure the leg with towel/pad to an armboard. Cleanse the site with antiseptic. 1% lidocaine may be injected. Grasp the posterior thigh, knee, & lower limb to stabilize the site. The needle/cannula must be directed 90° to the tibia. Angulation toward the tibia head risks injury to epiphyseal plate. Hand powered insertion requires a firm twisting/drilling motion. The needle is in the bone marrow cavity when there is a sudden decrease in resistance, the cannula can remain upright without support, aspiration returns bloody bone marrow, and a 10 mL saline flush encounters no resistance. Evacuate air from IV administration set and connect to cannula. Begin continuous infusion, and assess for signs of infiltration: Increased firmness of surrounding tissue Increased circumference of the soft tissue of the extremity Increased resistance to injection. Stabilize the cannula by supporting with a bulky dressing. If the cannula becomes obstructed, it can be replaced with a second cannula, as long as there is no evidence of infiltration. If infiltrated, remove cannula, select an alternative insertion site.
Complications:	Occur in < 1 % of patients, but include: Infiltration, Cellulitis, Fracture, Osteomyelitis, Skin necrosis, Compartment syndrome.

Pediatric Advanced Life Support (PALS)

American Heart Association, 2010

Kleinman ME, Chameides L, Schexnayder SM, et al. Part 14: Pediatric advanced life support: 2010 American Heart Association Guidelines for Cardiopulmonary Resuscitation and Emergency Cardiovascular Care. Circulation. 2010;122:S876 –S908.

	About IV, IO, ET medication administration in children:
IV:	Drugs given by peripheral IV should be given at the port closest to the catheter and should be followed by a bolus of at least 5 mL NS.
IO:	Rapid, safe, effective route. Can give meds, fluids, blood. Onset of drug action is the same as if given intravenously. Can also obtain samples for T & C, chemistry, and blood gases.
ET:	Only lipid-soluble drugs can be given ET and include Lidocaine, Epinephrine, Atropine, Naloxone ("LEAN"). ET administration requires doses that are 2 - 3 times higher than IV doses. Instill via catheter that is passed beyond the tip of the ET tube, follow with 2 - 5 mL NS, then give 5 positive pressure breaths.

After Advanced Airway Placement: Stop CPR cycles, 2 rescuers switch to 100 compressions/min and 8 - 10 breaths/minute, without pause for breaths.

With each algorithm, **search for and treat possible causes:**

Hypovolemia	Hypo/hyperkalemia	Toxins/poisons/drugs
Hypoxia	Hypoglycemia	Tamponade, cardiac
Hydrogen ion (acidosis)	Hypothermia	Tension pneumothorax
	Trauma	Thrombosis (coronary or pulmonary)

Tachycardia with Poor Perfusion

American Heart Association, 2010

Assess and maintain **airway, breathing, circulation.**
Administer 100 % **oxygen**
Attach monitor/pacer. Prepare for possible cardioversion.
Establish IV/IO access. Consider expert consultation.
Evaluate duration of the QRS:

Sinus Tachycardia QRS ≤ 0.09 sec.	**Supraventricular Tach** QRS ≤ 0.09 sec.	**Wide Complex SVT or Ventricular Tachycardia** QRS > 0.09 sec.
History suggests cause. P waves are present and upright in leads I, aVF. Physical activity affects the heart rate. Variable R-R interval. Constant P-R interval. Infant: HR usually < 220 Child: HR usually < 180	History is nonspecific, or there is history of abrupt changes in heart rate. Absent or negative P waves in leads II, III, and aVF. HR is unrelated to the patient's physical activity Infant: HR usually ≥ 220 Child: HR usually ≥ 180	**If the SVT is causing adverse effects** (acutely altered LOC, hypotension, signs of shock) proceed to synchronized cardioversion 0.5 - 1 joule/kg. If ineffective, increase to 2 joules/kg. Sedate if possible, but don't delay treatment.
Identify and manage possible causes. (Verapamil 0.1 - 0.3 mg/kg may be effective in treating SVT in older children, but in infants, is not used without first seeking expert opinion).	Consider vagal maneuvers, e.g., blow through a straw. Adenosine 0.1 mg/kg IV, (max of 6 mg) rapidly. If no response, Adenosine 0.2 mg/kg (max of 12 mg) rapidly. *or* **If hemodynamically unstable, proceed to** Synchronized cardioversion 0.5 - 1 joule/kg. If ineffective, increase to 2 joules/kg. Sedate if possible, but don't delay treatment.	**If the SVT is causing no adverse effects, the rhythm is regular, and the QRS is monomorphic:** Adenosine 0.2 mg/kg (max of 12 mg) rapidly. *or* Amiodarone 5 mg/kg IV over 20 - 60 minutes *or* Procainamide 15 mg/kg over 30 - 60 minutes. Expert consultation is strongly recommended.

Unstable Bradycardia with Pulse

American Heart Association, PALS 2010 for HCP's

Recognize:	There is a pulse, but there is hypotension, signs of shock, altered level of consciousness. Underlying cause must be found & treated.
Airway:	Maintain patency with chin-lift maneuver.
Breathing:	Supply oxygen.
Monitor:	Heart rate & rhythm, blood pressure, PaO2 with pulse oximetry. If available, 12-lead ECG, but do not delay treatment.
IV/IO:	Secure IV or intraosseous access.
Reevaluate in 2 minutes:	If signs of poor perfusion persist, give the following medications: **Epinephrine:** IV/IO: 0.01 mg/kg (0.1 mL/kg of a 1:10,000 solution) ***or*** ET: 0.1 mg/kg (0.1 mL/kg of a 1:1,000 solution). May repeat every 3 - 5 minutes. **Atropine?** For those patients with increased vagal tone or AV block. IV/IO: 0.02 mg/kg or ET: 0.04 - 0.06 mg/kg. May repeat once. Minimum single total dose is 0.1 mg. Maximum single total dose is 0.5 mg.
Pacing?	Transthoracic or Transvenous pacing may be considered for complete heart block or sinus node dysfunction, especially in the presence of heart disease. Remember: Pacing is ineffective for asystole. Pacing is ineffective for bradycardia following cardiac arrest or due to respiratory failure.
Pulseless?	Start CPR. Go to Cardiac Arrest Algorithm.
√ for Cause:	Recall the H's and T's.

Asystole /PEA

American Heart Association, PALS 2010 for HCP's

Recognize:	Unresponsive, pulseless, not breathing. ECG monitor displays Asystole or PEA.
Activate:	Emergency Response Team.
Compression:	at least 100/minute, at depth ≥ 1/3 of anterior-posterior diameter of the chest. Minimize interruptions. Focus on quality CPR.
Airway and Breathing:	Supply O2 to resuscitation bag. Avoid excessive ventilation. **If 1 rescuer + No artificial airway:** 1 Rescuer: 30:2 ratio of compressions to breath 2 Rescuers: 15:2 ratio of compressions to breath Compressions are paused for breaths. **If 2 rescuers + Artificial airway** is in place: 1 breath q 6 - 8 seconds (8 - 10 breaths/min.) Do not pause compressions for breaths.
IV/IO:	Secure IV or intraosseous access.
Epinephrine:	IV/IO: 0.01 mg/kg (0.1 mL/kg of a 1:10,000 solution). Maximum dose is 1 mg IV/IO. May repeat q 3 - 5 minutes. ***or*** ET: 0.1 mg/kg (0.1 mL/kg of a 1:1,000 solution). Maximum dose is 2.5 mg ET. Total dose of repeated meds should be calculated to avoid toxicity.
Rhythm √:	After 2 minutes of CPR, take < 10 seconds to check rhythm/pulse.
CPR:	If rhythm is identified as Asystole or PEA, immediately resume CPR. Minimize interruptions. Repeat sequences of CPR, epinephrine, rhythm √.
√ for Cause:	Recall the H's and T's.

VFib or Pulseless VTach

American Heart Association, PALS 2010 for HCP's

Recognize:	The patient is unresponsive, pulseless, not breathing or agonal. Monitor shows VFib or Pulseless VTach.
Activate:	Emergency response team.
Compression:	at least 100/minute, at depth ≥ 1/3 of anterior-posterior diameter of the chest. Minimize interruptions. Focus on quality CPR.
Airway and Breathing:	100% O2 to resuscitation bag. Avoid excessive ventilation, which increases intrathoracic pressure, impedes venous return, reducing cardiac output, as well as coronary and cerebral blood flow, and may cause harm to those with head injury. Also may cause air trapping, barotrauma, and stomach inflation followed by regurgitation and aspiration. **If No artificial airway + 1 rescuer:** 1 Rescuer: 30:2 ratio of compressions to breath. 2 Rescuers: 15:2 ratio of compressions to breath. Pause the compressions for breaths. **If Artificial airway + 2 rescuers:** 1 breath q 6 - 8 seconds (8 - 10 breaths/min.) Do not pause compressions for breaths.
1st Shock:	Use the appropriate size paddles or self-adhesive pads: • For infants < 10 kg: "Infant" size. • For children > 10 kg (older than approximately 1 year): "Adult" size (8 to 10 cm). Do not allow the pads to touch. First defibrillation dose is 2 joules/kg
CPR:	Immediately resume CPR for 2 minutes, while Epinephrine given.
Epinephrine:	IV/IO: 0.01 mg/kg (1:10,000 solution, give 0.1 mL/kg). ***or*** ET: 0.1 mg/kg (1:1,000 solution, give 0.1 mL/kg). May repeat Epinephrine every 3 - 5 minutes during CPR.
Rhythm √:	Take < 10 seconds to check rhythm and pulse. Rhythm is identified as VF/Pulseless VT.
2nd Shock:	4 joules/kg.
CPR:	Immediately resume CPR for 2 minutes.
Epinephrine:	Repeat Epinephrine every 3 - 5 minutes. Total dose of repeated meds should be calculated to avoid toxicity.
Rhythm √:	Take < 10 seconds to check rhythm and pulse. Rhythm is identified as VF/Pulseless VT.
3rd Shock:	≥ 4 joules/kg, up to 10 joules/kg, or adult dose.
CPR:	Immediately resume compressions for 2 minutes.
Amiodarone:	5 mg/kg bolus. May repeat up to 2 times for refractory VF or pulseless VT.
Monitor effectiveness:	Improve CPR if $PetCO_2$ < 10 mm Hg, or Diastolic BP < 20 mm Hg. Continuous ScvO2 monitoring may be helpful.
√ for causes:	Hypovolemia — Toxins Hypoxia — Tamponade, cardiac Hydrogen ion (acidosis) — Tension pneumothorax Hypo/hyperkalemia — Thrombosis (coronary or pulmonary) Hypothermia — Trauma (hypovolemia, increased ICP)
No Pacing:	Pacing (of any type) is not recommended in cardiac arrest.
ROSC:	After return of spontaneous circulation, reduce the FiO2 to a level that maintains the SpO2 ≥ 94%.

IV Push and Infusions

See the next topic, "Emergency IV Push Dose" for weight specific and volume specific dose.
Information on CV Meds, Analgesics, Antiemetics, Antagonists, Sedatives, and Neuromuscular Blocking Agents follow the "Emergency IV Push Dose" tables.

Medication	IV Push Dose	Mix for infusion pump	Concen tration per mL	Infusion Dose
Amiodarone (Cordarone)	5 mg/kg over 5 - 30 mins.	500 mg 250 mL D5W	2000 mcg	5 - 10 mcg/kg/min
Dobutamine (Dobutrex)	NA	250 mg 250 mL D5W, NS, or RL	1000 mcg	2 - 20 mcg/kg/min start 2 - 5 mcg/kg/min
Dopamine (Intropin)	NA	400 mg 250 mL D5W, NS, or RL	1600 mcg	2 - 20 mcg/kg/min begin 2-5 mcg/kg/min
Epinephrine	0.01 mg/kg	5 mg 250 mL D5W, NS, or RL	2 mcg	0.1 - 1 mcg/kg/min
Heparin	50 - 75 units/kg	25,000 units 500 mL NS, premixed	50 units	< 1 yo: 28 units/kg/hr ≥ 1 yo: 20 units/kg/hr max is 35 units/kg/hr
Insulin	NA	100 units 100 mL NS or 1/2NS	1 unit	0.01 - 0.1 units/kg/hr max is 0.2 units/kg/hr
Lidocaine	1 mg/kg	1000 mg 250 mL D5W, NS, or RL	4 mg	10 - 50 mcg/kg/min
Midazolam (Versed)	0.05 - 0.15 mg/kg (30 mg/kg for SCI)	10 mg 100 mL D5W or NS	0.1 mg	1 - 2 mcg/kg/min
Milrinone (Primacor)	50 mcg/kg over 10 - 30 mins.	40 mg 200 mL premixed	200 mcg	0.25-0.75 mcg/kg/min
Morphine	0.05-0.1 mg/kg	15 mg 30 mL D5W premixed	0.5 mg	0.01 - 0.1 mg/kg/hour
Naloxone (Narcan)	≤ 20 kg: 0.1 mg/kg > 20 kg: 2 mg total	1 mg 250 mL D5W or NS	0.004 mg	0.04 - 0.16 mg/kg/hr
Nitroglycerin	NA	50 mg 250 mL	200 mcg	0.5 - 5 mcg/kg/min Some pts have required 15 - 10 mcg/kg/min
Nitroprusside (Nipride)	NA	50 mg 250 mL D5W	200 mcg	0.5 - 1 mcg/kg/min, titrate to effect up to 5 mcg/kg/min max.
Norepi-nephrine	NA	10 mg 250 mL D5W or NS	40 mcg	0.05 - 2 mcg/kg/min, adjust to achieve desired BP
Pentobarbital (Nembutal)	1 - 3 mg/kg	5000 mg 100 mL D5NS	50 mg	for Pento coma: 1 - 5 mg/kg/hr
Phenylephrine (Neosyn-ephrine)	NA	20 mg 250 mL D5W	80 mcg	0.1 - 0.5 mcg/kg/min. 1 mcg/kg/min is the maximum dose.
Procainamide ((Pronestyl)	3 - 6 mg/kg over 5 mins.	500 mg 250 mL D5W	2 mg	20 - 50 mcg/kg/min

IV Push Dose for Pedi Patients 4 - 20 kg

*The lowest dose in the dose range was used to derive the weight-specific doses.

Medication	Dose range*	Use this mix	Dose	4 kg	6 kg	8 kg	10 kg	12 kg	14 kg	16 kg	18 kg	20 kg
Adenosine (Adenocard)	0.1 mg/kg rapidly; may repeat	dilute 3 mg in 3 mL NS = 1 mg/mL	pt's dose: mL to give:	0.4mg 0.4 mL	0.6 mg 0.6 mL	0.8 mg 0.8 mL	1 mg 1 mL	1.2 mL 1.2 mL	1.4 mg 1.4 mL	1.6 mg 1.6 mL	1.8 mg 1.8 mL	2 mg 2 mL
Amiodarone (Cordarone)	5 mg/kg over 5 - 30 mins.	50 mg/mL	pt's dose: mL to give:	20 mg 0.4 mL	30 mg 0.6 mL	40 mg 0.8 mL	50 mg 1 mL	60 mg 1.2 mL	70 mg 1.4 mL	80 mg 1.6 mL	90 mg 1.8 mL	100 mg 2 mL
Atropine sulfate	0.02 mg/kg (max = 0.5 mg if ≤ 12 yo; 1 mg if > 12 yo)	dilute 1 mg in 10 mL NS = 0.1 mg/mL	pt's dose: mL to give:	0.08 mg 0.8 mL	0.12 1.2 mL	0.16 mg 1.6 mL	0.2 mg 2 mL	0.24 mg 2.4 mL	0.28 mg 2.8 mL	0.32 mg 3.2 mL	0.36 mg 3.6 mL	0.4 mg 4 mL
Bicarbonate ($NaHCO_3$)	1 mEq/kg	1 mEq/mL	pt's dose: mL to give:	4 mEq 4 mL	6 mEq 6 mL	8 mEq 8 mL	10 mEq 10 mL	12 mEq 12 mL	14 mEq 14 mL	16 mEq 16 mL	18 mEq 18 mL	20 mEq 20 mL
CaCl 10 % Calcium Chloride	20 mg/kg	100 mg/mL	pt's dose: mL to give:	80 mg 0.8 mL	120 mg 1.2 mL	160 mg 1.6 mL	200 mg 2 mL	240 mg 2.4 mL	280 mg 2.8 mL	320 mg 3.2 mL	360 mg 3.6 mL	400 mg 4 mL
Dexamethasone (Decadron)	0.25* - 0.6 mg/kg (1 - 2 mg/kg for high ICP)	4 mg/mL	pt's dose: mL to give:	1 mg 0.3 mL	1.5 mg 0.4 mL	2 mg 0.5 mL	2.5 mg 0.6 mL	3 mg 0.8 mL	3.5 mg 0.9 mL	4 mg 1 mL	4.5 mg 1.1 mL	5 mg 1.3 mL
Diazepam (Valium)	0.1* - 0.3 mg/kg	5 mg/mL (do not dilute; precipitates)	pt's dose: mL to give:	0.4 mg 0.08 mL	0.6 mg 0.12 mL	0.8 mg 0.16 mL	1 mg 0.2 mL	1.2 mg 0.24 mL	1.4 mg 0.28 mL	1.6 mg 0.32 mL	1.8 mg 0.36 mL	2 mg 0.4 mL
Diphenhydramine (Benadryl)	1* - 2 mg/kg (maximum single dose is 50 mg)	dilute 50 mg in 10 mL = 5 mg/mL	pt's dose: mL to give:	4 mg 0.8 mL	6 mg 1.2 mL	8 mg 1.6 mL	10 mg 2 mL	12 mg 2.4 mL	14 mg 2.8 mL	16 mg 3.2 mL	18 mg 3.6 mL	20 mg 4 mL
Epinephrine (Adrenalin)	0.01 mg/kg	0.1 mg/mL (1:10,000 solution)	pt's dose: mL to give:	0.04 mg 0.4 mL	0.06 mg 0.6 mL	0.08 mg 0.8 mL	0.1 mg 1 mL	0.12 mg 1.2 mL	0.14 mg 1.4 mL	0.16 mg 1.6 mL	0.18 mg 1.8 mL	0.2 mg 2 mL
Etomidate (Amidate)	0.2* - 0.4 mg/kg over 30 - 60 seconds	2 mg/mL	pt's dose: mL to give:	0.8 mg 0.4 mL	1.2 mg 0.6 mL	1.6 mg 0.8 mL	2 mg 1 mL	2.4 mg 1.2 mL	2.8 mg 1.4 mL	3.2 mg 1.6 mL	3.6 mg 1.8 mL	4 mg 2 mL
Fentanyl (Sublimase)	0.5* - 2 mcg/kg	dilute 50 mcg in 5 mL = 10 mcg/mL	pt's dose: mL to give:	2 mcg 0.2 mL	3 mcg 0.3 mL	4 mcg 0.4 mL	5 mcg 0.5 mL	6 mcg 0.6 mL	7 mcg 0.7 mL	8 mcg 0.8 mL	9 mcg 0.9 mL	10 mcg 1 mL
Furosemide (Lasix)	1* - 2 mg/kg	10 mg/mL	pt's dose: mL to give:	4 mg 0.4 mL	6 mg 0.6 mL	8 mg 0.8 mL	10 mg 1 mL	12 mg 1.2 mL	14 mg 1.4 mL	16 mg 1.6 mL	18 mg 1.8 mL	20 mg 2 mL
Glucose 25% D25W	0.25* - 0.5 g/kg	0.25 g/mL	pt's dose: mL to give:	1 g 4 mL	1.5 g 6 mL	2 g 8 mL	2.5 g 10 mL	3 g 12 mL	3.5 g 14 mL	4 g 16 mL	4.5 g 18 mL	5 g 20 mL
Ketamine (Ketalar)	1* - 2 mg/kg for RSI	dilute 50 mg in 5 mL NS = 10 mg/mL	pt's dose: mL to give:	4 mg 0.4 mL	6 mg 0.6 mL	8 mg 0.8 mL	10 mg 1 mL	12 mg 1.2 mL	14 mg 1.4 mL	16 mg 1.6 mL	18 mg 1.8 mL	20 mg 2 mL

*The lowest dose in the dose range was used to derive the weight-specific doses.

IV Push Doses for Pedi Patients 4 - 20 kg

*The lowest dose in the dose range was used to derive the weight-specific doses.

www.kathywhite.com

Medication	Dose range*	Use this mix	Dose	4 kg	6 kg	8 kg	10 kg	12 kg	14 kg	16 kg	18 kg	20 kg
Lidocaine (Xylocaine)	1 mg/kg slowly	20 mg/mL	pt's dose:	4 mg	6 mg	8 mg	10 mg	12 mg	14 mg	16 mg	18 mg	20 mg
			mL to give:	0.2 mL	0.3 mL	0.4 mL	0.5 mL	0.6 mL	0.7 mL	0.8 mL	0.9 mL	1 mL
Lorazepam (Ativan)	0.05* - 0.1 mg/kg	dilute 4 mg in 4 mL = 1 mg/mL	pt's dose:	0.2 mg	0.3 mg	0.4 mg	0.5 mg	0.6 mg	0.7 mg	0.8 mg	0.9 mg	1 mg
			mL to give:	0.2 mL	0.3 mL	0.4 mL	0.5 mL	0.6 mL	0.7 mL	0.8 mL	0.9 mL	1 mL
Magnesium Sulfate 50 %	25 - 50 mg/kg over 10 - 20 mins.	500 mg/mL	pt's dose:	100 mg	150 mg	200 mg	250 mg	300 mg	350 mg	400 mg	450 mg	500 mg
			mL to give:	0.2 mL	0.3 mL	0.4 mL	0.5 mL	0.6 mL	0.7 mL	0.8 mL	0.9 mL	1 mL
Mannitol 25 %	0.25* - 0.5 g/kg	0.25 g /mL	pt's dose:	1 g	1.5 g	2 g	2.5 g	3 g	3.5 g	4 g	4.5 g	5 g
			mL to give:	4 mL	6 mL	8 mL	10 mL	12 mL	14 mL	16 mL	18 mL	20 mL
Methylprednisolone (Solu-medrol)	1* - 2 mg/kg (30 mg/kg for SCI)	dilute 40 mg in 4 mL = 10 mg/mL	pt's dose:	4 mg	6 mg	8 mg	10 mg	12 mg	14 mg	16 mg	18 mg	20 mg
			mL to give:	0.4 mL	0.6 mL	0.8 mL	1 mL	1.2 mL	1.4 mL	1.6 mL	1.8 mL	2 mL
Midazolam (Versed)	0.05* - 0.2 mg/kg	dilute 5 mg in 5 mL = 1 mg/mL	pt's dose:	0.2 mg	0.3 mg	0.4 mg	0.5 mg	0.6 mg	0.7 mg	0.8 mg	0.9 mg	1 mg
			mL to give:	0.2 mL	0.3 mL	0.4 mL	0.5 mL	0.6 mL	0.7 mL	0.8 mL	0.9 mL	1 mL
Milrinone (Primacor)	0.05 mg/kg over 10 - 30 mins.	1 mg/mL	pt's dose:	0.2 mg	0.3 mg	0.4 mg	0.5 mg	0.6 mg	0.7 mg	0.8 mg	0.9 mg	1 mg
			mL to give:	0.2 mL	0.3 mL	0.4 mL	0.5 mL	0.6 mL	0.7 mL	0.8 mL	0.9 mL	1 mL
Morphine	0.05* - 0.1 mg/kg	dilute 2 mg in 4 mL = 0.5 mg/mL	pt's dose:	0.2 mg	0.3 mg	0.4 mg	0.5 mg	0.6 mg	0.7 mg	0.8 mg	0.9 mg	1 mg
			mL to give:	0.4 mL	0.6 mL	0.8 mL	1 mL	1.2 mL	1.4 mL	1.6 mL	1.8 mL	2 mL
Naloxone (Narcan)	≤ 20 kg: 0.1 mg/kg > 20 kg: 2 mg total	1 mg/mL	pt's dose:	0.4 mg	0.6 mg	0.8 mg	1 mg	1.2 mg	1.4 mg	1.6 mg	1.8 mg	2 mg
			mL to give:	0.4 mL	0.6 mL	0.8 mL	1 mL	1.2 mL	1.4 mL	1.6 mL	1.8 mL	2 mL
Pentobarbital (Nembutal)	1* - 3 mg/kg	dilute 50 mg in 5 mL = 10 mg/mL	pt's dose:	4 mg	6 mg	8 mg	10 mg	12 mg	14 mg	16 mg	18 mg	20 mg
			mL to give:	0.4 mL	0.6 mL	0.8 mL	1 mL	1.2 mL	1.4 mL	1.6 mL	1.8 mL	2 mL
Phenobarbital (Luminal)	10* - 20 mg/kg (max of 1000 mg)	130 mg/mL	pt's dose:	40 mg	60 mg	80 mg	100 mg	120 mg	140 mg	160 mg	180 mg	200 mg
			mL to give:	0.3 mL	0.5 mL	0.6 mL	0.8 mL	0.9 mL	1.1 mL	1.2 mL	1.4 mL	1.5 mL
Phenytoin or Fosphenytoin	10* - 20 mg/kg	50 mg/mL	pt's dose:	40 mg	60 mg	80 mg	100 mg	120 mg	140 mg	160 mg	180 mg	200 mg
			mL to give:	0.8 mL	1.2 mL	1.6 mL	2 mL	2.4 mL	2.8 mL	3.2 mL	3.6 mL	4 mL
Succinylcholine (Anectine)	1* - 2 mg/kg for RSI	20 mg/mL	pt's dose:	4 mg	6 mg	8 mg	10 mg	12 mg	14 mg	16 mg	18 mg	20 mg
			mL to give:	0.2 mL	0.3 mL	0.4 mL	0.5 mL	0.6 mL	0.7 mL	0.8 mL	0.9 mL	1 mL
Thiopental (Pentothal)	2* - 6 mg/kg	dilute 250 mg in 10 mL NS = 25 mg/mL	pt's dose:	8 mg	12 mg	16 mg	20 mg	24 mg	28 mg	32 mg	36 mg	40 mg
			mL to give:	0.3 mL	0.5 mL	0.6 mL	0.8 mL	1 mL	1.1 mL	1.3 mL	1.4 mL	1.6 mL
Vecuronium (Norcuron)	0.1* - 0.2 mg/kg for RSI	1 mg/mL	pt's dose:	0.4 mg	0.6 mg	0.8 mg	1 mg	1.2 mg	1.4 mg	1.6 mg	1.8 mg	2 mg
			mL to give:	0.4 mL	0.6 mL	0.8 mL	1 mL	1.2 mL	1.4 mL	1.6 mL	1.8 mL	2 mL

*The lowest dose in the dose range was used to derive the weight-specific doses.

IV Push Dose for Pedi Patients 22 - 40 kg

*The lowest dose in the dose range was used to derive the weight-specific doses.

Medication	Dose range*	Use this mix	Dose	22 kg	24 kg	26 kg	28 kg	30 kg	32 kg	34 kg	36 kg	38 kg	40 kg
Adenosine (Adenocard)	0.1 mg/kg rapid IV push	3 mg/mL	pt's dose: mL to give:	2.2 mg 0.7 mL	2.4 mg 0.8 mL	2.6 mg 0.9 mL	2.8 mg 0.9 mL	3 mg 1 mL	3.2 mg 1.1 mL	3.4 mg 1.1 mL	3.6 mg 1.2 mL	3.8 mg 1.3 mL	4 mg 1.3 mL
Amiodarone (Cordarone)	5 mg/kg over 5 - 30 mins.	50 mg/mL	pt's dose: mL to give:	110 mg 2.2 mL	120 mg 2.4 mL	130 mg 2.6 mL	140 mg 2.8 mL	150 mg 3 mL	160 mg 3.2 mL	170 mg 3.4 mL	180 mg 3.6 mL	190 mg 3.8 mL	200 mg 4 mL
Atropine sulfate	0.02 mg/kg (maximum single dose is 1 mg)	1 mg/mL	pt's dose: mL to give:	0.4 mg 0.4 mL	0.5 mg 0.5 mL	0.5 mg 0.5 mL	0.5 mg 0.5 mL	0.6 mg 0.6 mL	0.6 mg 0.6 mL	0.7 mg 0.7 mL	0.7 mg 0.7 mL	0.8 mg 0.8 mL	0.8 mg 0.8 mL
Bicarbonate (NaHCO3)	1 mEq/kg	1 mEq/mL	pt's dose: mL to give:	22 mEq 22 mL	24 mEq 24 mL	26 mEq 26 mL	28 mEq 28 mL	30 mEq 30 mL	32 mEq 32 mL	34 mEq 34 mL	36 mEq 36 mL	38 mEq 38 mL	40 mEq 40 mL
CaCl 10 % Calcium Chloride	20 mg/kg (500 mg max)	100 mg/mL	pt's dose: mL to give:	440 mg 4.4 mL	480 mg 4.8 mL	500 mg 5 mL	500 mg 5 mL	500 mg 5 mL	500 mg 5 mL	500 mg 5 mL	500 mg 5 mL	500 mg 5 mL	500 mg 5 mL
Dexamethasone (Decadron)	0.25* - 0.5 mg/kg	4 mg/mL	pt's dose: mL to give:	5.5 mg 1.4 mL	6 mg 1.5 mL	6.5 mg 1.6 mL	7 mg 1.8 mL	7.5 mg 1.9 mL	8 mg 2 mL	8.5 mg 2.1 mL	9 mg 2.3 mL	9.5 mg 2.4 mL	10 mg 2.5 mL
Diazepam (Valium)	0.1* - 0.2 mg/kg	5 mg/mL	pt's dose: mL to give:	2.2 mg 0.4 mL	2.4 mg 0.5 mL	2.6 mg 0.5 mL	2.8 mg 0.6 mL	3 mg 0.6 mL	3.2 mg 0.6 mL	3.4 mg 0.7 mL	3.6 mg 0.7 mL	3.8 mg 0.8 mL	4 mg 0.8 mL
Diphenhydramine (Benadryl)	1* - 2 mg/kg (maximum single dose is 50 mg)	50 mg/mL	pt's dose: mL to give:	22 mg 0.4 mL	24 mg 0.5 mL	26 mg 0.5 mL	28 mg 0.6 mL	30 mg 0.6 mL	32 mg 0.6 mL	34 mg 0.7 mL	36 mg 0.7 mL	38 mg 0.8 mL	40 mg 0.8 mL
Epinephrine (Adrenalin)	0.01 mg/kg	0.1 mg/mL (1:10,000 solution)	pt's dose: mL to give:	0.22 mg 2.2 mL	0.24 mg 2.4 mL	0.26 mg 2.6 mL	0.28 mg 2.8 mL	0.3 mg 3 mL	0.32 mg 3.2 mL	0.34 mg 3.4 mL	0.36 mg 3.6 mL	0.38 mg 3.8 mL	0.4 mg 4 mL
Etomidate (Amidate)	0.2* - 0.4 mg/kg over 30 - 60 seconds	2 mg/mL	pt's dose: mL to give:	4.4 mg 2.2 mL	4.8 mg 2.4 mL	5.2 mg 2.6 mL	5.6 mg 2.8 mL	6 mg 3 mL	6.4 mg 3.2 mL	6.8 mg 3.4 mL	7.2 mg 3.6 mL	7.6 mg 3.8 mL	8 mg 4 mL
Fentanyl (Sublimase)	0.5* - 2 mcg/kg	dilute 50 mcg/5 mL = 10 mcg/mL	pt's dose: mL to give:	11 mcg 1.1 mL	12 mcg 1.2 mL	13 mcg 1.3 mL	14 mcg 1.4 mL	15 mcg 1.5 mL	16 mcg 1.6 mL	17 mcg 1.7 mL	18 mcg 1.8 mL	19 mcg 1.9 mL	20 mcg 2 mL
Furosemide (Lasix)	1* - 2 mg/kg	10 mg/mL	pt's dose: mL to give:	22 mg 2.2 mL	24 mg 2.4 mL	26 mg 2.6 mL	28 mg 2.8 mL	30 mg 3 mL	32 mg 3.2 mL	34 mg 3.4 mL	36 mg 3.6 mL	38 mg 3.8 mL	40 mg 4 mL
Glucose 25% D25W	0.25* - 0.5 g/kg	0.25 g/mL	pt's dose: mL to give:	5.5 g 22 mL	6 g 24 mL	6.5 g 26 mL	7 g 28 mL	7.5 g 30 mL	8 g 32 mL	8.5 g 34 mL	9 g 36 mL	9.5 g 38 mL	10 g 40 mL
Ketamine (Ketalar)	1* - 2 mg/kg for RSI	dilute 50 mg/ 5mL = 10 mg/mL	pt's dose: mL to give:	22 mg 2.2 mL	24 mg 2.4 mL	26 mg 2.6 mL	28 mg 2.8 mL	30 mg 3 mL	32 mg 3.2 mL	34 mg 3.4 mL	36 mg 3.6 mL	38 mg 3.8 mL	40 mg 4 mL

*The lowest dose in the dose range was used to derive the weight-specific doses.

IV Push Dose for Pedi Patients 22 - 40 kg

*The lowest dose in the dose range was used to derive the weight-specific doses.

Medication	Dose range*	Use this mix	Dose	22 kg	24 kg	26 kg	28 kg	30 kg	32 kg	34 kg	36 kg	38 kg	40 kg
Lidocaine (Xylocaine)	1 mg/kg slowly	20 mg/mL	pt's dose: mL to give:	22 mg 1.1 mL	24 mg 1.2 mL	26 mg 1.3 mL	28 mg 1.4 mL	30 mg 1.5 mL	32 mg 1.6 mL	34 mg 1.7 mL	36 mg 1.8 mL	38 mg 1.9 mL	40 mg 2 mL
Lorazepam (Ativan)	0.05* - 0.1 mg/kg	dilute 4 mg in 4 mL = 1 mg/mL	pt's dose: mL to give:	1.1 mg 1.1 mL	1.2 mg 1.2 mL	1.3 mg 1.3 mL	1.4 mg 1.4 mL	1.5 mg 1.5 mL	1.6 mg 1.6 mL	1.7 mg 1.7 mL	1.8 mg 1.8 mL	1.9 mg 1.9 mL	2 mg 2 mL
Magnesium Sulfate 50 %	25* - 50 mg/kg over 10 - 20 minutes	500 mg/mL	pt's dose: mL to give:	550 mg 1.1 mL	600 mg 1.2 mL	650 mg 1.3 mL	700 mg 1.4 mL	750 mg 1.5 mL	800 mg 1.6 mL	850 mg 1.7 mL	900 mg 1.8 mL	950 mg 1.9 mL	1 g 2 mL
Mannitol 25 %	0.25* - 1 g/kg	0.25 g/mL	pt's dose: mL to give:	5.5 mg 22 mL	6 mg 24 mL	6.5 mg 26 mL	7 mg 28 mL	7.5 mg 30 mL	8 mg 32 mL	8.5 mg 34 mL	9 mg 36 mL	9.5 mg 38 mL	10 mg 40 mL
Methylpredisolone (Solu-medrol)	1* - 2 mg/kg (30 mg/kg for SCI)	40 mg/mL	pt's dose: mL to give:	22 mg 0.6 mL	24 mg 0.6 mL	26 mg 0.7 mL	28 mg 0.7 mL	30 mg 0.8 mL	32 mg 0.8 mL	34 mg 0.9 mL	36 mg 0.9 mL	38 mg 1 mL	40 mg 1 mL
Midazolam (Versed)	0.05* - 0.1 mg/kg	dilute 5 mg in 5 mL = 1 mg/mL	pt's dose: mL to give:	1.1 mg 1.1 mL	1.2 mg 1.2 mL	1.3 mg 1.3 mL	1.4 mg 1.4 mL	1.5 mg 1.5 mL	1.6 mg 1.6 mL	1.7 mg 1.7 mL	1.8 mg 1.8 mL	1.9 mg 1.9 mL	2 mg 2 mL
Milrinone (Primacor)	0.05 mg/kg over 10-30 minutes.	1 mg/mL	pt's dose: mL to give:	1.1 mg 1.1 mL	1.2 mg 1.2 mL	1.3 mg 1.3 mL	1.4 mg 1.4 mL	1.5 mg 1.5 mL	1.6 mg 1.6 mL	1.7 mg 1.7 mL	1.8 mg 1.8 mL	1.9 mg 1.9 mL	2 mg 2 mL
Morphine	0.05* - 0.1 mg/kg	2 mg/mL	pt's dose: mL to give:	1.1 mg 0.6 mL	1.2 mg 0.6 mL	1.3 mg 0.6 mL	1.4 mg 0.7 mL	1.5 mg 0.7 mL	1.6 mg 0.8 mL	1.7 mg 0.8 mL	1.8 mg 0.9 mL	1.9 mg 0.9 mL	2 mg 1 mL
Naloxone (Narcan)	for pts > 20 kg: 2 mg total dose	1 mg/mL	pt's dose: mL to give:	2 mg 2 mL	2 mg 2 mL	2 mg 2 mL	2 mg 2 mL	2 mg 2 mL	2 mg 2 mL	2 mg 2 mL	2 mg 2 mL	2 mg 2 mL	2 mg 2 mL
Pentobarbital (Nembutal)	1* - 3 mg/kg	50 mg/mL	pt's dose: mL to give:	22 mg 0.44 mL	24 mg 0.48 mL	26 mg 0.52 mL	28 mg 0.56 mL	30 mg 0.6 mL	32 mg 0.64 mL	34 mg 0.68 mL	36 mg 0.72 mL	38 mg 0.76 mL	40 mg 0.8 mL
Phenobarbital (Luminal)	10* - 20 mg/kg	130 mg/mL	pt's dose: mL to give:	220 mg 1.7 mL	240 mg 1.8 mL	260 mg 2 mL	280 mg 2.2 mL	300 mg 2.3 mL	320 mg 2.5 mL	340 mg 2.6 mL	360 mg 2.8 mL	380 mg 2.9 mL	400 mg 3.1 mL
Phenytoin or Fosphenytoin	10* - 20 mg/kg	50 mg/mL	pt's dose: mL to give:	220 mg 4.4 mL	240 mg 4.8 mL	260 mg 5.2 mL	280 mg 5.6 mL	300 mg 6 mL	320 mg 6.4 mL	340 mg 6.8 mL	360 mg 7.2 mL	380 mg 7.6 mL	400 mg 8 mL
Succinylcholine (Anectine)	1* - 2 mg/kg for RSI	20 mg/mL	pt's dose: mL to give:	22 mg 1.1 mL	24 mg 1.2 mL	26 mg 1.3 mL	28 mg 1.4 mL	30 mg 1.5 mL	32 mg 1.6 mL	34 mg 1.7 mL	36 mg 1.8 mL	38 mg 1.9 mL	40 mg 2 mL
Thiopental (Pentothal)	2* - 5 mg/kg	dilute 250 mg in 10 mL NS = 25 mg/mL	pt's dose: mL to give:	44 mg 1.8 mL	48 mg 1.9 mL	52 mg 2.1 mL	56 mg 2.2 mL	60 mg 2.4 mL	64 mg 2.6 mL	68 mg 2.7 mL	72 mg 2.9 mL	76 mg 3 mL	80 mg 3.2 mL
Vecuronium (Norcuron)	0.1* - 0.2 mg/kg for RSI	1 mg/mL	pt's dose: mL to give:	2.2 mg 2.2 mL	2.4 mg 2.4 mL	2.6 mg 2.6 mL	2.8 mg 2.8 mL	3 mg 3 mL	3.2 mg 3.2 mL	3.4 mg 3.4 mL	3.6 mg 3.6 mL	3.8 mg 3.8 mL	4 mg 4 mL

*The lowest dose in the dose range was used to derive the weight-specific doses.

Stat CV Meds

Adenosine	
Action:	Slows AV conduction.
Indication:	Supraventricular tachycardia.
Dose:	A 2-syringe technique is preferred. The IV site closest to the patient's heart should be used. 0.1 mg/kg IV (maximum: 6 mg for first dose) as rapidly as possible, followed by immediate rapid flush with 5 – 10 mL of normal saline. If no AV block occurs and there is no response within 30 seconds of the first dose, the initial dose may be doubled (0.2 mg/kg, up to a maximum total dose of 12 mg for the second and subsequent doses) followed immediately by rapid saline flush. May be given intraosseously if IV access has not been achieved.
Caution:	Continuous ECG monitoring should be employed during use. A defibrillator must be immediately available. Contraindicated in patients who have had a heart transplant. Contraindicated in 2° and 3° AV block or sick-sinus syndrome, unless the patient has a pacemaker.

Amiodarone	
Action:	Antiarrhythmic, with vasodilatory and negative chronotropic effects.
Indication:	Pulseless ventricular fibrillation (VT).
Dose:	IV/IO: 5 mg/kg (maximum total dose of 300 mg) over 5 minutes. May be repeated up to a total daily dose of 15 mg/kg. In pulseless ventricular arrhythmias, Amiodarone is given when defibrillation and epinephrine have been unsuccessful. When considered for conditions other than cardiac arrest, cardiology service should be consulted.
Indication:	VT with a pulse, or SVT with a pulse.
Dose:	IV/IO: 5 mg/kg (maximum total dose 300 mg) over 20 – 60 min. Adjust administration rate according to urgency. May be followed by infusion of 5 mcg/kg per min, increased to maximum of 10 mcg/kg/min. Concentration of continuous infusion should not exceed 2 mg/mL and should be diluted with D5W.
Caution:	May cause hypotension, bradycardia, heart block, prolonged QT interval, and torsades de pointes. Contraindicated in severe sinus node dysfunction, marked sinus bradycardia, and 2° and 3° degree AV block. Expert consultation should be obtained before combining with procainamide or other drugs that prolong the QT interval.

Atropine	
Action:	Anticholinergic.
Indication:	Symptomatic bradycardia unresponsive to O_2 and ventilation.
Dose:	IV/IO: 0.02 mg/kg, up to a maximum single dose as follows: Child: 0.5 mg Adolescent: 1 mg IM: 0.02 – 0.04 mg/kg. ET: Neonates: 0.01 – 0.03 mg/kg. ET: Children and adolescents: 0.04 – 0.06 mg/kg. Follow with or dilute in saline flush (1 – 5 mL) based on patient size.
Indication:	Prevention of bradycardia associated with rapid sequence intubation
Dose:	IV/IO: 0.02 mg/kg IM: 0.02 - 0.04 mg/kg given before the paralytic agent.
Indication:	Anticholinesterase poisoning.
Dose:	IV: for children, 0.05 mg/kg (up to a total dose: 2 – 5 mg). Poisonings with anticholinesterase or nerve gas may require large doses of atropine (may double the dose and repeat every 10 – 20 minutes as needed to control pulmonary secretions).

Calcium Chloride	
Action:	Electrolyte; enhances myocardial contractility.
Indication:	Critical hypocalcemia; Calcium channel blocker toxicity.
Dose:	IV/IO: 20 mg/kg (0.2 mL/kg when using 10% CaCl), given slowly Maximum dose is 2 g. For indications other than cardiac arrest, infuse over 30 – 60 minutes. Monitor heart rate; may repeat dose as necessary. Stop injection if symptomatic bradycardia occurs. Do not give via endotracheal tube.
Caution:	Produces a more rapid increase in ionized calcium concentration than calcium gluconate and is preferred for the critically ill child. Used for cardiac resuscitation only for the indications listed above. Administer through a central venous line if possible; extravasation from a peripheral IV may cause severe soft tissue injury.

Dobutamine	
Action:	Inotrope, mild chronotrope, mild vasodilator.
Indication:	Cardiogenic shock, congestive heart failure.
Dose:	IV infusion: 2 – 20 mcg/kg per min, titrated to desired clinical effect.
Caution:	May cause arrhythmias and hypertension. Extravasation can result in severe skin injury. See Phentolamine for treatment of extravasation.

Dopamine	
Action:	Inotrope, chronotrope, and depending on dose, vasoactive activity.
Indication:	Cardiogenic shock, Distributive shock.
Dose:	IV infusion: 2 – 20 mcg/kg per min, titrated to desired clinical effect. Effects are dose dependent: low-dose (1 – 5 mcg/kg/min) usually stimulates dopaminergic and beta-adrenergic receptors. higher doses stimulate alpha-adrenergic receptors.
Caution:	May cause arrhythmias and hypertension. Infusion rates > 20 mcg/kg/min may cause peripheral, renal, and splanchnic vasoconstriction and ischemia. Extravasation can result in severe skin injury. See Phentolamine for treatment of extravasation.

Epinephrine	
Action:	Potent catecholamine with alpha and beta agonist effects.
Indication:	Cardiopulmonary resuscitation.
Dose:	Newborn: 0.01 – 0.03 mg/kg of 1:10 000 solution. Infants/children: 0.01 mg/kg of 1:10 000 solution (maximum: 1 mg), repeated every 3 – 5 minutes.
Indication:	Anaphylaxis.
Dose:	IM/SC: 0.01 mg/kg of 1:1000 solution (maximum: 0.3 - 0.5 mg), repeated q 5 – 20 min. if needed, or proceed to continuous infusion.
Indication:	Continued shock after volume resuscitation.
Dose:	IV infusion: 0.1 - 1 mcg/kg/min. Start at lowest dose, titrate to effect. Dose as high as 5 mcg/kg/min is sometimes necessary.
Indication:	Laryngotracheobronchitis (croup).
Dose:	0.5 mL/kg of 1:1000 solution (maximum: 5 mL = 5 mg) by nebulizer.
Caution:	Epinephrine is available in 2 concentrations: 1:1000 (1 mg/mL) and 1:10 000 (0.1 mg/mL). Use caution to ensure selection of the appropriate concentration for the route of administration and patient age and condition. In pts with perfusing rhythm, epinephrine causes increased HR and possibly ventricular ectopy, vasoconstriction, and increased BP. IV infiltration can result in severe skin/tissue injury. See Phentolamine for treatment of extravasation. No longer recommended for acute asthma.

Stat CV Meds

	Lidocaine
Action:	Antiarrhythmic
Indication:	Ventricular arrhythmias. Wide complex tachycardia.
Dose:	IV/IO: 1 mg/kg (maximum: 100 mg). Repeat every 5 – 10 min to desired effect, or total of 3 mg/kg. IV infusion: 20 – 50 mcg/kg/min. ET: 2 – 3 mg/kg, followed by saline (1 – 5 mL) based on patient size.
Caution:	Lidocaine is less effective than amiodarone. High concentrations may cause myocardial depression, hypotension, seizures. Contraindicated in complete heart block & wide complex tachycardia
	Magnesium Sulfate
Action:	An inorganic salt that is essential to all cells.
Indication:	Hypomagnesemia, torsades de pointes, refractory status asthmaticus
Dose:	IV/IO: 25 – 50 mg/kg (maximum: 2 g) over 10 - 20 minutes. For pulseless torsades, dose is given faster. For status asthmaticus, dose is given over 20 – 30 minutes.
Caution:	Rapid infusion may cause hypotension and bradycardia. Have CaCl available if needed to reverse magnesium toxicity.
	Milrinone
Action:	Phosphodiesterase inhibitor; Inotrope; Vasodilator.
Indication:	Myocardial dysfunction with increased SVR/PVR.
Dose:	IV/IO: loading dose of 50 mcg/kg given over 10 – 60 min. Infusion: 0.25 – 0.75 mcg/kg per min.
Caution:	May cause hypotension, ventricular arrhythmias, chest pain. Monitor BP and ECG continuously. Maintain intravascular volume. Longer infusion times reduce the risk of hypotension.
	Nitroprusside
Action:	Potent peripheral vasodilator
Indication:	Hypertensive crisis. Cardiogenic shock with high SVR.
Dose:	Start infusion at 0.5 - 1mcg/kg/min and titrate for the desired effect. Maximum dose is 5 mcg/kg/min.
Caution:	Cover bottle, burette, IV tubing, or syringe pump with foil. Can cause profound hypotension. Monitor BP with arterial line. Guard against too-rapid or accidental bolus injection. May cause cyanide/thiocyanate toxicity and metabolic acidosis.
	Norepinephrine
Action:	Inotrope. Peripheral vassoconstrictor
Indication:	Fluid resistant shock with low SVR (septic shock, neurogenic shock).
Dose:	IV/IO: 0.1 – 2 mcg/kg/min, titrated to desired effect.
Caution:	May cause tachycardia, bradycardia, arrhythmias, hypertension. Extravasation can result in severe skin injury.
	Phenylephrine
Action:	Alpha receptor stimulant, potent vasoconstrictor
Indication:	Shock due to vasodilation
Dose:	2-12 years old: 5 - 20 mcg/kg IV bolus, then 0.1 - 0.5 mcg/kg/min IV; Max: 3 - 5 mcg/kg/min IV
	Procainamide
Action:	Antiarrhythmic.
Indication:	Wide complex tachycardia with a pulse, atrial flutter/fib, supraventricular tachycardia resistant to other drugs.
Dose:	IV/IO loading dose: 15 mg/kg over 30 – 60 min.
Caution:	May cause hypotension, negative inotropic effect, prolonged QT, torsades de pointes, heart block, cardiac arrest. Stop administration if QRS widens ≥ 50% or hypotension occurs..

Analgesics

Analgesics		Dose
Acetaminophen	(Tylenol)	PO: 10 - 15 mg/kg/dose q 4 hrs
Buprenorphine	(Buprenex)	IM or IV: 2 - 12 yrs: 2 - 6 mcg/kg q 4 - 6 hrs ≥ 13 yrs: 0.3 mg q 6 hrs
Codeine		PO, SC, or IM: 0.5 - 1 mg/kg/dose q 4 - 6 hrs
Fentanyl	(Sublimase)	IVP: 0.5 - 1 mcg/kg/dose q 1 - 2 hrs. IV infusion: 0.5 - 1 mcg/kg/*hr*
Ibuprofen		PO: 4 - 10 mg/kg q 6 - 8 h, up to 40 mg/kg/d
Ketorolac	(Toradol)	IM: 1 mg/kg (max of 30 mg) IV: 0.5 mg/kg (max of 15 mg)
Meperidine	(Demerol)	SC, IM, IV: 1 - 1.5 mg/kg/dose q 3 - 4 hr
Methadone	(Dolophine)	PO: 0.1 mg/kg q 6 - 12 hrs IV: 0.1 mg/kg q 4 hr x 2, then q 6-12 h maximum dose is 10 mg
Morphine		IM: 50 - 100 mcg/kg/dose (max total is 10 mg) IVP: 50 - 100 mcg/kg/dose IV infusion: < 6 months: 10 - 15 mcg/kg/*hr* > 6 months: 25 - 30 mcg/kg/*hr*
Nalbuphine	(Nubain)	SC/IV/IM: 0.2 mg/kg (max dose is 20 mg)
Sufentanil	(Sufenta)	IVP: 1 - 2 mcg/kg

Antiemetics

Antiemetics		Dose
Chlorpromazine	(Thorazine)	IM/IV: (for ≥ 6 months of age): 0.5 - 1 mg/kg/dose q 6 - 8 hrs
Droperidol	(Inapsine)	IM/IV: 2 -12 yrs: 0.05 mg/kg/dose q 4 - 6 hrs > 12 yrs: 2.5 mg/dose q 4 hrs
Glycopyrrolate	(Robinul)	IM/IV: 5 - 10 mcg/kg/dose q 3 - 4 hrs (0.2 mg/dose max)
Granisetron	(Kytril)	IV: ≥ 2 yrs: 10 mcg/kg
Ondansetron	(Zofran)	IV: 4 - 11 yrs: 4 mg/dose, over 2 - 5 min., q 8 hr IV: ≥ 12 yrs: 8 mg/dose q 8 hr
Promethazine	(Phenergan)	IM/IV: > 2 yo: 0.25 - 1 mg/kg/dose q 6 hrs (25 mg maximum single dose)

Antagonists

Antagonists		Dose
Narcotic Antagonist	**Naloxone** (Narcan)	< 5 yo (< 20 kg): 0.1 mg/kg ≥ 5 yo (≥ 20 kg): 2 mg total Infusion: 0.04 - 0.16 mg/kg/hr
Benzodiazepine antagonist	**Flumazenil** (Romazicon)	0.01 mg/kg (max of 0.2 mg) repeat q 1 min, not to exceed a total cumulative dose of 0.05 mg/kg or 1 mg

Sedatives

Sedatives	Dose and Information
Diazepam (Valium)	0.1 mg/kg/dose. Given over 3 minutes. May be repeated after 15 - 30 min, not to exceed 10 mg/dose.
Ketamine (Ketalar)	1 - 1.5 mg/kg slow IV push (not to exceed 0.5 mg/kg/min). Additional doses may be given at 0.5 mg/kg IV q 10 - 15 min. Peak occurs is 30 seconds, duration of action is about 5 - 10 min. Preserved airway reflexes and respiratory drive, and bronchodilatory effects make it the sedative of choice for patients with bronchospasm.
Lorazepam (Ativan)	0.05 - 0.1 mg/kg (max of 4 mg/dose) for Status Epilepticus. May repeat the dose q 10 - 15 mins for continued seizures.
Midazolam (Versed)	< 6 months old: dose not established. 6 months to 12 years old: 0.05 - 0.1 mg/kg IV. > 12 years old: 0.01 - 0.05 mg/kg (0.5 - 4 mg). Max. single dose is 5 mg. Give slowly, over several minutes. May repeat q 10 - 15 min. Cumulative dose is 10 mg maximum.

Neuromuscular Blocking Agents

Warning from the American Academy of Pediatrics:
"Ventilatory support is necessary. Personnel with skills in airway management must be present and prepared to respond when (any of these agents) is administered. Age-appropriate equipment for suctioning, oxygenation, intubation, and ventilation should be immediately available."

- NMBA's do not alter consciousness or provide analgesia or amnesia.
- With any NMBA, a sedative must also be given, and if indicated, an analgesic for patients affected by pain.
- A peripheral nerve stimulator should be used to titrate NMBA dosage to the therapeutic level of paralysis, avoiding overdosage and its long term effects.
- In obese patients, the initial dose should be determined using the patient's **ideal** body weight, not actual body weight.
- Severe anaphylactic reactions to neuromuscular blocking agents have been reported. These reactions have in some cases been life-threatening and fatal.

Nondepolarizing NMBA's

Generic name (Brand name)	Dose and Information
Mivacurium (Mivacron)	0.15 - 0.3 mg/kg in patients older than 2 years of age. Onset in 1 minute, duration of 15 - 20 minutes. Dose-related hypotension. Reduce dose in patients with renal or hepatic impairment. To facilitate mechanical ventilation, continuous infusion dose in child older than 2 years: 11 - 14 mcg/kg/min.
Pancuronium (Pavulon)	0.1 mg/kg (in infants less than 1 month old, test the patient's response with initial dose of 0.02 mg/kg). Onset in 2 - 3 minutes, duration of 60 minutes. Can be used when succinylcholine is contraindicated, but has more CV side effects. Pancuronium is a long-acting neuromuscular blocker that requires ventilatory assistance for at least 1 hour.
Rocuronium (Zemuron)	1 mg/kg prior to intubation. 0.6 mg/kg to facilitate mechanical ventilation. Onset in 1 - 1.5 minutes, duration of 30 - 45 minutes. The preferred NMBA for Rapid Sequence Intubation, due to fast onset, short duration, minimal cardiovascular effects, and available premixed in a ready-to-use vial. Sugammadex is a new agent reported to rapidly reverse Rocuronium.
Vecuronium (Norcuron)	0.1 - 0.2 mg/kg to intubate. Onset in 2 minutes, duration of 45 - 90 minutes depending on the dose. Rocuronium or succinylcholine are preferred over Vecuronium for facilitating rapid intubation in emergency situations.

Depolarizing NMBA

Generic name (Brand name)	Dose and Information
Succinycholine also known as **Suxamethonium** (Anectine)	1 - 2 mg/kg to intubate. Onset in 1 minute, duration of 4 - 5 minutes. Has the shortest duration of all NMBA's. Contraindicated in patients with previous history of malignant hyperthermia, severe burns, spinal cord injury, neuromuscular disease, or myopathies (there have been cases of rapid muscle breakdown, arrhythmias, cardiac arrest, death). When contraindications exist, a fast-acting nondepolarizing muscle relaxant such as rocuronium is used. Also, repeated doses may cause bradycardia.

Submersion Injury

Facts:	• Of all drowning deaths in children, 75% are age 1 - 4 years. • Infant drownings most often occur in a bathtub, bucket, hot tub, or toilet. For toddlers, a residential swimming pool. • Children at high risk for drowning while swimming are those who have epilepsy, hyperventilation disorder, or hypoglycemia.
Drowning Timeline:	Immediate: After initial breath holding, presence of liquid in the pharynx or larynx triggers reflex laryngospasm. Hypoxia leads to release of the laryngospasm. 2 - 4 minutes: Loss of consciousness. 5 minutes: PO_2 as low as 4 mm Hg. CO_2 doubles, pH falls to < 7. 5 - 10 mins: Cardiac arrest
Patho-physiology:	• Aspiration is typically 3 - 4 mL/kg (but as much as 11-22 mL/kg). • Fresh water drowning: hypotonic and rapidly absorbed. Expect hypervolemia, hemodilution, RBC hemolysis, hyperkalemia. • Sea water drowning: hypertonic, induces fluid shift from the circulation, causing hypovolemia and elevated serum electrolytes. • Both fresh and sea water drowning cause functional loss of surfactant. Large areas of atelectasis result. • Hypoxemia, acidosis, CNS ischemia, and lung insult dominate. • Aspiration of vomitus, dirt, sewage results in bronchial occlusion, bronchospasm, pneumonia, abscess formation, and inflammatory damage to alveolar capillary membranes. • Profound hypoxemia causes capillary injury and leak, which culminate in hypovolemia, ARDS, and cerebral edema. • Airway bronchospasm and/or forced expiration against fluid filled bronchi may cause alveolar rupture and pneumothorax.
ABC:	100% O_2. CPR if pulseless. Many have bradycardia, PEA, asystole. Make no attempt to remove water from the airways. Beware that 50 - 80% vomit during CPR or endotracheal intubation. Cricoid pressure should be applied during intubation. Prepare to monitor SpO_2, ECG, BP, end-tidal CO_2, $ScvO_2$.
Fluids:	Almost all require fluids (crystalloid or colloid) 10 - 40 mL/kg.
Hemo-dynamics:	After ROSC, expect myocardial dysfunction. Dopamine 5 - 10 mcg/kg/min or Epinephrine 0.2 - 1 mcg/kg/min.
Arrhythmia	Core temp < 28° C: expect VFib, which is unresponsive to meds. Expect platelet dysfunction, coagulopathy. Aggressively rewarm pt.
Hypo-thermia:	• If pt. temp ≥ 33° C, use blankets, but no active warming measures. • If 28 - 32° C, heat the ventilator gases and warm the IV fluids. • If < 28 ° C, warm lavage of gastric, urinary, peritoneal catheters. Prevent over-warming, which increases CNS metabolism 7% for each degree Celsius, intensifying cerebral ischemia.
Acid-Base Balance:	Respiratory acidosis adversely affects neuro outcome and must be reversed. But also avoid hyperventilation ($PaCO_2$ < 30 mm Hg), which can cause cerebral ischemia. End-tidal CO_2 monitor is helpful Severe metabolic acidosis, with base deficits of greater than 10 should be corrected using 1 mEq/kg of sodium bicarbonate.
Neuro care:	Prevent: Hypoxia, Hypotension, Hyperthermia, Hyperglycemia. Prevent hyponatremia, which contributes to cerebral edema. Quickly and aggressively manage seizure activity. Use EEG monitoring if necessary to detect subclinical seizures.
Mechanical Ventilation:	Expect development of acute respiratory distress syndrome. Lung protective strategies include low tidal volumes, FiO_2 less than 60%, optimal PEEP. See the ARDS topic in this chapter for details.
Other injuries:	Cervical spine (c-spine) injuries are rare (less than 0.5% of victims). Protect neck until spinal cord has been cleared of injury.
ECMO:	For refractory hypoxemia, low cardiac output, and rewarming.
Outcome:	35% die despite emergency and critical care. 11% of those who survive have severe neurologic impairment.

Acute Respiratory Distress Syndrome

Description:	Acute onset of hypoxemia, tachypnea, and development of pulmonary infiltrates following direct or indirect lung injury. Severity and mortality risk is predicted by the Oxygenation Index. OI = (Mean Airway Pressure x FIO_2)/PaO_2 ≥ 13 is linked to a 36 % mortality rate ≤ 12 is linked to a 20 % mortality rate The duration of mechanical ventilation averages 10 - 16 days. Although the incidence of ARDS is lower in infants and children, the risk for ventilator-induced injury is greater.
Pathophysiology:	Direct injury due to aspiration or submersion injury or indirect injury due to infection, sepsis, exposure to cardiopulmonary bypass, or to blood transfusion. The results are: • Injury to the alveolar epithelium, resulting in impaired surfactant production, atelectasis, increased airway resistance, small airway collapse, alveolar flooding, and decreased lung compliance. • Injury to the pulmonary capillary endothelium, resulting in capillary leaking and flooding of interstitial spaces. • As work of breathing increases, the $PaCO_2$ will rise as respiratory muscle fatigue develops. • Inflammatory response deposits fibrin in interstitial spaces • The end result is reduced lung compliance (stiff lung) with escalating work of breathing, intrapulmonary shunting, and poor gas exchange. • Mechanical ventilation inflicts additional lung injury with alveolar over-distention (barotrauma), alveolar collapse and re-expansion, and O_2 toxicity.
Diagnostic criteria for ALI/ARDS:	• Acute onset of hypoxemia and tachypnea. • Severe arterial hypoxemia resistant to O_2 therapy, as evidenced by PaO_2/FIO_2 ratio < 200. • Diffuse pulmonary inflammation (bilateral infiltrates on chest radiograph). • No evidence of left atrial hypertension.
About ARDS in Infants and Small Children:	1. Compared to older children and adults, infants and small children have smaller airways, higher airway resistance, more compliant chest walls, lower residual capacity. 2. Infants and small children also have a lower hematocrit, as well as higher sedation requirements. 3. The risk for ARDS is higher, the onset is more rapid, and the hypoxemia lasts longer than in adults. 4. Infants and small children are also more vulnerable to the damaging effects of profound hypoxemia.
Mortality:	ARDS accounts for 30% of all Pedi ICU deaths. ARDS-related death rates in patients with: near-drowning: 54% cardiac disease: 39% sepsis: 31% pneumonia: 11% aspiration: 12% Factors that increase the mortality risk: pre-existing medical conditions, immunosuppression, higher ventilation requirements, the development of multiple-organ system failure.
Assessment Findings:	• Tachypnea, early hypoxemia, and hypocapnea. • Escalating work of breathing. Rise in $PaCO_2$. • Rales over the areas of atelectasis or alveolar congestion. • Decreased breath sounds over the areas of consolidation.
ET intubation is needed when:	• Hypoxemia is severe and unresponsive to O_2 therapy. • The work of breathing is excessive.

Cheifetz IM. Pediatric Acute Respiratory Distress Syndrome. Resp Care. 2011 Oct;56(10):1589-99.

Acute Respiratory Distress Syndrome

Treatment

Mechanical Ventilation:	• Cuffed endotracheal tube is usually required to ensure delivery of PEEP to noncompliant (stiff) lungs. • Arterial access should be secured early. • Titrate PEEP to achieve: SpO_2 = 88 - 95% on $FiO_2 \leq$ 50 - 60%. • Tidal volume is limited to 6 mL/kg ***ideal*** body weight. • Peak airway pressure should be limited to ≤ 30 cm H_2O. • Maintain arterial pH = 7.30 - 7.45. • Maintain PaO_2 60 - 80 torr. • Permit hypercapnea unless contraindicated (e.g., ↑ ICP) • Sedation and analgesia help aide mechanical ventilation. • Outcome is improved with a mean airway pressure < 17 cm H_2O, and oxygenation index is < 15 O_2 index= $\frac{FiO_2}{PaO_2}$ x Mean Airway Pressure • O_2 index > 40 indicates failure of conventional ventilation. ECMO (Extracorporeal Membrane Oxygenation) should be considered. Intravenous Nitrous Oxide may be used as a bridge to ECMO.
Additional Treatment:	• Early antibiotics for suspected infection. • Use Hgb = 10 g/dL as the PRBC transfusion threshold in unstable patients, and Hgb = 7 g/dL in stable patients. • Fluids to optimize hemodynamics and urinary output. • Titrate vasoactive agents to achieve age-appropriate BP. • Monitor CVP, organ function. For persistent hypervolemia and oliguria, Continuous Renal Replacement Therapy (CRRT) may be required • Prone positioning, surfactant replacement, nitrous oxide, may be considered in selected individuals. • Prevent stress ulcer development and GI bleeding (which is associated with high morbidity). • Tight glucose control in children with ARDS is not recommended until further trials confirm safety/efficacy. (24% of patients experienced accidental hypoglycemia). • Daily interruption of sedative and neuromuscular blockade. • Nutritional support must be provided. • Identify persistent triggers of the inflammatory cascade (e.g., infection, necrosis, pancreatitis).
If the patient suddenly deteriorates:	Remove the patient from the ventilator and ventilate with self-inflating bag. Assess for causes (look for **DOPE**): **D**isplaced tube **O**bstructed tube **P**neumothorax **E**quipment failure
Extubation:	Studies have reported extubation failure rates of 10% to 20%, most commonly associated with upper airway swelling. The PALISI Network (Pediatric Acute Lung Injury and Sepsis Investigators) used 3 extubation criteria: 1) minimal tidal volume of 5 mL/kg exhaled, measured at the endotracheal tube, 2) SpO_2 of ≥ 95% on PEEP of ≤ 5 cm H_2O, with $FIO_2 \leq$ 50%, and 3) a respiratory rate that is appropriate for age. These criteria produced an extubation failure rate of 15%.
Promising therapies:	High-frequency oscillatory ventilation Noninvasive ventilation High Flow humidified oxygen Corticosteroids for lung inflammation and fibrosis Use of restrictive fluid management

Randolph AG. Management of acute lung injury and acute respiratory distress syndrome in children. **Crit Care Med** 2009; 37:2448–2454.

Status Asthmaticus

Description:	When stimulated by infection or airborne allergen, hyper-reactive airways constrict, produce excess mucus, and become obstructed. Standard treatment (bronchodilator and steroid) fails. Progressive deterioration (which may be slow or fast) threatens life.
Patho-physiology:	A stimulus (allergen, infection, stress) triggers an inflammatory response by mast cells, lymphocytes, epithelial cells, resulting in: • Bronchial hypersensitivity, constriction, spasm, obstruction. • Mucosal edema and epithelial destruction. • Mucus hypersecretion progressing to mucus plugging. The clinical result is: • Severe alveolar air trapping, which can lead to ↑ lung volume, ↑ intra-thoracic pressure, ↓ venous return, ↓ cardiac output. • CO_2 retention and respiratory acidosis. • ↑ airway resistance -> ↑ work of breathing, prolonged expiration, diaphragmatic and respiratory muscle fatigue, exhaustion. • ↑ pulmonary vascular resistance -> right ventricular strain.
Pt History linked to Asthma-Related Death:	Hx of near fatal asthma requiring intubation, mechanical ventilation Hx of hospitalization or emergency visit for asthma in the past year. Hx of taking or recently stopped taking oral glucocorticosteroids. Dependent on rapid-acting beta-2 agonist (1 canister of salbutamol or equivalent monthly). Hx of sedative use, psychiatric disease or psychosocial problems. Hx of poor adherence to asthma meds and/or written asthma plan.
Signs of severe respiratory compromise	1. Resp. rate: ≥ 40 in a 2 - 3 year old; ≥ 36 in a 4 - 5 year old; ≥ 31 in a 6 - 12 year old; ≥ 28 in a pt > 12 years old (Warning: normal or ↓ respiratory rate may precede decompensation) 2. Inspiratory & expiratory wheezes, or decreased breath sounds. 3. Dyspnea, speaks in single words or short phrases or grunts.
Signs of imminent respiratory failure:	• Intercostal and/or sternal retractions, abdominal retractions. • Prolonged expiratory phase. $PaCO_2$ > 50 mm Hg. • Paradoxic Pulse > 10 mm Hg in children, > 18 mm Hg in teens. • Diaphoresis. Metabolic acidosis. Cyanosis. Decreased LOC. • Peak expiratory flow rate is < 20 % of predicted, and fails to improve with first-line therapy. • Prior to CV Failure: bradycardia, weak pulses, slow capillary refill
Treatment STAT:	1. O_2 by mask to achieve SaO_2 of ≥ 95% 2. Rapid acting inhaled beta2-agonist 3. Inhaled anticholinergic 4. Systemic glucocorticosteroids (but 4-6 hrs are required for effect) 5. Intravenous Magnesium to maintain serum Mg at 4 mg/dL. 6. Intubation and mechanical ventilation in patients with respiratory acidosis, refractory hypoxemia, exhaustion, ↓ LOC. Beware hypotension may follow intubation, the result of overly vigorous ventilation, hypovolemia, or pneumothorax. 7. If refractory to the above, theophylline may be considered. 8. Epinephrine (SQ or IM) is no longer recommended for SE.
Mechanical Ventilation:	• Ventilator TV = 4 - 7 mL/kg and rate of 10 - 14 bpm. • Moderate respiratory acidosis (pH = 7.2) is allowed. • Sedation is usually required. • Muscle relaxants are avoided (when given with the high doses of steroid, prolonged paralysis may result). • Beware of the high risk for barotrauma and pneumothorax. • Some use noninvasive positive pressure ventilation (NPPV). • Prevent bronchoconstriction with suctioning, by providing adequate sedation. Some recommend endotracheal administration of 2% Lidocaine 1 mg/kg prior to suctioning.

Global Strategy for Asthma Management and Prevention 2012. www.ginasthma.org
Pathophysiology and Pathogenesis of Asthma. www.nhlbi.nih.gov August 28, 2007.
Agarwal S, Kache S. **Status Asthmaticus.** Ped.Stanford.edu. Accessed July 2013.

Medications for Status Asthmaticus

	Class	Medication	Actions	Dose	Side Effects
1 (Beta-2 agonists)	*Nebulized* β2-agonist	**Albuterol** (Ventolin)	Relax smooth muscle, inhibit mast cells from releasing chemical mediators that cause bronchodilation.	Nebulize: 0.5 - 0.6 mg/kg/hr for 1 hr, with O_2 flow rate 10 - 12 LPM, then if pt ≤ 12 yrs old: 0.15 - 0.3 mg/kg q 1 - 4 hr. if pt > 12 yrs old: 2.5 - 10 mg q 1 - 4 hr.	Headache Tremors, anxiety, palpitation, restlessness Nausea/vomiting Tachycardia, ↑ BP
		Levalbuterol (Xopenex)	Relaxes smooth muscles of all airways, from the trachea to the terminal bronchioloes.	Metered dose inhaler: 2 inhalations q 4 - 6 hr. Warning: life-threatening bronchospasm may occur. Discontinue and seek alternative agent.	Flushing Hypokalemia Hyperglycemia
	Intravenous β2-agonists	**Salbutamol**	(Not available in the US).	IV: 10 mcg/kg over 10 minutes, then 0.2 - 4 mcg/kg/min (10 mcg/kg/min max).	Prolongation of QT interval Ventricular arrhythmias
	SC or IV B-2 agonist	**Terbutaline** (Brethine) 1:1000	B2-selective, with fewer side effects than Epinephrine, Isuprel, and Ephedrine.	SC: 0.01 mg/kg/dose (max of 0.3 mg/dose). May repeat q 15 - 20 min for up to 3 doses. IV: loading dose is 5 - 10 mcg/kg over 10 mins then continuous infusion 0.4 - 4 mcg/kg/min.	Allergic reaction
2	Corticosteroid	Methyl-prednisolone **(Solu-medrol)**	Anti-inflammatory effects. Reduces airway edema and mucus production.	IV: 1 - 2 mg/kg loading dose (max 125 mg) given slowly, then 0.5 mg/kg q 6 hrs for 48 hrs, then tapered.	Insomnia, increased appetite, change in mental status, hyperglycemia, peripheral edema.
3	Anticholinergic	**Ipratropium** (Atrovent)	Produces less bronchodilation; onset is more delayed than β-agonists, but duration of effect is longer.	Nebulize: 0.25 - 0.5 mg or 4 - 8 puffs q 20 mins up to 3 doses. Onset is slow (20 - 30 minutes). Peak effect in 60 - 90 minutes.	Few central nervous system side effects. Dry mouth, GI distress, nervousness, dizziness, tachycardia.
4	Inorganic salt	**Magnesium sulfate**	Bronchodilates by modulating movement of Ca ions into bronchial smooth muscle.	Given only if the above 3 agents fail. IV: 50 mg/kg (not to exceed 2 gm), over 20 minutes q 4 hr or continuously at 10 - 20 mg/kg/hr.	Weakness, hypotension, tachycardia, nausea, vomiting, arrhythmias. Monitor Mg level q 6 hr, maintain at 1.5 - 2 mg/dL.
5	Sedative, if mechanically ventilated	**Ketamine** (Ketalar)	Ideal because it has both bronchodilating and sedative effects.	1 mg/kg/hr, then titrate. Benzodiazepine is given to control increased secretions caused by Ketamine.	Increases sympathetic tone, preserving BP, but may depress myocardium, ↑ secretions. Hallucinations may occur when dc'd.

Septic Shock: Hour 1

See the Hemodynamic Chapter for the pathophysiology of, and the criteria for, "Sepsis, "Severe Sepsis," and "Septic Shock."

Facts:

- In pediatric severe sepsis, the hemodynamic picture is more often characterized by low CO, than by low SVR.
- Compared with adults, children are more likely to require:
  1. Proportionally larger quantities of fluid
  2. Both inotrope and vasodilator therapies
  3. Hydrocortisone for absolute adrenal insufficiency
  4. ECMO for refractory shock
- Treatment **must** begin when early signs of severe sepsis appear. Once hypotension occurs, cardiovascular collapse is imminent.

Signs of Septic Shock: Occur **with or without** hypotension. Look for the triad of:

1. Hypothermia or hyperthermia
2. Altered mental status (lack of interaction with parents, inconsolable, irritability, lethargy progressing to unarousable)
3. Cold shock (peripheral vasoconstriction): capillary refill > 2 sec, weak pulses, mottled and cool extremities, narrow pulse pressure

   or Warm shock (peripheral vasodilation): flash capillary refill, bounding peripheral pulses, wide pulse pressure.

	Goals that must be achieved in Hour 1	
	• Normal mental status • Minimal acceptable HR according to age • Normal blood pressure according to age • Capillary refill ≤ 2 seconds • Normal peripheral and central pulses • Warm extremities • Urinary output > 1 mL/kg/hr	
	Interventions that must be completed within Hour 1	**Clock**
Recognize:	Severe sepsis, particularly poor mental status, poor perfusion. Begin high flow O_2. Establish IV/IO access. Completed by minute 5.	5
O_2	If respiratory status is stable, give high flow O_2 by face mask. If there is respiratory distress and hypoxemia, however, intubation can cause instability. So high-flow nasal cannula oxygen or nasopharyngeal continuous positive airway pressure (CPAP) is used, and intubation delayed until IV access is secured, volume resuscitation is underway, and inotropic meds are considered. Monitor SpO_2.	
Fluids:	As long as rales are absent, large fluid deficits may exist. Push boluses of 20 mL/kg normal saline or albumin up to and over 60 mL/kg if needed, until perfusion improves or unless rales/hepatomegaly develop.	
BG, Ca^{++}, Antibiotic	Correct hypoglycemia and hypocalcemia. Begin Antiobiotic. If possible, obtain cultures before antibiotic is given, but <u>not</u> if it will cause significant delay (> 45 mins). Clindamycin is recommended to decrease toxins. By min. 15.	by min. 15
Inotropes:	If fluids fail to reverse shock, or fluid excess (rales) detected, a peripheral inotrope should be given while central access is achieved. Atropine and ketamine IV/IO are recommended for central line placement, intubation and ventilation. for Cold Shock: titrate central dopamine up to 10 mcg/kg/min or epinephrine 0.05 - 0.3 mcg/kg/min. for Warm Shock: titrate central norepinephrine. By min. 45	by min. 45
Intubate if:	Mental status is impaired Hypoventilating Work of breathing is increased Signs of fluid excess develop (rales or hepatomegaly).	
Hydro-cortisone:	Death from septic shock in pts with adrenal insufficiency can occur in < 8 hrs. Hydrocortisone infusion is given. By min. 60	by min. 60

Septic Shock: Hour 2

ICU Hemodynamic Goals that must be achieved in hour 2	
Normal MAP and CVP	CI = 3.3 - 6 L/min/m2
Hgb > 10 g/dL	$ScvO_2 \geq 70\%$

Treatment of 3 Different Types of Shock:

If **Cold** shock with **normal** BP, and ↓ CO, ↑ SVR	Titrate fluids and Epinephrine 0.05 - 0.3 mcg/kg/min. to maintain ScvO2 > 70%	If ScvO2 still < 70%, add vasodilator (nitroglycerin, nitroprusside, milrinone, enoximone, inamrinone, prostacyclin, fenoldopam) Consider levosimendan*
If **Cold** shock with **low** BP, and ↓ CO, ↑ SVR	Titrate fluids and Epinephrine 0.05 - 0.3 ug/kg/min. to maintain ScvO2 > 70%.	If still hypotensive, consider norepinephrine. If ScvO2 still < 70%, consider dobutamine, milrinone, enoximone. Consider levosimendan*
If **Warm** shock with **low** BP, and ↑ CO, ↓ SVR	Titrate fluids and norepinephrine to maintain ScvO2 > 70%.	If still hypotensive, vasopressin is considered (but safety is unclear). If ScvO2 still < 70%, low dose epinephrine is considered.

*levosimendan is a calcium sensitizer licensed in many countries, but not the US. (53% of patients had serious side effects: V Tach, hypotension, nausea/vomiting.)

Additional ICU Interventions that must be achieved in hour 2	
Hemoglobin:	Maintain Hgb > 10 g/dL for the first 72 hours. Then, if the patient is hemodynamically stable, Hgb > 7 g/dL is acceptable.
ScvO2:	If central venous oxygen saturation > 70 % is achieved within the first 6 hours, mortality rate is reduced by 40%. Achieving ScvO2 > 70 % requires: 1. Supporting adequate oxygen delivery (CO, Hgb, and SaO2). 2. Controlling tissue oxygen demands (managing agitation, increased work of breathing, fever, shivering). Accurate measurement of ScvO2 requires positioning the catheter tip close to the junction of the superior vena cava and right atrium, or the inferior vena cava and right atrium.
Mechanical Ventilation:	Decreases the high O2 demand of excess work of breathing. Mild hyperventilation may counterbalance metabolic acidosis. Beware the effect of excessive ventilation on CO, especially if the patient is hypovolemic. Additional volume is often needed. Sedation, given with a sedation goal, is recommended. Neuromuscular blocking agent should be considered.
Other Causes of ↓ BP:	If hypotension is refractory to treatment, look for other causes: pericardial effusion or tamponade, pneumothorax, bleeding, abdominal hypertension, endocrine crisis.
ECMO:	If shock continues to be refractory, exracorporeal membrane oxygenation has proven successful in children. Survival rates for neonates: 80%. For children: 50%.
Toxic Shock:	Children are more vulnerable to toxic shock due to lack of circulating antibodies. Immunoglobulin G may be considered.
Control BG:	Insulin to control hyperglycemia. Target a BG < 180 mg/dL. In infants and children, continuous D10W is also given to prevent inadvertant hypoglycemia and its neuro consequences.
FFP:	Fresh frozen plasma may be given to correct PT and PTT.
Meds to Avoid:	Propofol, benzodiazepines, thiopental, and inhalation agents can cause myocardial depression and vasodilation.
Find the Source in < 12 hours:	Within the first 12 hours, early and aggressive effort to identify and control the source of infection.

refer to: Dellinger RP, Levy MM, Rhodes A, et al. Surviving Sepsis Campaign: International Guidelines. Shock: 2012, **CritCareMed**, Feb 2014.41(2):613-620.
Brierley J, Carcillo JA, Choong K, et al. Clinical practice parameters for hemodynamic support of pediatric and neonatal patients. CCM, 2009;37(2):666-688.

Status Epilepticus

Description:	Seizure activity lasting ≥ 30 minutes. The seizures may be: 1. Generalized tonic and/or clonic convulsion, occurring continuously, or in repeated episodes, without full recovery of consciousness between episodes, or 2. Nonconvulsive, detectable only by electroencephalograph (EEG) SE is "refractory" when 2 doses of anticonvulsants have no effect. Mortality rate is 32% if seizures last > 60 minutes. Presence of a structured seizure protocol is highly recommended.
Causes:	Atypical febrile seizure; Infection (meningitis, encephalitis) Head Trauma; Drug toxicity (e.g., Theophylline) Narcotic withdrawal; Hypertensive crisis Anticonvulsant withdrawal; Brain Tumor Degenerative or progressive neurologic disorders Ischemic/anoxic insult (stroke, cerebral emboli, drowning)
Patho-physiology:	Convulsive seizures cause a 4-fold increase in oxygen demand, while airway compromise and abnormal diaphragmatic movement impair oxygenation and the elimination of CO_2. Respiratory and metabolic acidosis may produce a pH < 6.9. Acidosis results in ↑ K, which perpetuates seizure activity. Sustained muscle contraction/s may lead to rhabdomyolysis. Unrelenting electrical discharge increases cerebral metabolic rate, causing depletion of glucose stores, cerebral edema, loss of autoregulation, and eventually neuronal edema/injury/death. After the seizure ends, body temperature continues to rise.
Initial Approach:	While the care is implemented, medications must be given. Nothing should be placed in the pt's mouth to serve as a bite block. Ensure airway patency, prevent aspiration. Give supplemental O_2. Reliable IV access ASAP. Intraosseous route is an alternative. Presume hypoglycemia as inciting event, check Blood Glucose. Rapid sequence intubation if SpO_2 < 90%, hypoventilating, GCS < 8. For intubation, short acting NMBA such as rocuronium is used. For Temp > 40° C, passive cooling. Do not allow shivering.
EEG:	If Neuromuscular Blocking Agent is required, continuous EEG is needed to detect nonconvulsive SE.
Compli-cations:	Acidosis, Aspiration, Hypotension, Hypoglycemia, Hypoxemia, Cerebral edema or infarction, Rhabdomyolysis, Death.

STAT Meds for SE: Hour 1		
Minute 0	Lorazepam: or Midazolam:	0.1 mg/kg IV (total maximum dose is 4 mg), or if no IV access, then 0.2 mg/kg IM (total maximum dose is 10 mg)
Minute 5 seizure persists	Lorazepam:	0.1 mg/kg IV (max 4 mg) Peak effect of Lorazepam occurs in 15 mins, duration is 3 - 6 hours.
Minute 10 seizure persists	Fosphenytoin:	30 mg PE/kg IV or IO over 10 minutes. Effect peaks in 20 minutes.
Minute 20 - 30 Refractory	Phenobarbital:	If child is 1 month - 2 years: Phenobarbital 20 mg/kg IV over 10 minutes.
	Valproate:	If child is > 2 years: Valproate 20 mg/kg IV over 4 min, ***unless*** contraindicated by known or suspected liver disease, then levetiracetam 30 mg/kg IV (max 3 g) over 6 minutes.
Minute 45 Induce coma	Midazolam:	0.2 mg/kg IV bolus + infusion 0.1 mg/kg/hr Repeat bolus and increase infusion rate by 0.1 mg/kg/hr (max 2 mg/kg/hr) every 5 minutes until seizure stops.
Minute 60 Seizure persists	Pentobarbital:	10 mg/kg IV bolus, then infusion of 1 mg/kg/hr and wean midazolam.

Marmor A, Nash K. Pediatric Emergency Medicine. Pediatric Neurology 3/4/2011, sfghed.ucsf.edu

Trauma

See the *Fast Facts* specialty chapter "Trauma" for specific organ injuries and burns.

Facts:
Pediatric Trauma Score < 9 is linked to significant risk for death.
Blunt trauma to the head is the most common pediatric injury.
In children, shock is less obvious and respiratory failure is more likely, compared to adults with equivalent injuries.

Airway:
Give high flow 100% O_2 per nonrebreathing mask.
Use jaw thrust with manual stabilization of the cervical spine.
Infants are nasal breathers and are at greater risk for airway obstruction due to fractures, soft tissue injuries, nasogastric tube.
Nasal intubation is avoided, it requires too small an endotracheal tube and is dangerous in the presence of basilar skull fracture.
If endotracheal intubation fails, needle cricothyrotomy is attempted.

Breathing:
Central cyanosis is not an early or reliable indicator of hypoxemia.
If the patient has inadequate respiratory effort, respiratory distress, or is unresponsive, ventilate with bag-mask (volume 10 mL/kg).
Since infants and small children are mostly diaphragmatic breathers, any compromise of diaphragmatic function can severely limit the child's ability to ventilate.
If head injury is present, do not routinely hyperventilate.

Circulation:
Sympathetic-adrenal response to hemorrhage can maintain "normal" blood pressure. Often, hypotension does not occur until more than 1/3 of the circulating blood volume has been lost.
Look for signs of poor perfusion:

- ↓ Level of consciousness (LOC).
- Compensatory tachycardia (in children, heart rate is considered the most sensitive indicator of cardiac output).
- Capillary refill > 2 seconds, skin pallor, vasoconstriction.
- Weak peripheral pulses (progressively weakening pulses often precede impending cardiac arrest).
- Urinary output < 0.5 mL/kg/hr.

Control bleeding, secure vascular access, volume replace.
Estimate pt's blood volume (85 mL/kg) and % blood volume lost.
The best access is large bore peripheral catheterization.
Intraosseous infusion is a safe, rapid, and efficient method for delivering fluids/meds/blood. See page 5 for technique.
Give warmed isotonic fluid (RL or NS) 20 mL/kg bolus over 15 minutes; repeat according to patient response.
The 2/5 rule: 10 minutes after fluid bolus:
if CVP is < 2, continue fluids; if CVP > 5, slow the fluids.
If no improvement in HR, LOC, or perfusion, or if hypotension is severe (< 70 mm Hg + twice the age in years), warmed packed red cells 10 - 20 mL/kg should be given. Wrap extremities, cover head. Hypothermia can ↑ catecholamine secretion, depress myocardium, cause metabolic acidosis, contribute to coagulopathy.

Head Injury:
Head injury is the most common cause of death in pedi trauma.
Intracranial injuries often occur without skull fracture.
Open fontanelles or sutures do not preclude development of ↑ ICP.
In children, diffuse edema rather than focal space-occupying lesions predominate. The edema can develop slowly, unexpectedly, or begin hours after admission.
Quick neuro exam: LOC, pupillary light reflex, Glasgow Coma Scale, motor tone/movement, sensory ability, reflexes.
Keep PCO_2 = 35 - 40 mm Hg ($PaCO_2$ < 35 reduces cerebral flow).
Those with a GCS score of 8 or less or with a waning mental status should be intubated using rapid-sequence intubation, receive ICP monitoring, and should have immediate noncontrast CT.
Any child with a history of trauma and loss of consciousness longer than 5 minutes or an altered LOC should have CT.
Prevent secondary brain injury caused by ↓ BP, fever, hypoxemia, hypocapnea, hypo- or hyperglycemia, fluid overload, ↑ ICP.

Trauma

Thorax: Thoracic injury is the 2nd leading cause of death in pedi trauma.
Rib fractures are uncommon. Pliable rib cage and mediastinal mobility can allow significant injury with few external signs.
Hemo/pneumothoraces are common.
If present, multiple rib fractures are linked to a 40% mortality rate.
Chest tubes are placed mid-axillary line, 5th ICS (level of nipple).
If a stable patient suddenly deteriorates, suspect pneumothorax.
Tension pneumothorax may require immediate needle thoracentesis.
Any xray evidence of pulmonary contusion should be treated ASAP.
Suspect myocardial contusion if there is: chest pain, dysrhythmia, myocardial dysfunction, gallop rhythm, tachycardia, pulmonary edema. There is risk for sudden lethal arrhythmia, even if ECG is unremarkable. ICU admit if continuous ECG is required.
Emergency thoracotomy has dismal outcome, reserved for massive hemothorax (20 mL/kg) or ongoing bleed (2-4 mL/kg/hr), massive air leak, or food or salivary drainage from chest tube.
P/F ratio 200 - 300 is evidence of acute lung injury.

Spine: In all trauma pts, presume spine injury, immobilize head/spine.
SCIWORA (spinal cord injury without radiologic abnormality) can result from stretching of the cord or nerve roots, leaving little or no anatomic evidence of injury. Raise the index of suspicion for even minor neurologic deficit if: tenderness localized to the spine, paresthesia, weakness/paralysis, diaphragmatic breathing, urinary retention, hypotension while skin is flushed, warm, dry.
Steroid is no longer recommended, and may cause harm.

Abdomen: Minor force can cause major injury. Undeveloped abdominal muscles provide little protection for the major organs.
Solid organ injury (spleen, liver, kidney) are common.
Reassess often for abdominal pain or distention.
NG tube (which is placed orally in infants and children) is used to decompress stomach and prevent aspiration of gastric contents.
Abdominal distention that persists after NG tube placement suggests intraabdominal bleeding.
Endotracheal tube is placed orally in infants/small children.
Peritoneal signs may not develop until 24 hrs after injury.
Delayed bleeding (days to weeks later) may occur if splenic or hepatic hematomas expand and rupture.
Small diaphragmatic tear/s eventually progress to at least some herniation of abdominal contents into the chest.
Sonography is used to detect abdominal bleeding in unstable pts.
CT is the preferred imaging technique for stable patients.
Nonoperative management of blunt trauma has a 90% success rate and is the standard of care, but requires availability of a surgical team and frequent, careful monitoring for delayed bleeding.
Immediate surgery required if: massive or continued hemorrhage, suspected perforation of bowel or bladder, evisceration, disrupted pancreatic duct, diaphragmatic tear.

Extremities: Since immature bone is more elastic, fractures are often incomplete or non-displaced and are easy to miss during the initial assessment.
There is a high incidence of ischemic vascular injury in pedi fxs.
Injury to a major artery may result in ischemia and retarded growth in that limb. Need early diagnosis and aggressive management.
Be very alert for development of neurovascular impairment. 6 P's: Pain, Pallor, Paresthesia, Paralysis, Pulselessness, or Polar (cold).
Compartment syndrome occurs when tissue pressure > 40 cm H_2O.
Absence of a pulse for more than 6 hrs results in vessel thrombosis.

Pain: Pain relief can be provided with morphine 0.1 mg/kg or a combination of fentanyl 1 mcg/kg and midazolam 0.05 - 0.1 mg/kg.

Antibiotics and anti-coagulants: Fever, leukocytosis, other signs of inflammation are common during the acute phase. Routine antibiotics are not recommended.
DVT incidence is low. Routine anticoagulation is not recommended.

Treatment of ↑ ICP following Head Injury

ICP	Significance
< 7 mm Hg	Normal in children
> 20 mm Hg	Begin treatment
20 - 40 mm Hg	Moderate outcome, 28% mortality rate
> 40 mm Hg	100 % mortality
$PbtO_2$ (PO_2 of Brain Tissue)	
maintain > 15 mm Hg (normal = 25 - 35)	

CPP (cerebral perfusion pressure) CPP = MAP - ICP	
Infant/toddler:	maintain > 45 mm Hg
Child:	maintain > 50 mm Hg
Teenager:	maintain > 65 mm Hg
Adult:	maintain > 65 mm Hg
CPP < 40 - 50 mm Hg predicts poor outcome/death.	

Signs of ↑ ICP:	Early	Late	Very Late
	↓ LOC, ↓ GCS Vomiting Irritable Pupil dysfunction Cranial nerve (CN) dysfunction	↓ LOC, ↓ GCS, ↑ BP Bulging fontanelle ↓ Spontaneous movement Posturing Pupil dysfunction Papilledema	↓ BP Irregular breathing or hyperventilation. Absent movement Unreactive pupils

Tier I — **Severe TBI, ICP is unknown:**

1. If GCS < 8 or if CT indicates mass or swelling, intubation is needed. Even with a normal CT, 10 - 15% of patients with a GCS < 8 have increased ICP.
2. Keep PaO_2 > 80 - 100 mm Hg, SpO_2 > 92 %.
3. Maintain $PaCO_2$ = 35 - 38 mm Hg. $PaCO_2$ < 35 mm Hg causes cerebral vasoconstriction. $PaCO_2$ > 40 mm Hg causes cerebral vasodilation. Both cause insult to injured, as well as to uninjured brain tissue.
4. Maintain euvolemia. Raise HOB to 30° as long as the pt is euvolemic.
5. Support O_2 delivery by maintaining Hgb/Hct at least 10g/30%.
6. Prevent obstruction to jugular veins. Keep head in neutral position.
7. Maintain temperature between 35 - 38.5 ° C. Hyperthermia (T > 38.5 ° C) increases cerebral metabolic rate, oxygen demand, neuron stimulation and excitation, and cell death. Hypothermia (T < 35 ° C) causes increased SVR, decreased CO, impaired immune system function, metabolic acidosis, electrolyte imbalance (decreased K, Mg, Phos), and impaired coagulation.
8. Give adequate sedation and analgesia (e.g., fentanyl 1 - 2 mcg/kg/hr). Beware sedatives may cause hypotension, reducing cerebral perfusion. Propofol is **NOT** recommended (reports of hypoxia, rhabdomyolysis, fatal myocardial failure). Also, steroids make **NO** difference in outcome.
9. Post traumatic seizure occur in 1/3 of pedi pts with severe head injury. Prophylactic anticonvulsants, however, are not recommended.

Tier II — **There are signs of herniation and/or ICP is ≥ 20 mm Hg:**

1. Intraventricular catheterization is recommended for monitoring of ICP, calculation of cerebral perfusion pressure, and drainage of CSF.
2. Hyperosmolar therapy is used to reduce cerebral edema. Choices are:
   a. Mannitol 0.25 - 1 g/kg q 4-6 h as long as serum osmo is < 320 mOsm/L,
   b. Hypertonic (3%) Saline 0.1 - 1 mL/kg/hour via central line as long as serum osmo is < 370 mOsm/L. This achieves a lower ICP than Mannitol, but too-rapid increase in serum Na risks central pontine myelinolysis.
3. Increase ventilation to maintain $PaCO_2$ to 30 - 35 mm Hg.
4. Repeat CT to rule out surgical mass. Consider $SjvO_2$, $PbtO_2$ monitoring.

Tier III — **ICP > 30 mm Hg, Intracranial Hypertension is Refractory:**

1. If ventriculostomy is working, no CSF obstructions exist, and there is no major mass lesion, lumbar drain may be considered.
2. If EEG is active, the pt is hemodynamically stable and salvageable, and there are no contraindications, high dose barbiturate is an option. Pentobarbital: load 10 - 15 mg/kg over 30 minutes, then 1 - 5 mg/kg/hr for 3 hrs, then 1 - 3 mg/kg/hr titrated to achieve EEG burst suppression and a serum level of 3 - 4 mg/dL. Usual duration is 24 hrs, then taper.
3. If salvageable patient and diffuse swelling on CT and it is within 24 - 48 hrs of injury, decompressive craniectomy may be considered.
4. Transient use of hyperventilation ($PaCO_2$ < 30) is permissible.
5. Inducing moderate hypothermia (32 - 33° C) may be considered.

Assessment Scores

Glasgow Coma Scale

Assessment	Infant	Child	Score
Eye Opening	Spontaneously	Spontaneously	4
	To speech	To verbal command	3
	To pain only	To pain only	2
	No response	No response	1
Verbal Response	Coos and babbles	Oriented, appropriate	5
	Irritable cries	Confused, inappropriate	4
	Cries to pain, or inappropriate screams	Cries to pain, or inappropriate screams	3
	Moans to pain	Incomprehensible sounds	2
	No response	No response	1
Motor Response	Moves spontaneously	Obeys command	6
	Withdraws to touch	Localizes pain	5
	Withdraws to pain	Withdraws to pain	4
	Decorticates to pain	Decorticates to pain	3
	Decerebrates to pain	Decerebrates to pain	2
	No response	No response	1

Muscle Strength:

Moves against gravity and full resistance	5
Moves against gravity, can overcome some resistance	4
Moves against gravity, but cannot overcome resistance	3
Moves with gravity eliminated (moves limb on bed)	2
Some muscle contraction, but does not move joint	1
No evidence of muscle contraction. No movement	0

Trauma Score:

Category	Score +2 if:	Score +1 if:	Score -1 if:	Your pt's score
Weight (kg)	> 20	10 - 20	< 10	
Airway	Normal	O_2, mask, cannula	Intubated	
Systolic BP	> 90 Good peripheral pulses	50 - 90 Carotid & femoral pulses are palpable	< 50 Weak or no pulses	
LOC	Awake	Obtunded	Coma or Posturing	
Open Wound	No abnormality	Minor contusions, abrasions, laceration < 7 cm	Major or penetrating, through fascia	
Skeletal Trauma	None	Single closed fracture	Multiple or open fractures	
			Total Score:	

Total the scores for all of the categories.
The highest possible total score is +12,
the lowest possible total score is -6.

Adapted from: Tepas JJ, Mollitt DL, Talbert JL, Bryant M. The pediatric trauma score as predictor of injury severity. ***J Pediatr Surg*** 1987;22:14-18.

Pedi Hemodynamics and O_2 Transport

	Parameter	Normal Value	Formula
MAP	Mean arterial pressure	75 - 95 mm Hg	1/3(Sys - Dias) + Dias
CVP	Central venous pressure	1 - 5 mm Hg	
RVP	Right ventricular pressure	Sys: 14 - 38 mm Hg Dias: 0 - 5 mm Hg	
PAS	Pulmonary artery pressure systolic	20 - 30 mm Hg	
PAD	Pulmonary artery pressure diastolic	5 - 10 mm Hg	
PAM	Pulmonary artery mean pressure	15 mm Hg	
PCWP	Pulmonary capillary wedge pressure	5 - 10 mm Hg	
SvO_2	Mixed venous O_2 saturation	65 - 80 %	
CI	Cardiac index	2.5 - 4.2 $L/min/m^2$	CO /BSA
SV	Stroke volume	(see chart below) mL/beat	(CO x 1000)/HR
SVI	Stroke volume index	33 - 47 $mL/beat/m^2$	(CI x 1000)/HR
SVR	Systemic vascular resistance	Infant: 2800-4000 $dyne{\cdot}sec/cm^{-5}$ Toddler: 2000-2800 Child: 1200-2000	$\frac{(MAP - CVP)80}{CO}$
SVRI	Systemic vascular resistance index	Infant: 800-1200 $dyne{\cdot}sec/cm^{-5}/m^2$ Toddler: 1600 Child: 1200-2400	$\frac{(MAP - CVP)90}{CI}$
PVR	Pulmonary vascular resistance	40-320 $dyne{\cdot}sec/cm^{-5}$	$\frac{(PAM - PCWP)80}{CO}$
PVRI	Pulmonary vascular resistance index	80-240 $dyne{\cdot}sec/cm^{-5}/m^2$	$\underline{(PAM - PCWP)80}$
RVSWI	Right ventricular stroke work index	0.5 ± 0.06 $g\text{-}m/m^2$	SVI x PAM x .0136
LVSWI	Left ventricular stroke work index	56 ± 6 $g\text{-}m/m^2$	SVI x MAP x .0136
O2I	Oxygenation Index	> 40 indicates failure of mechanical ventilation	$\frac{FiO_2}{PaO_2}$ x Mean airway pressure
DO_2	Oxygen delivery	620 ± 50 $mL/min/m^2$	CI (1.39 x Hgb xSaO_2)10
VO_2	Oxygen consumption	120 - 200 $mL/min/m^2$	(SaO_2-SvO_2)xCIxHgbx13.9
CerPP	Cerebral Perfusion Pressure	40 - 60 mm Hg (minimum)	MAP - ICP
ICP	Intracranial pressure	Infant: 2 - 6 mm Hg Child: 3 - 7 mm Hg Older child: 0 - 10 mm Hg	
CBF	Cerebral Blood Flow	Neonate: 25 - 30 mL/100g brain/minute Child: 30 - 40 mL/100g brain/minute	Ischemia onset is CBF < 18 mL/100g brain/minute
$CerVO_2$	Cerebral tissue O_2 consumption	3.5 mL/100g brain/minute at rest	
$PbtO_2$	Partial pressure of O_2 in brain tissue	Normal $PbtO_2$ > 20 mm Hg	Ischemia onset is $PbtO_2$ < 15 mm Hg
$SjvO_2$	O_2 saturation of jugular venous blood	55 - 70%	

Age	Weight (kg)	BSA (m^2)	Cardiac output (mL/min)	Heart Rate (bpm)	Stroke volume (mL)	DO_2 ($mL/min/m^2$)	VO_2 ($mL/min/m^2$)
Newborn	3.2	0.2	700-800	145	5	665-1000	180-270
6 months	8	0.42	1000-1600	120	10	476-667	167-238
1 year	10	0.5	1300-1500	115	13	520-600	170-220
2 yr	13	0.59	1500-2000	115	18	508-678	154-208
4 yr	17	0.71	2300-2375	105	27	648-669	155-211
5 yr	19	0.77	2500-3000	95	31	649-779	149-221
8 yr	28	0.96	3400-3600	83	42	708-750	156-200
10 yr	35	1.1	3800-4000	75	50	690-727	122-227
15 yr	50	1.4	5000-6000	70	85	857	120-200

adapted from Hazinski MF. *Manual of Pediatric Critical Care,* St. Louis: Mosby, 1999, p. 112.

Body Surface Area (BSA) for Pedi

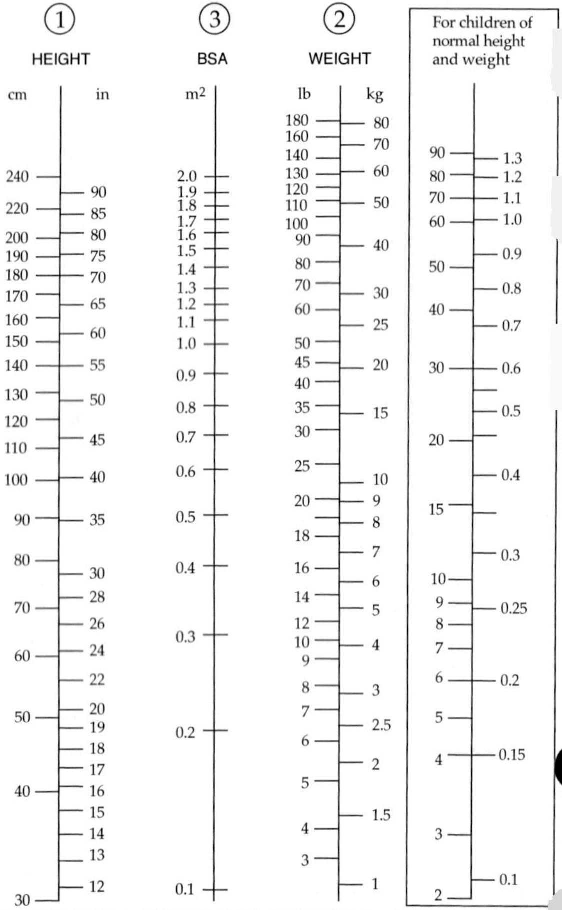

To determine the child's body surface area (BSA):
On bar 1, plot the child's height (in either cm or in.).
On bar 2, plot the child's weight (in either lbs or kg).
Connect the two points with a straight line.
Where the line intersects bar 3, read the child's BSA.

or

If the child has normal height and weight, use the graph above. Locate the child's weight in pounds on the left of the scale. Then read the BSA listed next to it on the right side of the scale.

$$\text{Body Surface Area (m}^2) = \sqrt{\frac{\text{Height (cm)} \times \text{Weight (kg)}}{3600}}$$

Graphs used with permission from: Behrman, Vaughn, Kleigman, and Arvin. ***Nelson's Textbook of Pediatrics***, 15th Edition. Philadelphia: WB Saunders Co. 1996: 2079.

Growth and Development

< 1 year Infant	1 month	holds chin up when prone
	2 months	raises chest up when prone
	4 months	sits up
	5 months	grasps object
	6 months	sits in high chair begins to have "stranger anxiety"
	7 months	sits alone
	8 months	stands with help
	9 months	stands holding onto furniture
	10 months	crawls
	11 months	walks when led; weaning to a cup
	Needs to feel physically safe, through close relationship with one care-taking person (usually the mother). Trust develops through needs being met consistently. Mistrust and anxiety develop when needs are met inconsistently.	
1 - 3 years Toddler	12 months	beginning bowel/bladder training
	13 months	pulls on furniture to stand
	14 months	climbs stairs
	15 months	stands alone
	18-24 months	fontanelles closed
	20 months	walks alone
	24 months	completing bowel/bladder training
	Discovers and explores self and surrounding world. Enjoys new mobility skills. Acquiring language. Develops egocentric thinking and need for parallel play. Tolerates short separations from mother. Transitional objects (security blanket, special toy) provide some comfort. Oppositional syndrome ("no" stage). Exerting independence. Separation anxiety an important problem in hospitalized toddlers aged 8 - 24 months, when separated from mother.	
4 - 6 years Preschool	Growth of self-awareness, conscience (guilt). Capable of being educated and being a part of a group. Magical thinking based on what the child would like to believe. Cannot always distinguish fantasy from reality. Forming the concepts of good and evil. Parents are extremely important in this phase. Fears intrusive procedures; Castration fears are common. Asserting some independence and mastering new skills. Learning to share. Gender aware.	
7 - 11 years Preadolescent	Struggles between mastering new skills and failure. Enjoys school, learning skills, games with rules. Learning social communication; appropriate sexual role. Competitive; Needs to succeed. Eager to please. Fears body mutilation; May feel need to be "brave." Can understand hospital rules. World expanding beyond family. Peers become important.	
12 - 18 years Adolescent	Vacillates between needs for independence and dependence. Learning to recognize limitations, while achieving emotional independence. Has adult cognitive abilities, deductive reasoning. Coping mechanisms: rationalization, intellectualization. Peer acceptance very important. Egocentric, rebellious at times, especially against parents and authority figures. Very concerned with body image, body changes, sexuality, role. Searching for "who I am."	

Normal Pediatric Lab Values

Blood

Albumin

Newborn:	2.6–3.6 g/dL
1–3 years:	3.4–4.2 g/dL
4–6 years:	3.5–5.2 g/dL
7–9 years:	3.7–5.6 g/dL
10–19 years:	3.7–5.6 g/dL

Ammonia

Newborns:	< 50 mmol/L
Thereafter:	0–35 mmol/L

Bicarbonate, Actual
Calculated from pH and $PaCO_2$

Newborns:	17.2–23.6 mmol/L
2 months–2 yrs:	19–24 mmol/L
Children:	18–25 mmol/L
Adult males:	20.1–28.9 mmol/L
Adult females:	18.4–28.8 mmol/L

Bleeding Time
2–9 min.

Calcium

Premature infants:	3.5–4.5 mEq/L (1.7–2.3 mmol/L)
Full-term infants:	4.0–5.0 mEq/L (2.0–2.5 mmol/L)
Thereafter:	4.4–5.3 mEq/L (2.2–2.7 mmol/L)

Carbon Dioxide (PCO_2)

Newborn:	27–40 mmHg (3.6–5.5 kPa)
Infant:	27–41 mmHg (3.6–5.5 kPa)
Children:	32–48 mmHg (4.3–6.4 kPa)

Chloride

1 year:	96–111 mmol/L
1–17 years:	102–112 mmol/L

Creatinine

Infant:	0.2-0.4 mg/dL
Child:	0.3-0.7 mg/dL
Adolescent:	0.5-1.0 mg/dL

Fibrinogen
200–500 mg/dL (5.9–14.7 mol/L)

Glucose

Premature infants:	20–80 mg/dL
Full-term infants:	30–100 mg/dL
Children and adults (fasting):	60–105 mg/dL

Hematocrit

Age	Males (%)	Females (%)
Newborns	43.4–56.1	37.4–55.9
6 months–2 yrs	30.9–37.0	31.2–37.2
2–6 years	31.7–37.7	32.0–37.1
6–12 years	32.7–39.3	33.0–39.6
12–18 years	34.8–43.9	34.0–40.7

Hemoglobin

Age	Males (g/dL)	Females (g/dL)
Newborns	14.7–18.6	12.7–18.3
6 months–2 yrs	10.3–12.4	10.4–12.4
2–6 years	10.5–12.7	10.7–12.7
6–12 years	11.0–13.3	10.9–13.3
12–18 years	11.5–14.8	11.2–13.6

Blood

Lactate Dehydrogenase (LDH)

1–3 days:	40–348 IU/L
1 month–5 yrs:	150–360 IU/L
5–8 years:	150–300 IU/L
8–12 years:	130–300 IU/L
12–14 years:	130–280 IU/L
14–16 years:	130–230 IU/L
Adult males:	70–178 IU/L
Adult females:	42–166 IU/L

Lead

0–15 years	10 g/dL (0.48 mol/L)

Magnesium mg/dL (mmol/L)

Age	Males
1–30 days	1.7–2.4 (0.70–0.99)
31–365 days	1.6–2.5 (0.66–1.03)
1–3 years	1.7–2.4 (0.70–0.99)
4–9 years	1.7–2.4 (0.70–0.99)
10–15 years	1.6–2.2 (0.66–0.91)
16–18 years	1.5–2.2 (0.62–0.91)

Age	Females
1–30 days	1.7–2.5 (0.70–1.03)
31–365 days	1.9–2.4 (0.78–0.99)
1–3 years	1.7–2.4 (0.70–0.99)
4–9 years	1.6–2.3 (0.66–0.95)
10–15 years	1.6–2.2 (0.66–0.91)
16–18 years	1.5–2.2 (0.62–0.91)

Osmolality

Birth–1 month:	275–305 mOsm/kg
Adults:	282–300 mOsm/kg

Partial Thromboplastin Time

Children:	42–54 sec

pH

0–6 months	7.18–7.50
6–12 months	7.27–7.49

Phenylalanine
0.7–3.5 mg/dL (0.04–0.21 mmol/L)

Phosphorus

Newborns:	5.0–7.8 mg/dL (1.61–2.52 mmol/L)
1 year:	3.8–6.2 mg/dL (1.23–2.0 mmol/L)
10 years:	3.6–5.6 mg/dL (1.16–1.81 mmol/L)
Adults:	3.1–5.1 mg/dL (1.0–1.65 mmol/L)

Platelet Count (Value x $10^3/mm^3$)

Age	Males	Females
Newborns	164–351	234–346
1–2 months	275–567	295–615
2–6 months	275–566	288–598
6 months–2 yrs	219–452	229–465
2–6 years	204–405	204–402
6–12 years	194–364	183–369
12–18 years	165–332	185–335

Potassium

Premature infants:	4.5–7.2 mEq/L
Full-term infants:	3.7–5.2 mEq/L
Children:	3.5–5.8 mEq/L
Adults:	3.5–5.5 mEq/L

Prothrombin Time
Children: 11–15 sec

adapted from NIH Clinical Center, Pediatric Services,www.cc.nih.gov/ccc/pedweb/pedsstaff/pedlab.html, Sept 2012

For monovalent ions:	1 meq = 1 mmol.
For divalent ions:	1 meq = 0.5 mmol.
For trivalent ions:	1 meq » 0.333 mmol

Normal Pediatric Lab Values

Blood

Total Protein g/dL

At birth	4.6–7.0
3 months	4.5–6.5
1 year	5.4–7.5
4 years	5.9–8.0

Red Blood Cell Count

Age	Males	Females
Newborns	4.2–5.5	3.4–5.4
6 months–2 yrs	4.1–5.0	4.1–4.9
2–12 years	4.0–4.9	4.0–4.9
12–18 years	4.2–5.3	4.0–4.9

Sedimentation Rate
< 2 years: 1–5 mm/hr
> 2 years: 1–8 mm/hr

Sodium
Newborns: 133–146 mmol/L
Children and adults: 135–148 mmol/L

Thrombin Time
Children: 12–16 seconds

Thyroid-stimulating Hormone (mU/L)

Age	Males	Females
1–30 days	0.52–16.00	0.72–13.10
1 month–5 yrs	0.55–7.10	0.46–8.10
6–18 years	0.37–6.00	0.36–5.80
12–18 years	4.5–10.0	4.8–10.1

Blood

Thyroxine g/dL (nmol/L).

Age	Males
1–30 days	5.9–21.5 (76–276)
1–12 months	6.4–13.9 (82–179)
1–3 years	7.0–13.1 (90–169)
4–6 years	6.1–12.6 (79–162)
7–12 years	6.7–13.4 (86–172)
13–15 years	4.8–11.5 (62–148)
16–18 years	5.9–11.5 (76–148)
Age	**Females**
1–30 days	6.3–21.5 (81–276)
1–12 months	4.9–13.7 (63–176)
1–3 years	7.1–14.1 (91–180)
4–6 years	7.2–14.0 (93–180)
7–12 years	6.1–12.1 (79–156)
13–15 years	5.8–11.2 (75–144)
16–18 years	5.2–13.2 (67–170)

Urea Nitrogen

1–3 years	5–17 mg/dL (1.8–6.0 mmol/L)
4–13 years	7–17 mg/dL (2.5–6.0 mmol/L)
14–19 years	8–21 mg/dL (2.9–7.5 mmol/L)

Uric Acid
Males:

0–14 years:	2–7 mg/dL (119–416 mol/L)
>14 years:	3–8 mg/dL (178–476 mol/L)

Females:

All ages:	2–7 mg/dL (119–416 mol/L)

White Blood Cell Count
Values x 10^3/μmL (μL = mm^3)

Age	Males	Females
Newborns	6.8–13.3	8.0–14.3
6 months–2 yrs	6.2–14.5	6.4–15.0
2–6 years	5.3–11.5	5.3–11.5
6–12 years	4.5–10.5	4.7–10.3

Urine

Albumin

First month:	1–100 mg/L
Second month:	0.2–34 mg/L
2–12 months:	0.5–19 mg/L

Ammonia

2–12 months:	4–20 mEq/min/m^2
1–16 years:	6–16 mEq/min/m^2

Calcium
4–12 years: 4–8 mEq/L (2–4 mmol/L)

Casts
(12-hr specimen): < 10,000

Creatinine Clearance

Newborns (1 day):	5–50 mL/min/1.73 m^2
Newborns (6 days):	15–90 mL/min/1.73 m^2
Adult males:	85–125 mL/min/1.73 m^2
Adult females:	75–115 mL/min/1.73 m^2

Osmolality

Infants:	50–600 mosm/L
Older children:	50–1400 mosm/L

Urine

Potassium
26–123 mmol/L

Protein
(12-hr specimen): < 55 mg

Red cells
(12-hr specimen): <1 million

Sodium
Infants: 0.3–3.5 mmol/24 hr (6–10 mmol/m^2)
Children and adults: 5.6–17 mmol/24 hr

Specific Gravity
1.010–1.030

Urea Clearance

Premature infants:	3.5–17.3 mL/min/1.73 m^2
Newborns:	8.7–33 mL/min/1.73 m^2
2–12 months:	40–95 mL/min/1.73 m^2
> 2 years:	> 52 mL/min/1.73 m^2

Urobilinogen
< 3 mg/24 hr (< 5.1 μmol/24 hr)

White cells
(12-hr specimen): < 2 million

Cerebrospinal Fluid

Protein	Newborns:	40–120 mg/dL
	< 1 month:	20–80 mg/dL
	> 1 month:	15–45 mg/dL
Glucose	All ages:	60%–80% of blood glucose

Broselow Pediatric Resuscitation Tape

Adapted from the ***2002 Broselow Pediatric Resuscitation Tape,*** Armstrong Medical Industries, Lincolnshire, IL. 1-800-323-4220. www.armstrongmedical.com.

	Newborn or Small Infant (3 - 5 kg)	Infant (6 - 9 kg)	Toddler (10 - 11 kg)	Small Child (12 - 14 kg)	Child (15 - 18 kg)	Child (19 - 22 kg)	Large Child (24 - 30 kg)	Adult (32+ kg)
Resuscitation bag	Child	Child	Child	Child	Child	Child	Child/adult	Adult
O_2 mask	Newborn	Newborn	Pediatric	Pediatric	Pediatric	Pediatric	Adult	Adult
Oral airway	Infant/small child	Infant/small child	Small child	Child	Child	Child/Sm. adult	Child/Sm adult	Medium adult
Laryngoscope blade size	0 - 1 straight	1 straight	1 straight	2 straight	2 straight or curved	2 straight or curved	2 - 3 straight or curvec	3 straight or curved
Tracheal tube	2.5 - 3.5 uncuffed	3.5 uncuffed	4.0 uncuffed	4.5 uncuffed	5.0 uncuffed	5.5 uncuffed	6.0 cuffed	6.5 cuffed
Tracheal tube length (cm at lip)	10 - 10.5	10 - 10.5	11 - 12	12.5 - 13.5	14 - 15	15.5 - 16.5	17 - 18	18.5 - 19.5
Stylet (Fr.)	6	6	6	6	6	14	14	14
Suction catheter	6 - 8	8	8 - 10	10	10	10	10	12
BP cuff	Newborn/Infant	Newborn/Infant	Infant/Child	Child	Child	Child	Child/adult	Adult
IV catheter	22 - 24	22 - 24	20 - 24	18 - 22	18 - 22	18 - 20	18 - 20	16 - 20
Butterfly	23 - 25	23 - 25	23 - 25	21 - 23	21 - 23	21 - 23	21 - 22	18 - 21
NG tube (Fr.)	5 - 8	5 - 8	8 - 10	10	10 - 12	12 - 14	14 - 18	18
Urinary cath (Fr.)	5 - 8	5 - 8	8 - 10	10	10 - 12	10 - 12	12	12
Paddles for Defib/Cardiovert	Infant paddles	Infant paddles until 1 yr or 10 kg	Adult paddles if ≥ 1 yr or ≥ 10 kg	Adult	Adult	Adult paddles	Adult paddles	Adult paddles
Chest tube (Fr.)	10 - 12	10 - 12	16 - 20	20 - 24	20 - 24	24 - 32	28 - 32	32 - 40